Organelle and Molecular Targeting

Organelle and Molecular Targeting

Edited by
Lara Scheherazade Milane and Mansoor M. Amiji

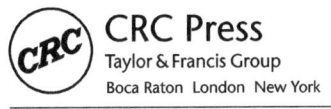

CRC Press
Taylor & Francis Group
Boca Raton London New York

CRC Press is an imprint of the
Taylor & Francis Group, an **informa** business

First edition published 2022
by CRC Press
6000 Broken Sound Parkway NW, Suite 300, Boca Raton, FL 33487-2742

and by CRC Press
2 Park Square, Milton Park, Abingdon, Oxon, OX14 4RN

Library of Congress Cataloging–in–Publication Data

Names: Scheherazade Milane, Lara, editor. | Amiji, Mansoor M, editor.
Title: Organelle and molecular targeting / edited by Lara Scheherazade Milane, Mansoor M Amiji.
Description: First edition. | Boca Raton : Taylor and Francis, 2022. | Includes bibliographical references and index.
Identifiers: LCCN 2021030913 (print) | LCCN 2021030914 (ebook) | ISBN 9780367551377 (hardback) | ISBN 9780367552831 (paperback) | ISBN 9781003092773 (ebook)
Subjects: LCSH: Drug targeting.
Classification: LCC RM301.63 .I585 2022 (print) | LCC RM301.63 (ebook) | DDC 615.1/9--dc23
LC record available at https://lccn.loc.gov/2021030913
LC ebook record available at https://lccn.loc.gov/2021030914

ISBN: 978-0-367-55137-7 (hbk)
ISBN: 978-0-367-55283-1 (pbk)
ISBN: 978-1-003-09277-3 (ebk)

DOI: 10.1201/9781003092773

Typeset in Times
by Deanta Global Publishing Services, Chennai, India

I dedicate this book to all who have had faith in me over the years, especially Mansoor Amiji; to the people I have loved and lost, Samantha Tari Jabr and Joshua David Milane; and to my brilliant daughter, Mirabella Samantha Milane, whose patience, love, and light enable me.

Lara Scheherazade Milane

I dedicate this book to the past and present research scientists, postdoctoral associates, graduate students, and all other trainees in my lab at Northeastern University. I owe all my success to these incredibly creative and hardworking individuals.

Mansoor M. Amiji

Contents

Preface

We are currently in the era of molecular therapeutics. Specific organelles and molecules have always been the desired drug targets but due to a lack of drug specificity and lack of directed drug delivery, most therapeutics to date are associated with off-target effects and non-specificity. The era of molecular therapeutics began recently when there was a shift in therapeutic design capabilities to achieve specificity at the molecular level. Pharmaceutical science, biomanufacturing, and clinical evaluation are finally established for targeting specific intracellular targets. The recent rapid design, development, and distribution of nanotechnology-based mRNA vaccines for SARS-CoV-2 demonstrated the capabilities and demand for molecular therapeutics; without the rapid sequencing and publication of the SARS-CoV-2 RNA genome, the current mRNA vaccines encoding the viral spike protein would not have been able to be designed, and without the use of lipid nanoparticles, the fragile mRNA constructs could not be administered as a vaccine. The glowing attribute of molecular therapeutics is specificity, an attribute that is largely lacking for classical small molecule drugs. An additional characteristic of molecular therapeutics is that they are often coupled to an advanced drug delivery system such as a nanoparticle. However, this is not always the case. Another key example that demonstrates the capabilities of molecular therapeutics is RNA interference (RNAi) drugs (also delivered via lipid particles) such as patisiran, givosiran, and lumasiran. However, even these drugs target specific mRNA constructs and silence translation; there are multiple barriers that must be overcome for appreciable efficacy of molecular therapeutics. The first section of this book discusses organism-level and tissue-level barriers and cellular localization, while the second section of this book discusses overcoming cellular barriers for specific organelle and molecular targeting.

In Chapter 1 of this text, Dr. Kim discuss the tissue challenges associated with specific routes of administration and how the route of administration dictates absorption and membrane transport. Overcoming the mucosal barrier is important for oral, intranasal, and pulmonary drug delivery. Strategies to overcome the mucosal barriers include mucus-penetrating coatings, mucoadhesive polymers, and mucolytic particles. Although oral drug delivery is ideal due to compliance and ease, oral delivery remains a challenge for peptides and proteins; protease inhibitors and nanoparticle encapsulation can aid in the oral delivery of these agents, yet this route is not yet optimized for macromolecule delivery. Intranasal administration is an ideal strategy for drug delivery to the brain via the olfactory epithelium and the trigeminal nerve pathway; however, the small surface area and limited volume of liquid (100–250 µl) and powder (20–50 mg) that can be administered are formulation considerations. Two additional important routes of administration that avoid the first pass effect are pulmonary and transdermal drug delivery. The large surface area of the lung is an opportunity for optimizing drug absorption; however, the mucosal barrier must be overcome and alveolar deposition must be achieved to optimize drug absorption. The skin also provides a large surface area for drug absorption, but here, the most significant barrier is the stratum corneum which consists of lipids integrated with keratinized cells.

As discussed by Dr. Vitorino in Chapter 2, nanotechnology-based approaches to drug delivery are excellent options for overcoming biological barriers. Although there are many approved nanomedicines that have studded the market since the first nanomedicine approval in 1995 (Doxil®), more recent nanomedicines have become more specialized and tailored per application. Nanomedicine approvals for cancer, infectious and immunological diseases, chronic kidney disease, and ocular disease have been the most common, and the formulations include lipid-based, polymer-based, metallic-based, and hybrid systems. Examples of more specialized systems include the anionic nanoemulsion of cyclosporine for treating dry eye disease and ultrasmall superparamagnetic iron oxide nanoparticles (SPION) for treating iron deficiency anemia. Lipid-based systems have dominated clinical approvals compared to metallic, polymer, and hybrid systems, and the advancements in lipid systems continue to dominate with recent triumphs. Important advancements in nanotechnology-based drug delivery systems include the development of transferosomes, self-assembled phospholipid-based vesicles containing lipid bilayer destabilizers called edge activators. Edge activators are single-chain surfactants with a high radius of curvature that allows the particle lipid bilayers to be highly flexible and deformable. Transferosomes are an important advancement in nanomedicines for transdermal drug delivery as the increased flexibility allows greater penetration through the skin without systemic absorption. Intricate liposome systems such as pharmacosomes have been developed with improved stability, even for oral delivery, which rely on formulation with a pre-complexed drug-phospholipid.

Although nanomedicine approaches are advancing significantly, nanomedicine design must also consider strategies to avoid recognition and clearance by the immune system. In Chapter 3 Dr. Peng discuss chemical and biological modifications to avoid immune clearance. Nanoparticles that are chemically modified to avoid immune clearance are often referred to as "stealth" nanoparticles; surface modifiers include polyethylene glycol (PEG; PEGylation) and poly(2-oxazoline) (POX). Biological strategies focus on carrier cells such as erythrocytes and stem cells or biomimetics such as coating nanoparticles with endogenous membrane components including dextrans and hyaluronic acid or coating with immunoglobulin proteins such as CD47 or CD200. An alternative and newer strategy being explored is to use ghost cells (cell membranes devoid of organelles) as drug delivery vehicles. Once the immune system is successfully diverted, the drug or biologic must reach its target site and be internalized (or bind to the cell surface receptor) to initiate activity. Chapter 4, discusses passive drug delivery approaches and the classical mechanisms of cellular uptake (micropinocytosis, phagocytosis, clathrin-mediated endocytosis, caveolae-mediated endocytosis, and clathrin-/caveolin-independent endocytosis).

Localizing therapeutics to specific systems and tissues is important for the activity of molecular therapeutics. Chapters 5 through 10 focus on targeting specific systems and tissues. In Chapter 5, Dr. Pan discusses the important advancements in tumor targeting; tumor targeting is particularly important as cancer is the second leading cause of death in the world and treatment is often interrupted or stopped due to off-target effects and toxicity, giving the patient time to recover but also giving a tumor time to develop more drug resistance. Targeted cancer therapies include hormone therapies, signal transduction inhibitors, angiogenesis inhibitors, immune checkpoint inhibitors, antibody-drug conjugates, and previously discussed nanotechnology-based approaches. In Chapter 6, Dr. Grabrucker provides a thorough update on strategies for localizing therapeutics to the brain. The blood–brain barrier, blood–cerebral spinal fluid barrier, and blood–tumor barrier are explained in depth. Strategies for crossing these barriers include intranasal drug delivery, nanoparticles, ultrasound, convection enhanced delivery, intra-arterial delivery, osmotic gradients, and prodrug approaches. In Chapter 7, Dr. Mansour details the advantages, strategies, and challenges of pulmonary drug delivery. In addition to surfactant, a significant barrier to pulmonary delivery is the requirement for a device, which adds to patient-to-patient variability in dose administration. Being the most perfused organ in the body, the lungs are prime organs for drug delivery but for drug absorption aerosol drug deposition must occur through inertial impact, sedimentation, or Brownian diffusion. To optimize deposition and minimize device variability, techniques such as particle replication in non-wetting templates (PRINT) are being explored to produce micro- and nanomedicines as API/excipient mixtures pressed into pre-made molds. In Chapter 8, Dr. Han offers a critical evaluation of cardiovascular disease pathophysiology, treatment strategies, and active targeting advancements. As cardiovascular disease remains the number one cause of death globally, advancements in cardiovascular disease targeting are critical to public health. Advancements include gene therapy for heart failure with adeno-associated viruses and polymeric nanoparticles. Exosomes, activated macrophages, and nanoparticle-coated stents are also being explored as cardiac drug delivery systems. The oral route of administration is the most common and most preferred method of drug administration to ensure patient compliance. However, the extreme pH of the stomach (from pH 1.5 to 5), the long transition times, and enzyme activity in the gastrointestinal tract are challenging barriers to oral drug delivery. In Chapter 9, Dr. Yang details a smart delivery technique for gastrointestinal drug delivery that optimizes pH, transition time, and ligand-rector interactions to achieve specific gastrointestinal delivery in the stomach, small intestine, or large intestine. The gastro-retentive drug delivery systems include floating low-density drug delivery systems, high-density sinking systems, expandable systems, and super porous hydrogels. Small intestine targeting approaches include pH-responsive systems, mucoadhesive polymers, and M-cell (specialized enterocyte) mediated transport. In the last system-specific chapter, Chapter 10, Dr. Milane discusses targeting immune cells and dysfunction as this strategy has applications to a range of pathologies from atherosclerosis to neurodegenerative disease. Reversing chronic inflammation is critical to resolving these pathologies. Advanced approaches to repolarizing macrophages, activating T cells, and activating B cells are discussed such as the application of checkpoint inhibitory peptide nanofibers in treating cancer. The implications of SARS-CoV-2 variants and efficacy of the nanoparticle-based COVID-19 mRNA vaccines are also discussed.

Section 2 of this book dives deeper into crossing cellular barriers for specific organelle and molecular targeting. Dr. Bernardes begin this section with Chapter 11 focusing on crossing the plasma membrane, exploiting specific mechanisms of cellular uptake such as transferrin receptor targeting of cancer cells and the use of cell-penetrating peptides. Dr. Bernardes uses azurin/p28 targeting of cancer cells as a case study of a specific, temperature-sensitive approach to targeting the plasma membrane of cancer cells. The mucosal barrier is a challenge for orally, respiratory, and nasally administer drugs. In Chapter 12, Dr. Nielsen discusses multiple strategies for improving drug delivery across mucosal barriers such as shape optimization and the slippery surface strategy of creating a dense cationic and anionic surface charge to increase mucosal diffusion. Lysosomes are important organelles for managing cellular debris, detoxifying cells, maintaining homeostasis, and autophagy. Lysosome dysfunction can have detrimental effects on the cell and lead to necrosis. Considering that lysosomes have the lowest pH of any intracellular organelle, it is easy to conceive how critical maintaining the integrity of lysosomes is for homeostasis. Lysosome dysfunction is linked to lysosome storage disorders, cancer, and neurodegenerative disease. Exploiting lysosomes is detailed by Dr. Torchilin in Chapter 13 with a discussion of macromolecular targeting residues and complexation strategies. Probing lysosomes as indicators of cell health is also discussed. Microtubules provide cytoskeletal support to a cell and exist as a vast highway for intracellular transport and movement. In Chapter 14 Dr. Chithrani discuss microtubules as a critical target for cancer therapy. Microtubule destabilizing and stabilizing drugs derived from natural sources are discussed along with synthetic microtubins, nanoparticle approaches to targeting, and combination therapy. The endoplasmic reticulum is the largest organelle that pans from the nuclear envelope to the plasma membrane and forms contact with multiple organelles including mitochondria, microtubules, endosomes, and the Golgi apparatus. The endoplasmic reticulum functions in protein synthesis, calcium balance, and autophagy. As the endoplasmic reticulum is the largest and most inter-connected organelle it can be thought of as one of the most critical intracellular communication pipelines within a cell. Through the endoplasmic reticulum, almost every cellular component (from DNA to mitochondria to the plasma membrane) is connected. Coupled with its critical cellular functions, this makes the endoplasmic reticulum a prime target for therapeutic manipulation. In Chapter 15, Dr. Milane discusses endoplasmic reticulum targeting strategies based on exploiting endogenous peptide-targeting approaches and applying these to nanomedicines. Mitochondria are also critical organelle targets; they produce cellular energy, regulate cell death, control mitophagy and autophagy, and maintain ROS levels. Mitochondria exist in a dynamic intracellular network that continually fuses together and fisses apart depending on cellular need. The fused network conformation is capable of higher energy production and is resistant to cell death, while separated individual mitochondria are sensitive to apoptotic signaling. Mitochondria also fuse with the endoplasmic reticulum coupling energy supply with the energy demand of protein synthesis. Mitochondrial targeting strategies are discussed by Dr. Milane in Chapter 16, and these include the use of mitochondrial leader sequences, mitochondrial penetrating peptides, delocalized cations, and DQAsomes. Mitochondria have the most negative membrane potential (–170 mV) of any organelle, and this can easily be exploited with lipophilic cations. Mitochondrial targeting has application to a range of pathologies from cancer to diabetes and neurodegenerative disease. Chapter 17, discusses the current therapies that target DNA and RNA with a highlight on the recently developed mRNA SARS-CoV-2 vaccines. In Chapter 18 Dr. Iyer summarize the benefits and approaches for organelle targeting. Molecular and organelle targeting is critical to the development of future therapeutics that have increased specificity, increased efficacy, and lower toxicity. The contributors to this book are experts in their respective fields who have worked together to create this fundamental resource in pharmaceutical science and drug delivery. As we continue through the beginning of the Molecular Therapeutics Era, our hope is that this text summarizing the current advancements and principles of molecular and organelle targeting will advance the future of this era.

Acknowledgments

We would like to thank all of the authors who worked hard to make great contributions to this book and the publishers for making this book a reality. We thank all of the scientists who have advanced the field of organelle and molecular targeting and those who established the foundation of drug delivery. Special thanks to the wonderful staff at CRC Press including Hilary Lafoe, Danielle Zarfati, and Jessica Poile who made the idea of this book into reality. We express our hope and gratitude for the future scientists who will continue to advance the field and who will continue to improve therapeutic outcomes for future patients.

Editors

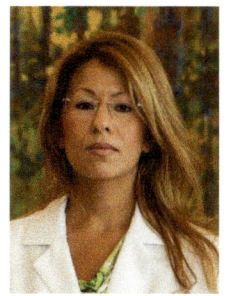 **Dr. Lara Scheherazade Milane** is the Bouvé College of Health Sciences Distinguished Educator (2021) and Assistant Teaching Professor in the Department of Pharmaceutical Sciences, Northeastern University, Boston, MA, USA. Her research interests include mitochondrial nanomedicine and developing nanotechnology-based solutions to manipulate cell communication. Dr. Milane is particularly interested in applications for treating multidrug-resistant cancer and neurodegenerative diseases. Dr. Milane is also an advocate for women in science, and has published 21 peer-reviewed articles, 3 white papers, and 5 book chapters.

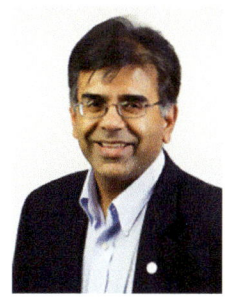 **Dr. Mansoor M. Amiji** is the University Distinguished Professor, Professor of Pharmaceutical Sciences, and Professor of Chemical Engineering at Northeastern University in Boston, MA, USA. His primary areas of research interest are in the development of targeted therapeutic solutions for chronic diseases such as cancer, neurodegenerative diseases, and inflammatory diseases. Dr. Amiji has edited 10 books including *Applied Physical Pharmacy* (now in its 3rd edition), *Nanotechnology for Cancer Therapy* (Taylor & Francis, 2007), *Handbook of Materials for Nanomedicine* (Pan Stanford Publishing, 2010), and *Diagnostic and Therapeutic Applications of Exosomes in Cancer* (Elsevier, 2018) along with over 70 published book chapters, and over 360 peer-reviewed articles.

Contributors

Wafaa Alabsi
Skaggs Pharmaceutical Sciences Center
College of Pharmacy
and
Department of Chemistry and Biochemistry
University of Arizona
Tucson, AZ, USA

Abdulaziz Alhussan
Department of Physics and Astronomy
University of Victoria
Victoria, BC, Canada

Esmael M. Alyami,
Department of Chemical and Biological
    Engineering
University of Idaho
Moscow, ID, USA

Ayatakshi Barari
Use-Inspired Biomaterials and Integrated Nano
    Delivery (U-BiND) Systems Laboratory,
    Department of Pharmaceutical Sciences
Wayne State University
Detroit, MI, USA

Nuno Bernardes
Institute for Bioengineering and Biosciences (iBB)
    and Department of Bioengineering
Instituto Superior Técnico, Universidade de Lisboa
and
Associate Laboratory i4HB—Institute for Health
    and Bioeconomy
Instituto Superior Técnico, Universidade de Lisboa
Lisbon, Portugal

Ketki Bhise
Use-Inspired Biomaterials and Integrated Nano
    Delivery (U-BiND) Systems Laboratory,
    Department of Pharmaceutical Sciences
Wayne State University
Detroit, MI, USA

Stephen M. Black
Departments of Cellular Biology & Pharmacology
    and Environmental Health Sciences
Florida International University
Miami FL, USA

Devika B. Chithrani
Department of Physics and Astronomy
and
Division of Medical Sciences
and
Centre for Advanced Materials and Related
    Technologies (CAMTEC)
and
Centre for Biomedical Research
University of Victoria
and
Department of Computer Science, Mathematics,
    Physics and Statistics
Okanagan Campus, University of British Columbia
Victoria, BC, Canada

Melis Debreli Coskun
Department of Biomedical and Nutritional
    Sciences
University of Massachusetts Lowell
Lowell, MA, USA

Eoghan Cunnane
Department of Materials
and
Department of Bioengineering
and
Institute of Biomedical Engineering
Imperial College London
London, UK

Somrita Dey
Use-Inspired Biomaterials and Integrated Nano
    Delivery (U-BiND) Systems Laboratory,
    Department of Pharmaceutical Sciences
Wayne State University
Detroit, MI, USA

Sarah Eaton
Department of Physics and Astronomy
University of Victoria
Victoria, BC, Canada

Basanth Babu Eedara
Skaggs Pharmaceutical Sciences Center
College of Pharmacy
University of Arizona
Tucson, AZ, USA

David Encinas-Basurto
Skaggs Pharmaceutical Sciences Center
College of Pharmacy
University of Arizona
Tucson, AZ, USA

Arsenio M Fialho
Institute for Bioengineering and Biosciences (iBB)
and Department of Bioengineering, Instituto
Superior Técnico
and
Associate Laboratory i4HB—Institute for Health
and Bioeconomy at Instituto Superior Técnico
Universidade de Lisboa
Lisbon, Portugal

Nina Filipczak
Center for Pharmaceutical Biotechnology and
Nanomedicine
Northeastern University
Boston, MA, USA

Parisa Foroozandeh
USM-RIKEN International Centre for Ageing
Science (URICAS), School of Biological
Science
Universiti Sains Malaysia
Penang, Malaysia

Mitali Ghose
Department of Pharmaceutical Sciences
Northeastern University
Boston, MA, USA
and
KSQ Therapeutics Inc.
Boston, MA, USA

Andreas M. Grabrucker
BioScience and BioEngineering Research
(BioSciBer), Bernal Bio Materials Research
Cluster, Bernal Institute
and
Cellular Neurobiology and Neuro-Nanotechnology
Lab, Department of Biological Sciences
and
Health Research Institute (HRI)
University of Limerick
Limerick, Ireland

Jena B. Goodman
Vascular Biology Section, Department of
Medicine, Whitaker Cardiovascular Research
Institute
Boston University
Boston, MA, USA

Jingyan Han
Vascular Biology Section, Department of Medicine,
Whitaker Cardiovascular Research Institute
Boston University
Boston, MA, USA

Sakshi Hans
BioScience and BioEngineering Research
(BioSciBer), Bernal Bio Materials Research
Cluster, Bernal Institute
and
Cellular Neurobiology and Neuro-Nanotechnology
Lab, Department of Biological Sciences
University of Limerick
Limerick, Ireland

Don Hayes Jr
Division of Pulmonary Medicine
Cincinnati Children's Hospital Medical Center
and
Division of Pulmonary, Critical Care, and Sleep
Medicine
University of Cincinnati Medical Center
and
Department of Pediatrics and Internal
Medicine
University of Cincinnati College of Medicine
Cincinnati, OH, USA

Stine Harloff-Helleberg
Center for Biopharmaceuticals and Biobarriers
   in Drug Delivery, Department of Pharmacy,
   Faculty of Health and Medical Sciences
University of Copenhagen
Copenhagen, Denmark

Arun K. Iyer
Use-Inspired Biomaterials and Integrated Nano
   Delivery (U-BiND) Systems Laboratory,
   Department of Pharmaceutical Sciences
Wayne State University
and
Molecular Imaging Program
Karmanos Cancer Institute
Detroit, MI, USA

Aubrey Johnson
Smilow Cancer Hospital of Yale-New Haven
   Health
New Haven, CT, USA

Siti Asmaa Mat Jusoh
USM-RIKEN International Centre for Ageing
   Science (URICAS), School of Biological
   Science
Universiti Sains Malaysia
Penang, Malaysia
and
School of Health Sciences
Universiti Sains Malaysia Health Campus
Kelantan, Malaysia

Jonghan Kim
Department of Biomedical and Nutritional Sciences
University of Massachusetts Lowell
Lowell, MA, USA

Zhaoyuan Li
Vascular Biology Section, Department of
   Medicine, Whitaker Cardiovascular Research
   Institute
Boston University
Boston, MA, USA

Xiang Li
Center for Pharmaceutical Biotechnology and
   Nanomedicine
Northeastern University
Boston, MA, USA
and

State Key Laboratory of Innovative Drug and
   Efficient Energy-Saving Pharmaceutical
   Equipment
Jiangxi University of Traditional Chinese Medicine
Nanchang, China

Carla M. Lopes
FP-I3ID, CEBIMED
Universidade Fernando Pessoa
Porto, Portugal

Marlene Lúcio
CF-UM-UP/CBMA, Centro de Física das
   Universidades do Minho e Porto e Centro de
   Biologia Molecular e Ambiental
Universidade do Minho, Escola de Ciências,
   Campus de Gualtar
Braga, Portugal

Heidi M. Mansour
Skaggs Pharmaceutical Sciences Center, College of
   Pharmacy
and
Department of Medicine, Division of Translational
   and Regenerative Medicine, College of
   Medicine
and
BIO5 Institute
University of Arizona
Tucson, AZ, USA

Karrina McNamara
BioScience and BioEngineering Research
   (BioSciBer), Bernal Bio Materials Research
   Cluster, Bernal Institute
University of Limerick
Limerick, Ireland

Didier Merlin
Institute for Biomedical Sciences, Digestive
   Disease Research Group
Georgia State University
Atlanta, GA, USA
and
Atlanta Veterans Affairs Medical Center
Decatur, GA, USA

Lara Scheherazade Milane
Department of Pharmaceutical Sciences
Northeastern University
Boston, MA, USA

Janni Støvring Mortensen
Center for Biopharmaceuticals and Biobarriers
 in Drug Delivery, Department of Pharmacy,
 Faculty of Health and Medical Sciences
University of Copenhagen
Copenhagen, Denmark

John J.E. Mulvihill
BioScience and BioEngineering Research
 (BioSciBer), Bernal Bio Materials Research
 Cluster, Bernal Institute
and
School of Engineering
and
Health Research Institute (HRI)
University of Limerick
Limerick, Ireland

Hanne Mørck Nielsen
Center for Biopharmaceuticals and Biobarriers
 in Drug Delivery, Department of Pharmacy,
 Faculty of Health and Medical Sciences
University of Copenhagen
Copenhagen, Denmark

Nicholas Palmerley
Department of Physics and Astronomy
University of Victoria
Victoria, BC, Canada

Eva Y. Pan
Smilow Cancer Hospital of Yale-New Haven
 Health
New Haven, CT, USA

Ching-An Peng
Department of Chemical and Biological Engineering
University of Idaho
Moscow, ID, USA

Robin Polt
Professor of Chemistry and Biochemistry
Pharmacology and Toxicology, BIO5
University of Arizona
Tucson, AZ, USA

Aisling M. Ross
BioScience and BioEngineering Research
 (BioSciBer), Bernal Bio Materials Research
 Cluster, Bernal Institute
and
Education and Health Sciences
University of Limerick
Limerick, Ireland

Samaresh Sau
Use-Inspired Biomaterials and Integrated
 Nano Delivery (U-BiND) Systems Laboratory,
 Department of Pharmaceutical Sciences
Wayne State University
Detroit, MI, USA

Shaharum Shamsuddin
USM-RIKEN International Centre for Ageing
 Science (URICAS), School of Biological
 Science
Universiti Sains Malaysia
Penang, Malaysia
and
School of Health Sciences,
Universiti Sains Malaysia Health Campus
Kelantan, Malaysia

Mai Bay Stie
Center for Biopharmaceuticals and
 Biobarriers in Drug Delivery, Department
 of Pharmacy, Faculty of Health and Medical
 Sciences
University of Copenhagen
Copenhagen, Denmark

Ammar Tarar
Department of Chemical and Biological
 Engineering
University of Idaho
Moscow, ID, USA

Katyayani Tatiparti
Use-Inspired Biomaterials and Integrated
 Nano Delivery (U-BiND) Systems
 Laboratory, Department of Pharmaceutical
 Sciences
Wayne State University
Detroit, MI, USA

Vladimir Torchilin
Center for Pharmaceutical Biotechnology and
 Nanomedicine
Northeastern University
Boston, MA, USA
and
Department of Oncology, Radiotherapy and Plastic
 Surgery
I.M. Sechenov First Moscow State Medical
 University (Sechenov University)
Moscow, Russia

Kushal Vanamala
Use-Inspired Biomaterials and Integrated Nano
    Delivery (U-BiND) Systems Laboratory,
    Department of Pharmaceutical Sciences
Wayne State University
Detroit, MI, USA

Carla Vitorino
FFUC/CCC, Faculty of Pharmacy
and
Coimbra Chemistry Centre, Department of
    Chemistry
University of Coimbra
Coimbra, Portugal

Chunhua Yang
Institute for Biomedical Sciences, Digestive
    Disease Research Group
Georgia State University
Atlanta, GA, USA
and
Atlanta Veterans Affairs Medical Center
Decatur, GA, USA

Satya Siva Kishan Yalamarty
Center for Pharmaceutical Biotechnology and
    Nanomedicine
Northeastern University
Boston, MA, USA

Mo Zhang
Vascular Biology Section, Department of
    Medicine, Whitaker Cardiovascular Research
    Institute
Boston University
Boston, MA, USA

Jennifer Zhao
Smilow Cancer Hospital of Yale-New Haven
    Health
New Haven, CT, USA

SECTION ONE

Introduction: Organ, Tissue, and Cellular Localization

There are barriers to drug delivery at multiple levels from the whole body to the organ, tissue, cell, and subcellular levels. One of the first considerations in effective drug delivery is selecting the appropriate route of administration. This is dictated by the pathology as well as the formulation. The route of administration is a contributing factor to the biodistribution which in turn contributes to efficacy as well as toxicity. Although there are multiple drug delivery approaches such as pro-drug formulations and exploiting albumin binding, nanomedicine is an important and highly relevant drug delivery approach. Nanotechnology based solutions enable the delivery of otherwise undeliverable cargo such as peptides and nucleic acids. The importance of nanomedicine is demonstrated by the SARS-CoV-2 vaccines; many of these vaccines use nanoparticles to deliver RNA, DNA, and proteins. Without the use of nanoparticles, these vaccines would not be in the clinic. The use of nanoparticles can also decrease the clearance of drugs by the immune system, increasing the efficacy of a system. Escaping immune clearance is an important aspect of drug delivery that must be optimized in relevant immune-competent *in vivo* models.

The mechanism of cell uptake (active, passive, receptor-mediated, etc.) and internalization determines the sub-cellular fate of a drug and/or drug delivery system. Drug delivery systems can be designed to be internalized via specific uptake mechanisms including direct targeting of specific cell surface receptors. Important organs and pathologies for targeting include tumors, the brain, the lungs, the cardiovascular system, the gastrointestinal system, and the immune system. Section one of this book covers molecular targeting of each of these organ systems. Section two dives deeper into subcellular targeting.

DOI: 10.1201/9781003092773-1

Route of Administration, Distribution, and Tissue-Specific Challenges

1

Melis Debreli Coskun and Jonghan Kim

Contents

DOI: 10.1201/9781003092773-2

1.1 INTRODUCTION

For effective drug therapies, it is crucial to develop treatment strategies that ensure the delivery of the drug to the target sites (the sites of drug action), such as specific organs, tissues, and cells. Therapeutic agents that are effective *in vitro* often fail *in vivo* due to a number of challenges, including biological barriers that prevent site-specific delivery. Nanoparticles (NPs) provide a promising approach for overcoming physiological barriers in the body (Thomas and Weber 2019). Some barriers are inherent to all tissues and others are organ-specific such that various factors and conditions, including administration routes and NPs' physicochemical properties, should be considered for efficient drug delivery (Busatto et al. 2019). The optimal drug delivery systems should be stable in biological fluids, maintain the intrinsic properties of drugs, localize the target sites, be capable of crossing biological barriers, ensure specific routes of administration, reduce side or adverse effects of drugs, and prolong drug interactions with the target molecules. These characteristics help maintain the required drug levels in plasma and target sites, thereby preventing off-target effects and any damage to the normal tissue/cells induced by the drug (Dhanasekaran and Chopra 2016). These can be achieved and optimized by different drug delivery systems as well as various routes of administration. In addition to the traditional approaches (e.g., oral, injectable, transdermal, inhalation, suppository, and ophthalmic dosage forms), novel drug delivery systems, including targeted delivery and drug–nanocarrier combinations, have attracted great attention in biopharmaceutics and drug development. Various drug delivery approaches can be used to maximize therapeutic efficacy and minimize toxicity, by altering the absorption, distribution, metabolism, and excretion (ADME) of drug compounds (Wen, Jung, and Li 2015). In this chapter, we provide a brief review of the impact of the route of administration and transport on the distribution of drug products and discuss tissue- and cell-specific challenges in drug delivery.

1.2 DRUG ADMINISTRATION AND MEMBRANE TRANSPORT

Different routes of administration significantly alter the bioavailability as well as biodistribution of drugs and NPs. The rate and extent of these processes are determined not only by the distinct physiochemical characteristics of drugs or NPs, but by the properties of the biological barriers and physiological status of the body. Membrane transport is a fundamental process required for ADME of bioactive substances and drugs. To exert pharmacological effects, drug molecules must cross the cell membrane either by passive or active transport. Hence, drug delivery approaches have been divided into (i) passive and (ii) active targeting strategies. As passive targeting is entirely reliant on diffusion-based transport, the physicochemical properties (e.g., size, shape, and surface chemistry/charge) of nanocarriers are critically important for cell entry (Kumar Khanna 2012). To some extent, passive targeting can achieve site-specific delivery of therapeutics and increase their local concentrations and thereby therapeutic efficacy, while reducing the drug's undesirable side effects. The ideal nanocarrier size should be 10–100 nm. For efficient extravasation from the fenestrations in leaky vasculature, the size of the nanocarriers could be <400 nm. To avoid renal filtration by the kidneys, nanocarriers need to be >10 nm in size, and to avoid the specific capture by the liver, nanocarriers need to be <100 nm. The charge of the particles should be neutral or anionic for efficient evasion of the renal elimination. For effective delivery, the nanocarriers must avoid the RES uptake, which results in opsonization and phagocytosis (Danhier, Feron, and Préat 2010).

Active targeting can be achieved by surface modification of nanocarriers with biological ligands, such as proteins, polysaccharides, aptamers, peptides, and small molecules, which facilitate the cellular uptake in cell type-specific manners (Yoo et al. 2019). Targeting ligands are attached at the surface of the nanocarrier to allow for binding to appropriate receptors expressed at the target site. Moreover, the target receptors should be expressed homogeneously on all targeted cells. These requirements ultimately decrease the unwanted non-specific interactions and localization of the drug in non-target tissues (Danhier, Feron, and Préat 2010). Various physicochemical characteristics of nanocarriers, including the formation of stable interactions with ligands, different size and shape, high carrier capacity, and ability to deliver both hydrophilic and hydrophobic substances, make them favorable platforms for target-specific and controlled delivery of micro- and macromolecules in therapies (Yetisgin et al. 2020). Various nanocarrier platforms have been developed to overcome several *in vivo* transport issues, such as limited solubility, drug aggregation, low bioavailability, poor biodistribution, and lack of selectivity, and to reduce the side effects of therapeutic drugs. These include (i) organic-based NPs (liposomes or lipid NPs, dendrimers, polymeric NPs, micelles, nanogels, and solid lipid nanoparticles (SLNPs)), (ii) inorganic-based NPs (iron oxide nanoparticles IONPs, gold nanoparticles AuNPs, ceramic NPs, semiconductor nanocrystals, silica NPs, quantum dots (QDs), and carbon nanotubes CNTs), and (iii) hybrid NPs (lipid-core/polymer-shell hybrid NPs, PEGS-core/HA-shell hybrid NPs, polymeric-micellar hybrid NPs, porous silica-based magnetic hybrid NPs) (Chenthamara et al. 2019; Li et al. 2019; Sailor and Park 2012).

1.3 DRUG ABSORPTION/DISTRIBUTION AND CHALLENGES THROUGH MUCOSAL TRANSPORT

1.3.1 Mucosal Transport

The barrier function of the mucosal layer protects the gastrointestinal (GI) tract, urinary bladder, reproductive tracts, lung airways, nose, eyes, and other mucosal surfaces. Most foreign particulates, including nano- and micro-sized objects, viruses, and bacteria, are efficiently trapped in mucus layers by steric obstruction and/or adhesion that limit their penetration to the epithelium (Lai, Wang, and Hanes 2009). The mucus is not just a steric barrier to deposited particulates; it is also an effective adhesive that can immobilize particles by hydrophobic and electrostatic interactions as well as hydrogen bonding (Čabanová et al. 2020). The uptake and transport of NPs across the epithelial cells under the mucus layer take place via two main epithelial drug transport mechanisms: (i) passive transport (paracellular and transcellular transport) and (ii) active transport (carrier-mediated transport and endo-transcytosis) (Lee 2001). Paracellular transport occurs through the tight junctions between epithelial cells in the gut (enterocytes) by diffusion, whereas transcellular transport occurs through the epithelial cells by crossing the apical and basolateral membranes (Karasov 2017). NPs that are smaller than 50 nm in size are transported paracellularly, and they can be taken up by enterocytes (50–200 nm in size) and/or the lymphoid tissues in Peyer's patches (200 nm–5 μm in size) through endocytosis (Barua and Mitragotri 2014; Shakweh et al. 2005). Strategies to overcome the mucus barrier include the development of nanocarriers with special physical and chemical properties, such as mucoadhesive and/or mucus-penetrating activity, improved solubility, enhanced permeation and uptake, improved pH-sensitive delivery capability with controlled drug release, and prolonged drug retention in mucus to delay intestinal clearance (Wang et al. 2018; Laffleur and Bernkop-Schnürch 2013).

1.3.2 Oral Administration

Oral delivery is the most common method of drug administration with greater convenience, efficacy, safety, no pain, high patient compliance, a reduction in the risk of infection from needle stick injuries, and cost-effectiveness (Chenthamara et al. 2019). The challenges in oral drug delivery include the poor aqueous solubility of drugs, chemical and enzymatic instability of drugs in variable pHs of the biological environment in the GI tract, and a protective mucus layer (Gaucher et al. 2010). The human GI tract consists of the stomach, small intestine, and large intestine. The main process of drug absorption occurs in the small intestine. The mucus layer is the first layer of defense in the epithelium, and underlying intestinal epithelial cells (IECs) have specific functions in the maintenance of the physical barrier. These cells include absorptive cells (colonocytes, enterocytes), mucus secretory goblet cells, the M cells, enteroendocrine cells, Paneth cells, and tuft cells (Ali, Tan, and Kaiko 2020). Drugs can penetrate the intestinal epithelium through several pathways, including (i) paracellular passive transport through diffusion (e.g., small molecules, hydrophilic macromolecules), (ii) transcellular passive and/or active transport (e.g., low molecular weight lipophilic drugs), (iii) facilitated diffusion, (iv) receptor-mediated endocytosis, and (v) fluid-phase endocytosis (pinocytosis) (Gaucher et al. 2010). For example, active transport is mediated by membrane transporters (e.g., P-glycoprotein) expressed on the apical (luminal) membrane of GI epithelial cells, which transport drugs back into the GI lumen after cellular uptake into enterocytes (Ma and Williams 2018). Although oral delivery works well for small molecules, the absorption of macromolecules (e.g., insulin, peptides/proteins) has been limited due to high molecular weight, the acidic environment of the stomach (e.g., high or low pH) and enzymatic degradation by intestinal proteases in the GI tract, and low permeability across the intestinal epithelium, thereby decreasing the therapeutic efficacy (Kumar, Soppimath, and Nachaegari 2006). Therefore, several approaches, including mucus-penetrating coatings, mucoadhesive polymers, polymeric nanoparticles, liposomal encapsulation, protease inhibitors, paracellular permeation enhancers, and transcellular permeation enhancers, have been used to enhance the stability of protein- or peptide-based drugs and increase their absorption (Brown, Whitehead, and Mitragotri 2020; Ibrahim et al. 2020; Plapied et al. 2011).

1.3.3 Intranasal and Pulmonary Administration

Intranasal drug delivery is an efficient, non-invasive, easily accessible route for local and systemic delivery of drugs with other advantages, including a reasonably large surface area for drug absorption, rapid onset of action and avoidance of hepatic first-pass metabolism and/or drug degradation in the GI tract (Grassin-Delyle et al. 2012). The nasal cavity is comprised of vestibules, an olfactory region, a respiratory region, and a nasopharynx (Illum 2003). To develop a drug delivery system through the nasal mucosa, drugs must cross the mucus layer and the epithelium by two different routes: the transcellular route (receptor-, carrier-, or vesicular-mediated transport) (e.g., lipophilic molecules) and the paracellular route (molecular weight <1000 Da polar drugs such as small peptides and proteins) (McMartin et al. 1987). In contrast, larger peptides and proteins are able to pass through the nasal membrane via endocytosis with limited amounts (Inagaki et al. 1985). Intranasal drug delivery is an attractive strategy for brain-targeted drug delivery via olfactory neuroepithelium and trigeminal nerve pathways that do not require transport through the blood–brain barrier (BBB) (Kumar et al. 2017; Misra and Kher 2012; Pardeshi and Belgamwar 2013).

The human respiratory system (lung) mainly consists of two vital regions: the conducting airways (trachea, bronchi, and bronchioles) and the respiratory region (respiratory bronchioles, alveolar ducts, and alveolar sacs), characterized by high vascularization and endothelial permeability that favor systemic and/or local drug delivery (Kuzmov and Minko 2015). Drug delivery through the lungs can be performed by inhalation. The mucus layer in the lung is composed of the periciliary (sol) layer and the luminal (gel) layer, which are quite different with respect to composition and function. The sol layer is watery, less viscous, and close to the bronchial wall epithelium, whereas the gel layer contains cilia to propel pathogens and inhaled particles trapped in the mucous layer out of the airways. A lot of inhaled materials are trapped in the respiratory mucus that lines the respiratory epithelium from the nose to the terminal bronchioles (Patil and Sarasija 2012). Strategies to overcome mucosal barriers include mucoadhesive, mucus-penetrating, and mucolytic particles (Wu et al. 2018).

1.3.4 Transdermal and Topical Administration

Transdermal drug delivery across the skin achieves many advantages, such as non-invasiveness, absence of first-pass hepatic metabolism, improved patient compliance, enhanced drug permeation, reduced dosing frequency, ease of self-administration, maintenance of plasma drug concentrations, extended duration of action, and low cost of the system (Qindeel et al. 2020). The skin is composed of three layers: the epidermis, dermis, and hypodermis layers, and all layers provide an effective defensive barrier to the external environment. The major barrier for diffusion through the skin is the outermost layer of the epidermis, the stratum corneum, which is composed of lipids including ceramides, triglycerides, cholesterol, and free fatty acids, which fill the spaces between dead keratin-filled cells (corneocytes) (Yang et al. 2017). The micro- and macromolecules enter the skin through three pathways: (i) the intercellular pathway (through the lipid matrix occupying the intercellular spaces of the keratinocytes, allowing for the diffusion of lipophilic or non-polar solutes), (ii) the intracellular pathway (through the keratinocytes for the transport of hydrophilic or polar solutes), and (iii) transappendageal pathway across the hair follicles through sebaceous glands and sweat glands (Desai, Patlolla, and Singh 2010; Alkilani, McCrudden, and Donnelly 2015). Since most of the molecules applied onto the skin undergo diffusion along the lipid bilayers in the intercellular regions, different nanocarriers, such as nanoemulsions, vesicular forms (transfersomes, flexosomes, ethosomes, niosomes, vesosomes), and micro- and nanoparticles are developed to overcome the stratum corneum barrier (Neubert 2011). Many studies have been focused on the lipid composition and organization in the stratum corneum and the changes involved in this lipid organization as a consequence of the topical application of drugs in formulations and patches (Bouwstra and Honeywell-Nguyen 2002; Pierre et al. 2001; İzgü et al. 2017).

1.3.5 Others

Sublingual drug delivery has been shown to be an effective alternative to the traditional oral route, especially when fast onset of action is required. Unlike oral administration, the sublingual route affords rapid drug entry into the systemic circulation via venous drainage to the superior vena cava, thereby bypassing the hepatic first-pass effect. Therefore, the sublingual route is useful for drugs that undergo high hepatic clearance or degradation in the GI tract and for patients who have swallowing difficulties (Hua 2019). Intravesical (local) drug administration is specifically used for the treatment of urinary bladder diseases, such as bladder cancer, interstitial cystitis/painful bladder syndrome, and overactive bladder, which would cause acute damage to the bladder wall and cannot be effectively treated by the systemic administration of drugs (Nirmal et al. 2012). The urothelium, the epithelial layer of the urinary bladder, serves as the primary barrier to the permeation of molecules into the bladder wall. It is composed of three cell types, including the outermost umbrella (also known as superficial facet cells that are connected with high-resistance tight junctions), intermedia, and basal cell layers (Khandelwal, Abraham, and Apodaca 2009). Intravesical drug delivery involves the administration of dosage forms directly into the bladder through a catheter, which has proven to be an effective method to ensure maximal delivery of therapeutic agents at the site of the disease and minimize systemic side effects. It is therefore important to develop a novel delivery system that not only prolongs the residence time of drugs inside the bladder, but also enables drugs to attach onto the urinary bladder wall (GuhaSarkar and Banerjee 2010). The use of polymeric hydrogels and nano/microcarriers is a major development in the field of intravesical drug delivery systems that enable prolonged drug exposure in the bladder and ultimately eliminate the need for frequent administration and target-cell specificity (Yoon et al. 2020).

1.4 DRUG ABSORPTION/DISTRIBUTION AND CHALLENGES AFTER PARENTERAL ADMINISTRATION

1.4.1 Subcutaneous and Intramuscular Administration

The subcutaneous (SC) drug delivery route provides great advantages such as low cost, self-administration, and slow/sustained absorption. SC injections are widely utilized as an effective delivery route for compounds that have limited oral bioavailability or that require an extended-release profile. The SC route is more robust relative to oral delivery because it does not undergo extensive first-pass metabolism by the liver (Chen et al. 2018). Drug administration by SC injection results in delivery to the interstitial matrix underlying the dermis of the skin and above the muscle or fat and from the interstitium to the systemic circulation either by blood or by lymphatic capillaries (Richter, Bhansali, and Morris 2012). This transport process depends on the properties of drugs or NPs, especially size and molecular weight. Small molecules (<1 kDa) are preferentially absorbed by the blood capillaries due to their largely unrestricted permeability across the vascular endothelium with the high rate of filtration and reabsorption of fluid across the vascular capillaries, whereas the transport of small particulates (<100 nm) and macromolecules into the blood is restricted by their limited permeability across the vascular endothelium. Thus, the lymphatic capillaries provide an alternative absorption pathway from the interstitial space (McLennan, Porter, and Charman 2005). To improve SC drug delivery, several methods have attracted growing interest, including long-acting formulations to maintain high plasma concentrations (Chen et al. 2018), high-concentration solutions, the use of infusion pumps, and coadministration of the dispersion enhancer hyaluronidase (Bittner, Richter, and Schmidt 2018).

Intramuscular (IM) injection is a common technique used to deliver medications into the striated muscle which has good vascularity, and IM-injected drug diffuses into the systemic circulation rapidly and thereafter into the specific region of action, bypassing first-pass metabolism. The most commonly used sites for IM injection are the deltoid, dorsogluteal, rectus femoris, vastus lateralis, and ventrogluteal muscles. IM-injected water-soluble drugs (e.g., insulin for diabetes) diffuse more rapidly, whereas drugs dissolved in an oil-based vehicle diffuse more slowly (Bolger 2018).

1.4.2 Intrathecal or Intraspinal Administration

The intrathecal drug delivery system is typically used for the treatments of chronic non-malignant pain, muscle spasticity, and cancer-related pain. It consists of two parts, a pump that serves as a drug reservoir and an intrathecal catheter that is surgically placed under the abdominal skin to deliver pain or spasticity medications directly into the cerebrospinal fluid (CSF) in the intrathecal space (Shah 2021). Intrathecally delivered drugs in the CSF permeate across the pia-arachnoid and white matter of the spinal cord to access the target dorsal horn receptors and ion channels engaged in nociceptive processing and transmission (Kroin 1992).

1.5 DRUG DISTRIBUTION/ELIMINATION AND CHALLENGES AFTER VASCULAR ADMINISTRATION

The intravascular (IV) injection is the most effective administration route for the delivery of drugs which are poorly absorbed by the GI tract and thus overcomes first-pass elimination. IV drug delivery displays the most rapid onset of action (immediate response) since the drug enters directly into the systemic circulation without delay in the absorption processes and presents complete bioavailability of drugs even with low doses. However, there are some drawbacks of the IV route, including (i) direct systemic drug exposure at high concentrations that could increase drug-related toxicity, (ii) requirement of the assistance of experienced healthcare personnel and tools for safe injection, (iii) potential contamination, (iv) injection-related pain, and (v) high costs (Sábio et al. 2021).

When NPs are present in the bloodstream, the barriers against targeted drug delivery (Figure 1.1) manifest in the form of (i) immune clearance by the reticuloendothelial system (RES), including the liver and spleen, especially by the resident macrophages in these organs, (ii) renal clearance for nanoparticles of <5 nm in size (Choi et al. 2007), (iii) permeation across the vascular endothelium into target tissues,

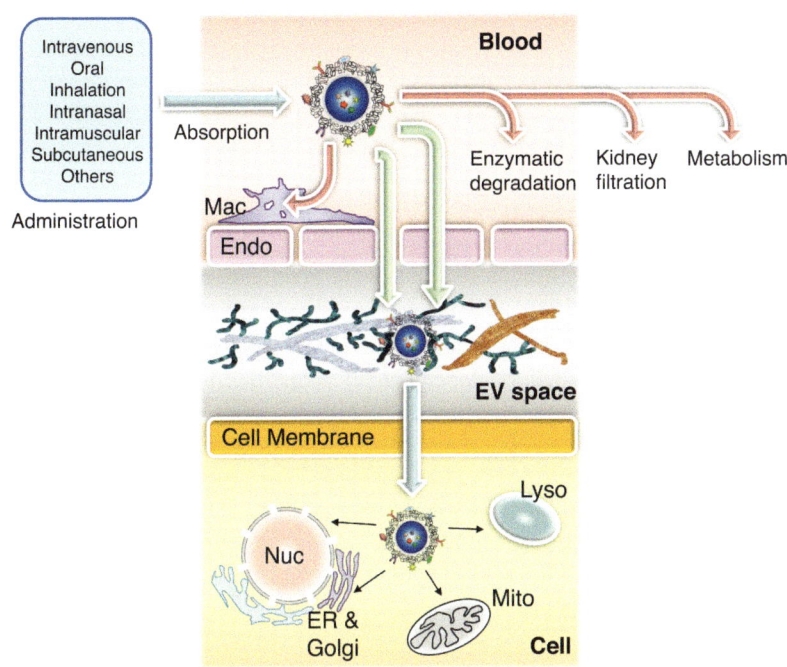

FIGURE 1.1 Drug delivery and transport. The absorption, biodistribution, intracellular transport, and elimination of NPs are shown, following different routes of administration. The fate of the NPs depends on the physicochemical properties of NPs, the route of administration, physiological status, and biological barriers. Abbreviations: Endo, endothelial cells; ER, endoplasmic reticulum; EV, extravascular; Lyso, lysosomes; Mac, macrophages; Mito, mitochondria; Nuc, nucleus.

(iv) diffusion through the dense extracellular matrix, (v) penetration into target tissue through endocytosis, (vi) cellular internalization into endosomes and endosomal escape to release the active drug cargo, (vii) diffusion through the cytoplasm, and (viii) entry into the nucleus or other organelles (Barua and Mitragotri 2014).

1.5.1 Transport from Vascular Space to Extravascular Space

NPs that are not cleared by the RES arrive at the vasculature via blood-borne transport and interact with the vascular endothelium. The endothelium is an important barrier to the free passage of NPs from blood to interstitium (Ozcelikkale, Ghosh, and Han 2013). Under healthy conditions, NPs cannot cross the vascular endothelium because tight junctions (paracellular pathway) between endothelial cells act as a barrier that limits NP transport from circulation to normal tissues. However, in certain pathological conditions (e.g., tumor neovasculature, inflammation, oxidative stress, and thrombosis) and during the activation of pro-inflammatory cytokines, endothelial cells lose their cellular integrity and the gap between the endothelial cells is increased. Consequently, NPs can extravasate from the circulation to the diseased site (e.g., solid tumor) through gaps (Galley and Webster 2004). Physiological and pathological conditions of vascularized solid tumors make their vasculature highly permeable to NPs, and therefore NPs can efficiently enter the tumor; this phenomenon is termed the enhanced permeation and retention (EPR) effect (Matsumura and Maeda 1986; Izci et al. 2021). EPR-based drug delivery depends on circulation time, targeting, and other features, such as the barrier composition and function, and these properties are also modulated by altering various factors, including size, shape, and surface properties of the drug particles. (Koren and Torchilin 2011). If NPs escape from the vascular endothelium, NPs face another barrier: interstitial space or extravascular space. The interstitial space is composed of collagen and an elastic fiber network of glycosaminoglycans and other proteins that form the extracellular matrix (ECM) (Barua and Mitragotri 2014). In certain diseases (e.g., liver fibrosis and cancer), the collagen content is higher than that of the normal tissue. This excessive rigidity and increased interstitial pressure of the ECM poses a barrier to interstitial transport of NPs from the capillaries to the target cells (Jain 1987) (Figure 1.1).

1.5.2 Transport from Extracellular Space to Intracellular Compartment

The next barrier for NP transport is the plasma membrane, and NPs are internalized by the target cell via different mechanisms, including phagocytosis, endocytosis, and pinocytosis (Jhaveri and Torchilin 2016). Specific targeting and internalization depend on NP properties (e.g., shape, size, surface properties, structure) and targeted cell types. The surface-modified NPs enter the cells mainly via receptor-mediated endocytosis. Following internalization, NPs move into vesicles from early endosomes to late endosomes, followed by digestion in lysosomes. If NPs escape the endosome or lysosome, they diffuse in the cytoplasm and could enter the nucleus, mitochondria, or other cellular organelles (Ozcelikkale, Ghosh, and Han 2013). The barriers against organelle-specific delivery as well as the targeting strategies to overcome such challenges are comprehensively discussed in other chapters.

1.6 TISSUE-SPECIFIC TRANSPORT

NP-based targeted drug therapies aim to deliver drugs to the target (diseased) site, which holds promise in reducing off-target effects, decreasing unwanted toxicities, and thereby enhancing the therapeutic efficacy of the drug. For example, brain-targeted drug delivery is required for the successful treatment of many CNS diseases (e.g., Alzheimer's disease, Parkinson's disease, multiple sclerosis, stroke, brain tumors) (Altinoglu and Adali 2020; Bourganis et al. 2018; Liu, Yang, and Ho 2018). Chronic liver diseases (e.g., viral hepatitis, liver cirrhosis, and hepatocellular carcinoma) will benefit from liver-targeted drug delivery (hepatocytes and nonparenchymal cells) (Mishra et al. 2013). However, tissue- and cell type-specific barriers hamper the access of systemically administered drugs to the target cells. Therefore, carrier molecules are designed for their selective cellular uptake by taking advantage of specific receptors or binding sites present on the surface membrane of the target cell (Zhao et al. 2020). Several important tissues are discussed below with a focus on transport and challenges, while readers are encouraged to consult more comprehensive reviews for detailed information on tissue targeting (Cheng et al. 2020; Ghosh et al. 2019; Alsaggar and Liu 2018).

1.6.1 Liver

The liver is a vital organ with a wide range of functions in the body including detoxification of numerous substances, protein synthesis, and bile production, which is necessary to digest food. Therefore, patients with chronic liver diseases, such as viral hepatitis, liver cirrhosis, or hepatocellular carcinoma, need immediate attention because they often receive prolonged drug treatments. Existing issues in liver therapies include a lack of site-specific delivery of drugs to the hepatocytes and/or nonparenchymal cells and adverse effects associated with their off-target interactions. Therefore, liver-targeted drug delivery can decrease the side effects of the drugs by reducing drug distribution in non-target cells and improve the therapeutic efficacy of the drugs by concomitantly increasing the drug concentration in target cells (Mishra et al. 2013). Different types of receptors are found on the surface of different cells present in the liver (i.e., hepatocytes, Kupffer cell, hepatic stellate cell, sinusoidal endothelial cells, bile duct epithelial cells), and these receptors can be used to achieve selective liver targeting since they bind to different types of ligands, including galactose ligands, lactobionic acid, asialofetuin, glycyrrhetinic acid, lactoferrin, and soybean-derived sterylglucoside (Rohilla et al. 2016).

1.6.1.1 Hepatocytes

Hepatocytes are vulnerable to various liver diseases, like viral hepatitis (hepatitis A, B, or C), alcohol-induced steatohepatitis (ASH), non-alcohol-induced steatohepatitis (NASH), and some genetic disorders (e.g., Wilson's disease, hemochromatosis, α-1 antitrypsin deficiency) (Mishra et al. 2013). Liver hepatocytes express asialoglycoprotein receptors (ASGPR) which exhibit high affinity for carbohydrates specifically galactose, N-acetylgalactosamine, and glucose (Fallon and Schwartz 1988; D'Souza and Devarajan 2015). ASGPR binds to terminal non-reducing galactose residues and N-acetyl-galactosamine residues of desialated tri- or tetra-antennary N-linked glycans, and therefore plays a role in the clearance of drugs from the circulation by receptor-mediated endocytosis (Meier et al. 2000). New ligands have been designed for the ASGPR mediated delivery of drugs to hepatocytes for liver diseases, including galactose-modified chitosan NPs (Zheng et al. 2012; Wang et al. 2010; Zhou et al. 2013), glycyrrhizin-modified chitosan NPs (Lin et al. 2008; Mishra et al. 2014), glycyrrhetinic acid-modified NPs (Chen et al. 2017; Li et al. 2020; Tian et al. 2010), lactosylceramide-conjugated liposomes (Spanjer and Scherphof 1983), and asialofetuin-conjugated liposomes (Wu et al. 1998; Detampel et al. 2014). In recent years, N-acetylgalactosamine (GalNAc) has shown compelling successes in the development of oligonucleotide drugs, including siRNAs, anti-miRs, and antisense oligonucleotides (ASOs) (Huang 2017). GalNAc-small interfering RNAs (siRNA) are a simple solution for the targeted delivery of siRNA to liver hepatocytes; the prototypical siRNA conjugate is a trimer of GalNac, which avidly binds to the ASGPR that is highly expressed on liver hepatocytes, resulting in rapid endocytosis (Prakash et al. 2014, 2016; Migawa et al. 2016). Subcutaneous administration of siRNA-GalNAc conjugates resulted in robust RNAi-mediated gene silencing in liver hepatocytes (Rajeev et al. 2015; Matsuda et al. 2015; Nair et al. 2014).

1.6.1.2 Kupffer Cells

Liver Kupffer cells, the resident liver macrophages, are located inside the sinusoid capillaries at the luminal side of the hepatic sinusoidal endothelium, which are responsible for phagocytic activity of the liver. After IV administration, nanocarriers can be recognized by RES; since liver Kupffer cells play a major role in phagocytosis (>85% of injected dose), while splenic macrophages contribute less (<15% of injected dose), strategies that avoid the uptake of nanocarriers by Kupffer cells can enhance spleen delivery (Jindal 2016). Macrophages recognize the drug delivery systems via the recognition of opsonins present over them or through interaction with multiple scavenger receptors (e.g., toll-like, mannose, and Fc receptors) that are expressed on the Kupffer cell membrane (Mishra et al. 2013). There are several NP uptake mechanisms by cells, including phagocytosis, macropinocytosis (allows internalization of 0.5–5 μm nanosystems), clathrin-mediated endocytosis (100–350 nm size), caveolin-mediated endocytosis (20–100 nm size), and additional endocytotic pathways. The internalization process is also modulated by the size and shape of the NPs as well as other characteristics such as surface charge and functionalization (Sousa de Almeida et al. 2021). Liposomes of which surfaces are modified by cetylmannoside could be useful for targeting to Kupffer cells (Chikamasa et al. 1991). Liposomes are also suitable vehicles for the targeting of anti-inflammatory compounds such as dexamethasone (Melgert et al. 2001; Bartneck et al. 2015), curcumin (Maradana et al. 2018), or calcitriol (Rafique et al. 2019) to the Kupffer cells.

1.6.1.3 Liver Sinusoidal Endothelial Cells

Liver sinusoids are composed of sinusoidal endothelial and Kupffer cells. Liver sinusoidal endothelial cells (LSEC) constitute the sinusoidal wall (also called endothelium), representing the interface between blood cells and hepatocytes/hepatic stellate cells (Tsutsui and Nishiguchi 2014). Blood circulates within the liver sinusoids which can be regarded as unique capillaries because of the presence of open pores or fenestrae (100 to 200 nm in diameter, membrane bound round cytoplasmic holes) that lack a diaphragm and a basal lamina underneath the endothelium. The capillary endothelium plays a role in regulating the exchange of macromolecules, solutes, and fluid between the blood and the surrounding tissues. Some substances are directly delivered to the endothelial cells by endocytosis, whereas others are transported across the endothelium to the surrounding tissues by transcytosis (Braet and Wisse 2002). LSECs do not simply form a barrier within the hepatic sinusoids but have vital physiological and immune functions, including filtration, endocytosis, antigen presentation, and leukocyte recruitment. LSECs play an essential role in immune homeostasis within the liver (e.g., regulation of the vascular tone, inflammation, and thrombosis) and in controlling the immune response during acute and chronic liver injury (Shetty, Lalor, and Adams 2018; Wilkinson, Qurashi, and Shetty 2020; Gracia-Sancho et al. 2021). LSECs have a very high endocytic capacity aided by scavenger receptors (SR), such as SR-A, SR-B, CD-36, SR-E (Lox-1 and mannose receptors), SR-H (stabilins), and SR-L (LRP-1), and along with other SRs, LSECs co-express two surface lectins called LSECtin and L-SIGN (Pandey, Nour, and Harris 2020). In the liver, interleukin-1 (IL-1) up-regulates the endocytic activity of the mannose receptor (ManR) expressed by LSECs (Asumendi et al. 1996). Besides the ManR, stabilin-1 and stabilin-2 are the major scavenger receptors expressed by LSEC. Stabilin-1 and -2 together provide proper hepatic clearance of potentially noxious agents in the blood and maintain tissue homeostasis not only in the liver but also distant organs (Schledzewski et al. 2011). Both stabilin-1 and stabilin-2 were highly expressed in the LSECs and involved in the LSEC endocytosis of oxLDLs (oxidized form of low-density lipoprotein), but experiments with stabilin-transfected cells pointed to stabilin-1 as the most important receptor for mildly oxLDL (Li et al. 2011). LSECs also play a key role in the initial uptake of viral pathogens (hepatitis B virus) into the liver; at later stages, the viruses leave the LSEC and enter the hepatocytes (Breiner, Schaller, and Knolle 2001).

1.6.1.4 Hepatic Stellate Cells

Hepatic stellate cells (HSCs) are located in the space of Disse, an anatomical space between hepatocytes and the sinusoid, and maintain close interactions with LSECs and hepatocytes. HSCs are liver-specific mesenchymal cells and store vitamin A in the body. When the liver is injured due to viral infection or hepatic toxins, HSCs receive signals secreted by injured hepatocytes and immune cells that transdifferentiate them into activated myofibroblast-like cells to promote fibrosis, leading to cirrhosis and hepatocellular carcinoma (Barry et al. 2020). At the site of injury, activated HSCs generate a temporary scar to protect the liver from further damage and also secrete cytokines and growth factors that promote the regeneration of hepatic epithelial cells (Yin et al. 2013). Targeted delivery of coupled mycophenolic acid (immunosuppressive drug) to the HSC-selective drug carrier mannose-6-phosphate (M6P) modified human serum albumin (HSA) results in decreased activation of HSC, making it the first drug that is successfully delivered to this cell type (Greupink et al. 2005). In a rat model of liver fibrosis, M6P-HSA-liposomes can be efficiently targeted to non-parenchymal cells, including HSCs (Adrian et al. 2007). More detailed information about targeted drug delivery to hepatic stellate cells for the treatment of liver fibrosis is found elsewhere (Chen et al. 2019; Mishra et al. 2013).

1.6.2 Kidney

Direct targeting to the kidneys is a promising strategy to improve the treatment of kidney diseases. A variety of engineered NPs, liposomes, macromolecular carriers (low molecular weight proteins (LMWPs), lysozyme, low molecular weight chitosan (LMWC), poly(vinylpyrrolidone-co-dimethyl maleic acid-PVD, G3-C12 peptide), and prodrugs (sugar-, amino acid-, folate-modified drugs) have been developed for nanomedicine (Zhou, Sun, and Zhang 2014). In addition to the organs of the RES, the kidneys are the second major organ for NPs clearance, which filter NPs from the blood, ensure that essential plasma proteins are retained in the blood, and quickly remove unnecessary small molecules from the body. Kidney filtration is carried out by the glomerular filtration membrane (GFM), which is supported by mesangial cells (or mesangium) in the mesangial matrix. The glomerular filtration barrier consists of an endothelial glycocalyx, fenestrated endothelial cells, the glomerular basement membrane (GBM), and highly specialized podocytes (Du, Yu, and Zheng 2018; Arif and Nihalani 2013).

Targeting drug delivery strategies to the renal glomerulus and proximal renal tubule (receptor-mediated internalization pathway) provides new therapeutic approaches for the treatment of kidney diseases (Liu et al. 2019). Various studies describe the targeting of NPs to the glomerulus (Zuckerman and Davis 2013). Within the glomerulus, NPs have been shown to target the GBM (Zuckerman et al. 2012) and mesangial cells (Choi et al. 2011; Yuan et al. 2019). The size, shape, surface charge, flexibility, and deformability are the primary properties of NP deposition within the glomerulus regardless of NP composition, including gold nanoparticles, siRNA nanoparticles, and polymer-drug nanoparticles. All these three nanoparticles are sub-100 nm and readily accumulate within the glomerulus, although siRNA nanoparticles lead them to deposit in the GBM, whereas gold- and polymer-drug NPs only deposit in the mesangium (Zuckerman et al. 2012). Recent preclinical studies demonstrated selective renal targeting and renal tubular localization of NPs (Williams et al. 2018). NPs that are small enough to pass through the glomerular filtration barrier could subsequently be taken up by highly endocytic epithelial cells of the proximal tubule (Liu et al. 2007; Choi et al. 2007). Accumulation of these particles in the proximal tubules may adversely affect the function of the nephron segment and consequently the entire kidney (Nair et al. 2015). Macromolecular carriers are useful for targeting drugs to the kidney; in particular, low-molecular-weight proteins (LMWP, MW < 66 kDa) undergo glomerular filtration, followed by reabsorption by renal proximal tubules (Zhou, Sun, and Zhang 2014), whereas the structure of glomerular filtration barrier prevents the abnormal passage of albumin (MW = 66 kDa) (Tojo and Kinugasa 2012; Lawrence et al. 2017) and high-molecular-weight proteins (MW > 66 kDa) (Raila, Forterre, and Schweigert 2005). Conversely, ultrasmall NPs can be used to target proximal tubule cells for therapeutic drug delivery. Interestingly, mesoscale NPs (~400 nm in diameter) unexpectedly and selectively localized in renal proximal tubules and up to seven times more efficiently in the kidney than other organs (Williams et al. 2015).

1.6.3 Brain

Multiple approaches have been attempted to deliver drugs into the brain, including direct access routes via invasive methods (e.g., intracerebral or intraventricular injections and implants), intranasal administration, and the intravenous route (Bellettato and Scarpa 2018). Drug delivery to the brain is particularly challenging due to the unique barrier system: the blood–brain barrier (BBB), which is formed by endothelial tight junctions that maintain a continuous, nonfenestrated basal lamina and interact with astrocytes, pericytes, microglia, and perivascular macrophages (Wong et al. 2013). For CNS delivery, drugs must traverse the endothelium and partition into the aqueous environment of the cerebrospinal fluid (CSF) and/or brain interstitial fluid. Molecules may cross the BBB by two pathways: (i) paracellular transport (e.g., small hydrophilic molecules) and (ii) transcellular transport (e.g., small lipophilic molecules), which involves passing across the luminal side of the endothelial cell, the cytoplasm, and the abluminal side of the endothelial cell and entering the brain interstitium. However, for almost all other substances, carrier-mediated transport (e.g., glucose, amino acids, nucleosides), receptor-mediated transcytosis (e.g., insulin, transferrin), or adsorptive transcytosis (e.g., albumin and other positively charged plasma proteins) is required to pass the BBB (Pardridge 2012; Hersh et al. 2016; Gawdi and Emmady 2021; Chen and Liu 2012). Small-molecule drugs can be synthesized for carrier-mediated transport (CMT) systems, whereas large-molecule drugs can be reengineered with molecular Trojan horse delivery systems to access receptor-mediated transport (RMT) systems (Pardridge 2012). The BBB permeability can also be altered by physiological factors, such as brain-to-blood efflux transporters (e.g., P-glycoprotein), enzymatic activity, plasma protein binding, and cerebral blood flow (Dong 2018). Strategies for the delivery of therapeutics across the BBB include osmotic/chemical disruption, enhanced transcytosis, nanoparticles/nanotubes, cell-mediated delivery, and ultrasound-mediated BBB opening. Interstitial wafers/microchips and catheter-enhanced local delivery bypass the BBB (Hersh et al. 2016). Current delivery strategies to the brain using NPs rely on conjugation with ligands which bind to target proteins associated with the BBB (e.g., LRP1, TfR1, Glut1, and SLC7A5). However, these strategies have significant limitations against brain specificity since protein expression is not limited to the BBB. For instance, LRP1/TfR1, Glut1, and SLC7A5 are also highly expressed on the lung, kidney, and intestine epithelium/endothelium, respectively, leading to high off-target accumulation of functionalized NPs into peripheral organs (Gonzalez-Carter et al. 2020).

Intranasal administration is one of the promising options to bypass the BBB and blood–CSF barrier. Intranasal delivery is a noninvasive and convenient route into the brain since the olfactory region of the nasal cavity provides direct access to the CNS via the neuroepithelial layer where the CNS has direct exposure to the environment. The permeable nasal epithelium allows rapid drug absorption to the brain due to high blood flow, porous endothelial membrane, reasonable surface area, and avoidance of first-pass metabolism (Bahadur et al. 2020). Intranasal delivery does not necessarily require any modification to therapeutic agents and allows drugs to be delivered to the CNS within minutes with minimal systemic exposure and thereby decreased systemic side effects (Dhuria, Hanson, and Frey 2010; Godfrey et al. 2018). More recently, the contribution made by the trigeminal pathway to intranasal delivery to the CNS has also been recognized, especially to caudal brain regions and the spinal cord (Hanson and Frey 2008; Bahadur et al. 2020; Keller, Merkel, and Popp 2021; Veronesi et al. 2020; Erdő et al. 2018). There are some limitations associated with the nose-to-brain route, including small volume for drug administration (for liquids of 100–250 µl and powders 20–50 mg), limited surface area of the olfactory epithelium (especially in humans), short retention time for drug absorption, enzymatic degradation in the nasal cavity, and irritation in the nasal cavity, which must be acknowledged when developing new therapeutics to be administered via this route (Wang et al. 2019). Recently, intranasal delivery of luciferase-nonviral mRNA capsulated in cationic liposomes demonstrated significantly higher luciferase activity in the cortex, striatum, and midbrain regions in the brain (Dhaliwal et al. 2020). Combined, these efforts suggest that intranasal nanocarriers can efficiently deliver not only small-molecule drugs, but different types of proteins and nucleic acids that can treat various neurological disorders.

1.7 CONCLUDING REMARKS

The overall theme of this chapter is to discuss different routes of nanocarrier administration, and the challenges associated with each drug delivery method to provide improved understanding of the biological barriers and their impact on drug delivery and distribution. These efforts will help researchers and biomedical scientists design and develop nanocarriers that can overcome various physiological barriers and deliver the drugs selectively to the target sites in higher concentrations, while minimizing the toxic effects of the drugs. The physiochemical properties of nanocarriers can be tuned by altering their compositions (organic, inorganic, or hybrid), optical property, magnetic property, particle sizes, morphology (sphere, rod, or cube), and surface properties (surface charge, functionalized groups, PEGylation or other coating, attachment of targeting moieties), which can effectively deliver drugs and therapeutic genes to certain locations, provide protection against enzymatic degradation, avoid RES clearance, minimize immunogenicity (e.g., by preventing opsonization), enhance plasma stability and solubility, improve the pharmacological profile, allow for controlled and sustained release of the drug, and reduce the side effects of drugs. The physicochemical factors related to delivery systems and their pharmacokinetic behavior are the primary determinants for the improved targeting and therapeutic effectiveness. Therefore, the optimization of these factors during formulation development can lead to more promising and effective treatments for diseases.

REFERENCES

Adrian, Joanna E., Jan A. A. M. Kamps, Gerrit L. Scherphof, and Dirk K. F. Meijer, A. M. van Loenen-Weemaes, C. Reker-Smit, P. Terpstra, and K. Poelstra, Anne-miek van Loenen-Weemaes, Catharina Reker-Smit, Peter Terpstra, and Klaas Poelstra. "A Novel Lipid-based Drug Carrier Targeted to the Non-parenchymal Cells, Including Hepatic Stellate Cells, in the Fibrotic Livers of Bile Duct Ligated Rats." *Biochimica & Biophysica Acta (BBA)* 1768, no. 6 (2007): 1430–39.

Ali, Ayesha, HuiYing Tan, and Gerard E. Kaiko. "Role of the Intestinal Epithelium and Its Interaction with the Microbiota in Food Allergy." *Frontiers in Immunology* 11 (2020).

Alkilani, Ahlam Zaid, Maelíosa T. C. McCrudden, and Ryan F. Donnelly. "Transdermal Drug Delivery: Innovative Pharmaceutical Developments Based on Disruption of the Barrier Properties of the Stratum Corneum." *Pharmaceutics* 7, no. 4 (2015): 438–70.

Alsaggar, Mohammad, and Dexi Liu. "Organ-Based Drug Delivery." *Journal of Drug Targeting* 26, no. 5–6 (2018): 385–97.

Altinoglu, G., and T. Adali. "Alzheimer's Disease Targeted Nano-Based Drug Delivery Systems." *Current Drug Targets* 21, no. 7 (2020): 628–46.

Arif, Ehtesham, and Deepak Nihalani. "Glomerular Filtration Barrier Assembly: An Insight." *Postdoc Journal: a Journal of Postdoctoral Research & Postdoctoral Affairs* 1, no. 4 (2013): 33–45.

Asumendi, A., A. Alvarez, I. Martinez, B. Smedsrød, and F. Vidal-Vanaclocha. "Hepatic Sinusoidal Endothelium Heterogeneity with Respect to Mannose Receptor Activity Is Interleukin-1 Dependent." *Hepatology* 23, no. 6 (1996): 1521–9.

Bahadur, S., D. M. Pardhi, J. Rautio, J. M. Rosenholm, and K. Pathak. "Intranasal Nanoemulsions for Direct Nose-to-Brain Delivery of Actives for CNS Disorders." *Pharmaceutics* 12, no. 12 (2020): 1230–57 .

Barry, Anna E., Rajkumar Baldeosingh, Ryan Lamm, Keyur Patel, Kai Zhang, Dana A. Dominguez, Kayla J. Kirton, Ashesh P. Shah, and Hien Dang. "Hepatic Stellate Cells and Hepatocarcinogenesis." *Frontiers in Cell & Developmental Biology* 8 (2020): 709–25.

Bartneck, M., K. M. Scheyda, K. T. Warzecha, L. Y. Rizzo, K. Hittatiya, T. Luedde, G. Storm, C. Trautwein, T. Lammers, and F. Tacke. "Fluorescent Cell-Traceable Dexamethasone-Loaded Liposomes for the Treatment of Inflammatory Liver Diseases." *Biomaterials* 37 (2015): 367–82.

Barua, S., and S. Mitragotri. "Challenges Associated with Penetration of Nanoparticles Across Cell and Tissue Barriers: A Review of Current Status and Future Prospects." *Nano Today* 9, no. 2 (2014): 223–43.

Bellettato, Cinzia M., and Maurizio Scarpa. "Possible Strategies to Cross the Blood–Brain Barrier." *Italian Journal of Pediatrics* 44, no. Suppl 2 (2018): 131.

Bittner, B., W. Richter, and J. Schmidt. "Subcutaneous Administration of Biotherapeutics: An Overview of Current Challenges and Opportunities." *BioDrugs* 32, no. 5 (2018): 425–40.

Bolger, Gordon T. "Routes of Drug Administration☆." In *Reference Module in Biomedical Sciences*. Amsterdam: Elsevier, 2018.

Bourganis, Vassilis, Olga Kammona, Aleck Alexopoulos, and Costas Kiparissides. "Recent Advances in Carrier Mediated Nose-to-Brain Delivery of Pharmaceutics." *European Journal of Pharmaceutics & Biopharmaceutics* 128 (2018): 337–62.

Bouwstra, J. A., and P. L. Honeywell-Nguyen. "Skin Structure and Mode of Action of Vesicles." *Advanced Drug Delivery Reviews* 54 Suppl. 1 (2002): S41–S55.

Braet, Filip, and Eddie Wisse. "Structural and Functional Aspects of Liver Sinusoidal Endothelial Cell Fenestrae: A Review." *Comparative Hepatology* 1, no. 1 (2002): 1–18.

Breiner, K. M., H. Schaller, and P. A. Knolle. "Endothelial Cell-Mediated Uptake of a Hepatitis B Virus: A New Concept of Liver Targeting of Hepatotropic Microorganisms." *Hepatology* 34, no. 4 Pt 1 (2001): 803–8.

Brown, Tyler D., Kathryn A. Whitehead, and Samir Mitragotri. "Materials for Oral Delivery of Proteins and Peptides." *Nature Reviews Materials* 5, no. 2 (2020): 127–48.

Busatto, Sara, Anthony Pham, Annie Suh, Shane Shapiro, and Joy Wolfram. "Organotropic Drug Delivery: Synthetic Nanoparticles and Extracellular Vesicles." *Biomedical Microdevices* 21, no. 2 (2019): 46.

Čabanová, Kristina, Oldřich Motyka, Lenka Čábalová, Kamila Hrabovská, Hana Bielniková, Ľubomíra Kuzníková, Jana Dvořáčková, Karol Zeleník, Pavel Komínek, and Jana Kukutschová. "Metal Particles in Mucus and Hypertrophic Tissue of the Inferior Nasal Turbinates from the Human Upper Respiratory Tract." *Environmental Science & Pollution Research* 27, no. 22 (2020): 28146–54.

Chen, Jing, Yuchao Chen, Yi Cheng, Youheng Gao, Pinjing Zheng, Chuangnan Li, Yidan Tong, Zhao Li, Wenhui Luo, and Zhao Chen. "Modifying Glycyrrhetinic Acid Liposomes with Liver-Targeting Ligand of Galactosylated Derivative: Preparation and Evaluations." *Oncotarget* 8, no. 60 (2017): 102046–66.

Chen, Wei, Bryant C. Yung, Zhiyong Qian, and Xiaoyuan Chen. "Improving Long-Term Subcutaneous Drug Delivery by Regulating Material-Bioenvironment Interaction." *Advanced Drug Delivery Reviews* 127 (2018): 20–34.

Chen, Yan, and Lihong Liu. "Modern Methods for Delivery of Drugs Across the Blood–Brain Barrier." *Advanced Drug Delivery Reviews* 64, no. 7 (2012): 640–65.

Chen, Z., A. Jain, H. Liu, Z. Zhao, and K. Cheng. "Targeted Drug Delivery to Hepatic Stellate Cells for the Treatment of Liver Fibrosis." *Journal of Pharmacology & Experimental Therapeutics* 370, no. 3 (2019): 695–702.

Cheng, Qiang, Tuo Wei, Lukas Farbiak, Lindsay T. Johnson, Sean A. Dilliard, and Daniel J. Siegwart. "Selective Organ Targeting (SORT) Nanoparticles for Tissue-Specific mRNA Delivery and CRISPR–Cas Gene Editing." *Nature Nanotechnology* 15, no. 4 (2020): 313–20.

Chenthamara, Dhrisya, Sadhasivam Subramaniam, Sankar Ganesh Ramakrishnan, Swaminathan Krishnaswamy, Musthafa Mohamed Essa, Feng-Huei Lin, and M. Walid Qoronfleh. "Therapeutic Efficacy of Nanoparticles and Routes of Administration." *Biomaterials Research* 23 (2019): 20.

Chikamasa, Yamashita, Matsuo Hirotami, Akiyama Kazue, and Kiwada Hiroshi. "Enhancing Effect of Cetylmannoside on Targeting of Liposomes to Kupffer Cells in Rats." *International Journal of Pharmaceutics* 70, no. 3 (1991): 225–33.

Choi, C. H., J. E. Zuckerman, P. Webster, and M. E. Davis. "Targeting Kidney Mesangium by Nanoparticles of Defined Size." *Proceedings of the National Academy of Sciences of the United States of America* 108, no. 16 (2011): 6656–61.

Choi, H. S., W. Liu, P. Misra, E. Tanaka, J. P. Zimmer, B. Itty Ipe, M. G. Bawendi, and J. V. Frangioni. "Renal Clearance of Quantum Dots." *Nature Biotechnology* 25, no. 10 (2007): 1165–70.

D'Souza, A. A., and P. V. Devarajan. "Asialoglycoprotein Receptor Mediated Hepatocyte Targeting: Strategies and Applications." *Journal of Controlled Release* 203 (2015): 126–39.

Danhier, F., O. Feron, and V. Préat. "To Exploit the Tumor Microenvironment: Passive and Active Tumor Targeting of Nanocarriers for Anti-Cancer Drug Delivery." *Journal of Controlled Release* 148, no. 2 (2010): 135–46.

Desai, Pinaki, Ram R. Patlolla, and Mandip Singh. "Interaction of Nanoparticles and Cell-Penetrating Peptides with Skin for Transdermal Drug Delivery." *Molecular Membrane Biology* 27, no. 7 (2010): 247–59.

Detampel, P., D. Witzigmann, S. Krähenbühl, and J. Huwyler. "Hepatocyte Targeting Using Pegylated Asialofetuin-Conjugated Liposomes." *Journal of Drug Targeting* 22, no. 3 (2014): 232–41.

Dhaliwal, Harkiranpreet Kaur, Yingfang Fan, Jonghan Kim, and Mansoor M. Amiji. "Intranasal delivery and transfection of mRNA therapeutics in the brain using cationic liposomes." *Molecular Pharmaceutics* 17, no. 6 (2020): 1996–2005.

Dhanasekaran, Sugapriya, and Sumitra Chopra. "Getting a Handle on Smart Drug Delivery Systems: A Comprehensive View of Therapeutic Targeting Strategies." In *Smart Drug Delivery System*. 2016.

Dhuria, S. V., L. R. Hanson, and W. H. Frey, 2nd. "Intranasal Delivery to the Central Nervous System: Mechanisms and Experimental Considerations." *Journal of Pharmaceutical Sciences* 99, no. 4 (2010): 1654–73.

Dong, Xiaowei. "Current Strategies for Brain Drug Delivery." *Theranostics* 8, no. 6 (2018): 1481–93.

Du, Bujie, Yu Mengxiao, and Jie Zheng. "Transport and Interactions of Nanoparticles in the Kidneys." *Nature Reviews Materials* 3, no. 10 (2018): 358–74.

Erdő, Franciska, Luca Anna Bors, Dániel Farkas, Ágnes Bajza, and Sveinbjörn Gizurarson. "Evaluation of Intranasal Delivery Route of Drug Administration for Brain Targeting." *Brain Research Bulletin* 143 (2018): 155–70.

Fallon, R. J., and A. L. Schwartz. "Asialoglycoprotein Receptor Phosphorylation and Receptor-Mediated Endocytosis in Hepatoma Cells. Effect of Phorbol Esters." *Journal of Biological Chemistry* 263, no. 26 (1988): 13159–66.

Galley, H. F., and N. R. Webster. "Physiology of the Endothelium." *British Journal of Anaesthesia* 93, no. 1 (2004): 105–13.

Gaucher, Geneviève, Prashant Satturwar, Marie-Christine Jones, Alexandra Furtos, and Jean-Christophe Leroux. "Polymeric Micelles for Oral Drug Delivery." *European Journal of Pharmaceutics & Biopharmaceutics* 76, no. 2 (2010): 147–58.

Gawdi, R., and P. D. Emmady. "Physiology, Blood Brain Barrier." In *Stat Pearls*. Treasure Island, FL: StatPearls Publishing LLC, 2021.

Ghosh, Dipanjana, Neeraj Upmanyu, Tripti Shukla, and Tarani P. Shrivastava. "Chapter 1: Cell and Organ Drug Targeting." In *Nanomaterials for Drug Delivery and Therapy*, edited by Alexandru Mihai Grumezescu. William Andrew Publishing, 2019.

Godfrey, Lisa, Antonio Iannitelli, Natalie L. Garrett, Julian Moger, Ian Imbert, Tamara King, Frank Porreca, Ramesh Soundararajan, Aikaterini Lalatsa, Andreas G. Schätzlein, and Ijeoma F. Uchegbu. "Nanoparticulate Peptide Delivery Exclusively to the Brain Produces Tolerance Free Analgesia." *Journal of Controlled Release* 270 (2018): 135–44.

Gonzalez-Carter, Daniel, Xueying Liu, Theofilus A. Tockary, Anjaneyulu Dirisala, Kazuko Toh, Yasutaka Anraku, and Kazunori Kataoka. "Targeting Nanoparticles to the Brain by Exploiting the Blood–Brain Barrier Impermeability to Selectively Label the Brain Endothelium." *Proceedings of the National Academy of Sciences of the United States of America* 117, no. 32 (2020): 19141–50.

Gracia-Sancho, Jordi, Esther Caparrós, Anabel Fernández-Iglesias, and Rubén Francés. "Role of Liver Sinusoidal Endothelial Cells in Liver Diseases." *Nature Reviews. Gastroenterology & Hepatology* 18, no. 6 (2021): 411–31.

Grassin-Delyle, S., A. Buenestado, E. Naline, C. Faisy, S. Blouquit-Laye, L. J. Couderc, M. Le Guen, M. Fischler, and P. Devillier. "Intranasal Drug Delivery: An Efficient and Non-Invasive Route for Systemic Administration: Focus on Opioids." *Pharmacology & Therapeutics* 134, no. 3 (2012): 366–79.

Greupink, R., H. I. Bakker, C. Reker-Smit, A. M. van Loenen-Weemaes, R. J. Kok, D. K. Meijer, L. Beljaars, and K. Poelstra. "Studies on the Targeted Delivery of the Antifibrogenic Compound Mycophenolic Acid to the Hepatic Stellate Cell." *Journal of Hepatology* 43, no. 5 (2005): 884–92.

GuhaSarkar, Shruti, and R. Banerjee. "Intravesical Drug Delivery: Challenges, Current Status, Opportunities and Novel Strategies." *Journal of Controlled Release* 148, no. 2 (2010): 147–59.

Hanson, Leah R., and William H. Frey, 2nd. "Intranasal Delivery Bypasses the Blood-Brain Barrier to Target Therapeutic Agents to the Central Nervous System and Treat Neurodegenerative Disease." *BMC Neuroscience* 9 Suppl. 3 (2008): S5–S.

Hersh, David S., Aniket S. Wadajkar, Nathan Roberts, Jimena G. Perez, Nina P. Connolly, Victor Frenkel, Jeffrey A. Winkles, Graeme F. Woodworth, and Anthony J. Kim. "Evolving Drug Delivery Strategies to Overcome the Blood Brain Barrier." *Current Pharmaceutical Design* 22, no. 9 (2016): 1177–93.

Hua, Susan. "Advances in Nanoparticulate Drug Delivery Approaches for Sublingual and Buccal Administration." *Frontiers in Pharmacology* 10 (2019): 1328–28.

Huang, Y. "Preclinical and Clinical Advances of GalNAc-Decorated Nucleic Acid Therapeutics." *Molecular Therapy: Nucleic Acids* 6 (2017): 116–32.

Ibrahim, Yousif H. E. Y., Géza Regdon, Elnazeer I. Hamedelniel, and Tamás Sovány. "Review of Recently Used Techniques and Materials to Improve the Efficiency of Orally Administered Proteins/Peptides." *DARU: Journal of Pharmaceutical Sciences* 28, no. 1 (2020): 403–16.

Illum, Lisbeth. "Nasal Drug Delivery: Possibilities, Problems and Solutions." *Journal of Controlled Release* 87, no. 1–3 (2003): 187–98.

Inagaki, M., Y. Sakakura, H. Itoh, K. Ukai, and Y. Miyoshi. "Macromolecular Permeability of the Tight Junction of the Human Nasal Mucosa." *Rhinology* 23, no. 3 (1985): 213–21.

Izci, Mukaddes, Christy Maksoudian, Bella B. Manshian, and Stefaan J. Soenen. "The Use of Alternative Strategies for Enhanced Nanoparticle Delivery to Solid Tumors." *Chemical Reviews* 121, no. 3 (2021): 1746–803.

İzgü, F., G. Bayram, K. Tosun, and D. İzgü. "Stratum Corneum Lipid Liposome-Encapsulated Panomycocin: Preparation, Characterization, and the Determination of Antimycotic Efficacy Against Candida spp. Isolated from Patients with Vulvovaginitis in an In Vitro Human Vaginal Epithelium Tissue Model." *International Journal of Nanomedicine* 12 (2017): 5601–11.

Jain, R. K. "Transport of Molecules in the Tumor Interstitium: A Review." *Cancer Research* 47, no. 12 (1987): 3039–51.

Jhaveri, A., and V. Torchilin. "Intracellular Delivery of Nanocarriers and Targeting to Subcellular Organelles." *Expert Opinion on Drug Delivery* 13, no. 1 (2016): 49–70.

Jindal, A. B. "Nanocarriers for Spleen Targeting: Anatomo-Physiological Considerations, Formulation Strategies and Therapeutic Potential." *Drug Delivery & Translational Research* 6, no. 5 (2016): 473–85.

Karasov, William H. "Integrative Physiology of Transcellular and Paracellular Intestinal Absorption." *Journal of Experimental Biology* 220, no. 14 (2017): 2495.

Keller, Olivia Merkel Lea-Adriana, and Andreas Popp. "Intranasal Drug Delivery: Opportunities and Toxicologic Challenges During Drug Development." *Drug Delivery & Translational Research* (2021).

Khandelwal, Puneet, Soman N. Abraham, and Gerard Apodaca. "Cell Biology and Physiology of the Uroepithelium." *American Journal of Physiology. Renal Physiology* 297, no. 6 (2009): F1477–FF501.

Koren, E., and V. P. Torchilin. "Drug Carriers for Vascular Drug Delivery." *IUBMB Life* 63, no. 8 (2011): 586–95.

Kroin, J. S. "Intrathecal Drug Administration. Present Use and Future Trends." *Clinical Pharmacokinetics* 22, no. 5 (1992): 319–26.

Kumar, H., G. Mishra, A. K. Sharma, A. Gothwal, P. Kesharwani, and U. Gupta. "Intranasal Drug Delivery: A Non-Invasive Approach for the Better Delivery of Neurotherapeutics." *Pharmaceutical Nanotechnology* 5, no. 3 (2017): 203–14.

Kumar Khanna, Vinod. "Targeted Delivery of Nanomedicines." *ISRN Pharmacology* 2012 (2012): 571394.

Kumar, T. R., K. Soppimath, and S. K. Nachaegari. "Novel Delivery Technologies for Protein and Peptide Therapeutics." *Current Pharmaceutical Biotechnology* 7, no. 4 (2006): 261–76.

Kuzmov, Andriy, and Tamara Minko. "Nanotechnology Approaches for Inhalation Treatment of Lung Diseases." *Journal of Controlled Release* 219 (2015): 500–18.

Laffleur, F., and A. Bernkop-Schnürch. "Strategies for Improving Mucosal Drug Delivery." *Nanomedicine* 8, no. 12 (2013): 2061–75.

Lai, S. K., Y. Y. Wang, and J. Hanes. "Mucus-Penetrating Nanoparticles for Drug and Gene Delivery to Mucosal Tissues." *Advanced Drug Delivery Reviews* 61, no. 2 (2009): 158–71.

Lawrence, Marlon G., Michael K. Altenburg, Ryan Sanford, Julian D. Willett, Benjamin Bleasdale, Byron Ballou, Jennifer Wilder, Feng Li, Jeffrey H. Miner, Ulla B. Berg, and Oliver Smithies. "Permeation of Macromolecules into the Renal Glomerular Basement Membrane and Capture by the Tubules." *Proceedings of the National Academy of Sciences of the United States of America* 114, no. 11 (2017): 2958–63.

Lee, V. H. "Mucosal Drug Delivery." *Journal of the National Cancer Institute Monographs* 2001, no. 29 (2001): 41–4.

Li, Chong, Jiancheng Wang, Yiguang Wang, Huile Gao, Gang Wei, Yongzhuo Huang, Yu Haijun, Yong Gan, Yongjun Wang, Lin Mei, Huabing Chen, Haiyan Hu, Zhiping Zhang, and Yiguang Jin. "Recent Progress in Drug Delivery." *Acta Pharmaceutica Sinica B* 9, no. 6 (2019): 1145–62.

Li, Min, Yan Wang, Shuai Jiang, Yang Gao, Weijie Zhang, Shaobo Hu, Xiang Cheng, Chen Zhang, Ping Sun, Wenbo Ke, Guoliang Wang, Zifang Song, Yong Zhang, and Qi Chang Zheng. "Biodistribution and Biocompatibility of Glycyrrhetinic Acid and Galactose-Modified Chitosan Nanoparticles as a Novel Targeting Vehicle for Hepatocellular Carcinoma." *Nanomedicine* 15, no. 2 (2020): 145–61.

Li, Ruomei, Ana Oteiza, Karen Kristine Sørensen, Peter McCourt, Randi Olsen, Bård Smedsrød, and Dmitri Svistounov. "Role of Liver Sinusoidal Endothelial Cells and Stabilins in Elimination of Oxidized Low-Density Lipoproteins." *American Journal of Physiology. Gastrointestinal & Liver Physiology* 300, no. 1 (2011): G71–G81.

Lin, Aihua, Yiming Liu, Yu Huang, Jingbo Sun, Zhifeng Wu, Xian Zhang, and Qineng Ping. "Glycyrrhizin Surface-Modified Chitosan Nanoparticles for Hepatocyte-Targeted Delivery." *International Journal of Pharmaceutics* 359, no. 1–2 (2008): 247–53.

Liu, C. P., Y. Hu, J. C. Lin, H. L. Fu, L. Y. Lim, and Z. X. Yuan. "Targeting Strategies for Drug Delivery to the Kidney: From Renal Glomeruli to Tubules." *Medicinal Research Reviews* 39, no. 2 (2019): 561–78.

Liu, Shanshan, Shili Yang, and Paul C. Ho. "Intranasal Administration of Carbamazepine-Loaded Carboxymethyl Chitosan Nanoparticles for Drug Delivery to the Brain." *Asian Journal of Pharmaceutical Sciences* 13, no. 1 (2018): 72–81.

Ma, Xiangyu, and Robert O. Williams. "Polymeric Nanomedicines for Poorly Soluble Drugs in Oral Delivery Systems: An Update." *Journal of Pharmaceutical Investigation* 48 (2018): 61–75.

Maradana, M. R., S. K. Yekollu, B. Zeng, J. Ellis, A. Clouston, G. Miller, M. Talekar, Z. A. Bhuyan, S. Mahadevaiah, E. E. Powell, K. M. Irvine, R. Thomas, and B. J. O'Sullivan. "Immunomodulatory Liposomes Targeting Liver Macrophages Arrest Progression of Nonalcoholic Steatohepatitis." *Metabolism* 78 (2018): 80–94.

Matsuda, S., K. Keiser, J. K. Nair, K. Charisse, R. M. Manoharan, P. Kretschmer, C. G. Peng, V. Kel'in, A. P. Kandasamy, J. L. Willoughby, A. Liebow, W. Querbes, K. Yucius, T. Nguyen, S. Milstein, M. A. Maier, K. G. Rajeev, and M. Manoharan. "siRNA Conjugates Carrying Sequentially Assembled Trivalent N-acetylgalactosamine Linked Through Nucleosides Elicit Robust Gene Silencing In Vivo in Hepatocytes." *ACS Chemical Biology* 10, no. 5 (2015): 1181–7.

Matsumura, Y., and H. Maeda. "A New Concept for Macromolecular Therapeutics in Cancer Chemotherapy: Mechanism of Tumoritropic Accumulation of Proteins and the Antitumor Agent Smancs." *Cancer Research* 46, no. 12 Pt 1 (1986): 6387–92.

McLennan, Danielle N., Christopher J. H. Porter, and Susan A. Charman. "Subcutaneous Drug Delivery and the Role of the Lymphatics." *Drug Discovery Today: Technologies* 2, no. 1 (2005): 89–96.

McMartin, Colin, Lusie E. F. Hutchinson, Robert Hyde, and Gill E. Peters. "Analysis of Structural Requirements for the Absorption of Drugs and Macromolecules from the Nasal Cavity." *Journal of Pharmaceutical Sciences* 76, no. 7 (1987): 535–40.

Meier, M., M. D. Bider, V. N. Malashkevich, M. Spiess, and P. Burkhard. "Crystal Structure of the Carbohydrate Recognition Domain of the H1 Subunit of the Asialoglycoprotein Receptor." *Journal of Molecular Biology* 300, no. 4 (2000): 857–65.

Melgert, B. N., P. Olinga, J. M. Van Der Laan, B. Weert, J. Cho, D. Schuppan, G. M. Groothuis, D. K. Meijer, and K. Poelstra. "Targeting Dexamethasone to Kupffer Cells: Effects on Liver Inflammation and Fibrosis in Rats." *Hepatology* 34, no. 4 Pt 1 (2001): 719–28.

Migawa, M. T., T. P. Prakash, G. Vasquez, W. B. Wan, J. Yu, G. A. Kinberger, M. E. Østergaard, E. E. Swayze, and P. P. Seth. "A Convenient Synthesis of 5'-Triantennary N-Acetyl-Galactosamine Clusters Based on Nitromethanetrispropionic Acid." *Bioorganic & Medicinal Chemistry Letters* 26, no. 9 (2016): 2194–7.

Mishra, D., N. Jain, V. Rajoriya, and A. K. Jain. "Glycyrrhizin Conjugated Chitosan Nanoparticles for Hepatocyte-Targeted Delivery of Lamivudine." *Journal of Pharmacy & Pharmacology* 66, no. 8 (2014): 1082–93.

Mishra, Nidhi, Narayan Prasad Yadav, Vineet Kumar Rai, Priyam Sinha, Kuldeep Singh Yadav, Sanyog Jain, and Sumit Arora. "Efficient Hepatic Delivery of Drugs: Novel Strategies and Their Significance." *BioMed Research International* 2013 (2013): 382184.

Misra, A., and G. Kher. "Drug Delivery Systems from Nose to Brain." *Current Pharmaceutical Biotechnology* 13, no. 12 (2012): 2355–79.

Nair, Anil V., Edmund J. Keliher, Amanda B. Core, Dennis Brown, and Ralph Weissleder. "Characterizing the Interactions of Organic Nanoparticles with Renal Epithelial Cells In Vivo." *ACS Nano* 9, no. 4 (2015): 3641–53.

Nair, Jayaprakash K., Jennifer L. S. Willoughby, Amy Chan, Klaus Charisse, Md. Rowshon Alam, Qianfan Wang, Menno Hoekstra, Pachamuthu Kandasamy, Alexander V. Kel'in, Stuart Milstein, Nate Taneja, Jonathan O'Shea, Sarfraz Shaikh, Ligang Zhang, Ronald J. van der Sluis, Michael E. Jung, Akin Akinc, Renta Hutabarat, Satya Kuchimanchi, Kevin Fitzgerald, Tracy Zimmermann, Theo J. C. van Berkel, Martin A. Maier, Kallanthottathil G. Rajeev, and Muthiah Manoharan. "Multivalent N-Acetylgalactosamine-conjugated siRNA Localizes in Hepatocytes and Elicits Robust RNAi-Mediated Gene Silencing." *Journal of the American Chemical Society* 136, no. 49 (2014): 16958–61.

Neubert, Reinhard H. H. "Potentials of New Nanocarriers for Dermal and Transdermal Drug Delivery." *European Journal of Pharmaceutics & Biopharmaceutics* 77, no. 1 (2011): 1–2.

Nirmal, Jayabalan, Yao-Chi Chuang, Pradeep Tyagi, Michael B. Chancellor, and M. B. Chancellor. "Intravesical Therapy for Lower Urinary Tract Symptoms." *Urological Science* 23, no. 3 (2012): 70–7.

Ozcelikkale, Altug, Soham Ghosh, and Bumsoo Han. "Multifaceted Transport Characteristics of Nanomedicine: Needs for Characterization in Dynamic Environment." *Molecular Pharmaceutics* 10, no. 6 (2013): 2111–26.

Pandey, Ekta, Aiah S. Nour, and Edward N. Harris. "Prominent Receptors of Liver Sinusoidal Endothelial Cells in Liver Homeostasis and Disease." *Frontiers in Physiology* 11 (2020): 873–73.

Pardeshi, C. V., and V. S. Belgamwar. "Direct Nose to Brain Drug Delivery via Integrated Nerve Pathways Bypassing the Blood-Brain Barrier: An Excellent Platform for Brain Targeting." *Expert Opinion on Drug Delivery* 10, no. 7 (2013): 957–72.

Pardridge, W. M. "Drug Transport Across the Blood-Brain Barrier." *Journal of Cerebral Blood Flow & Metabolism* 32, no. 11 (2012): 1959–72.

Patil, J. S., and S. Sarasija. "Pulmonary Drug Delivery Strategies: A Concise, Systematic Review." *Lung India: Official Organ of Indian Chest Society* 29, no. 1 (2012): 44–9.

Pierre, M. B., A. C. Tedesco, J. M. Marchetti, and M. V. Bentley. "Stratum Corneum Lipids Liposomes for the Topical Delivery of 5-Aminolevulinic Acid in Photodynamic Therapy of Skin Cancer: Preparation and In Vitro Permeation Study." *BMC Dermatology* 1 (2001): 5–11.

Plapied, Laurence, Nicolas Duhem, Anne des Rieux, and Véronique Préat. "Fate of Polymeric Nanocarriers for Oral Drug Delivery." *Current Opinion in Colloid & Interface Science* 16, no. 3 (2011): 228–37.

Prakash, T. P., M. J. Graham, J. Yu, R. Carty, A. Low, A. Chappell, K. Schmidt, C. Zhao, M. Aghajan, H. F. Murray, S. Riney, S. L. Booten, S. F. Murray, H. Gaus, J. Crosby, W. F. Lima, S. Guo, B. P. Monia, E. E. Swayze, and P. P. Seth. "Targeted Delivery of Antisense Oligonucleotides to Hepatocytes Using Triantennary N-Acetyl Galactosamine Improves Potency 10-Fold in Mice." *Nucleic Acids Research* 42, no. 13 (2014): 8796–807.

Prakash, T. P., J. Yu, M. T. Migawa, G. A. Kinberger, W. B. Wan, M. E. Østergaard, R. L. Carty, G. Vasquez, A. Low, A. Chappell, K. Schmidt, M. Aghajan, J. Crosby, H. M. Murray, S. L. Booten, J. Hsiao, A. Soriano, T. Machemer, P. Cauntay, S. A. Burel, S. F. Murray, H. Gaus, M. J. Graham, E. E. Swayze, and P. P. Seth. "Comprehensive Structure-Activity Relationship of Triantennary N-Acetylgalactosamine Conjugated Antisense Oligonucleotides for Targeted Delivery to Hepatocytes." *Journal of Medicinal Chemistry* 59, no. 6 (2016): 2718–33.

Qindeel, Maimoona, Muhammad Hameed Ullah, Din Fakhar ud, Naveed Ahmed, and Asim ur Rehman. "Recent Trends, Challenges and Future Outlook of Transdermal Drug Delivery Systems for Rheumatoid Arthritis Therapy." *Journal of Controlled Release* 327 (2020): 595–615.

Rafique, A., A. Etzerodt, J. H. Graversen, S. K. Moestrup, F. Dagnæs-Hansen, and H. J. Møller. "Targeted Lipid Nanoparticle Delivery of Calcitriol to Human Monocyte-Derived Macrophages In Vitro and In Vivo: Investigation of the Anti-Inflammatory Effects of Calcitriol." *International Journal of Nanomedicine* 14 (2019): 2829–46.

Raila, J., S. Forterre, and F. J. Schweigert. "Physiologic and Pathophysiologic Fundamentals of Proteinuria: A Review." *Berliner & Munchener Tierarztliche Wochenschrift* 118, no. 5–6 (2005): 229–39.

Rajeev, K. G., J. K. Nair, M. Jayaraman, K. Charisse, N. Taneja, J. O'Shea, J. L. Willoughby, K. Yucius, T. Nguyen, S. Shulga-Morskaya, S. Milstein, A. Liebow, W. Querbes, A. Borodovsky, K. Fitzgerald, M. A. Maier, and M. Manoharan. "Hepatocyte-Specific Delivery of siRNAs Conjugated to Novel non-Nucleosidic Trivalent N-acetylgalactosamine Elicits Robust Gene Silencing In Vivo." *ChemBioChem* 16, no. 6 (2015): 903–8.

Richter, Wolfgang F., Suraj G. Bhansali, and Marilyn E. Morris. "Mechanistic Determinants of Biotherapeutics Absorption Following SC Administration." *AAPS Journal* 14, no. 3 (2012): 559–70.

Rohilla, Raman, Tarun Garg, Amit K. Goyal, and Goutam Rath. "Herbal and Polymeric Approaches for Liver-Targeting Drug Delivery: Novel Strategies and Their Significance." *Drug Delivery* 23, no. 5 (2016): 1645–61.

Sábio, Rafael Miguel, Andréia Bagliotti Meneguin, Aline Martins dos Santos, Andreia Sofia Monteiro, and Marlus Chorilli. "Exploiting Mesoporous Silica Nanoparticles as Versatile Drug Carriers for Several Routes of Administration." *Microporous & Mesoporous Materials* 312 (2021): 110774.

Sailor, Michael J., and Ji-Ho Park. "Hybrid Nanoparticles for Detection and Treatment of Cancer." *Advanced Materials* 24, no. 28 (2012): 3779–802.

Schledzewski, K., C. Géraud, B. Arnold, S. Wang, H. J. Gröne, T. Kempf, K. C. Wollert, B. K. Straub, P. Schirmacher, A. Demory, H. Schönhaber, A. Gratchev, L. Dietz, H. J. Thierse, J. Kzhyshkowska, and S. Goerdt. "Deficiency of Liver Sinusoidal Scavenger Receptors stabilin-1 and −2 in Mice Causes Glomerulofibrotic Nephropathy via Impaired Hepatic Clearance of Noxious Blood Factors." *Journal of Clinical Investigation* 121, no. 2 (2011): 703–14.

Shah, N., and D. Padalia 2021. "Intrathecal Delivery System" In *StatPearls* [Internet]. Treasure Island, FL: StatPearls. https://www.ncbi.nlm.nih.gov/books/NBK538237/.

Shakweh, Monjed, Madeleine Besnard, Valérie Nicolas, and Elias Fattal. "Poly (Lactide-Co-Glycolide) Particles of Different Physicochemical Properties and Their Uptake by Peyer's Patches in Mice." *European Journal of Pharmaceutics & Biopharmaceutics* 61, no. 1–2 (2005): 1–13.

Shetty, Shishir, Patricia F. Lalor, and David H. Adams. "Liver Sinusoidal Endothelial Cells: Gatekeepers of Hepatic Immunity." *Nature Reviews. Gastroenterology & Hepatology* 15, no. 9 (2018): 555–67.

Sousa de Almeida, Mauro, Eva Susnik, Barbara Drasler, Patricia Taladriz-Blanco, Alke Petri-Fink, and Barbara Rothen-Rutishauser. "Understanding Nanoparticle Endocytosis to Improve Targeting Strategies in Nanomedicine." *Chemical Society Reviews* 50, no. 9 (2021): 5397–434.

Spanjer, Halbe H., and Gerrit L. Scherphof. "Targeting of Lactosylceramide-Containing Liposomes to Hepatocytes In Vivo." *Biochimica & Biophysica Acta (BBA)* 734, no. 1 (1983): 40–7.

Springer, Aaron D., and Steven F. Dowdy. "GalNAc-siRNA Conjugates: Leading the Way for Delivery of RNAi Therapeutics." *Nucleic Acid Therapeutics* 28, no. 3 (2018): 109–18.

Subhan, Md Abdus, Satya Siva Kishan Yalamarty, Nina Filipczak, Farzana Parveen, and Vladimir P. Torchilin. "Recent Advances in Tumor Targeting via EPR Effect for Cancer Treatment." *Journal of Personalized Medicine* 11, no. 6 (2021): 571–98.

Thomas, Oliver S., and Wilfried Weber. "Overcoming Physiological Barriers to Nanoparticle Delivery: Are We There Yet?." *Frontiers in Bioengineering & Biotechnology* 7 (2019): 415–36.

Tian, Q., C. N. Zhang, X. H. Wang, W. Wang, W. Huang, R. T. Cha, C. H. Wang, Z. Yuan, M. Liu, H. Y. Wan, and H. Tang. "Glycyrrhetinic Acid-Modified Chitosan/Poly(Ethylene Glycol) Nanoparticles for Liver-Targeted Delivery." *Biomaterials* 31, no. 17 (2010): 4748–56.

Tojo, Akihiro, and Satoshi Kinugasa. "Mechanisms of Glomerular Albumin Filtration and Tubular Reabsorption." *International Journal of Nephrology* 2012 (2012): 481520.

Tsutsui, H., and S. Nishiguchi. "Importance of Kupffer Cells in the Development of Acute Liver Injuries in Mice." *International Journal of Molecular Sciences* 15, no. 5 (2014): 7711–30.

Veronesi, M. C., M. Alhamami, S. B. Miedema, Y. Yun, M. Ruiz-Cardozo, and M. W. Vannier. "Imaging of Intranasal Drug Delivery to the Brain." *American Journal of Nuclear Medicine & Molecular Imaging* 10, no. 1 (2020): 1–31.

Wang, L., Y. Zhou, M. Wu, M. Wu, X. Li, X. Gong, J. Chang, and X. Zhang. "Functional Nanocarrier for Drug and Gene Delivery via Local Administration in Mucosal Tissues." *Nanomedicine* 13, no. 1 (2018): 69–88.

Wang, Qin, Liang Zhang, Wei Hu, Zhan-Hong Hu, Yong-Yan Bei, Jing-Yu Xu, Wen-Juan Wang, Xue-Nong Zhang, and Qiang Zhang. "Norcantharidin-Associated Galactosylated Chitosan Nanoparticles for Hepatocyte-Targeted Delivery." *Nanomedicine: Nanotechnology, Biology & Medicine* 6, no. 2 (2010): 371–81.

Wang, Zian, Guojun Xiong, Wai Chun Tsang, Andreas G. Schätzlein, and Ijeoma F. Uchegbu. "Nose-to-Brain Delivery." *Journal of Pharmacology & Experimental Therapeutics* 370, no. 3 (2019): 593.

Wen, Hong, Huijeong Jung, and Xuhong Li. "Drug Delivery Approaches in Addressing Clinical Pharmacology-Related Issues: Opportunities and Challenges." *AAPS Journal* 17, no. 6 (2015): 1327–40.

Wilkinson, Alex L., Maria Qurashi, and Shishir Shetty. "The Role of Sinusoidal Endothelial Cells in the Axis of Inflammation and Cancer Within the Liver." *Frontiers in Physiology* 11 (2020): 990–1015.

Williams, R. M., J. Shah, B. D. Ng, D. R. Minton, L. J. Gudas, C. Y. Park, and D. A. Heller. "Mesoscale Nanoparticles Selectively Target the Renal Proximal Tubule Epithelium." *Nano Letters* 15, no. 4 (2015): 2358–64.

Williams, Ryan M., Janki Shah, Helen S. Tian, Xi Chen, Frederic Geissmann, Edgar A. Jaimes, and Daniel A. Heller. "Selective Nanoparticle Targeting of the Renal Tubules." *Hypertension* 71, no. 1 (2018) (1979): 87–94.

Wong, Andrew D., Mao Ye, Amanda F. Levy, Jeffrey D. Rothstein, Dwight E. Bergles, and Peter C. Searson. "The Blood-Brain Barrier: An Engineering Perspective." *Frontiers in Neuroengineering* 6 (2013): 7.

Wu, Jian, Pei Liu, Jian-Liang Zhu, Sivaramaiah Maddukuri, and Mark A. Zern. "Increased Liver Uptake of Liposomes and Improved Targeting Efficacy by Labeling with Asialofetuin in Rodents." *Hepatology* 27, no. 3 (1998): 772–78.

Wu, Lei, Wei Shan, Zhirong Zhang, and Yuan Huang. "Engineering Nanomaterials to Overcome the Mucosal Barrier by Modulating Surface Properties." *Advanced Drug Delivery Reviews* 124 (2018): 150–63.

Yang, Rong, Tuo Wei, Hannah Goldberg, Weiping Wang, Kathleen Cullion, and Daniel S. Kohane. "Getting Drugs Across Biological Barriers." *Advanced Materials* 29, no. 37 (2017): 1606596–621.

Yetisgin, A. A., S. Cetinel, M. Zuvin, A. Kosar, and O. Kutlu. "Therapeutic Nanoparticles and Their Targeted Delivery Applications." *Molecules* 25, no. 9 (2020): 2193–224.

Yin, Chunyue, Kimberley J. Evason, Kinji Asahina, and Didier Y. R. Stainier. "Hepatic Stellate Cells in Liver Development, Regeneration, and Cancer." *Journal of Clinical Investigation* 123, no. 5 (2013): 1902–10.

Yoo, Jihye, Changhee Park, Gawon Yi, Donghyun Lee, and Heebeom Koo. "Active Targeting Strategies Using Biological Ligands for Nanoparticle Drug Delivery Systems." *Cancers* 11, no. 5 (2019): 640.

Yoon, Ho Yub, Yang Hee Mang, Chang Hyun Kim, Yoon Tae Goo, Myung Joo Kang, Sangkil Lee, and Young Wook Choi. "Current Status of the Development of Intravesical Drug Delivery Systems for the Treatment of Bladder Cancer." *Expert Opinion on Drug Delivery* 17, no. 11 (2020): 1555–72.

Yuan, Zhenghui Shang Zhi-xiang, Jian Gu, and Lili He. "Renal Targeting Delivery Systems." *Future Medicinal Chemistry* 11, no. 17 (2019): 2237–40.

Zhao, Z., A. Ukidve, J. Kim, and S. Mitragotri. "Targeting Strategies for Tissue-Specific Drug Delivery." *Cell* 181, no. 1 (2020): 151–67.

Zheng, D., C. Duan, D. Zhang, L. Jia, G. Liu, Y. Liu, F. Wang, C. Li, H. Guo, and Q. Zhang. "Galactosylated Chitosan Nanoparticles for Hepatocyte-Targeted Delivery of Oridonin." *International Journal of Pharmaceutics* 436, no. 1–2 (2012): 379–86.

Zhou, Nuo, Xiaoli Zan, Zheng Wang, Hua Wu, Dengke Yin, Chunyan Liao, and Ying Wan. "Galactosylated Chitosan–Polycaprolactone Nanoparticles for Hepatocyte-Targeted Delivery of Curcumin." *Carbohydrate Polymers* 94, no. 1 (2013): 420–29.

Zhou, Peng, Xun Sun, and Zhirong Zhang. "Kidney-Targeted Drug Delivery Systems." *Acta Pharmaceutica Sinica B* 4, no. 1 (2014): 37–42.

Zuckerman, J. E., C. H. Choi, H. Han, and M. E. Davis. "Polycation-siRNA Nanoparticles Can Disassemble at the Kidney Glomerular Basement Membrane." *Proceedings of the National Academy of Sciences of the United States of America* 109, no. 8 (2012): 3137–42.

Zuckerman, J. E., and M. E. Davis. "Targeting Therapeutics to the Glomerulus with Nanoparticles." *Advances in Chronic Kidney Disease* 20, no. 6 (2013): 500–7.

Nanomedicine and Drug Delivery Approaches

2

Carla Vitorino, Carla M. Lopes, and Marlene Lúcio

Contents

2.1 INTRODUCTION

While nanotechnology is a relatively new science, we have been using it for over a thousand years. One of the most ancient examples of nanotechnology known in history is the Lycurgus Cup made by Roman artisans around the 4th century (AD) (Freestone et al. 2007). An interesting aspect about the cup is its dichroic effect – it changes color according to the light source. With the reflected light, the cup has a greenish-yellow tone, but when the light is transmitted through glass, the color of the cup changes to red (Freestone et al. 2007). At the end of the 1980s, it was possible to prove that these peculiar optical properties were due to the glass containing nanoparticles (50–100 nm in diameter) of silver: gold (7:3) alloy. In one of the most well-known examples of ancient nanotechnology, medieval stained glass, a similar optical effect is observed (Molina et al. 2013). This glass also contained silver/gold nanoparticles that confer a ruby red

DOI: 10.1201/9781003092773-3

or a deep yellow color to the glass. It is currently understood that the color variation is determined by the size of nanoparticles (and not by the gold or silver composition). This color shift example is a demonstration of the drastic change in nanoscale material properties. The Roman and medieval artisans were the first nanotechnologists, but they were unaware of the rationale behind the optical effects obtained. In this context, controlling matter locally and intentionally on the atomic molecular scale has become a major goal of natural science (Riehemann et al. 2009). This goal began to be achieved in 1959 with the famous lecture "There's Plenty of Room at the Bottom, An Invitation to Enter a New Field of Physics" given by Richard Feynman at the annual meeting of the American Physical Society, where he developed the vision of manipulating and controlling mater on a small scale (Feynman 1960). Feynman's talk can also be considered the earliest vision of nanotechnology applied to medicine as he raised the question of the "manufacture of an object that can maneuver at the level of biological cells". Fifteen years after Feynman discovered this emerging area of science that drew the attention of many scientists, Norio Taniguchi, a Japanese scientist, was the first to use and describe the word "nanotechnology" in 1974 as: "nanotechnology mainly consists of the processing of separation, consolidation, and deformation of materials by one atom or one molecule" (Taniguchi 1974). As a consequence, nanotechnology has become one of the most promising technologies of the 21st century and it is described as a science, engineering, and technology conducted at the nanoscale (1 to 100 nm), where unique phenomena enable novel applications in a wide range of fields, from chemistry, physics, and biology, to medicine, engineering, and electronics (Bayda et al. 2019, Riehemann et al. 2009). This description implies the existence of two important aspects of nanotechnology. The first is the scale: nanotechnology concerns the use of structures by manipulating their form and size on a nanometric scale. The second has to do with taking advantage of the special properties that occur at the nanoscale (Bayda et al. 2019, Riehemann et al. 2009).

In spite of Feynman's early allusions to the use of nanotechnology in medicine, the term "nanomedicine" was first introduced only after the publication of the book *Unbounding the Future: The Nanotechnology Revolution* by Drexler, Peterson, and Pergamit, in which they used the word "nanobots" or "assemblers" for nanoprocesses in medical applications (Drexler, Peterson, and Pergamit 1991). Nanomedicine is a research and technology area related to the diagnosis, treatment, and prevention of serious trauma and diseases. It aims to ease human pain and preserve human health using molecular tools and molecular knowledge of the human body. The early and accurate diagnosis of pathologies and capacity to provide an effective therapy without secondary effects has long been the purpose and major priority of medicine. The accomplishment of this purpose appears closer than ever with the advent of nanotechnology. Nanotechnology allied to medicine can reach different areas: diagnosis (nanodiagnosis), controlled drug delivery (nanotherapy), combined therapy and diagnostics (theranostics), and tissue engineering and regenerative medicine. In the area of nanotherapy in particular, the advancement of drug delivery nanosystems (DDNs) poses exciting developments in clinical practice that have allowed classical medical limitations to be addressed by several strategies: (i) carrying and delivering efficient molecules that may not otherwise be used due to their high toxicity (e.g., anticancer drugs), (ii) exploring several modes of therapeutic action (e.g., hyperthermia, photodynamic therapy (PDT)), (iii) optimizing the efficiency of the therapeutic agent (e.g., by improving its pharmacokinetic profile) while reducing dose and toxicity, (iv) directing drugs specifically to the target tissues avoiding off-target distribution and improving transport across biological barriers, and (v) providing a triggered and controlled release of the drug at the target site (Faria et al. 2019, Fernandes et al. 2018, Soares et al. 2018a, Viseu et al. 2018). Owing to the progressive ageing of the population, nanomedicine is becoming much more significant, contributing to facing the rise in age-related diseases (e.g., neurodegenerative diseases, age-related retinopathy), which in the coming years is expected to have a remarkably high socioeconomic effect. In this respect, nanotherapy provides benefits over traditional therapy that is not successful in addressing biological obstacles that limit the effectiveness of therapeutic agents (e.g., the brain–blood barrier, ocular barriers) (Madni et al. 2017, Gote et al. 2019, Teixeira et al. 2020a, b, Soares et al. 2018b).

This chapter focuses on the application of nanomedicine and drug delivery approaches to meet the emerging problems of classical medicine. In the following pages, we offer an overview of the existing concepts of nanomaterials and nanomedicine by regulatory authorities and the safety, quality, and efficacy strategies of the design methods that can be used in the production of nanomedicine. In addition, the chapter points out a series of literature descriptions of DDNs produced as nanomedicines at different stages of development: in the research stage or pre-clinical and commercially approved stages. Finally, there is a critical perspective on the achievements of nanomedicine and the big problems that have yet to come.

2.2 NANOMEDICINE: DEFINITION AND APPLICATION

2.2.1 Definition

From a regulatory perspective, several definitions have been attempted aiming at setting forth harmonized assumptions. According to the European Commission recommendation, nanomaterial refers to a natural, incidental, or manufactured material comprising particles, either in an unbound state or as an aggregate wherein one or more external dimensions is in the size range of 1–100 nm for 50% of the particles, based on the number size distribution. In cases of environmental, health, safety, or competitiveness concern, the number size distribution threshold of 50% may be replaced by a threshold between 1 and 50%. Structures, such as fullerenes, graphene flakes, and single wall carbon nanotubes, with one or more external dimensions below 1 nm, should be considered as nanomaterials. Materials with a surface area by volume exceeding 60 m^2/cm^3 are also included (EC 2011). This defines a nanomaterial in terms of legislation and policy in the European Union. Based on this definition, the regulatory bodies have issued their own guidance to support drug product development (Saleh 2020, Soares et al. 2018a).

The European Medicines Agency (EMA) working group introduces the concept of nanomedicines as purposely designed systems for clinical applications, comprising at least one component at nanoscale range. It results in programmable properties and characteristics, which are interlinked to the specific nanotechnology application and characteristics for the devised use (e.g., route of administration, dose), being also associated with the expected clinical advantages of the nano-engineering (e.g., preferential organ/tissue distribution) (Ossa 2014). The regulation of nanomedicines relies on the documentation of material intrinsic properties as well as the biological behavior of the materials (Fadeel and Alexiou 2020).

The Food and Drug Administration (FDA) has not established its own definition for "nanotechnology", "nanomaterial", "nanoscale", or other related concepts, but rather endorsed the meanings commonly employed in relation to the engineering of materials that have at least one dimension in the size range of approximately 1 to 100 nm (FDA 2017). In addition, given their potential impact on subjects related to safety, effectiveness, performance, quality, public health impact, or regulatory status of products, FDA advises to verify any unique properties and behaviors that the application of nanotechnology may impart. Note that nanoscale materials can display distinct chemical or physical properties, or biological effects when compared to larger-scale equivalents. For instance, dimension-dependent properties or phenomena may confer an enhanced bioavailability, decreased dosage, increased potency, or reduced toxicity of a drug product. These effects may stem from changes in chemical, biological, or magnetic properties, variations in the electrical or optical activity, augmented structural integrity, or other specific characteristics of materials in the nanoscale form not usually evidenced or expected in larger-scale materials with similar chemical composition (FDA 2014).

2.2.2 Applications

Nanoscale medicines can be deemed highly beneficial, assuming that many biological significant molecules, e.g., antibodies, proteins, glucose, enzymes, and receptors, are included within this range (Seigneuric et al. 2010). A wide spectrum of applications of nanotechnology in the field of medicine has been witnessed, with the possibility of exerting a revolutionary impact on healthcare (Foulkes et al. 2020).

Nanomedicine is rapidly gaining recognition in the management of several domains including the way diseases are detected and/or treated. The nanoscale manipulation opens avenues in the targeting and delivery ability, also enabling the controlled release of drugs or imaging agents (Shi et al. 2010). For that reason, drug delivery mediated by nanosystems has been pointed out as a subtle strategy to overcome pharmaceutical development issues. The small size of the nanosystems can assist in the transport through biological barriers, improve the bioavailability of poorly water-soluble drugs, reduce dose and adventitious toxicity, assemble multiple mechanisms of action in a single structure, or even afford protection against drug degradation. Technological problems, such as low solubility or stability, may be bypassed. Also, the functionalization of their surface, whether by using specific ligands (Shen et al. 2016b) or triggering moieties, sensitive to specific environments (Li et al. 2020a), clearly enlarges the portfolio of potential solutions towards more specific and selective therapies (Couvreur 2019, Su and Kang 2020). This assumes particular relevance when it comes to the oncology area, owing to the balance between the toxicity required and the very challenging tumor landscape, which hinders effective drug treatment (Foulkes et al. 2020). Considerable efforts are also being made in the development of nanomedicines for the treatment of cardiovascular and neurodegenerative conditions (Arias 2016), as well as for metabolic and infectious diseases (Jackman, Lee, and Cho 2016), or even for prevention, like the recently issued COVID-19 vaccines that became the first prophylactic measure against severe acute respiratory syndrome coronavirus 2 (SARS-CoV-2) infection (Editorial 2020).

The role of nanotechnology is not limited to treatment. Other biomedical areas have benefitted from the current scientific and technical understanding of nanomaterials and their characteristics. This is the case of the disease diagnosis – nanodiagnostics – or its joint approach with nanotherapy – nanotheranostics. The former features an improved sensitivity and integration of analytical methods to render a more reliable outcome (Tekade et al. 2017). The latter results from the integration of diagnostic and therapeutic functions in a unique system, resorting to the benefits of nanotechnology. This is considered a one-size-fits-all approach. By serving the dual purpose of identifying biomarkers to obtain insights on the diagnosis and treating the specific disorder on the basis of the precise diagnosis, it leads the way to the highly desired personalized medicine (Kim, Lee, and Chen 2013). For example, these advanced nanoplatforms may be helpful in brain cancer diagnosis at early stages, therefore enabling the timely initiation of first-line therapy, continuous monitoring, and if required, the rapid introduction of ensuing treatments (Mendes et al. 2018). Many nanodevices have been investigated, under the umbrella of the joint alliance signed by the National Cancer Institute (NCI) and EMA, so as to provide fine-tuned and early detection, diagnosis, and ultimate treatment of various diseases like cancer, human immunodeficiency virus (HIV) infection, cardiac and respiratory illnesses, and depression (Tekade et al. 2017).

Nanotechnology has also been applied into multiple research areas related to regenerative medicine. This concerns methods aiming to regrow, repair, or replace damaged or diseased cells, tissues, or organs grounded on integrated approaches of tissue engineering, molecular biology, biomaterials, and stem cell biology (Yang et al. 2019). Given the similarity in terms of nanoscale and the intrinsic ability to mimic human tissues, many functional biomimetic nanomaterials have been employed to deliver drugs, proteins, and genes for tissue regeneration (Alarçin et al. 2016). Several studies have reported that nanotechnology has the ability to speed up many regenerative therapies, including those directed to the bone, vascular, heart, cartilage, bladder, and brain tissues (Khang et al. 2010).

2.3 DRUG DELIVERY NANOSYSTEMS

2.3.1 Drug Delivery Nanosystems and the Magic Bullet Concept

More than a century ago, Paul Ehrlich had the vision that, in the future, scientists would be able to develop a therapeutic arsenal that would act as "magic bullets" as they could be specifically administered to target cells, tissues, or organs (Houshmand et al. 2020, Strebhardt and Ullrich 2008). Generations of researchers working in nanomedicine and nanotherapy have interpreted Ehrlich's vision of a magic bullet to develop DDNs consisting of drugs loaded in nanosystems designed to overcome a number of biological and physicochemical barriers in order to direct the drug to a single target in a highly specific way (Houshmand et al. 2020). Depending on the route of administration of DDNs and their target tissue, these nanosystems follow various biological pathways and can encounter different barriers. For example, when administered intravenously, DDNs should undergo a five-step "CAPIR" cascade (circulation, accumulation, penetration, internalization, and release), i.e., DDNs enter the systemic circulation and should be kept circulating long enough to be distributed and accumulated in the target tissues (Xu et al. 2019). In order to accumulate in the target tissues, DDNs are also needed to penetrate these tissues, and if the target is intracellular, cell internalization is also required. Finally, when the target is reached, the drug should be released from the nanosystem to exert its effect. The optimum performance of DDNs at each stage of the CAPIR cascade is of great importance in achieving improved final therapeutic benefits and overall survival (Xu et al. 2019). In this respect, different strategies need to be put in place for DDNs to increase the chances of successful delivery of the drug to the target. These strategies have also progressed with the advancement of nanotherapy (Couvreur 2019). The first generation of DDNs (e.g., liposomes and polymer nanoparticles) produced in the 1970s did not contain any coating, but still effectively protected drugs from degradation (Couvreur 2019). Once in circulation, these naked DDNs are quickly opsonized by serum proteins (Figure 2.1 A) that promote their recognition by the mononuclear phagocytic system (MPS). Consequently, the DDNs are signalized for elimination and are targeted to the liver in a passive way (Couvreur 2019). Therefore, if the liver or the cells from MPS were the target of the drugs carried, the naked DDNs would be effective. However, the opsonization of DDNs and early MPS recognition decreased their circulation times and thus their chances of reaching other target tissues. Hence, in the

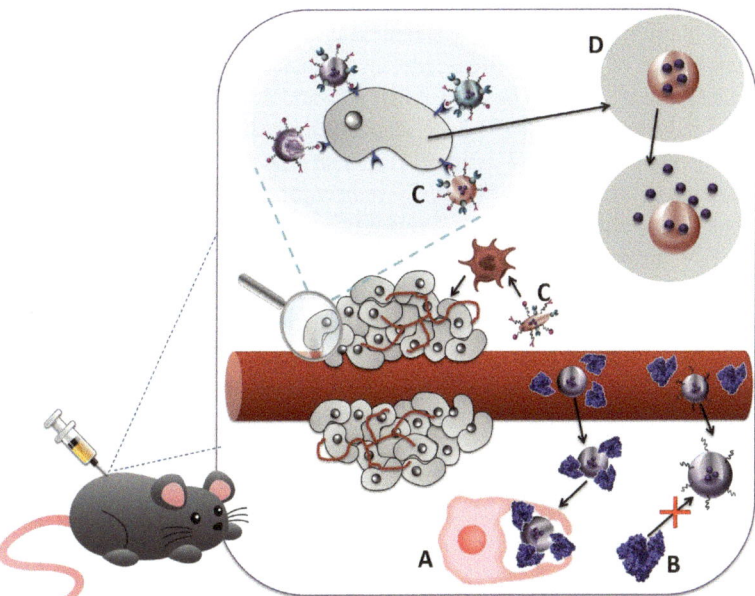

FIGURE 2.1 Schematic representation of drug delivery nanosystems (DDNs) overcoming circulation, accumulation, penetration, internalization, and release (CAPIR) barriers. When in circulation naked DDNs are opsonized by serum proteins and phagocyted and eliminated (A). PEGylated DDNs (coated with PEG polymers) have longer circulation times as they avoid binding to serum proteins. The DDNs can accumulate in the target tissues either passively by EPR that occurs at highly vascularized cancer cells, or actively binding to target cells receptors (C). Once internalized in target cells DDNs, physiological stimuli such as pH and temperature could trigger the intracellular drug delivery (D).

1990s, stealth strategies based on the physicochemical principle of steric repulsion were employed. These stealth strategies consisted of coating DDNs' surface with hydrophilic chains (e.g., polyethylene glycol, PEG) to improve the stability of DDNs against aggregation (Couvreur 2019). Moreover, PEGylation, i.e., coating with PEG, minimizes DDNs detection and removal by MPS and increases their circulation time by reducing the opsonization of DDNs by serum proteins (Figure 2.1 B) (Amoozgar and Yeo 2012, Fam et al. 2020). The advent of PEGylation originated surface decorated DDNs that can have long circulation times on the CAPIR cascade and are therefore more likely to be distributed and accumulated in the target tissues (Xu et al. 2019). However, if the DDNs could only recur to stealth strategies, they would not be able to be directed to specific tissues. Instead, DDNs would be passively targeted at tumors and other inflammatory diseases due to their leaky vasculature and endothelial fenestration, which consequently increase accumulation at these sites through the so-called "enhanced permeability and retention" (EPR) effect (Nehoff et al. 2014, Shi et al. 2020). Subsequent developments in bioconjugate chemistry have made it possible to functionalize the surface of DDNs with specific ligands (e.g., monoclonal antibodies, sugar moieties, peptide fragments, or other ligands) that are involved in recognizing and binding to the target tissue signal receptors, thereby facilitating effective drug targeting, also known as active targeting strategies (Fu et al. 2020, Yoo et al. 2019). Such strategies facilitate the delivery of DDNs to the target areas (Figure 2.1 C), while preventing their accumulation in non-target tissues. In addition, target ligands such as cell-penetrating peptides can enhance the penetration into target tissues of DDNs and increase cellular uptake (Xie et al. 2020). For example, the peptide derived from the human immunodeficiency virus trans-activator transcription (TAT) is a cell-penetrating peptide that promotes the transport of DDNs by an adsorptive-mediated transcytosis mechanism across the blood–brain barrier (BBB), thereby improving penetration into brain tissues (Lúcio et al. 2021, Soares et al. 2018b). Furthermore, the positive charges of CPPs readily adsorb to negatively charged cell surface glycosaminoglycans which facilitates cellular intake and the uptake of DDNs (Xie et al. 2020). Consequently, CPP-functional DDNs are expected to be internalized in cells by a lipid raft-mediated macropinocytosis process that is independent of the receptors and transporters that all cells conduct (Xie et al. 2020). In conclusion, the active targeting strategies favor the accumulation step of the CAPIR cascade, also enhancing the penetration and internalization of DDNs in target cells (Xu et al. 2019). The last CAPIR step is the release of the drug from the DDS, which should ideally occur only when the DDNs have reached the target (Xu et al. 2019). To accomplish this aim of being able to trigger drug release, stimuli-responsive DDNs have been developed in recent years (Couvreur 2019). Therefore, triggering strategies have been implemented and consist of the use of DDNs with stimuli-responsive moieties to cause drug release (Figure 2.1 D) following exposure to an internal or external stimulus (Wang and Kohane 2017, Sun et al. 2017). Most of the preclinical research on local stimuli-triggered drug release is focused on internal changes occurring in pathological zones, such as cellular (e.g., acidic pH of intracellular lysosomes) or tissue level (e.g., in tumor tissues there is elevated temperature, acidic environment, and the over-expression of specific enzymes or over-production of radical oxygen species) (Sun et al. 2017). However, external stimuli (e.g., ultrasound, magnetic waves, and light) that are introduced from outside the body to the pathological tissues are also studied to trigger the release of drugs (Wang and Kohane 2017).

Figure 2.1 illustrates the stealth strategies, targeting strategies, and stimuli-responsive triggering strategies and their correlation with a successful CAPIR cascade. For a more complete description of stealth strategies, targeting strategies, and stimuli-responsive triggering strategies, please refer to reviews on the subject (Bhardwaj et al. 2015, Torchilin 2018, Zhao et al. 2020, Attia et al. 2019, Salmaso and Caliceti 2013, Fam et al. 2020).

2.3.2 Types of Drug Delivery Nanosystems

In terms of chemical composition, DDNs can be broadly classified into organic, composed of carbon-based nanomaterials; inorganic, composed of inorganic elements; or hybrid DDNs (Table 2.1). The inclusion of nanostructured-based systems composed of allotropes of carbon (e.g., fullerenes, carbon nanotubes, graphite oxide sheets, or graphene quantum dots) (Viseu et al. 2018) in the organic or inorganic DDNs classification is not so evident, and these systems can be considered as a separate group (Pirzada and Altintas 2019) or can be used as hybrid materials for the functionalization of organic or inorganic DDNs (Yan et al. 2019).

Organic DDNs are composed of natural and/or synthetic organic molecules, i.e., carbon-based nanomaterials, such as lipids (e.g., stearic acid, phospholipids) and polymers (e.g., chitosan and poly(lactic acid-co-glycolic acid) (PLGA)). In terms of physiological behavior, as carbon is a main component of the human body, organic nanosystems are the most appealing DDNs due to their biocompatibility, biodegradability, non-immunogenicity, low toxicity, and stability, and they can protect molecules from the hostile environment, enzymatic degradation, and blood plasma proteins (Gupta et al. 2019, Lombardo, Kiselev, and Caccamo 2019, Lúcio et al. 2021, Rout et al. 2018). Moreover, these types of DDNs can improve the loading capacity of a variety of hydrophilic/lipophilic drugs and can control their delivery. The surfaces of organic DDNs can be simply functionalized with specific biomolecules which is a relevant advantage for the development of targeted drug delivery systems (Rout et al. 2018). Nevertheless, organic DDNs also possess disadvantages, for example the production process of some types of these nanosystems is not easy, leading to less standardization and batch-to-batch variability (Lombardo, Kiselev, and Caccamo 2019, Lúcio et al. 2021). The most used organic DDNs include micelles, liposomes, solid lipid-based nanoparticles, polymeric nanoparticles, dendrimers, and nano/microemulsions.

Inorganic DDNs, such as magnetic nanoparticles, quantum dots, mesoporous silica nanoparticles (MSNs), and gold nanoparticles, possess unique mechanical, optical, structural, magnetic, and electrical properties that can be attributed to their inorganic components, which explain their advantages in relation to organic DDNs in terms of shape and size control and ease of production and functionalization (Saraiva et al. 2016). Additionally, inorganic DDNs are easier to track using microscopy and analytical techniques than organic DDNs (Lúcio et al. 2021). Considering these advantages together, inorganic DDNs present promising strategies for delivery, diagnostic, and theranostic applications. Nevertheless, these DDNs also present some intrinsic drawbacks related to the limited amounts of drug carried and to the degree of biotoxicity (Conde et al. 2014). Based on their inability to biodegrade, the use of inorganic DDNs presents critical issues concerning biocompatibility and biosafety. Therefore, the addition of a biocompatible surface to inorganic DDNs that protect from unwanted physical-chemical interactions with the biological microenvironment is often required (Lombardo, Kiselev, and Caccamo 2019, Lúcio et al. 2021).

Both organic and inorganic DDNs have been related with some limitations that can be overcome using the combinatorial approach of hybrid DDNs. In recent years, these hybrid DDNs have been the focus of much research with relevant improvements in drug targeting. Hybrid DDNs combine the benefits of both DDNs into a single drug delivery system (Torres-Ortega et al. 2021).

All the self-assembly/synthetic methods for the preparation of organic and inorganic DDNs have been widely described in a number of previous review papers (Salas, Costo, and Morales 2012, Has and Sunthar 2019, Akbarzadeh et al. 2013, Patravale, Upadhaya, and Jain 2019, Ganesan and Narayanasamy 2017, Rao and Geckeler 2011, Pelegri-O'Day, Lin, and Maynard 2014, Salome Amarachi, Kenechukwu, and Attama 2014, Avgoustakis 2004, Crucho and Barros 2017, Lefley, Waldron, and Becer 2020, Naseri, Valizadeh, and Zakeri-Milani 2015). Therefore, we will only briefly introduce some common organic and inorganic DDNs, their schematic representation, and their advantages and disadvantages as summarized in Table 2.1.

2.3.3 Drug Delivery Nanosystems: Current Applications in Nanomedicine

Before any DDNs enter the market, they have been explored by researchers to develop improved, efficient, and biocompatible structures with a wide range of applications in nanomedicine: nanotherapy, nanodiagnosis, theranostics, tissue engineering, and regenerative medicine. Table 2.2 presents some examples of

TABLE 2.1 Different Types of Drug Delivery Nanosystems (DDNs): Their Schematic Representation and Their Main Advantages and Disadvantages

Organic DDNs

Vesicles

TYPE OF DDNS AND SCHEMATIC REPRESENTATION	DESCRIPTION	ADVANTAGES	DISADVANTAGES	REFERENCES
Liposomes PHOSPHOLIPID WATER OIL 	• Synthetic vesicles formed by self-assembly of lipid bilayers containing aqueous phases in their core and surroundings. • According to the number of lipid bilayers can be classified in unilamellar (1 bilayer), oligolamellar (2–4 bilayers), or multilamellar (> 4 bilayers). • According to size can be classified as small (<100nm), large (100–500nm), or giant (>500nm).	• Encapsulate hydrophilic, hydrophobic, or amphiphilic drugs. • Biocompatible and biodegradable. • Flexible, able to penetrate tissues. • The majority of marketed approved DDNs are liposomes.	• Low stability *in vivo* and in storage conditions. • Administration routes are limited (mainly intranasal and IV). • Production processes are difficult to scale.	(Farjadian et al. 2019, Lúcio et al. 2021, Lopes et al. 2018, Soares et al. 2018b)
Ethosomes PHOSPHOLIPID ETHANOL WATER OIL 	• Self-assembled phospholipid-based vesicles with high ethanol content (20–45%). This is the main way they are different from liposomes.	• Similar to the advantages of liposomes. • More flexible than liposomes. Increase the penetration of drugs in skin and brain. Ability to cross the BBB.	• Similar to the disadvantages of liposomes. • More toxic than liposomes due to high content of ethanol. • Less stable than liposomes.	(Zylberberg and Matosevic 2016, Lopes et al. 2018, Lúcio et al. 2021, Soares et al. 2018b)
Transfersomes PHOSPHOLIPID EDGE ACTIVATOR WATER OIL 	• Self-assembled phospholipid-based vesicles containing lipid bilayer destabilizers called edge activators (i.e., single-chain surfactants with a high radius of curvature). • Due to the edge activators the lipid bilayers are deformable and highly flexible.	• Similar to the advantages of liposomes. • More flexible than liposomes and ethosomes. Increase the penetration of drugs in the skin. • Used in transdermal drug delivery: local action, avoids undesirable systemic absorption, avoids first-pass metabolism, and reduces side-effects.	• Similar to the disadvantages of liposomes. • More toxic than liposomes due to the lipid bilayer destabilizers that also function as cell membrane destabilizers. • Less stable than liposomes, as the lipid bilayer is easily destabilized.	(Rajan et al. 2011, Duangjit et al. 2011, Zylberberg and Matosevic 2016, Lopes et al. 2018)

(Continued)

TABLE 2.1 (Continued) Different Types of Drug Delivery Nanosystems (DDNs): Their Schematic Representation and Their Main Advantages and Disadvantages

Vesicles

TYPE OF DDNS AND SCHEMATIC REPRESENTATION	DESCRIPTION	ADVANTAGES	DISADVANTAGES	REFERENCES
Pharmacosomes DRUG – PHOSPHOLIPID CONJUGATE WATER OIL	• Self-assembled vesicles in which the phospholipid components result from a previous complexation with the drug by covalent, electrostatic or hydrogen bonding.	• Similar to the advantages of liposomes. • Compared to liposomes they have improved stability due to linkage with the drug and reduced leakage of entrapped drug. • Can be administered orally, topically, extra- or intravascularly.	• More laborious assembly techniques of production that require previous complexation steps in order to achieve the necessary lipid-drug complex.	(Semalty et al. 2009, Pandita and Sharma 2013, Zylberberg and Matosevic 2016)
Polymersomes POLYMER WATER OIL	• Self-assembled vesicles formed in aqueous solution of amphiphilic block copolymers resultant from adjacent hydrophobic and hydrophilic blocks. • Structurally, polymersomes are analogous to liposomes, once they present an aqueous core and surrounding there is a polymer membrane. The core of this membrane is formed from hydrophobic blocks of copolymer which are associated to diminish their interaction with water and are separated from the inner and outer aqueous phases by two interfaces of hydrophilic blocks.	• More versatile and suitable for functionalization for targeting or destabilization compared to liposomes. • Encapsulate hydrophilic, hydrophobic, or amphiphilic drugs. • Enhanced mechanical and chemical stability and robustness compared to liposomes. • Controlled therapeutic release kinetics. • Can be composed by stimuli-responsive polymers to trigger the release of drug. • Appealing tunable properties depending on the amphiphilic block copolymers and preparation methods.	• Therapeutic release is dependent on polymer degradability which can be difficult or prolong the therapeutic effect over time. • Many preparation methods require complex procedures and use of toxic organic solvents. • Higher toxicity than lipid-based nanosystems. • Block copolymers are polydisperse, resulting in lack of reproducibility. • Concerns related to the long-term use of polymer-somes due to their constitution and durability. • Some of new polymers used for polymersome preparation are currently not approved by the FDA.	(Müller and Landfester 2015, Lúcio et al. 2021, Discher et al. 1999)

(Continued)

TABLE 2.1 (Continued)   Different Types of Drug Delivery Nanosystems (DDNs): Their Schematic Representation and Their Main Advantages and Disadvantages

Micelles

TYPE OF DDNS AND SCHEMATIC REPRESENTATION	DESCRIPTION	ADVANTAGES	DISADVANTAGES	REFERENCES
Lipid micelles **PHOSPHOLIPID** **WATER** **OIL** 	• Spherical self-assembly aggregates (5–50 nm) of phospholipids in aqueous media which occur above a well-defined concentration, i.e., critical micelle concentration (CMC). • Unlike vesicles that contain an aqueous core, micelles possess hydrophilic portions turned to aqueous media and a hydrophobic core made by the phospholipids' acyl groups.	• Encapsulate hydrophilic, hydrophobic, or amphiphilic drugs. • Biocompatible and biodegradable. • Easier to produce than liposomes.	• Require concentrations above the CMC and can release the loaded drug upon dilution. • Stability problems upon dilution in the bloodstream or in the presence of plasma and tissue components that can bind to the phospholipids.	(Lopes et al. 2018, Lúcio et al. 2021, Soares et al. 2018b)

(Continued)

TABLE 2.1 (Continued)   Different Types of Drug Delivery Nanosystems (DDNs): Their Schematic Representation and Their Main Advantages and Disadvantages

TYPE OF DDNS AND SCHEMATIC REPRESENTATION	DESCRIPTION	ADVANTAGES	DISADVANTAGES	REFERENCES
Polymeric micelles WATER OIL	• Spherical self-assembly of amphiphilic block copolymers in aqueous media above CMC. • Core-shell structure with hydrophilic portions turned towards aqueous surroundings and a hydrophobic core composed by the hydrophobic portions of the amphiphilic polymers. • Despite the use of the same type of amphiphilic block copolymers, the final structure of the self-assembly aggregates (i.e., micelle or polymersome) depends on diverse parameters such as concentration, molecular weight, geometry of the amphiphilic block copolymers, or the ratio of the different blocks.	• Tunable self-assembly. • Encapsulate hydrophilic, hydrophobic, or amphiphilic drugs. • Higher therapeutic-loading capacity than lipidic micelles. • Superior tissue-penetration capability. • Good biocompatibility and stability in blood. • High circulation half-life due to the low rate of phagocytosis by the RES – passive targeting.	• Stability problems upon dilution in the bloodstream or in the presence of plasma and tissue components that can bind the individual amphiphilic polymers. • Physicochemical heterogeneity resulting in lack of reproducibility. • Higher toxicity than lipid-based nanosystems.	(Ahmad et al. 2014, Jhaveri and Torchilin 2014, Croy and Kwon 2006)

(Continued)

TABLE 2.1 (Continued)   Different Types of Drug Delivery Nanosystems (DDNs): Their Schematic Representation and Their Main Advantages and Disadvantages

Nanoparticles

TYPE OF DDNS AND SCHEMATIC REPRESENTATION	DESCRIPTION	ADVANTAGES	DISADVANTAGES	REFERENCES
Lipid nanoparticles	• Colloidal self-assembled dispersions comprising a hydrophobic matrix covered by a surfactant layer that favors its dispersion in aqueous media. Lipid nanoparticles are solid at body and room temperatures. • Lipid nanoparticles with hydrophobic matrices composed by solid lipids are named SLNs. When the hydrophobic matrices contain solid lipids and liquid lipids (oils), they are designated as NLCs.	• Composed of physiological lipids and GRAS excipients. • Biocompatible, biodegradable. • Good blood stability. • Encapsulates hydrophobic drugs. • Can cross BBB via receptor mediated transcytosis (target low-density lipoproteins receptors). • Easy scalable production methods.	• Not adequate for encapsulation of hydrophilic and amphiphilic drugs. • Less toxic than polymeric DDNs but more toxic than liposomes and toxicity depends on the surfactant content and composition.	(Duan et al. 2020, Müller, Radtke, and Wissing 2002, Naseri, Valizadeh, and Zakeri-Milani 2015, Lopes et al. 2018, Lúcio et al. 2021, Soares et al. 2018b) (Continued)

TABLE 2.1 (Continued)   Different Types of Drug Delivery Nanosystems (DDNs): Their Schematic Representation and Their Main Advantages and Disadvantages

TYPE OF DDNS AND SCHEMATIC REPRESENTATION	DESCRIPTION	ADVANTAGES	DISADVANTAGES	REFERENCES
Polymeric nanoparticles WATER OIL	• Solid colloidal self-assembled particles composed of a polymer material with diameters ranging usually from 100 to 300 nm. • They can be prepared as nanocapsules – i.e., the polymeric matrix membrane includes the drug within its core acting as reservoir form – or nanospheres – i.e., the drug is dissolved, dispersed, entrapped, or attached to the surface of the nanoparticle. • Proteins (e.g., gelatin, albumin, elastin), polysaccharides (e.g., dextran, chitosan, hyaluronic acid), and synthetic polymers (e.g., polyanhydrides, polyesters, polyamides) have been used in the composition of polymeric nanoparticles alone or in conjugation with other materials or functional moieties.	• Mostly composed by polymers that are biodegradable, biocompatible, low/nontoxic, and nonimmunogenic. • High loading capacity of hydrophilic and hydrophobic drugs. • Stability, chemical structure, and size can be tuned (i.e., selecting polymer and monitoring self-assembly conditions) to control the kinetic release of drugs. Production methods can be scaled up. • Higher stability compared to other DDNs (e.g., liposomes). • Can be administered by different routes such as parenteral, oral, ocular, topical.	• Bioactive release dependent on polymer degradability. • Toxicity issues regarding the residues of organic solvents used in some manufacturing processes as well as in catalysts for chemistry functionalization. • Physicochemical heterogeneity resulting in lack of reproducibility.	(Zielinska et al. 2020, Lúcio et al. 2021, Schaffazick et al. 2003).

(Continued)

TABLE 2.1 (Continued)   Different Types of Drug Delivery Nanosystems (DDNs): Their Schematic Representation and Their Main Advantages and Disadvantages

Emulsions

TYPE OF DDNS AND SCHEMATIC REPRESENTATION	DESCRIPTION	ADVANTAGES	DISADVANTAGES	REFERENCES
Micro/nanoemulsions 	• Colloidal dispersion composed of immiscible liquid phases, usually comprising aqueous phase and oily phase, one dispersed as droplets in the other (continuous phase), stabilized by a surfactant agent or a mixture of surfactant and co-surfactant agents. • Can be categorized in w/o or o/w, each designating the composition of the dispersed phase (droplets) in the continuous phase. • Microemulsions are thermodynamically stable self-assembled dispersions that require only the application of low external energy (e.g., heating or stirring) to be generated. Usually, the droplet sizes of the dispersed phase range from 10 to 100 nm, resulting in optically clear dispersion.	• Use of safe materials such as edible oils and biocompatible surfactants. • Increased solubilization of lipophilic drugs. • Improved drug transport and delivery due to large interfacial areas. • Easy to produce and scale up. • Various routes of administration like topical, oral, and IV can be used. Are especially interesting to increase oral bioavailability of drugs. • Can be applied as substitutes of liposomes because they are much more stable. • In particular, SDEDDS may prolong the release of drugs because, if they are located in the inner phases, they are forced to disperse in a number of phases prior to release at the target site.	• High concentrations of surfactants and cosurfactants are used particularly in microemulsions to stabilize nanodroplets. This fact may increase their toxicity and reduce their biocompatibility. • Although the preparation methods are simple, they may also be expensive. • Stability is affected by external factors such as pH and temperature, and nanoemulsions are the most prone to instability over time. • Limited solubility capacity for substances with high melting points.	(Salome Amarachi, Kenechuk-wu, and Attama 2014, Lúcio et al. 2021, Soares et al. 2018b)

(Continued)

TABLE 2.1 (Continued)   Different Types of Drug Delivery Nanosystems (DDNs): Their Schematic Representation and Their Main Advantages and Disadvantages

TYPE OF DDNS AND SCHEMATIC REPRESENTATION	DESCRIPTION	ADVANTAGES	DISADVANTAGES	REFERENCES
	• Nanoemulsions are thermodynamically unstable self-assembled dispersions that require the application of high external energy (e.g., high-pressure homogenization or ultrasonication) to be generated. Usually, the droplet sizes of the dispersed phase range from 20 to 500 nm. Nanoemulsions are more susceptible instability phenomena over time. • Current nanoemulsions used as DDNs include the self-nanoemulsifying drug delivery systems (SNDDS) that originate o/w nanoemulsions and self-double-emulsifying drug delivery systems (SDEDDS) that can be w/o/w, o/o/w, or o/w/o.			

(Continued)

TABLE 2.1 (Continued)   Different Types of Drug Delivery Nanosystems (DDNs): Their Schematic Representation and Their Main Advantages and Disadvantages

Other Forms

TYPE OF DDNS AND SCHEMATIC REPRESENTATION	DESCRIPTION	ADVANTAGES	DISADVANTAGES	REFERENCES
Polymer–therapeutic conjugates **POLYMER** **DRUG** 	• Water-soluble polymers are used to produce a conjugate with both protein-based therapeutics and small-molecule drugs. • Almost all the marketed approved protein conjugates are covalently linked to PEG. • Other natural and synthetic polymers such as polysaccharides (e.g., dextran, hyaluronic acid, and polysialic acid), polypeptides, polycarbonates, are also being evaluated for therapeutic agent conjugation. • Biologically active polymers (e.g., peptide molecular carriers) are also being explored as therapeutic conjugate carriers.	• Similar to the advantages of polymeric nanoparticles. • Good blood stability. • Reduce renal clearance and extend plasma circulation half-life. • Reduce frequent dosing. • Active intracellular delivery. • Can control the biodistribution, release profile, and activity of therapeutic molecules. • Minimize protein immunogenicity. • Particularly useful as carrier for small-molecule anticancer agents enhancing their safety and efficacy due to the passive accumulation/targeting in tumor tissues.	• Similar to the disadvantages of polymeric nanoparticles. • In case of biological active polymers, many conjugates exhibit decreased biological activity compared with the native polymer. • The use of high molecular mass of water-soluble polymers and its subsequent use in therapeutics could result in the accumulation of non-biodegradable polymers.	(Ekladious, Colson, and Grinstaff 2019, Pelegri-O'Day, Lin, and Maynard 2014, Tsai, Wang, and Darensbourg 2016, Wang, Cheetham, et al. 2017, Zhang et al. 2013)

(Continued)

TABLE 2.1 (Continued)   Different Types of Drug Delivery Nanosystems (DDNs): Their Schematic Representation and Their Main Advantages and Disadvantages

Other Forms

TYPE OF DDNS AND SCHEMATIC REPRESENTATION	DESCRIPTION	ADVANTAGES	DISADVANTAGES	REFERENCES
Dendrimers 	• Synthetic three-dimensional, hyperbranched globular-shaped polymeric structures. • Structurally, dendrimers contain polymeric branching repeat units covalently attached to a central nucleus (single atom or group of atoms), organized in concentric layers (known as generations – represented with different colors in the figure) and that terminate with functional surface groups that may have positive, negative, or neutral charges. • Can be classified according to the type of core and peripheral groups as polyamidoamine dendrimer, poly (propylene imine) dendrimer, glycodendrimer, liquid crystalline dendrimer, and peptide dendrimer.	• Can encapsulate hydrophilic, hydrophobic, or amphiphilic drugs. • Highly homogenous and monodisperse DDNs (compared to self-assembled nanosystems). • Monodisperse DDNs with uniform shape and defined molecular weight, which improve its bioavailability and biodistribution. • Dendrimers composed by small molecules or containing PEG or dendrimers having PEGylated surface show low immunogenicity. • High and easy control of surface functionalization, optimizing cellular recognition. • Can be administered by different routes such as parenteral, oral, topical, and transdermal. • Versatile properties due to the presence of multiple active groups on the surface of the dendrimer. • Versatile carriers for therapeutic, diagnostic, and transfection agents.	• Complex synthesis. • Toxicity and biocompatibility depend on the generation (i.e., size) of the dendrimer and the functional groups on the surface. • Lower generation dendrimers are better than higher generations regarding cytotoxicity, immunogenicity, and biocompatibility. • The positively charged dendrimers are more toxic than the negatively charged, PEGylated, or neutral dendrimers. • Fast clearance from system circulation. • Nonspecific drug delivery. • For covalent therapeutic-dendrimer conjugates, an abrupt release of drug can occur after exposure to the biological fluids due to absence of interactive forces with the DDNs.	(Duncan and Izzo 2005, Edgar and Wang 2017, Lombardo, Kiselev, and Caccamo 2019, Patel et al. 2020, Zhu, Liu, and Pang 2019)

(Continued)

TABLE 2.1 (Continued)   Different Types of Drug Delivery Nanosystems (DDNs): Their Schematic Representation and Their Main Advantages and Disadvantages

TYPE OF DDNS AND SCHEMATIC REPRESENTATION	DESCRIPTION	ADVANTAGES	DISADVANTAGES	REFERENCES
	• As DDNs, dendrimers can load drugs within the dendritic architecture by physical entrapment (e.g., electrostatic, hydrophobic, and hydrogen bond interactions) and covalent dendrimer-therapeutic conjugates.			
Inorganic DDNs **Magnetic nanoparticles**	• Structurally, magnetic nanoparticles are composed of a magnetic core, such as Fe_3O_4, $\gamma\text{-}Fe_2O_3$, cobalt ferrite, chromium dioxide, carbonyl iron, nickel, cobalt, neodymium-iron-boron, with a polymeric or inorganic material coating, or with magnetic nanoparticles precipitated inside the pores of a polymeric matrix.	• Adjustable and uniform sizes between 1 and 100 nm. • Possibility of easy functionalization and the potential to carry a high dose of therapeutics. • Can be detected and manipulated by remote magnetic fields. • Accumulation at desired sites through delivery guided by magnetic fields. • A promising strategy for MRI application.	• Surface disorder • Nanotoxicity resulting from the accumulation of nanoparticles and the production of excess ROS, such as free radicals (anion superoxide, hydroxyl radicals and non-radical hydrogen peroxide).	(Adibfar et al. 2018, Bárcena, Sra, and Gao 2009, Estelrich et al. 2015, Lombardo, Kiselev, and Caccamo 2019, Namdeo et al. 2008,

(Continued)

TABLE 2.1 (Continued)   Different Types of Drug Delivery Nanosystems (DDNs): Their Schematic Representation and Their Main Advantages and Disadvantages

TYPE OF DDNS AND SCHEMATIC REPRESENTATION	DESCRIPTION	ADVANTAGES	DISADVANTAGES	REFERENCES
	• Among all magnetic components, magnetite is the most widely investigated due to its high stability, high biocompatibility, and low cost. • Magnetic iron oxide nanoparticles with a diameter lower than 30 nm present a super para-magnetism effect (superparamagnetic iron oxide nanoparticles – SPION), i.e., magnetization of the nanoparticles up to their saturation in the presence of an applied field; however, no residual magnetism is detected upon removal of the magnetic field.			Pankhurst et al. 2003, Sensenig et al. 2012, Wu et al. 2019)

(Continued)

TABLE 2.1 (Continued)   Different Types of Drug Delivery Nanosystems (DDNs): Their Schematic Representation and Their Main Advantages and Disadvantages

TYPE OF DDNS AND SCHEMATIC REPRESENTATION	DESCRIPTION	ADVANTAGES	DISADVANTAGES	REFERENCES
	• Ideally, magnetic DDNs should be superparamagnetic to prevent agglomeration, avoiding embolism. • These DDNs respond to magnetic fields, which can produce an on-site triggered drug release based on direct structural rearrangements induced magnetically or as a byproduct of the hyperthermic effect of the magnetic field.			
Quantum dots 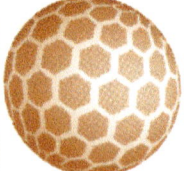	• Quantum dots are semiconductor nanocrystals with a quasi-spherical structure that regulates the fluorescence emission. • The nanocrystal can be any inorganic entity that displays a crystalline arrangement of atoms. Their diameter ranges from 2 to 10 nm and contain approximately 200–10,000 atoms.	• Small size and monodisperse. • Good chemical/photo-stability. • Near infrared (>650 nm) emission (advantage over organic fluorophores). • Excellent bioimaging properties: intense fluorescence (high quantum yield) with low photobleaching, and size-tunable light emission. • Good intracellular uptake and therapeutic release. • Easy surface modifications. • PEGylation produces higher permeation and retention (EPR) effect.	• Cytotoxicity due to: (i) toxic effects of the core inorganic elements (e.g., heavy metals like cadmium, tellurium, selenium, and mercury); (ii) remaining organic solvents used in synthesis processes; (iii) aggregation on the cell surface due to the stabilizing effect of surface ligands; (iv) induced formation of ROS. • Toxicity can be decreased by functionalizing the surface of quantum dots with biocompatible molecules. • Their metabolism, degradation, accumulation, and clearance inside the body are still basically unknown.	(Hild, Breunig, and Goepferich 2008, Krishnaswamy and Orsat 2017, Smith et al. 2008, Smith and Nie 2010)

(Continued)

TABLE 2.1 (Continued) Different Types of Drug Delivery Nanosystems (DDNs): Their Schematic Representation and Their Main Advantages and Disadvantages

TYPE OF DDNS AND SCHEMATIC REPRESENTATION	DESCRIPTION	ADVANTAGES	DISADVANTAGES	REFERENCES
	• These DDNs offer exceptional optical, semiconductor, photochemical, and catalytic properties due to their quantum confinement dictated by their structure, chemical composition, and size. • Surface coating with biomolecules is required after their synthesis, because the resulting quantum dots are insoluble in water.			
Gold nanoparticles 	• Gold nanoparticles are metallic nanoparticles comprised of a gold atom nucleus surrounded by negative reactive groups on the surface that can be simply modified and attached with several molecules.	• Small size and monodisperse. • High therapeutic loading capacity. • High cell permeability. • Amphiphilic properties. • Easy synthesis and surface functionalization. • Inert, non-cytotoxic, excellent biocompatibility. • Tunable stability. • Optical properties. • Ability to form heterogeneous biointeraction.	• Their interaction with cells must be clarified. • Can contribute to high production of ROS, which is not beneficial for cells.	(Lombardo, Kiselev, and Caccamo 2019, Kong et al. 2017)

(Continued)

TABLE 2.1 (Continued) Different Types of Drug Delivery Nanosystems (DDNs): Their Schematic Representation and Their Main Advantages and Disadvantages

TYPE OF DDNS AND SCHEMATIC REPRESENTATION	DESCRIPTION	ADVANTAGES	DISADVANTAGES	REFERENCES
Mesoporous silica nanoparticles 	• Silica nanoparticles are frequently termed as MSNs because structurally, MSNs present a solid framework containing pores with controlled diameters ranging from 2 to 50 nm (with narrow pore size distribution) and a great surface area. • Chemically, these MSNs have a honeycomb-like structure and an active surface with silanol groups. • The large surface area covered with silanol groups is easily functionalized, favoring drug loading and the capability to interact with the target molecules.	• Simple synthesis • Specific particle sizes with tunable features such as diameter, shape, porosity, and both core and surface features. • High loading of hydrophilic and lipophilic drugs. • PEGylation increases EPR effect. • Good thermal and chemical stability. The strong Si–O bond makes MSNs more stable to degradation and mechanical stress (compared to liposomes, and dendrimers). • Low toxicity (silica is recognized as safe for use by the FDA). • Stability *in vivo*. • Good biocompatibility and biodegradability. • Can be used as coating material.	• Without surface modification, silica nanoparticles can cause toxicity by two mechanisms: • Hemolysis resulting from the surface density of silanol groups that interacts with the surface of the phospholipids of the red blood cell membranes. • Siloxane groups on the surface can form three-membered siloxane rings, such as silanol groups, which are unstable and reactive and can cause lysis of membrane. • Metabolic changes induced by porous silica nanoparticles can promote melanoma.	(Bharti et al. 2015, Downing and Jain 2020," Lombardo, Kiselev, and Caccamo 2019, Mahmoodi, Ghavidast, and Amirmahani 2016)

Abbreviations: BBB – blood brain barrier; CMC – critical micelle concentration; DDNs – drug delivery nanosystems; EPR – enhanced permeability and retention; FDA – Food and Drug Administration; γ-Fe$_2$O$_3$ – maghemite; Fe$_3$O$_4$ – magnetite; GRAS – generally recognized as safe; MRI – magnetic resonance imaging; MSNs – mesoporous silica nanoparticles; NLCs – nanostructured lipid carriers; nm – nanometer; o/w – oil-in-water; PEG – polyethylene glycol; RES – reticuloendothelial system; ROS – reactive oxygen species; SDEDDS – self-double-emulsifying drug delivery systems; SLNs – solid lipid nanoparticles; SNDDS – self-nanoemulsifying drug delivery systems; SPION – superparamagnetic iron oxide nanoparticles; w/o – water-in-oil.

TABLE 2.2   Nanomedicine Applications of Organic and Inorganic Nanosystems

NANOSYSTEMS	APPLICATIONS IN NANOMEDICINE	MAIN OUTCOMES	REFERENCES
Liposomes	**Therapeutic delivery**	• Their amphiphilic nature, biocompatibility, biodegradation, and flexibility make liposomes suitable to encapsulate and deliver several bioactives, such as drugs, natural compounds, enzymes, hormones, nucleic acids, peptides. • Developed for a wide range of applications: ocular diseases like glaucoma and retinopathy; pain management and anesthesia; skin disorders and cosmetic applications; cancer; infections; cardiovascular and neurodegenerative diseases. In these pathological conditions, the efficiency of liposomes is enhanced by targeting and stimulus triggering release of drugs. • Good and effective carriers for ophthalmic drugs, because they allow a drug to pass through the barrier of the eye, and their lipidic nature allows them to adhere to the cornea. Therefore, liposomes are especially important for the improvement of intravitreal half-life and selective retinal delivery in the posterior eye segment diseases. • In skin disorders and in cosmeceutics, liposomes act as penetration enhancers, to promote the transport of compounds that cannot otherwise penetrate the skin. Liposomes minimize skin inflammation by maintaining drug release and skin hydration. They are not only used to treat hair follicle disorders, but also able to target new drugs into the pilosebaceous structures. • In neurodegenerative diseases, liposomes accumulate in the brain by using targeting ligands to receptors found in brain endothelial cells resulting in BBB-mediated receptor transcytosis. The use of cationic liposomes that interact with the polyanions of the BBB is another way of getting into the brain by adsorptive mediated transcytosis. • In cancer, liposomes can accumulate in tumors by EPR and by surface functionalization with ligands that target receptors overexpressed in cancer cells, or receptors present in the extracellular matrix of tumor cells or even receptors in organelles like mitochondria. • In addition to the therapeutic delivery, liposomes can also be used to produce novel vaccines, as they may be engineered for the delivery of antigens.	(Pujol-Autonell et al. 2017, Zakrewsky, Kumar, and Mitragotri 2015, Beiranvand and Moradkhani 2018, Beltrán-Gracia et al. 2019, Saraf et al. 2020, Lalu et al. 2017, Vieira and Gamarra 2016, Rahimpour and Hamishehkar 2012, Nisini et al. 2018, de Leeuw et al. 2009, Sun et al. 2017, Farjadian et al. 2019)

(Continued)

TABLE 2.2 (Continued)   Nanomedicine Applications of Organic and Inorganic Nanosystems

NANOSYSTEMS	APPLICATIONS IN NANOMEDICINE	MAIN OUTCOMES	REFERENCES
	Diagnosis and theranostic purposes	• Control of composition and surface functionalization has enabled progress in using liposomes for diagnosis of diseases or detection of biomarkers relevant to early detection of diseases. • Diagnostic applications are based on fluorescence imaging (e.g., by encapsulating near infrared absorbers such as graphene quantum dots); magnetic resonance imaging (by encapsulating MRI contrasting agents); nuclear imaging by functionalization with small molecule radioactive tracers; biomarker detection (e.g., by functionalizing liposomes with recognition ligands like peptides and DNA that specifically bind to the biomarker, triggering the rupture of the vesicle and releasing the encapsulated reporting agent). • Used for theranostic purposes by loading with various imaging agents and drugs together.	(Zhou, Wang, and Zhang 2013, Bally et al. 2010, Ogawa et al. 2014, Mikhaylov et al. 2011, Xing, Hwang, and Lu 2016)
	Tissue engineering and regenerative medicine	• Combination of liposomes with scaffolds can sequester liposomes at the tissue site and induce growth/differentiation of stem cells. Liposomes sequestered at tissue site can also be stimuli-responsive and used to monitor *in situ* formation of mineral, polymers, or mineral/polymers composite biomaterials. • Used to control the release of growth factors, avoiding their side-effects. Examples of growth factors delivered are bone morphogenic protein 2 (BMP-2) which induces osteogenic differentiation and TGF-β which promotes chondrogenic differentiation. • Used to deliver genes encoding BMP-2 and TGF-β that initiate bone and cartilage stem cell differentiation and coordinate the pathways of new bone ossification and cartilage maturation. Delivery of genes encoding for VEGF using bone marrow stromal cells is another use of liposomes to improve tissue vascularization. • Hybrid DDNs made of cationic liposomes containing magnetite nanoparticles can be injected and accumulated in the target tissue by using an external stimulus (magnetic field) to promote cell seeding in the inner space of the scaffolds.	(Ito et al. 2005b, Liu et al. 2004, Monteiro et al. 2015, Pederson, Ruberti, and Messersmith 2003, Collier and Messersmith 2001, Monteiro et al. 2014)

(Continued)

TABLE 2.2 (Continued)   Nanomedicine Applications of Organic and Inorganic Nanosystems

NANOSYSTEMS	APPLICATIONS IN NANOMEDICINE	MAIN OUTCOMES	REFERENCES
Ethosomes	**Therapeutic delivery**	• Much more effective in delivering drugs, bioactives, or cosmetic agents to the skin in terms of quantity and depth than liposomes. Ethosomes increase the residence time of drugs and cosmetic agents in the skin. • Used for transdermal delivery of antigens (e.g., hepatitis B), hormones (e.g., testosterone), psychoactive drugs, anti-psoriatic drugs (e.g., methotrexate), anti-inflammatory drugs (e.g., celecoxib). Because of improved permeation of BBB, ethosomes are also used for oral and transdermal delivery of natural compounds to the brain (e.g., catechin and ligustrazine). • Delivery of minoxidil for alopecia, azelaic acid for acne treatment, anti-cellulite agents, and antioxidants to prevent oxidative injury throughout the skin.	(Verma and Pathak 2010, Dayan and Touitou 2000, Dubey et al. 2007, Ainbinder and Touitou 2005, Mishra et al. 2008, Koli 2010, Esposito, Menegatti, and Cortesi 2004, Bragagni et al. 2012, Soares et al. 2018b)
Transfero-somes	**Therapeutic delivery**	• Their ultra-deformable properties allow the transferosome to penetrate deeper layers of the skin. They therefore show major advantages over liposomes for the delivery of drugs and other bioactives by transdermal delivery. • A large range of drugs, such as sinomenine (rheumatoid arthritis) and apigenine (leukemia), small hydrophobic drugs, and labile biomacromolecules like insulin (diabetes), have successfully been encapsulated within transferosomes. • It is possible to load transferosomes with low doses of potent drugs (e.g., tretinoin for acne treatment at 0.05%) or with high drug loads up to 20% (e.g., sinomenine). However, drug loading above 20% is challenging given the amount of lipids and edge activators required to generate stable transferosomes. Therefore, it is more likely that potent drugs at low doses become clinically translatable. • The first transferosomal formulation to enter the market (2007) indicated as a painkiller in knee osteoarthritis was Diractin®. Ketoprofen loaded in this formulation has been able to penetrate deeper tissues, including muscle, relative to other anti-inflammatory gels. However, because of the higher production costs, the profit was not significant enough to warrant the commercialization of the formulation and it was withdrawn six months later.	(Fernández-García et al. 2020, Wang et al. 2017a, Rother et al. 2009, Marwah et al. 2016, Kneer et al. 2013, Werner et al. 2009, Jangdey et al. 2017, Ascenso et al. 2014, Ahad et al. 2012)

(Continued)

TABLE 2.2 (Continued) Nanomedicine Applications of Organic and Inorganic Nanosystems

NANOSYSTEMS	APPLICATIONS IN NANOMEDICINE	MAIN OUTCOMES	REFERENCES
Pharmaco-somes	**Therapeutic delivery**	• Binding of lipids to drugs provides stability and enables the controlled release of various drugs, such as acyclovir (anti-viral), furosemide (diuretic), diclofenac, and ketoprofen (anti-inflammatory). • Minimize gastrointestinal toxic effects of anti-inflammatory drugs, as their loading in pharmacosomes increases absorption and reduces gastrointestinal residence time. • Improve bioavailability of biomacromolecules, such as insulin and calcitonin, and of biopolymers like hyaluronic acid. • Improve bioavailability of phytoactives (e.g., flavonoids, glycosides, xantones).	(Kamalesh et al. 2014, Chatap, Patil, and Patil 2014, Huang, Ling, and Zhang 2007, Cui et al. 2006, Taskintuna et al. 1997, Sang Yoo and Gwan Park 2004, Khazaeinia and Jamali 2003, Semalty et al. 2009, Pandita and Sharma 2013)
Polymersomes	**Therapeutic delivery**	• Controlled therapeutic release kinetics, prolonged circulation time and accumulation at the targeted site of drugs, such as anticancer agents, reducing their cytotoxicity. • Controlled nucleic acid binding and release, resulting in high transfection efficiency and reduced toxicity. • Encapsulated hemoglobin for blood substitutes. • Antibodies have been conjugated to polymersomes for targeted delivery. • Controlled and targeted *in vitro* and *in vivo* drug release in response to specific triggers, such as pH, temperature, redox environment, magnetic field, and other stimuli.	(Arifin and Palmer 2005, Chen et al. 2006, Kim et al. 2009, Li et al. 2007, Lin et al. 2006, Liu, Yaszemski, and Lu 2016, Lomas et al. 2007, Lomas et al. 2010, Lomas et al. 2008, Murdoch et al. 2010, Oliveira et al. 2013, Rameez, Alosta, and Palmer 2008, Rameez et al. 2012, Spain et al. 2011, Tan et al. 2018, Tuguntaev et al. 2016, Zhang and Zhang 2017)
	Diagnosis purposes	• Polymersomes can be loaded with imaging agents.	(Liu et al. 2017, Tanisaka et al. 2008, Makino et al. 2009, Leong et al. 2018, Meerovich and Dash 2019).

(Continued)

TABLE 2.2 (Continued)   Nanomedicine Applications of Organic and Inorganic Nanosystems

NANOSYSTEMS	APPLICATIONS IN NANOMEDICINE	MAIN OUTCOMES	REFERENCES
	Tissue engineering and regenerative medicine	• Efficient penetration and retention of polymersomes for intra-epithelial and/or trans-epithelial delivery of therapeutic compounds cross tissue engineered human oral mucosa.	(Hearnden et al. 2009)
Lipid micelles	**Therapeutic delivery**	• Integral lipid micelles are not used for therapeutic delivery, since their critical micelle concentration (CMC) is quite high, and their stability can be compromised by dilution in biological fluids. Instead, hybrid micelles with a phospholipid core conjugated with polymers (e.g., PEG-PE, or chitosan-PEG-oleic acid) are more interesting. • Lipid-core micelles are effective in the encapsulation and delivery of poorly soluble chemotherapeutics for cancer therapy (e.g., paclitaxel, camptothecin). Drug accumulation at cancer tissues is achieved either by EPR or ligand-mediated active targeting. • When positively charged, this hybrid micelles are capable of escaping endosomes delivering incorporated drugs directly into the cell cytoplasm.	(Torchilin 2005, Sawant and Torchilin 2010)
	Diagnosis purposes	• Lipid-core micelles can carry various reporter (contrast) agents for diagnostic imaging modalities.	
Polymeric micelles	**Therapeutic delivery**	• Increased aqueous solubility, dissolution rate, and oral bioavailability of poorly water-soluble therapeutic compounds. • Controlled therapeutic release kinetics, extended plasma half-life, and accumulation at the targeted site, such as anticancer agents, reducing their cytotoxicity. • Delivery of nucleic acids, enhancement of their stability in physiological media, and facilitation of their cellular internalization. • Enhance drug delivery and reduce side-effects by increasing the selective uptake by targets.	(Cabral and Kataoka 2014, Matsumura et al. 2004, Hu et al. 2015, Mochida et al. 2014, Hamaguchi et al. 2005, Banga et al. 2017, Chiappetta et al. 2011, Craparo et al. 2014, Kataoka et al. 2005, Movassaghian, Merkel, and Torchilin 2015, Savić, Eisenberg, and Maysinger 2006, Sawant et al. 2014, Yang et al. 2014).

(Continued)

TABLE 2.2 (Continued)   Nanomedicine Applications of Organic and Inorganic Nanosystems

NANOSYSTEMS	APPLICATIONS IN NANOMEDICINE	MAIN OUTCOMES	REFERENCES
	Diagnosis purposes	• Can be loaded with imaging agents providing enhanced effective contrast for cancer-recognition.	(Yang et al. 2013, Torchilin, Frank-Kamenetsky, and Wolf 1999).
	Tissue engineering and regenerative medicine	• Delivery of therapeutic agents (e.g., dexamethasone; apocynin (APO) prodrug) for improvement of the intracellular release and enhancement of tissue regeneration.	(Santo et al. 2015, Wang et al. 2020)
Lipid nanoparticles: solid lipid nanoparticles (SLNs) and nanostructured lipid carriers (NLCs)	**Therapeutic delivery**	• Suitable for encapsulation of drugs positioned in the biopharmaceutical classification system (BCS) class II and class IV, i.e., hydrophobic drugs with low aqueous solubility and low bioavailability. • Many different drugs have been incorporated in SLNs and NLCs, namely anticancer drugs, antimicrobial drugs, cardiovascular drugs (anti-hyperlipidemic and antihypertension), anti-diabetic drugs, and drugs that act in the central nervous system. • Suitable for gene therapy. The barriers to cell transfection, including nuclease degradation, cell internalization, and intracellular trafficking, can easily be overcome by complexes established between cationic charged SLNs/NLCs and nucleic acids. • Therapeutically important peptides (e.g., calcitonin, cyclosporine A, insulin, luteinizing hormone-releasing hormone, LHRH, somatostatin) and protein antigens (e.g., hepatitis B and malaria antigens) can be administered as the lipid matrix increases the stability of proteins, prevents proteolytic degradation after administration, and releases the protein in a controlled manner. • Capable of selectively targeting drugs or genes to a particular type of cell upon surface functionalization. In the case of cancer, active targeting strategies may be used in addition to EPR passive targeting. In the case of brain diseases, effective strategies include functionalization with angiopep-2 that specially binds to the LRP1 overexpressed at the BBB or functionalization with apolipoprotein E that has high affinity receptors along the BBB.	(Mendes et al. 2013, Vitorino et al. 2014, Barone et al. 2019, Iqbal, Vitorino, and Taylor 2017, Souto et al. 2019, Tupal et al. 2016, Bhalekar et al. 2017, Alsulays et al. 2019, González-Paredes et al. 2019, Ravi et al. 2014, Senthil Kumar et al. 2020, Rajpoot and Jain 2020, Costa, Sarmento, and Seabra 2018, Dal Magro et al. 2017, Müller, Radtke, and Wissing 2002, Attama 2011, Scioli Montoto, Muraca, and Ruiz 2020)

(Continued)

TABLE 2.2 (Continued)   Nanomedicine Applications of Organic and Inorganic Nanosystems

NANOSYSTEMS	APPLICATIONS IN NANOMEDICINE	MAIN OUTCOMES	REFERENCES
		• Versatile delivery systems for different routes of administration: parenteral, oral, cutaneous, and transdermal, nasal, ocular, pulmonary, and rectal. Recently, non-invasive routes have become increasingly important for the delivery of drugs, proteins, peptides, and biopharmaceuticals, by nasal, buccal, vaginal, and transdermal routes. • Hold eminent potential in dermopharmaceutical and cosmetic market because of SLNs/NLCs benefits: skin hydration, occlusion, and enhanced penetration.	
	Diagnosis and theranostic purposes	• SLN can carry several types of diagnostic agents such as superparamagnetic nanoparticles (for MRI), radiolabeled agents (for scintigraphy and positron emission tomography), and quantum dots (for *in situ* fluorescence imaging of the intracellular uptake of SLNs into cancer cells). In the latter case, the combination of quantum dots with anticancer drug paclitaxel in the same SLNs' formulation is an example of the suitability of these nanoparticles for theranostic purposes.	(Andreozzi et al. 2011, Bae et al. 2013, Videira et al. 2002, Peira et al. 2003, Shuhendler et al. 2012, Mussi and Torchilin 2013)
	Tissue engineering and regenerative medicine	• Suitable to be used as a scaffold for the stem cell attachment, to retain stemness, and for inducing stem cell differentiation. • Combined with biomaterials are used for tissue healing (e.g., fibrin-agarose biomaterials functionalized with NLCs loaded with antibiotics to treat infected wounds). • Suitable to carry growth factors that promote tissue regeneration and to enable their sustained release. For example, epidermal growth factor (EGF) in wounds after topical administration improves the proliferation of keratinocytes and fibroblasts and promotes healing and maturation in terms of chronic wounds and re-epithelization grade.	(Chato-Astrain et al. 2020, Gainza et al. 2014, Wang, Wang, et al. 2017, Zhu et al. 2016, Zhao et al. 2014, Chabra et al. 2011, Sussman et al. 2008)
Polymeric nanoparticles	**Therapeutic delivery**	• Enhancement of the permeability and bioavailability of therapeutic agents, including poorly water-soluble compounds, peptides/proteins, nucleic acids, in different membranes, such as gastrointestinal mucosa, buccal mucosa, vaginal mucosa, ocular membranes, or other barriers, such as skin layers and blood–brain barrier. • Protect therapeutic compounds from degradation caused by internal factors, such as intrinsic enzymes.	(Chan et al. 2010, Wang and Zhang 2012, das Neves et al. 2013, Frank et al. 2014, Lin et al. 2015, Ramyadevi et al. 2016, Shah et al. 2016, *(Continued)*

TABLE 2.2 (Continued)   Nanomedicine Applications of Organic and Inorganic Nanosystems

NANOSYSTEMS	APPLICATIONS IN NANOMEDICINE	MAIN OUTCOMES	REFERENCES
			El-Nahas et al. 2017, Kalam and Alshamsan 2017, Sun et al. 2017, Takeuchi et al. 2017, Castro et al. 2018, Fatima et al. 2018, Wen et al. 2018, Cayero-Otero et al. 2019, Pinto and Fernandes 2019, Ha-Lien Tran et al. 2020, Jiang et al. 2020, Lee et al. 2020, Silva et al. 2020, Rata et al. 2021)
	Diagnosis and theranostic purposes	• Used for theranostic purposes by loading with various imaging agents and drugs together.	(Luk and Zhang 2014)
	Tissue engineering and regenerative medicine	• Can be used to incorporate and to sustain the release of growth factors (e.g., BMP-2, SDF-1α) as chemoattractant for the homing of bone marrow resident mesenchymal stem cells. • Tuned release behavior from both smart polymeric nanoparticles alone, or incorporated into delivery scaffolds, such as hydrogels, fibers, is another way to deliver bioactive growth factors (e.g., VEGF, basic fibroblast growth factor, bFGf, PDGF-BB) with spatiotemporal adjustable character, suitable for different applications, such as angiogenic/osteogenic differentiations, promoting the vasculature within bone tissue engineered constructs, and promoting angiogenesis for wound healing and for cardiac tissue regeneration. • Surface modification of hybrid nanosystems – polymer replica particles templated from degradable mesoporous silica – can provide a facile means to tailor the interactions of nanostructure with biological systems, namely their aggregation in the major organs of the phagocyte mononuclear system, for tissue engineering applications.	(BaoLin and Ma 2014, Smith et al. 2009, Adibfar et al. 2018, Izadifar, Kelly, and Chen 2016, Song et al. 2017, Vrana et al. 2014, Wang et al. 2016, Xie et al. 2013, Yilgor et al. 2009, Zhang et al. 2018)

(Continued)

TABLE 2.2 (Continued)   Nanomedicine Applications of Organic and Inorganic Nanosystems

NANOSYSTEMS	APPLICATIONS IN NANOMEDICINE	MAIN OUTCOMES	REFERENCES
Polymer therapeutic conjugates	**Therapeutic delivery**	• Improvement of protein therapeutic characteristics, namely extended plasma half-life, prolonged dosing intervals, reduced renal clearance, enhanced pharmacokinetic profile, reduced immunogenicity, sustained immune stimulation, and protein binding selectivity. • Extend plasma half-life, enhance safety profile, and provide greater tumor accumulation and passive tumor targeting than unconjugated cytotoxic chemotherapeutic agents. • Modulating polymer molecular mass, architecture and linker chemistry can endow optimized therapeutic release profile and, subsequently, enhanced therapeutic efficacy.	(Graham 2003, Curran and McCormack 2008, Wang et al. 2002, Yang and Kido 2011, Naing et al. 2015, Charych et al. 2017, Charych et al. 2016, Etrych et al. 2012, Hoch et al. 2014, Jameson et al. 2013, Quan et al. 2014, Stirland et al. 2013)
Nanoemul-sions	**Therapeutic delivery**	• Suitable as DDNs via various routes of administration: topical, transdermal, ocular, oral, nasal/pulmonary, and parenteral. • Improve bioavailability of lipophilic drugs by optimizing their absorption through the skin. The surfactant component that provides interface between the aqueous and oily phases may enhance penetration throughout the skin. The small size and low surface tension of the nanoemulsions can boost the drug permeation rate. • Adequate for ocular drug delivery through the cornea, but in this case the type and concentration of the dispersed oily phase should be selected carefully to assure the correct refractive index, viscosity, and transparency. Can be used to prevent neovascularization and treat retinopathy when carrying antisense oligonucleotides (gene therapy). • Increase absorption and efficacy of orally administered lipophilic drugs by prolonging residency in the gastrointestinal tract and activating the intestinal lymphatic pathway, thereby preventing liver first pass metabolism. • Act as a solution with a large fine particle fraction, thus presenting high aerosolization efficiency after nebulization when compared to suspensions. For these DDNs, pulmonary route administration may therefore be further explored.	(Hörmann and Zimmer 2016, Comfort et al. 2015, O'Konek et al. 2015, Pandey et al. 2016, Boche and Pokharkar 2017, Das et al. 2012, Nasr, Nawaz, and Elhissi 2012, Pandey et al. 2017, Lim et al. 2016, Hagigit et al. 2012, Khandavilli and Panchagnula 2007, Salim et al. 2016, Tayeb and Sainsbury 2018)

(Continued)

TABLE 2.2 (Continued)   Nanomedicine Applications of Organic and Inorganic Nanosystems

NANOSYSTEMS	APPLICATIONS IN NANOMEDICINE	MAIN OUTCOMES	REFERENCES
		• Intranasal route is painless and noninvasive, and nanoemulsions can be used to distribute drugs locally or systemically. Local delivery includes vaccination by delivery of influenza vaccine to mucosal immune cells and small molecule delivery for psychological and neurological disorders. Systemic delivery through the nose includes aerosolized nanoemulsions for the treatment of migraine and for immunization with inactivated respiratory syncytial virus. • Parenteral delivery of nanoemulsions as DDNs has been developed to treat many health conditions including sepsis, hypertension, erectile dysfunction, epilepsy, cancer (using active and passive EPR targeting strategies), and nutritional therapy.	
	Diagnosis purposes	• Nanoemulsions for perfluorocarbons delivery could track particular cell types or target certain areas of the body for imaging. Nanoemulsions are also used as platforms for metallic MRI contrast agents and fluorescence-based imaging.	(Simion et al. 2016, Kislukhin et al. 2016, Tayeb and Sainsbury 2018) (Yang, Wang, et al. 2014, Patel et al. 2015, Ganta et al. 2015)
	Theranostic purposes	• Theranostic nanoemulsions have also been developed, e.g., to deliver anticancer drug with folate-targeting ovarian cancer cells while their surface was functionalized with an MRI contrasting agent.	
	Tissue engineering and regenerative medicine	• Nanoemulsions and cell-based therapies are being applied for regenerative ophthalmological medicine in ocular diseases.	(Mclaughlin et al. 2016)
Dendrimers	**Therapeutic delivery**	• Enhance solubility of hydrophobic compounds. • Can be administered by different routes, such as IV, oral, dermal, pulmonary, intranasal (nose-to-brain), intravitreal. • Controlled delivery of drugs, peptides, and oligonucleotides and used as permeability enhancers across different physiological barriers, such as skin layers, oral mucosa, pulmonary epithelium, and BBB. • Dendriplexes (positively charged dendrimers complexed with nucleic acids) are promising for gene therapy. An amphiphilic type of polyamidoamine dendrimer for gene transfection is commercially available (Superfect® from Qiagen).	(Manikkath et al. 2017, Teow et al. 2013, Venuganti and Perumal 2009, Mutalik et al. 2014, Bharatwaj et al. 2015, Mishra et al. 2014, Kannan et al. 2012, Hussain et al. 2004, Kojima et al. 2009, Na et al. 2006, Iezzi et al. 2012, Katare et al. 2015, *(Continued)*

TABLE 2.2 (Continued) Nanomedicine Applications of Organic and Inorganic Nanosystems

NANOSYSTEMS	APPLICATIONS IN NANOMEDICINE	MAIN OUTCOMES	REFERENCES
		• Efficient peptides and oligonucleosides vaccine delivery. • Extended circulation time and tumor accumulation and drug triggering at tumor cells. • Ability to modulate and develop an optimum PDT.	Xie et al. 2019, Bai, Thomas, and Ahsan 2007, Dave and Venuganti 2017, Kambhampati et al. 2014, Liu, Tee, and Chiu 2015, Choudhary et al. 2017, Ooya, Lee, and Park 2004, Chauhan 2018, Kesharwani, Jain, and Jain 2014, Patel et al. 2020)
	Diagnosis purposes	• Can be conjugated with contrasting or diagnosis agents, such as contrasting MRI agents to retain them in the blood for a prolonged period and provide more effective visualization and detection. • Can improve the diagnosis agents, such as fluorescent probes due to their ability to increase tissue permeation, promote accumulation, and enhance imaging parameters, e.g., fluorescence intensity.	(Thomas et al. 2004, Wang and Imae 2004, Kim et al. 2013, D'Emanuele et al. 2004, Kobayashi et al. 2003, Rai et al. 2020, Ye et al. 2013).
	Tissue engineering and regenerative medicine	• Act as a linker to the scaffold and as a carrier of bioactive molecules. E.g., cholecystic-derived extracellular matrix (CEM) was incorporated within G1-PAMAM dendrimer. • Can be used for biomineralized hard tissues such as bone and teeth.	(Wu et al. 2013, Zhang, Yang, et al. 2015, Oliveira et al. 2010, Lin, Xie, et al. 2017, Boduch-Lee et al. 2004, Chan et al. 2008, Gorain et al. 2017, Joshi and Grinstaff 2008, Pramanik and Imae 2012).
Magnetic nanoparticles	**Therapeutic delivery**	• Magnetically mediated delivery of drugs, overcoming different cellular barriers, such as BBB and endothelial luminal layer underlying the walls of blood vessels. • Surface functionalization for controlled therapeutic delivery in different targeted sites, such as tumor tissues, BBB, and brain, and for nucleic acid transfection (gene therapy).	(Hayashi et al. 2010, Rezaei et al. 2017,

(Continued)

TABLE 2.2 (Continued)   Nanomedicine Applications of Organic and Inorganic Nanosystems

NANOSYSTEMS	APPLICATIONS IN NANOMEDICINE	MAIN OUTCOMES	REFERENCES
		• Hyperthermia agents used in magnetic fluid hyperthermia (MFH) for cancer treatment, destroying the surrounding cells by heating through the application of a high-frequency alternating magnetic field.	Farjadian, Ghasemi, and Mohammadi-Samani 2016, Aghanejad et al. 2018, Shen et al. 2016, Chen et al. 2014, Majidi et al. 2016, McBain et al. 2008, Dowaidar et al. 2017, Wang et al. 2014, Alonso et al. 2016, Guibert et al. 2015, Hayek 2019, Chorny et al. 2010, Polyak et al. 2008, Chertok et al. 2008, Grillo et al. 2016, Tietze et al. 2009, Anderson, Gwenin, and Gwenin 2019)
	Diagnosis and theranostic purposes	• Used for theranostic purposes in oncology. • Used for stem cell and molecular/cellular tracking. • Used as magnetic contrast agents for MRI.	(Singh, Dilnawaz, and Sahoo 2011, Shevtsov et al. 2015, Tian et al. 2018, Ding et al. 2017, Hong et al. 2016, Chen et al. 2017, Anderson, Gwenin, and Gwenin 2019).
	Tissue engineering and regenerative medicine	• Can be used as magnetic scaffold to which growth factor or other biologically active molecules bind and can control the distribution of the cells within the scaffold. • Can be delivered on demand by means of an externally applied magnetic field.	(Ito et al. 2004, Ito et al. 2007, Ishii et al. 2011, Santos, Sofia Silva, and Mano 2020, *(Continued)*

TABLE 2.2 (Continued) Nanomedicine Applications of Organic and Inorganic Nanosystems

NANOSYSTEMS	APPLICATIONS IN NANOMEDICINE	MAIN OUTCOMES	REFERENCES
		• Applying magnetic force-based tissue engineering technique that involves the use of magnetite cationic liposomes containing magnetite nanoparticles which electrostatically interact with cell membranes, for different tissue-engineering processes, such as to generate artificial skeletal muscles, small-diameter vascular tissue for graft survival retinal pigment epithelium for choroidal neovascularization, bone tissue for repair of defects, to generate coculture system of different cells (e.g., hepatocytes, aortic endothelial cells, mesenchymal stem cell).	Lee et al. 2014, Sato et al. 2013, Bock et al. 2010, Thevenot et al. 2008, Perea et al. 2006, Ito et al. 2006, Ito et al. 2005a, Shimizu, et al. 2007a,b, 2006, Shimizu et al. 2007, Sensenig et al. 2012, Yamamoto et al. 2009)
Quantum dots	**Therapeutic delivery**	• Powerful tool for labeling therapeutics (e.g., drugs, nucleic acids) in the investigation of diverse cellular processes, such as cellular uptake, receptor trafficking, nuclear trafficking mechanisms, cell nuclear processes, and intracellular nanocarriers delivery, which can be improved by combined quantum dots with cell-specific biomolecules, such as proteins or peptides. • PEGylation produces accumulation of quantum dots in tumor sites by an EPR effect. • Application of quantum dots and photosensitizer complexes is used in PDT. • Can be use as targeting and triggering nanosystems for drug delivery.	(Chen and Gerion 2004, Young and Rozengurt 2006, Wu et al. 2003, Schipper et al. 2009, Kim et al. 2017, Lin, Chen, et al. 2017, Bentolila 2015, Qi and Gao 2008, Samia, Chen, and Burda 2003, Ahirwar, Mallick, and Bahadur 2020, Daou et al. 2009, Zheng et al. 2015)
	Diagnosis and theranostic purposes	• Used for theranostic purposes for simultaneous sensing, imaging (diagnosis), tracking drug delivery, and for therapy. • Biological optical (photophysical) properties allow long-term tracking of cells in intact and diseased tissue, which is useful for cancer diagnosis. • *In vitro* diagnosis for serum biomarkers or detection of diseases like brucellosis and cancer.	(Michalet et al. 2005, Yao et al. 2018, Derfus, Chan, and Bhatia 2004, Ballou et al. 2004, Wang et al. 2015, Cai et al. 2016, Farias et al. 2017, Li, Rong, et al. 2020, Olerile et al. 2017, Lv et al. 2017)

(*Continued*)

TABLE 2.2 (Continued)   Nanomedicine Applications of Organic and Inorganic Nanosystems

NANOSYSTEMS	APPLICATIONS IN NANOMEDICINE	MAIN OUTCOMES	REFERENCES
	Tissue engineering and regenerative medicine	• Used for labelling, tracking purposes, and delivery of different types of stem cells where cell self-renewal, differentiation, and integration can potentially be monitored for diverse tissue regeneration such as bone, teeth, skin.	(Hsieh et al. 2006, Shah and Mao 2011, Li et al. 2016, Saulite et al. 2017, Dapkute et al. 2017, Tao et al. 2017, Kundrotas et al. 2019, Jahed et al. 2020, Rafieerad et al. 2019)
Gold nanoparticles	**Therapeutic delivery**	• Used in cancer therapy, neurodegenerative diseases, diabetes mellitus, collagen arthritis, heart failure. • Can deliver multiple drugs, nucleotides and nucleic acids, proteins, antigens (in vaccines) by passive targeting (EPR effect) or into their targets by active strategies and can control drug release via stimuli internal or external activation. • Used in cancer PDT.	(Barathmani-kanth et al. 2010, Bonoiu et al. 2009, Brown et al. 2010, Chen et al. 2007, Deyev et al. 2017, Gholipour-malekabadi et al. 2017, Huang, Ling, and Zhang 2007, Kim et al. 2012, Leonavičienė et al. 2012, Liao et al. 2012, Obaid et al. 2015, Rosi et al. 2006, Saha et al. 2007, Schäffler et al. 2014, Shiang et al. 2013, Spivak et al. 2013, Sreejivungsa et al. 2016)
	Diagnosis and theranostic purposes	• Used as cancer biomarker trackers, or as molecular nanoprobes for diagnostic applications in tissue imaging. • Used for SERS as intracellular probes to monitor intracellular drug release as well as to target drugs to cellular compartments (e.g., endosomes, mitochondria, nucleus), combining specific tumor targeting and SERS-based detection in living cells.	(Dixit et al. 2015, Guo et al. 2016, Huefner et al. 2014, Indrasekara et al. 2013, Kong et al. 2011, Park et al. 2015, Xie et al. 2009, Zhang, Li, et al. 2015)

(Continued)

TABLE 2.2 (Continued) Nanomedicine Applications of Organic and Inorganic Nanosystems

NANOSYSTEMS	APPLICATIONS IN NANOMEDICINE	MAIN OUTCOMES	REFERENCES
		• Can form conjugates with molecular probes for computed tomography imaging applied to cancer diagnosis and to dual mode or multimode imaging. • Used for theranostic purposes by combining their optical properties with drug delivery.	
	Tissue engineering and regenerative medicine	• Used as nano-platforms to deliver siRNA for tissue regeneration therapy. • Can be used to enhance stem cell differentiation for bone tissue engineering. • Can be incorporated into scaffolds to improve biomaterials properties and to promote cell proliferation and differentiation (e.g., in wound healing, hernia repair, and cardiac tissue regeneration).	(Cozad, Bachman, and Grant 2011, Fleischer et al. 2014, Goreham et al. 2013, Heo et al. 2014, Patel et al. 2014, Ravichandran et al. 2014, Whelove et al. 2011, Yi et al. 2010)
Mesoporous silica nanoparticles (MSNs)	**Therapeutic delivery**	• Nucleic acids (e.g., plasmid DNA, siRNA) and peptides have been successfully delivered using MSNs. • Efficient delivery of anticancer drugs, alone or alongside siRNA, as well as small molecules (e.g., nitric oxide (NO) and carbon monoxide (CO)) which can be used in combined cancer therapy. • Coating the surface of MSNs with therapeutic agents (e.g., antimicrobial lysosome enzymes) is used as an alternative delivery mechanism. • Can be functionalized with photosensitizer and used in PDT. • Can be functionalized with ligands for targeting diseases (e.g., brain-based diseases, such as Alzheimer's disease). • Can use triggering strategies to release drugs carried in response to various stimuli, such as pH, enzymes, redox reactions. • MSNs can be used as potent adsorbers for antidote indication	(Ahir et al. 2020, Alvarez-Berríos and Vivero-Escoto 2016, Bharti et al. 2015, Chakraborty and Mascharak 2016, Farjadian et al. 2017, Ferreira et al. 2018, Gao et al. 2009, Geng et al. 2012, Goel et al. 2016, Gong et al. 2015, Kamkaew et al. 2016, Kwon et al. 2017, Li and Wang 2013, Martínez-Carmona et al. 2018, Möller et al. 2016, Montoya Mira et al. 2020, Wang, Liu, and Wu 2017c, Zhou et al. 2016)

(Continued)

TABLE 2.2 (Continued)   Nanomedicine Applications of Organic and Inorganic Nanosystems

NANOSYSTEMS	APPLICATIONS IN NANOMEDICINE	MAIN OUTCOMES	REFERENCES
	Diagnosis and theranostic purposes	• Used for theranostic purposes by combining loaded imaging agents with drug delivery. • Different bioimaging techniques can use MSNs: (i) tomography and MRI in which MSNs protect the radionucleotides during systemic circulation, which increases the quantity of contrast agents delivered to the target tissues; (ii) ultrasound imaging, in which the delivery of hollow MSNs to the target tissues adds "bubbles" to improve HIFU imaging resolution; (iii) time-gated fluorescence imaging, in which MSNs improve the signal to background contrast ratio.	(Cha and Kim 2019, Chu, Cheng, and Chen 2019, Ellison et al. 2017, Gu et al. 2013, Jeong et al. 2019, Liu et al. 2011, Lu, Zhao, and Zhang 2019, Luo et al. 2015, Wang et al. 2012)
	Tissue engineering and regenerative medicine	• Use of scaffolding system containing MSNs for effective delivery of bioactive factors or drugs to the target site for regulating cellular responses and accelerating the repair process, such as growth factors, dexamethasone, and siRNA. • MSNs possess inherent bioactivities in tissue engineering, namely the osteogenic capacity of MSNs, osteogenic differentiation and ectopic ossification of Ca/Mg-doped mesoporous silica scaffolds; metal ion-doped MSNs could act as a promising immunomodulatory agent for inducing osteogenesis. • MSNs with imaging capacity can be used for stem cell labelling. • Ability of MSNs to alter properties of scaffold. • Application of MSNs in bone tissue engineering and other fields, such as vascular tissue engineering and wound healing.	(Chen, Ma, et al. 2017, Chen and Zhou 2019, Cui et al. 2018, Dai et al. 2011, Guo et al. 2019, Kempen et al. 2015, Kim et al. 2014, Nie et al. 2018, Pinese et al. 2018, Qiu et al. 2016, Ren et al. 2018, Rosenbrand et al. 2018, Shi et al. 2016, Shi et al. 2017, Shi et al. 2015, Wang et al. 2019, Wang, Chen, et al. 2017, Wu et al. 2017, Wu et al. 2018, Zhou et al. 2018)

Abbreviations: APO – apocynin; BBB – blood–brain barrier; BCS – biopharmaceutical classification system; bFGF – basic fibroblast growth factor; BMP-2 – bone morphogenetic protein-2; BMP-7 – bone morphogenetic protein-7; CEM – cholecystic-derived extracellular matrix; CMC – critical micelle concentration; CO – carbon monoxide; DNA – desoxyribonucleic acid; DDNs – drug delivery nanosystems; EGF – epidermal growth factor; EPR – enhanced permeability and retention; FDA – Food and Drug Administration; G1-PAMAM – generation-1 polyamidoamine; HIFU – high intensity focused ultrasound; LHRH – luteinizing hormone-releasing hormone; LRP1 – low-density lipoprotein receptor related protein 1; MFH – magnetic fluid hyperthermia; MSNs – mesoporous silica nanoparticles; MRI – magnetic resonance imaging; NLCs – nanostructured lipid carriers; NO – nitric oxide; PAMAM – polyamidoamine; PDGF-BB – platelet-derived growth factor-BB; PDT – photodynamic therapy; PEG – polyethylene glycol; PEG-PE – polyethylene glycol-phosphatidyl ethanolamine conjugate; RES – reticuloendothelial system; ROS – reactive oxygen species; siRNA – small interfering ribonucleic acid; SDF-1α – stromal cell-derived factor-1α; SERS – surface-enhanced Raman spectroscopy; SLNs – solid lipid nanoparticles; TGF-β – transforming growth factor β; VEGF – vascular endothelial growth factor.

organic and inorganic nanosystems and their applications in nanomedicine, either in therapeutic applications as DDNs or as nanosystems applied in diagnostics and tissue engineering.

2.4 PAVING THE WAY TOWARDS NANOMEDICINE DEVELOPMENT BASED ON REGULATORY STANDARDS

Despite the unique set of opportunities offered by nanomedicine, its deployment has yet to be fully realized. Whilst nanoscale formulation has remarkable advantages for effective drug delivery , many safety concerns remain unaddressed. In the battle to translate nanotechnologies from the bench to the clinic, scientists have been struggling to decode fundamental aspects of engineered nanomaterial interactions with biological systems. General issues arise early at several levels of the development of nanomedicine products. These include physicochemical characterization, biocompatibility and nanotoxicology evaluation, pharmacokinetics and pharmacodynamics assessment, process control, and scale up-reproducibility (Soares et al. 2018a).

From a physicochemical perspective, the characterization of a nanomedicine is necessary to understand the respective behavior in the human body (e.g., how can particle size and shape be tailored for improved hemodynamics or how to modulate the innate immunity to reduce nanoparticle clearance), and to provide guidance for the process control and safety assessment. This characterization is not uniform in the number of parameters required for a correct and complete characterization. Internationally standardized methodologies and the use of reference nanomaterials are seen as the key to harmonize all the different opinions about this topic (Lin et al. 2014, Bursten 2016). Ideally, the characterization of a nanomaterial should be carried out at different stages throughout its life cycle, from the design to the evaluation of its *in vitro* and *in vivo* performance. It is worth noting that the interaction with the biological system or even the sample preparation or extraction procedures may modify some properties and interfere with some measurements. In addition, the determination of the *in vivo* and *in vitro* physicochemical properties is important for the understanding of the potential risk of nanomaterials, as well as to anticipate their *in vivo* distribution (Lin et al. 2014, Bursten 2016).

Another challenge in pharmaceutical development is the control of the manufacturing process by the identification of the critical parameters and technologies required to analyze them (Sainz et al. 2015, Gaspar 2010, Gaspar et al. 2014). The manufacturing process may impair many physicochemical characteristics of nanomaterials, therefore compromising the quality and safety of the final nanomedicine.

Pre-clinical assessment of nanomaterials involves a thorough biocompatibility testing program, which typically comprises *in vivo* studies complemented by selected *in vitro* assays to prove safety. If the biocompatibility of nanomaterials cannot be warranted, potentially advantageous properties of nanosystems may raise toxicological concerns.

Several initiatives, including scientific opinions, guidelines, and specific European regulations and Organization for Economic Co-operation and Development (OECD) guidelines, such as those for cosmetics, food-contact materials, and medical devices, and FDA regulations, as well as European Commission scientific projects specifically address nanomaterials safety (Juillerat-Jeanneret et al. 2015). In this context, it is important to identify the properties, to understand the mechanisms by which nanomaterials interact with living systems, and thus to comprehend exposure, hazards, and their possible risks.

The lack of clarity over regulation for clinical use is also greatly hindering their translation. This is partly ascribed to the complexity of addressing the diversity of innovative and existing nanomedicines. For that reason, it is critical to solve the scientific and regulatory gaps in order to guarantee that nanomedicine drives the next generation of biomedical innovation (Tinkle et al. 2014, Soares et al. 2018a).

Many boxes still need to be ticked to accelerate the process of nanomedicine development and approval from the regulatory authorities.

What is the right regulatory pathway for the approval of drug products containing nanomedicines? How can the pharmaceutical development of nanomedicines be designed in a more efficient way? How to determine Critical Quality Attributes (CQAs) for nanomedicines?

Some of these questions were already debated in international forums, such as the AAPS Guidance Forum on September 11, 2018, that brought together participants from industry, academia, and regulatory bodies to discuss assumptions to guide the developement of innovative and generic drug products that contain nanomaterials; this forum yielded the recently issued FDA draft guideline "Drug Products, Including Biological Products, That Contain Nanomaterials" (de Vlieger et al. 2019).

Methodological approaches that can be used in deciding how to define, structure, and implement quality, safety, and efficacy through design have been pointed out, rerouting the nanomedicine development. Also, from discovery and development and through the entire product lifecycle, artificial intelligence (AI) is starting to shake up the nanopharmaceutical companies.

2.4.1 QbD, SbD, and EbD Approaches: An Outlook

Quality by design (QbD) is one of the pharmaceutical development approaches that is recognized for the systematic evaluation and control of nanomedicines (Gaspar 2009, Rogério et al. 2014, Sainz, Conniot, Matos, Peres, Zupanöiö et al. 2015). The implementation of the quality by design approach is to be set forth using International Council for Harmonization of Technical Requirements for Pharmaceuticals for Human Use (ICH) Q8 elements, supported on computational frameworks for the establishment of factorial planning methodologies and process analytical technologies (PAT) (ICHQ8 2017). Briefly, it includes the definition of the quality target product profile (QTPP) and critical quality attributes (CQAs) of the drug product, the accomplishment of risk assessment (ICH Q9 2017) to identify critical material attributes (CMAs) and critical process parameters (CPPs), the definition of a design space through design of experiments (DoEs), the establishment of a control strategy (PAT, among others), and continual improvement and innovation throughout the product life cycle (ICH Q10, Q12); see Figure 2.2 (ICHQ9 2015, ICHQ12 2020, ICHQ10 2017).

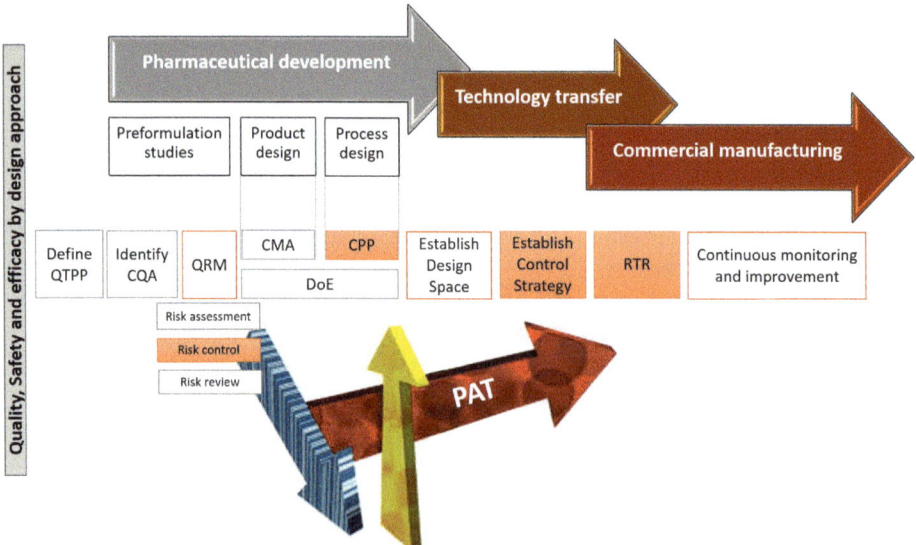

FIGURE 2.2   Qbd, SbD, EbD planning roadmap to the pharmaceutical development of nanomedicines. Key: QTTP, quality target product profile; CQA, critical quality attributes; QRM, quality risk management; CMA, critical material attributes; CPP, critical process parameters; DoE, design of experiments; RTR, real time release.

The deployment of QbD defends the idea that the quality should not be tested in nanomedicine, but built on it (by design) instead, by the understanding of the therapeutic purpose, pharmacological, pharmacokinetic, toxicological, chemical, and physical properties of the medicine, process formulation, packaging, and the design of the manufacturing process. This approach allows better focus on the relevant relationships between the characteristics, parameters of the formulation, and process, in order to develop effective processes to ensure the quality of the nanomedicines (FDA 2004). Likewise, it postulates that development must be oriented by considering the patient's point of view and intended clinical performance. This opens room for an integrated intervention with other domains, namely in safety and efficacy.

The increasing application of nanomaterials and the notion that their distinct features compared to larger sized counterparts should be considered in safety assessment have led to the development of risk assessment frameworks that are specific to nanomaterials, underlying the concept of safety by design (SbD). These frameworks aim to prioritize, rank, or assess the safety of a nanomaterial efficiently by targeting critical information in order to conserve resources. In particular, some issues such as exposure (stable dispersions, relevance of high-dose studies, and assessment of internalized dose), bioaccumulation, *in vitro-in vivo* comparison, and long-term effects deserve special attention (Oomen et al. 2018).

To this end, activities to standardize and develop protocols and guidance documents, including several functional assays, as well as suitable controls and reference materials have been actively pursued (Oomen et al. 2018). Benchmark frameworks already reported (e.g., NANoREG (NANoREG 2017, Gaspar 2010), DF4nanoGrouping (Landsiedel et al. 2017)), have combined information retrieved from non-testing tools such as prediction tools (e.g., qualitative or quantitative structure-activity relationship), and testing tools such as *in vitro* models (e.g., cytotoxicity, reactive oxygen species (ROS), and cytokines, among others) and *in vivo* assays (Arts et al. 2015). For that, several physicochemical properties need to be previously assigned for the risk assessment, including composition, shape, particle size (distribution), surface charge, surface coating, hydrophobicity, solubility/dissolution, and reactivity, among others (Lynch, Weiss, and Valsami-Jones 2014). European Union (EU)-funded projects, such as REFINE (REFINE 2019), BIORIMA (Giubilato et al. 2020), and PROSAFE (Steinhäuser and Sayre 2017), have been also recently kicked off, pertaining to the development and validation of methods that support the regulatory review of nanomedicines, as well as to develop an overarching nanobiomaterial risk management framework.

Considering now efficacy, it demands taking into account the potential targets or sites of action and designing the appropriate drug delivery strategies to provide the desired therapeutic outcome, i.e., a fit-for-purpose, or efficacy-by-design (EbD) approach. From a technological perspective, it means that, by making use of the right excipients, delivery nanocarriers, or functionalization strategies, formulators may control when, where, and how an active pharmaceutical ingredient (API) is released from the nanomedicine. Particular attention should be also given to the interaction in the biological environment (by interrogating, e.g., what is the impact of the biomolecule adsorption layer, known as "corona", that forms on the surface of colloidal nanoparticles, on their distribution, or if the nanocarrier can escape the immune system, given that its activation might potentially lead to severe side-effects), since it can alter the properties of the nanomedicine, ultimately compromising the therapeutic efficacy.

The endorsement of QbD, coupled to SbD and EbD approaches, will bring several advantages: (i) deep knowledge and understanding of the process, (ii) efficient scale-up, (iii) reduced product end-testing, (iv) enhanced control of variables and product quality, (v) the possibility of preventive actions, (vi) increased manufacturing efficiency, (vii) regulatory flexibility, and (viii) continual improvement (Henriques et al. 2019).

Such integrated approaches will dictate a structured product development, further reflected in the organization of the marketing authorization applications that will facilitate communication with the authorities (Figure 2.3).

2.4.2 The Role of Artificial Intelligence in Nanomedicine

Aligned with QbD (SbD and EbD) assumptions, AI methods may be integrated throughout nanomedicine development essentially to boost profit in nanotherapeutics or gain insights into nanotoxicology.

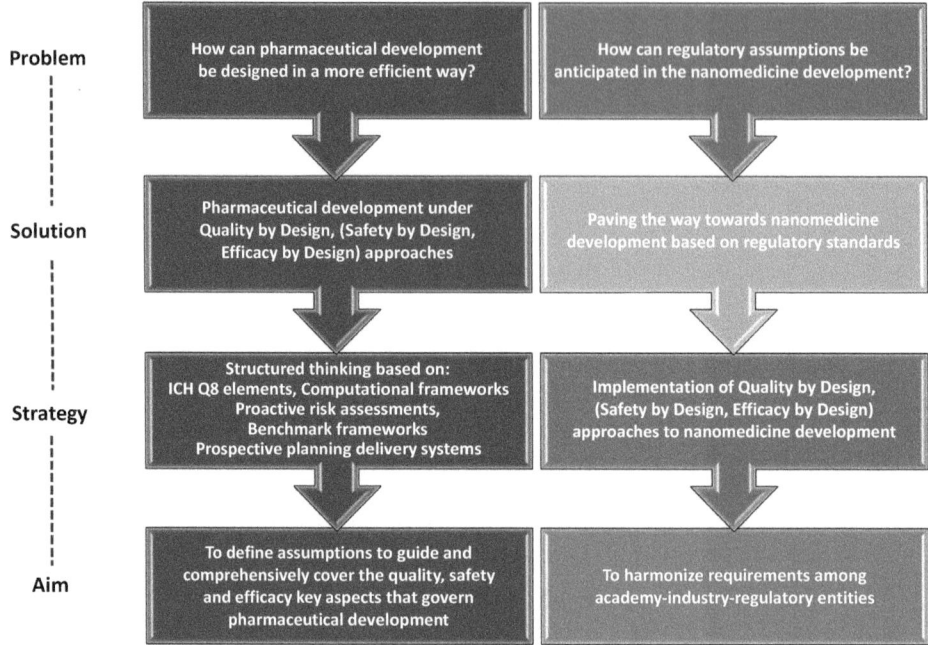

FIGURE 2.3   Application of QbD (SbD and EbD) to nanomedicine development.

Specifically, data mining and machine learning can be used to develop methods to predict both functional and structural properties of nanoparticles, and subsequently to refine medical treatments. Recent studies have reported several methods attempting to predict several nanoparticle properties, such as nanoparticle size, and polydispersity, molecular loading, molecular release, nanoparticle adherence, cellular uptake, and cytotoxicity (Dimitri and Talamo 2018). Among other applications, AI-driven platforms could assist in (i) drug discovery/development, by optimizing drug and dose parameters in combinatorial nanomedicine administration (Ho, Wang, and Kee 2019, Khong et al. 2020), or (ii) the optimization of formulation design in terms of drug delivery, or in designing safer nanoparticles by predicting bio-nanointeractions in the context of reactivity and nanotoxicity (Singh et al. 2020). The retrieved outcomes will clearly facilitate the translation of nanomedicines towards a broader clinical impact.

2.5 FROM THE BENCH TO THE MARKET

Currently, a significant number of DDNs with a variety of therapeutic activities are in different phases of clinical trials, whereas some are already approved by the FDA and/or the EMA (Table 2.3).

From a general point of view, lipid-based DDNs are best accepted by pharmaceutical companies, as their lipid components are generally recognized as safe (GRAS). In addition, lipid-based DDNs are biodegradable and are thus deemed not to accumulate in the body and are considered risk-free (Qi et al. 2017). Polymeric-based DDNs, particularly polymer-therapeutic conjugates, are also highly expressive given the number of clinical approved nano-based pharmaceutical products. Although in academic research, there is intensive research on active targeting and triggering strategies of DDNs, in the market these strategies are scarce, and the approved products are naked DDNs given the complexity of scaling up the functionalization processes.

TABLE 2.3 List of Clinical Approved Nano-Based Pharmaceutical Products According to the Therapeutic Indication or Diagnosis Purposes

PRODUCT DESIGNATION (MANUFACTURER)	GENERIC NAME (API)	TYPE OF NANOCARRIERS (COMPOSITION)	THERAPEUTIC INDICATION(S)	FUNCTION OF THE NANOCARRIER	ROUTE OF ADMINISTRATION	REGULATORY AUTHORITY APPROVAL (DATE)
CANCERS AND CONTROL OF ADVERSE EFFECTS CAUSED BY CANCER TREATMENT						
SMANCS® (Astellas Pharma, Inc.)	Zinostation Stimalaner (neocarzinosta-tin)	**Polymer therapeutic conjugate** (Poly(styrene-maleic acid) copolymer-neocarzinostatin)	• Hepatocellular carcinoma	• Accumulates in tumor tissue – passive targeting – due to enhanced permeability and retention (EPR) effect.	• IV administration.	• Japan (1993)
Oncaspar® (USA – Enzon Pharmaceuticals Inc.) (Europe – Les laboratoires Servier)	Pegaspargase (L-asparagi-nase)	**Polymer therapeutic conjugate** (PEG–L-asparaginase)	• Acute lymphoblastic leukemia and chronic myelogenous leukemia	• Improve protein stability and prolong plasma half-life: 357 hours compared to 20 hours for the unmodified enzyme (higher half-life of the API due to PEGylation). • Reduce the dosing frequency from 2–3 times/week to a single biweekly dose. • Reduce protein immunogenicity.	• IM injection. • IV injection.	• FDA (1994) • EMA (2016)
Neulasta® (Amgen, Inc.)	Filgrastim (r-metHuG-CSF)	**Polymer therapeutic conjugate** (PEG-r-metHuG-CSF protein conjugate)	• Chemotherapy induced neutro-penia	• Improve protein stability, prolong plasma half-life from 3.5–3.8 hours up to 42 hours. • Equivalent efficacy as a single administration/ chemotherapy cycle, rather than the multiple daily injections of unconjugated r-metHuG-CSF.	• Subcutaneous (SC) injection.	• FDA (2002) • EMA (2002)

(Continued)

TABLE 2.3 (Continued)   List of Clinical Approved Nano-Based Pharmaceutical Products According to the Therapeutic Indication or Diagnosis Purposes

CANCERS AND CONTROL OF ADVERSE EFFECTS CAUSED BY CANCER TREATMENT

PRODUCT DESIGNATION (MANUFACTURER)	GENERIC NAME (API)	TYPE OF NANOCARRIERS (COMPOSITION)	THERAPEUTIC INDICATION(S)	FUNCTION OF THE NANOCARRIER	ROUTE OF ADMINISTRATION	REGULATORY AUTHORITY APPROVAL (DATE)
				• Prevent the high clearance via internalization of the receptor ligand complex in neutrophil cells. • Decrease rate of aggregation under physiological conditions and no detectable insoluble precipitation with loss of activity in relation to native molecule.		
Eligard® (Tolmar, Inc.)	Leuprolide acetate	**Polymeric nanoparticles** (poly(lactic acid-co-glycolic acid (PLGA))	• Prostate cancer	• Longer circulation time. • Slowly releases the drug over 1 month due to biodegradation.	• Subcutaneous (SC) injection.	• FDA (2002)
Abraxane® (Celgene Pharmaceutical Co. Ltd)	Paclitaxel (ABI-007)	**Protein nanoparticles** (albumin)	• Metastatic breast cancer • Non-small cell lung cancer • Metastatic pancreatic cancer	• Increase site-specific delivery (tumor) and solubility. • Maintain the therapeutic benefits of paclitaxel while removing the toxicity of Cremophor (e.g., Taxol).	• IV administration.	• FDA (2005 – Metastatic breast cancer) • FDA (2012 – Non-small cell lung cancer) • FDA (2013 – Metastatic Pancreatic cancer) • EMA (2008)

(Continued)

TABLE 2.3 (Continued) List of Clinical Approved Nano-Based Pharmaceutical Products According to the Therapeutic Indication or Diagnosis Purposes

CANCERS AND CONTROL OF ADVERSE EFFECTS CAUSED BY CANCER TREATMENT

PRODUCT DESIGNATION (MANUFACTURER)	GENERIC NAME (API)	TYPE OF NANOCARRIERS (COMPOSITION)	THERAPEUTIC INDICATION(S)	FUNCTION OF THE NANOCARRIER	ROUTE OF ADMINISTRATION	REGULATORY AUTHORITY APPROVAL (DATE)
Genoxol® (Samyang Biopharmaceuticals)	Paclitaxel	**Polymeric micelles** mPEG-PDLLA	• Non-small cell lung cancer • Breast and ovarian cancers	• Improve solubility. • Reduce toxicity. • Improve efficacy. • Reduce hypersensitivity.	• IV injection.	• South Korea (2007)
Doxil® in the USA Caelyx® outside the USA (Janssen)	Doxorubicin	**PEGylated liposome** (HSPC:cholesterol: DSPE-PEG(2000) (56:39:5))	• Ovarian cancer • Multiple myeloma • HIV Kaposi's sarcoma	• Longer circulation time. • Improve delivery to tumor site. • Lower systemic toxicity and thus fewer toxic side-effects.	• IV administration.	• FDA (1995 – HIV Kaposi's sarcoma • FDA (2005 – Ovarian cancer) • FDA (2008 – Myeloma)
Mepact® (Takeda)	Mifamurtide	**Liposome** (POPC:DOPS)	• Non-metastatic resectable osteo-sarcoma	• Improve delivery to tumor site. • Lower systemic toxicity and thus fewer toxic side-effects.	• IV administration.	• EMA (2000)
Myocet® (Elan Pharmaceuticals)	Doxorubicin	**Liposome** (EPC:cholesterol (55:45))	• Metastatic breast cancer • Used in combination with Cyclophospha-mide	• Significantly improved therapeutic index compared with free doxorubicin. • Less cardiotoxic and better tolerated than free doxorubicin.	• IV administration.	• EMA (2000) • Canada (2001)
Marqibo® (Talon therapeutics)	Vincristine sulfate	**Liposome** (Sphingomyelin:cholesterol (60:40))	• Acute lymphoid leukemia	• Higher drug delivery to tumor. • Superior antitumor activity. • Higher maximum tolerated dose, lower systemic toxicity, and fewer toxic side-effects.	• IV administration.	• FDA (2012)

(Continued)

TABLE 2.3 (Continued)   List of Clinical Approved Nano-Based Pharmaceutical Products According to the Therapeutic Indication or Diagnosis Purposes

			CANCERS AND CONTROL OF ADVERSE EFFECTS CAUSED BY CANCER TREATMENT			
PRODUCT DESIGNATION (MANUFACTURER)	GENERIC NAME (API)	TYPE OF NANOCARRIERS (COMPOSITION)	THERAPEUTIC INDICATION(S)	FUNCTION OF THE NANOCARRIER	ROUTE OF ADMINISTRATION	REGULATORY AUTHORITY APPROVAL (DATE)
Lipo-Dox® (generic of Doxil®/ Caelyx®) (Sun Pharmaceutical Industries Ltd. (SPIL))	Doxorubicin	**PEGylated liposome** (HSPC:cholesterol:PEG 2000-DSPE (56:39:5))	• Ovarian cancer • Breast cancer • HIV Kaposi's sarcoma	• Longer circulation time. • Improve delivery to tumor site. • Lower systemic toxicity and thus fewer toxic side-effects.	• IV administration.	• FDA (2013)
Onivyde® (Merrimack Pharmaceuticals)	Irinotecan	**PEGylated liposome** (DSPC:cholesterol: DSPE-PEG(2000) (3:2:0.015)) (folic acid as active targeting ligand)	• Post gemcitabine metastatic pancreatic cancer • Use in combination with Fluouracile	• Longer circulation time. • Improve delivery to tumor site by enhanced permeability and retention (EPR) and active targeting. • Lower systemic toxicity and thus fewer toxic side-effects.	• IV administration.	• FDA (2015) • EMA (2016)
Vyxeos® (Jazz Pharma)	Daunorubicin + Cytarabin	**Liposome** (DSPC:DSPG:cholesterol (7:2:1)) (Daunorubicin:Cytarabin (5:1)	• Newly diagnosed therapy-related acute myeloid leukemia (AML) and AML with myelodysplasia-related change	• Improve delivery to tumor site. • Lower systemic toxicity and thus fewer toxic side-effects. • Controlled release of the drugs. • Synergic anticancer effect of co-loaded anticancer drugs.	• IV administration.	• FDA (2017) • EMA (2018)
NanoTherm® therapy (MagForce)	Superparamagnetic iron oxide nanoparticles	**Magnetic nanoparticles** Aminosilane-coated superparamagnetic iron oxide nanoparticles	• Glioblastoma • Prostate cancer • Pancreatic cancer	• Thermotherapy for destroy tumor cells or sensitized tumor cells or sensitized for additional therapies.	• Intratumorally administration.	• EMA (2013)

(Continued)

TABLE 2.3 (Continued)   List of Clinical Approved Nano-Based Pharmaceutical Products According to the Therapeutic Indication or Diagnosis Purposes

CANCERS AND CONTROL OF ADVERSE EFFECTS CAUSED BY CANCER TREATMENT

PRODUCT DESIGNATION (MANUFACTURER)	GENERIC NAME (API)	TYPE OF NANOCARRIERS (COMPOSITION)	THERAPEUTIC INDICATION(S)	FUNCTION OF THE NANOCARRIER	ROUTE OF ADMINISTRATION	REGULATORY AUTHORITY APPROVAL (DATE)
Infectious, Immunological Diseases						
Adagen® (Enzon Pharmaceuticals, Inc.)	Pegademase bovine (adenosine deaminase derive from bovine intestine)	**Polymer therapeutic conjugate** (Monomethoxy PEG-bovine adenosine deaminase enzyme conjugate)	• Severe immune-deficiency caused by an inherited deficiency of the adenosine deaminase enzyme	• Favorable pharmacokinetics and pharmacodynamics support once-weekly administration. • Less plasma clearance, increase of circulation time, and reduced immunogenicity compared to nonconjugated therapeutic agent.	• IM injection.	• FDA (1990)
Copaxone® (Teva)	Glatopa (glatiramer acetate – an immunomodulator)	**Polymer therapeutic conjugate** Random copolymer of l-glutamate, l-alanine, l-lysine and l-tyrosine	• Multiple sclerosis	• Large amino acid-based polymer with controlled molecular weight and clearance characteristics.	• SC injection.	• FDA (1996)
PegIntron® (Merck Sharp & Dohme Corp.)	Peginterferon α-2b (interferon α-2b)	**Polymer therapeutic conjugate** PEG- interferon α-2b conjugate	• Chronic hepatitis C	• Increase protein stability. • Longer serum half-life. • Lower elimination. • Greater efficacy via 1 dose/week compared to 3 dose/week of free interferon α-2b.	• SC injection.	• EMA (2000) • FDA (2001)

(Continued)

TABLE 2.3 (Continued)   List of Clinical Approved Nano-Based Pharmaceutical Products According to the Therapeutic Indication or Diagnosis Purposes

CANCERS AND CONTROL OF ADVERSE EFFECTS CAUSED BY CANCER TREATMENT

PRODUCT DESIGNATION (MANUFACTURER)	GENERIC NAME (API)	TYPE OF NANOCARRIERS (COMPOSITION)	THERAPEUTIC INDICATION(S)	FUNCTION OF THE NANOCARRIER	ROUTE OF ADMINISTRATION	REGULATORY AUTHORITY APPROVAL (DATE)
Pegasys® (Hoffmann-La Roche Inc. and currently Genentech USA, Inc.,)	Peginterferon α-2a (interferon α-2a)	**Polymer therapeutic conjugate** PEG- interferon α-2a conjugate	• Chronic hepatitis C • HBeAg positive • Chronic hepatitis B	• Higher protein stability • Enhanced protein serum half-life • Greater efficacy by 1 dose/week compared to 3 dose/week of free interferon α-2a, without losing tolerability.	• SC injection.	• FDA (2002) • EMA (2002)
Plegridy® (Biogen Idec Inc.)	Peginterferon β-1a (recombinant interferon β-1a)	**Polymer therapeutic conjugate** Methoxi PEG- interferon β–1a conjugate	• Relapsing forms of multiple sclerosis	• Increase protein stability and circulation time. • Less frequent dosing and reduce the relapse rate.	• SC injection.	• FDA (2014) • EMA (2014)
Infectious, Immunological Diseases						
Cimzia® (UCB Pharma)	Certolizumab pegol (Fab' fragment of humanized anti-tumor necrosis factor (TNF)-α antibody)	**Polymer therapeutic conjugate** PEG- anti-TNF-α Fab'antibody conjugate	• Crohn's disease • Rheumatoid arthritis • Psoriatic arthritis • Ankylosing spondylitis	• Greater stability in vivo. • Longer circulation time, half-life of 14 days, and administration as a single biweekly dose. • Reduce immunogenicity.	• SC injection.	• FDA (2008 – Crohn's disease) • EMA (2009 – rheumatoid arthritis, discontinued for Crohn's disease) • FDA (2013 – psoriatic arthritis) • EMA (2018 – psoriasis) • EMA (2020 –spondyloar-thritis) *(Continued)*

TABLE 2.3 (Continued)   List of Clinical Approved Nano-Based Pharmaceutical Products According to the Therapeutic Indication or Diagnosis Purposes

PRODUCT DESIGNATION (MANUFACTURER)	GENERIC NAME (API)	TYPE OF NANOCARRIERS (COMPOSITION)	THERAPEUTIC INDICATION(S)	FUNCTION OF THE NANOCARRIER	ROUTE OF ADMINISTRATION	REGULATORY AUTHORITY APPROVAL (DATE)
CANCERS AND CONTROL OF ADVERSE EFFECTS CAUSED BY CANCER TREATMENT						
VivaGel BV® (Starpharma) Different brand names: Betafem® BV Gel (UK), Betadine BVTM (Europe), BetadineTM BV Gel (Asia) and Fleurstat BVgel (Australia, New Zealand)	SPL7013 – macromolecular dendrimer itself is the API	**Dendrimer** Water-based vaginal gel containing the poly(l-lysine) dendrimer	• Treatment and symptomatic relief of bacterial vaginosis	• A non-antibiotic therapy that is not absorbed into the bloodstream.	• Intravaginal application.	Approved for marketing in Europe
Abelcet® (Sigma-tau Pharma)	Amphothericin B	**Liposome** (DMPC: DMPG (7:3))	• Invasive fungal infection	• Lower systemic toxicity and thus fewer toxic side-effects.	• IV administration.	• FDA (1995)
AmBisome® (Gilead Sciences)	Amphothericin B	**Liposome** (HSPC: DSPG:cholesterol: amphotericin B (2:0.8:1:0.4))	• Fungal infection • Protozoal infection (e.g., visceral leishmaniosis)	• Reduced nephrotoxicity. • Better pharmacokinetic properties and stability in circulation.	• IV administration.	• FDA (1997)
Vaccines						
Inflexal V® (Crucell)	Inactivated hemagglutinin of Influenza virus A, B	**Liposome** (DOPC: DSPE (75:25))	• Vaccine against influenza	• Influenza virus antigens are functionalized on the surface of the liposomes.	• IM administration.	• FDA (1997)

(Continued)

TABLE 2.3 (Continued)   List of Clinical Approved Nano-Based Pharmaceutical Products According to the Therapeutic Indication or Diagnosis Purposes

CANCERS AND CONTROL OF ADVERSE EFFECTS CAUSED BY CANCER TREATMENT

PRODUCT DESIGNATION (MANUFACTURER)	GENERIC NAME (API)	TYPE OF NANOCARRIERS (COMPOSITION)	THERAPEUTIC INDICATION(S)	FUNCTION OF THE NANOCARRIER	ROUTE OF ADMINISTRATION	REGULATORY AUTHORITY APPROVAL (DATE)
Epaxal® (Crucell)	Inactivated hepatitis A virus	**Liposome** (PC: Cephalin (PE) (80:20)) These liposomes are called Virosomes	• Vaccine against hepatitis A	• Hepatitis virus antigens, fusion active influenza hemagglutinin, and the neuraminidase are functionalized on the surface of the liposomes.	• IM administration.	• FDA (1997)
BNT162b2 (BioNTech and Pfizer)	mRNA coding for SARS-CoV-2 antigen	**Liposome** (ALC-0315, ALC-0159, DSPC, and cholesterol)	• Vaccine against COVID-19	• Lipoplexes formed by condensation of liposomes and mRNA encoding for SARS-CoV-2 antigen. Once inside the cell mRNA is released and temporarily induces the cell to produce the viral protein coded. • The protein is recognized by immune cells (T-cell and B-cell) as a foreign antigen. This elicits responses to generate neutralizing antibodies against COVID-19.	• IM administration.	• FDA (2020) • EMA (2020)

(Continued)

TABLE 2.3 (Continued)   List of Clinical Approved Nano-Based Pharmaceutical Products According to the Therapeutic Indication or Diagnosis Purposes

PRODUCT DESIGNATION (MANUFACTURER)	GENERIC NAME (API)	TYPE OF NANOCARRIERS (COMPOSITION)	THERAPEUTIC INDICATION(S)	FUNCTION OF THE NANOCARRIER	ROUTE OF ADMINISTRATION	REGULATORY AUTHORITY APPROVAL (DATE)
CANCERS AND CONTROL OF ADVERSE EFFECTS CAUSED BY CANCER TREATMENT						
mRNA-1273 (Moderna and US government)	mRNA coding for SARS-CoV-2 spike (S) protein	**Liposome** (lipid SM-102, cholesterol, DSPC, DMG-PEG(2000))	• Vaccine against COVID-19	• Lipoplexes are formed by condensation of liposomes and mRNA encoding for SARS-CoV-2 spike (S) protein. Once inside the cell mRNA is released and temporarily induces the cell to produce the viral protein coded. • The protein is recognized by immune cells (T-cell and B-cell) as a foreign antigen. This elicits responses to generate neutralizing antibodies against COVID-19.	• IM administration.	• FDA (2020) • EMA (2020)
Chronic Kidney Disease and Associated Anemia						
Renagel® (sevelamer hydrochloride) Renvela® (sevelamer carbonate) (Genzyme Corporation)	Sevelamer hydrochloride or Sevelamer carbonate	**Polymeric nanoparticles** (cross-linked polyallylamine hydrochloride while the cross-linking agent is epichlorohydrin)	• Chronic kidney disease	• Increase circulation time. • Site-specific delivery.	• Oral administration.	• FDA (2000) • EMA (2000)

(Continued)

TABLE 2.3 (Continued)   List of Clinical Approved Nano-Based Pharmaceutical Products According to the Therapeutic Indication or Diagnosis Purposes

CANCERS AND CONTROL OF ADVERSE EFFECTS CAUSED BY CANCER TREATMENT

PRODUCT DESIGNATION (MANUFACTURER)	GENERIC NAME (API)	TYPE OF NANOCARRIERS (COMPOSITION)	THERAPEUTIC INDICATION(S)	FUNCTION OF THE NANOCARRIER	ROUTE OF ADMINISTRATION	REGULATORY AUTHORITY APPROVAL (DATE)
Mircera® (Hoffmann-La Roche)	Epoetin beta (genetically recombinant form of erythropoietin)	**Polymer therapeutic conjugate** Methoxy PEG-epoetin beta conjugate	• Renal anemia in patients with chronic kidney disease	• Increase aptamer stability, prolong plasma half-life of around 135 hours compared with other erythropoiesis-stimulating agents which have plasma half-lives of <25 hours. • Extend dosing intervals (0.6 μg/kg every 2 weeks).	• IV administration. • SC injection.	• FDA (2007) • EMA (2007) • Swissmedic (2007)
Feraheme® (AMAG Pharmaceuticals, Inc.) (FDA approval)	Ferumoxytol	**Magnetic nanoparticles** Ultrasmall SPION coated with poly-glucose sorbitol carboxymethylether	• Iron deficiency anemia (IDA) in adult patients with chronic kidney disease	• Prolonged steady release and decreased number of doses.	• IV injection.	FDA (2009) Note: EMA approved Rienso® product in 2012, but now is discontinued

(Continued)

TABLE 2.3 (Continued)   List of Clinical Approved Nano-Based Pharmaceutical Products According to the Therapeutic Indication or Diagnosis Purposes

CANCERS AND CONTROL OF ADVERSE EFFECTS CAUSED BY CANCER TREATMENT

PRODUCT DESIGNATION (MANUFACTURER)	GENERIC NAME (API)	TYPE OF NANOCARRIERS (COMPOSITION)	THERAPEUTIC INDICATION(S)	FUNCTION OF THE NANOCARRIER	ROUTE OF ADMINISTRATION	REGULATORY AUTHORITY APPROVAL (DATE)
Ocular Disease						
Visudyne® (CHEPLAPHARM Arzneimittel GmbH Europe) (Parkedale Pharmaceutics and Novartis, USA)	Verteporphine	**Liposome** (DMPC: EPG)	• Age-related macular degeneration • Myopia • Ocular histoplasmosis	• Higher delivery to diseased vessels. • Light triggered drug release. • Under the light the photosensitizer produces reactive oxygen species that destroy newly formed leaky blood vessels, thus preventing or restoring the loss of vision.	• IV administration followed by shining a red light into the eye.	• FDA (2002) • EMA (2000)
Ocular Disease						
Restasis® (Allergan)	Ciclosporin	**Nanoemulsion (o/w)** (oily phase: castor oil; aqueous phase: glycerine, carbopolymer, water; surfactant: polysorbate 80)	• Treatment of severe keratitis in adult patients with dry eye disease	• Enhanced encapsulation of the corticosteroid drug with no systemic absorption. • Is an anionic emulsion, thus compared with Ikervis® is less efficient in binding to the cornea.	• Topical administration (eye emulsion drops).	• FDA (2003)

(Continued)

TABLE 2.3 (Continued)   List of Clinical Approved Nano-Based Pharmaceutical Products According to the Therapeutic Indication or Diagnosis Purposes

PRODUCT DESIGNATION (MANUFACTURER)	GENERIC NAME (API)	TYPE OF NANOCARRIERS (COMPOSITION)	THERAPEUTIC INDICATION(S)	FUNCTION OF THE NANOCARRIER	ROUTE OF ADMINISTRATION	REGULATORY AUTHORITY APPROVAL (DATE)
CANCERS AND CONTROL OF ADVERSE EFFECTS CAUSED BY CANCER TREATMENT						
Macugen® (Eyetech Pharmaceuticals, Inc./ Pfizer Inc.)	Pegaptanib sodium (anti-VEGF) RNA aptamer with 28 nucleotides)	**Polymer therapeutic conjugate** PEG – anti-VEGF RNA aptamer conjugate	• Neovascular age-related macular degeneration	• Improve aptamer stability. • Prolong the time that anti-VEGF remain in the tissue and the plasma half-life. • Administration of the appropriate dosage every 6 weeks. • Slow diffusion out of the vitreous humor, maximizing efficacy and minimizing systemic exposure.	• Intravitreal injection.	• FDA (2004) • Brazil (2005) • Canada (2006) Note: EMA approved in 2005; however, this medicine is now withdrawn from use in the European Union
Durezol® (Sirion therapeutics)	Difluprednate	**Nanoemulsion (o/w)** (oily phase: castor oil; aqueous phase: glycerine, water; surfactant: polysorbate 80)	• Ocular surgery pain and inflammation • Endogenous anterior uveitis	• Enhanced encapsulation of the corticosteroid drug with no systemic absorption. • Requires less frequent dosing than prednisolone acetate.	• Topical administration (eye emulsion drops).	• FDA (2008)
Ikervis® (Santen SAS)	Ciclosporin	**Nanoemulsion (o/w)** (oily phase: middle chain triglycerides; aqueous phase: glycerine, water; surfactant: tyloxapol, poloxamer 188, Cetalkonium chloride)	• Treatment of severe keratitis in adult patients with dry eye disease	• Emulsion optimizes cornea hydration. • Cationic emulsion establishes an electrostatic interaction with the negatively charged cells of the ocular surface which improves ciclosporin delivery.	• Topical administration (eye drops).	• EMA (2015)

(Continued)

TABLE 2.3 (Continued) List of Clinical Approved Nano-Based Pharmaceutical Products According to the Therapeutic Indication or Diagnosis Purposes

CANCERS AND CONTROL OF ADVERSE EFFECTS CAUSED BY CANCER TREATMENT

PRODUCT DESIGNATION (MANUFACTURER)	GENERIC NAME (API)	TYPE OF NANOCARRIERS (COMPOSITION)	THERAPEUTIC INDICATION(S)	FUNCTION OF THE NANOCARRIER	ROUTE OF ADMINISTRATION	REGULATORY AUTHORITY APPROVAL (DATE)
Other Therapeutic Indications						
Estrasorb™ (Novavax)	17β-estradiol	**Nanoemulsion (o/w)** (oily phase: soybean oil; aqueous phase: ethanol, water; surfactant: polysorbate 80)	• Menopause hormone therapy (menopause induced mild vaso-motor symptoms	• Sustained delivery of estradiol.	• Topical administration.	• FDA (2003)
Somavert® (Pfizer Pharmaceuticals)	Pegvisomant (B2036-PEG – analog of hGH receptor antagonist)	**Polymer therapeutic conjugate** PEG- B2036 conjugate	• Acromegaly	• Improve protein stability. • Reduce clearance and increase half-life of approximately 6 days after administration (PEG causes a steric hindrance at the level of the membrane receptor).	• SC injection.	• FDA (2003)
Movantik® (AstraZeneca Pharmaceuticals LP) (FDA approval) Moventig® (AstraZeneca) (EMA approval)	Naloxegol (naloxone)	**Polymer therapeutic conjugate** PEG-naloxone conjugate	• Opioid-induced constipation in patients with chronic pain	• Lower permeability and penetration into the central nervous system compared to free naloxone. • Higher opioid-related constipation and less naloxone counter-action of opioid analgesia.	• Oral administration.	• FDA (2014) • EMA (2014)

(Continued)

TABLE 2.3 (Continued) List of Clinical Approved Nano-Based Pharmaceutical Products According to the Therapeutic Indication or Diagnosis Purposes

PRODUCT DESIGNATION (MANUFACTURER)	GENERIC NAME (API)	TYPE OF NANOCARRIERS (COMPOSITION)	THERAPEUTIC INDICATION(S)	FUNCTION OF THE NANOCARRIER	ROUTE OF ADMINISTRATION	REGULATORY AUTHORITY APPROVAL (DATE)
			CANCERS AND CONTROL OF ADVERSE EFFECTS CAUSED BY CANCER TREATMENT			
Adynovate® (Baxalta US Inc.) (FDA approval) Adynovi® (Baxalta Innov.GmbH) (EMA approval)	Rurioctocog alfa pegol (recombinant anti-hemophilic factor VIII)	**Polymer therapeutic conjugate** PEG- recombinant anti-hemophilic factor VIII conjugate	• Hemophilia A (congenital factor VIII deficiency)	• Greater stability. • Prolong circulation time and longer drug half-life. • Reduce frequency of injection.	• Lyophilized powder for solution for IV injection.	• FDA (2015) • EMA (2018)
Rebinyn® (Novo Nordisk Inc.) (FDA approval) Refixia ® (Novo Nordisk A/S) (EMA approval)	Nonacog beta pegol (DNA-derived coagulation Factor IX (recombinant))	**Polymer therapeutic conjugate** GlycoPEG- recombinant coagulation Factor IX	• Control and prevention of bleeding episodes (e.g., in the perioperative setting for hemophilia B patients)	• Effective control in 95% of bleeding episodes; 98% of bleeds were treated with 1–2 infusions.	• Lyophilized powder for solution for IV injection.	• FDA (2017) • EMA (2017)
Other Therapeutic Indications						
Jivi® (Bayer Healthcare, Inc.)	Damoctocog alfa pegol (recombinant anti-hemophilic factor VIII)	**Polymer therapeutic conjugate** PEG- recombinant anti-hemophilic factor VIII conjugate	• Hemophilia A (congenital factor VIII deficiency)	• Prolong half-life that allows for twice-weekly initial dosing and may be adjusted to every five days and further individually adjusted to less or more frequent dosing.	• Lyophilized powder for solution for IV injection.	• FDA (2018) • EMA (2018)

(Continued)

TABLE 2.3 (Continued)   List of Clinical Approved Nano-Based Pharmaceutical Products According to the Therapeutic Indication or Diagnosis Purposes

PRODUCT DESIGNATION (MANUFACTURER)	GENERIC NAME (API)	TYPE OF NANOCARRIERS (COMPOSITION)	THERAPEUTIC INDICATION(S)	FUNCTION OF THE NANOCARRIER	ROUTE OF ADMINISTRATION	REGULATORY AUTHORITY APPROVAL (DATE)
		CANCERS AND CONTROL OF ADVERSE EFFECTS CAUSED BY CANCER TREATMENT				
Krystexxa® (Savient Pharmaceuticals)	Pegloticase (uricase)	**Polymer therapeutic conjugate** PEG-recombinant porcine-like uricase aptamer conjugate	• Refractory chronic gout	• Improve solubility of Pegloticase which removes risks of precipitates. • Increase protein stability and half-life to about 10 days (in comparison to Rasburicase which is 8 hours). Reduce immunogenicity.	• IV injection.	• FDA (2010) Note: EMA approved in 2013; however, this medicine is now withdrawn from use in the European Union
Palynziq® (BioMarin Pharmaceutical Inc.)	Pegvaliase-pqpz (phenylalanine ammonia lyase)	**Polymer therapeutic conjugate** PEG- phenylalanine ammonia lyase conjugate	• Phenylketonuria	• Improve circulation times and stability.	• SC injection.	• FDA (2018) • EMA (2019)
Diprivan® (AstraZeneca)	Propofol	**Nanoemulsion (o/w)** (oily phase: soybean oil; aqueous phase: glycerol, water; surfactant: egg lecithin)	• Sedative hypnotic agent for induction and maintenance of anesthesia	• Controlled and sustained drug release. • Superior pain relief and extended analgesia for 48 hours with less need for supplemental analgesia.	• IV injection.	• FDA (2001) Approved in some EU countries
Depodur® (Skypharma Inc)	Morphine sulfate	**Liposomes** (DOPC, DPPG, cholesterol, Triolein)	• Analgesia (chronic pain and postoperative pain)	• Controlled and sustained drug release. • Superior pain relief and extended analgesia for 48 hours with less need for supplemental analgesia.	• Epidural injection.	• EMA (2004) • FDA (2014) but now is discontinued

(Continued)

TABLE 2.3 (Continued)   List of Clinical Approved Nano-Based Pharmaceutical Products According to the Therapeutic Indication or Diagnosis Purposes

CANCERS AND CONTROL OF ADVERSE EFFECTS CAUSED BY CANCER TREATMENT

PRODUCT DESIGNATION (MANUFACTURER)	GENERIC NAME (API)	TYPE OF NANOCARRIERS (COMPOSITION)	THERAPEUTIC INDICATION(S)	FUNCTION OF THE NANOCARRIER	ROUTE OF ADMINISTRATION	REGULATORY AUTHORITY APPROVAL (DATE)
Other Therapeutic Indications						
Exparel® (Pacira Pharmaceuticals, Inc)	Bupivacaine	**Liposomes** (DEPC, DPPG, cholesterol, Tricaprylin) The multivesicular liposomal formulation is patented as DepoFoam	• Analgesia (chronic pain and postoperative pain)	• Controlled and sustained drug release. • Superior pain relief and extended analgesia for 72 hours after wound infiltration in patients.	• Local injection infiltration.	• FDA (2011) • EMA (2020)
Diagnosis Purposes						
Stratus CS acute care diagnostic system (Siemens Healthcare Diagnostics)	Tecto-dendrimer that functions as a cardiac marker.	**Dendrimers** PAMAM dendrimer-coupled antibody reagents	• Measurement of cardiac biomarkers	• Dendrimer enhanced radial partition immunoassay.	• Not indicated (*in vitro* diagnostic use).	• Not indicated (medical device)
GastroMARK™ (AMAG Pharmaceuticals	Ferumoxsil (poly [N-(2-aminoethyl)-3-aminopropyl] siloxane coated non-stoichiometric magnetite (FeO$_x$[C$_5$H$_{13}$N$_2$SiO$_2$]$_y$)	**Magnetic nanoparticles** Silicone-coated SPION	• Imaging agent (MRI)	• Superparamagnetic character – MRI contrast media	• Oral administration.	• FDA (1996)
Diagnosis Purposes						
Resovist® (Bayer Healthcare)	Ferucarbotran	**Magnetic nanoparticles** SPION coated with carboxydextran	• Imaging agent (MRI)	Superparamagnetic character – MRI contrast media.	• IV administration.	• EMA (2001) • Japan (2002) Note: product currently available in only limited countries, such as Japan *(Continued)*

TABLE 2.3 (Continued) List of Clinical Approved Nano-Based Pharmaceutical Products According to the Therapeutic Indication or Diagnosis Purposes

		CANCERS AND CONTROL OF ADVERSE EFFECTS CAUSED BY CANCER TREATMENT			
PRODUCT DESIGNATION (MANUFACTURER)	GENERIC NAME (API)	TYPE OF NANOCARRIERS (COMPOSITION)	THERAPEUTIC INDICATION(S)	FUNCTION OF THE NANOCARRIER	ROUTE OF ADMINISTRATION	REGULATORY AUTHORITY APPROVAL (DATE)
Verigene® System NanoGrid Technology (Luminex)	Depending upon the application, each nanoparticle is functionalized with nucleic acids or an antibody specific to the protein of interest	**Gold nanoparticles** Oligonucleotide-conjugated gold nanoparticle	• Detection of enteric pathogens	• Increased sensitivity by several orders of magnitude compared to fluorophores. Light emitted from one nanoparticle is equivalent to the light emitted from 500,000 fluorophores. • Enables high specificity for both nucleic acid and protein detection. • Reduces background noise, enhancing the emitted signal. • Extremely stable, with a long shelf-life. • Non-toxic.	• Not indicated.	• Not indicated (medical device)

Abbreviations: ALC-0315 – 4-hydroxybutyl)azanediyl)bis(hexane-6,1-diyl)bis(2-hexyldecanoate). It is a physiological pH cationic synthetic lipid; ALC-0159 – 2-[(polyethylene glycol)-2000]-N,N-ditetradecylacetamide). It is a non-ionic PEGylated surfactant; AML – acute myeloid leukemia; API – active pharmaceutical ingredient; DEPC – 1,2-dierucoyl-sn-glycero-3-phosphocholine; DMG-PEG(2000) – 1,2-dimyristoyl-rac-glycero-3-methoxypolyethylene glycol-2000; DMPC – 1,2-dimyristoyl-sn-glycero-3-phosphocholine; DMPG – 1,2-dimyristoyl-sn-glycero-3-phosphorylglycerol; DOPC – 1,2-dioleoyl-sn-glycero-3-phosphocholine; DOPS – 1,2-dioleoylsn-glycero-3-phospho-L-serine; DPPC – 1,2-dipalmitoyl phosphatidylcholine; DPPG – 1,2-dipalmitoyl-sn-glycero-3-phosphorylglycerol; DSPC – 1,2-distearoyl-sn-glycero-3-phosphocholine; DSPE – 1,2-distearoyl-sn-glycero-3-phosphorylethanolamine; DSPE-PEG(2000) – 1,2-distearoyl-sn-glycero-3-phosphoethanolamine-N-[amino(polyethylene glycol)-2000]; DSPG – 1,2-distearoyl-sn-glycero-3-phosphoglycerol; EMA – European Medicines Agency; EPC – L-α-phosphatidylcholine from egg; EPG – L-α-phosphatidylglycerol from egg; EPR – enhanced permeability and retention; Fab' – antigen-binding fragment; FDA – United States Food and Drug Administration; FeOx[C5H13N2SiO2]y – poly [N-(2-aminoethyl)-3-aminopropyl] siloxane coated non-stoichiometric magnetite; HBeAg – hepatitis B e-Antigen; hGH – human growth hormone; HIV – human immunodeficiency virus; HSPC – hydrogenated soybean phosphatidylcholine; IDA – iron deficiency anemia; IM – intramuscular; IV – intravenous; mPEG-PDLLA – monomethoxy-poly (ethylene glycol)-block-poly (D,L-lactide); mRNA – messenger RNA; o/w – oil-in-water; PC – phosphatidylcholine; PE – phosphatidylethanolamine (cephalin); PEG – polyethylene glycol; PLGA – poly(lactic acid-co-glycolic acid; POPC – 1-palmitoyl-2-oleoyl-sn-glycero-3-phosphocholine; r metHuG-CSF – recombinant methionyl human granulocyte colony-stimulating factor; SARS-CoV-2 – Severe Acute Respiratory Syndrome Coronavirus 2; SC – subcutaneous; SM-102 – (heptadecan-9-yl 8-((2-hydroxyethyl) (6-oxo-6-(undecyloxy) hexyl) amino) octanoate). It is a proprietary ionizable lipid used to form lipid nanoparticles in the Moderna COVID-19 vaccine; SPION – superparamagnetic iron oxide nanoparticle; SPL7013 – astodrimer sodium; TNF-α – tumor necrosis factor-alpha; VEGF – vascular endothelial growth factor.

References: (Patel et al. 2020, Patra et al. 2018, Ekladious, Colson, and Grinstaff 2019, Greish et al. 2018, Lombardo, Kiselev, and Caccamo 2019, Veronese and Mero 2008, Shetab Boushehri, Dietrich, and Lamprecht 2020, Farjadian et al. 2019, Zylberberg and Matosevic 2016, Beltrán-Gracia et al. 2019, Forni et al. 2021, Anselmo and Mitragotri 2019, Richard et al. 2012, Eroglu 2017, Foster et al. 2010, Bovier 2008).

2.6 CONCLUDING REMARKS AND FUTURE PROSPECTS

Nanomedicine, the application of nanotechnology to medicine, has harnessed the use of nanoscale materials for a wide spectrum of applications, including the diagnosis, monitoring, control, prevention, and treatment of diseases. Indeed, nanoscale technology is now widely used in medical devices and medicine where manipulations are made at the molecular level, benefiting from the novel properties a material acquires. The primary demand of this field in medicine is in making improvements in the delivery of treatments and healthcare outcomes. Signs of this progress are the sequential generations of DDNs that are reported in the literature and already strengthen the research and development programs.

Historically termed the magic bullets, DDNs have witnessed a remarkable expansion both in terms of nature and strategies to address the intended target(s) and purpose of application. The oncologic area is the area that has most profited from DDV advantages; however, the treatment of other pathologies and infections, such as SARS-CoV-2 infection, has clearly benefited from the applications of nanotechnology. Apart from this trend, ca. 50 nanomedicines/nanovaccines/nanodevices are currently available in the market, and hundreds of nano-based drug products are in the clinical trial programs.

Which nanosystem should one choose? This choice essentially relies on the issues that are framed and on the advantages sought. Whenever applied, the one-size-fits-all approach should be privileged, envisioning a multipurpose application. Irrespective of their nature or category, a sustained development under the umbrella of quality (safety and efficacy) by design premises is highly encouraged. It is worth noting that apart from quality, prospectively including safety and efficacy concerns in the design of a nanomedicine should be assumed as a priority. Such an integrative approach must be duly planned, always envisioning the patient as the ultimate user, and involving efforts at distinct levels, including the contribution from AI to comply and align with the regulatory standards.

The development of specific nanomedicine guidelines and regulatory affairs will lead to faster submission and approval processes and an increase in the pipeline of nanomedicine products.

ACKNOWLEDGMENTS

Carla Vitorino acknowledges Fundação para a Ciência e a Tecnologia (FCT), the Portuguese Agency for Scientific Research for the financial support assigned to the Coimbra Chemistry Centre (CQC) through the Project UID/QUI/00313/2020. Marlene Lúcio acknowledges FCT in the framework of the Strategic Funding [UID/FIS/04650/2019], and for the project CONCERT [POCI-01-0145-FEDER-032651 and PTDC/NAN-MAT/326512017], co-financed by the European Regional Development Fund (ERDF), through COMPETE 2020, under Portugal 2020, and FCT I.P.

LIST OF ABBREVIATIONS

AI	artificial intelligence
ALC-0315	4-hydroxybutyl)azanediyl)bis(hexane-6,1-diyl)bis(2-hexyldecanoate)
ALC-0159	2-[(polyethylene glycol)-2000]-N,N-ditetradecylacetamide)
AML	acute myeloid leukemia
API	active pharmaceutical ingredient
APO	apocynin

BBB	blood–brain barrier
BCS	biopharmaceutical classification system
bFGF	basic fibroblast growth factor
BMP-2	bone morphogenetic protein-2
BMP-7	bone morphogenetic protein-7
CEM	cholecystic-derived extracellular matrix
"CAPIR" cascade	circulation, accumulation, penetration, internalization, and release
CMAs	critical material attributes
CMC	critical micelle concentration
CO	carbon monoxide
CPPs	critical process parameters
CQAs	critical quality attributes
DEPC	1,2-dierucoyl-sn-glycero-3-phosphocholine
DMG-PEG(2000)	1,2-dimyristoyl-rac-glycero-3-methoxypolyethylene glycol-2000
DMPC	1,2-dimyristoyl-sn-glycero-3-phosphocholine
DMPG	1,2-dimyristoyl-sn-glycero-3-phosphorylglycerol
DDNs	drug delivery nanosystems
DNA	desoxyribonucleic acid
DoEs	design space through design of experiments
DOPC	1,2-dioleoyl-sn-glycero-3-phosphocholine
DOPS	1,2-dioleoylsn-glycero-3-phospho-L-serine
DPPC	1,2-dipalmitoyl phosphatidylcholine
DPPG	1,2-dipalmitoyl-sn-glycero-3-phosphorylglycerol
DSPC	1,2-distearoyl-sn-glycero-3-phosphocholine
DSPE	1,2-distearoyl-sn-glycero-3-phosphorylethanolamine
DSPE-PEG(2000)	1,2-distearoyl-sn-glycero-3-phosphoethanolamine-N-[amino(polyethylene glycol)-2000]
DSPG	1,2-distearoyl-sn-glycero-3-phosphoglycerol
EbD	efficacy by design
EGF	epidermal growth factor
EMA	European Medicines Agency
EPC	L-α-phosphatidylcholine from egg
EPG	L-α-phosphatidylglycerol from egg
EPR	Enhanced Permeability and Retention
Fab$'$	antigen-binding fragment
FDA	United States Food and Drug Administration
FeO$_x$[C$_5$H$_{13}$N$_2$SiO$_2$]$_y$	poly [N-(2-aminoethyl)-3-aminopropyl] siloxane coated non-stoichiometric magnetite
γ-Fe$_2$O$_3$	maghemite
Fe$_3$O$_4$	magnetite
G1-PAMAM	generation-1 polyamidoamine
GRAS	generally recognized as safe
HBeAg	hepatitis B e-Antigen
hGH	human growth hormone
HIFU	high intensity focused ultrasound
HIV	human immunodeficiency virus
HSPC	hydrogenated soybean phosphatidylcholine
ICH	International Council for Harmonisation of Technical Requirements for Pharmaceuticals for Human Use

IDA	iron deficiency anemia
IM	intramuscular
IV	intravenous
LHRH	luteinizing hormone-releasing hormone
LRP1	low-density lipoprotein receptor related protein 1
MFH	magnetic fluid hyperthermia
mPEG-PDLLA	monomethoxy-poly (ethylene glycol)-block-poly (D,L-lactide)
MPS	mononuclear phagocytic system
MRI	magnetic resonance imaging
mRNA	messenger RNA
MSNs	mesoporous silica nanoparticles
NCI	National Cancer Institute
NLCs	nanostructured lipid carriers
nm	nanometer
NO	nitric oxide
OECD	Organization for Economic Co-operation and Development
o/w	oil-in-water
PAMAM	polyamidoamine
PAT	process analytical technologies
PC	phosphatidylcholine
PDGF-BB	platelet-derived growth factor-BB
PDT	photodynamic therapy
PE	phosphatidylethanolamine (cephalin)
PEG	polyethylene glycol
PEG-PE	polyethylene glycol-phosphatidyl ethanolamine conjugate
PLGA	poly(lactic acid-co-glycolic acid)
POPC	1-palmitoyl-2-oleoyl-sn-glycero-3-phosphocholine
QbD	quality by design
QTPP	quality target product profile
RES	reticuloendothelial system
r-metHuG-CSF	recombinant methionyl human granulocyte colony-stimulating factor
ROS	reactive oxygen species
SARS-CoV-2	Severe Acute Respiratory Syndrome Coronavirus 2
SbD	safety by design
SC	subcutaneous
SDEDDS	self-double-emulsifying drug delivery systems
SDF-1α	stromal cell-derived factor-1α
SERS	surface-enhanced Raman spectroscopy
siRNA	small interfering RNA
SLNs	solid lipid nanoparticles
SM-102	heptadecan-9-yl 8-((2-hydroxyethyl) (6-oxo-6-(undecyloxy) hexyl) amino) octanoate
SNDDS	self-nanoemulsifying drug delivery systems
SPION	superparamagnetic iron oxide nanoparticles
SPL7013	astodrimer sodium
TAT	trans-activator transcription
TGF-β	transforming growth factor-β
TNF-α	tumor necrosis factor-α
VEGF	vascular endothelial growth factor
w/o	water-in-oil

REFERENCES

Adibfar, A., G. Amoabediny, M. B. Eslaminejad, J. Mohamadi, F. Bagheri, and B. Z. Doulabi. "VEGF Delivery by Smart Polymeric PNIPAM Nanoparticles Affects Both Osteogenic and Angiogenic Capacities of Human Bone Marrow Stem Cells." *Materials Science & Engineering. Part C* 93 (2018): 790–9. doi:10.1016/j.msec.2018.08.037.

Aghanejad, A., H. Babamiri, K. Adibkia, J. Barar, and Y. Omidi. "Mucin-1 Aptamer-Armed Superparamagnetic Iron Oxide Nanoparticles for Targeted Delivery of Doxorubicin to Breast Cancer Cells". 2, no. 8 (2018): 117–27. doi:10.15171/bi.2018.14.

Ahad, A., M. Aqil, K. Kohli, Y. Sultana, M. Mujeeb, and A. Ali. "Formulation and Optimization of Nanotransfersomes Using Experimental Design Technique for Accentuated Transdermal Delivery of Valsartan." *Nanomedicine* 8, no. 2 (2012): 237–49. doi:10.1016/j.nano.2011.06.004.

Ahir, M., P. Upadhyay, A. Ghosh, S. Sarker, S. Bhattacharya, P. Gupta, S. Ghosh, S. Chattopadhyay, and A. Adhikary. "Delivery of Dual miRNA Through CD44-Targeted Mesoporous Silica Nanoparticles for Enhanced and Effective Triple-Negative Breast Cancer Therapy." *Biomaterials Science* 8, no. 10 (2020): 2939–54. doi:10.1039/D0BM00015A.

Ahirwar, S., S. Mallick, and D. Bahadur. "Photodynamic Therapy Using Graphene Quantum Dot Derivatives." *Journal of Solid State Chemistry* 282 (2020). doi:10.1016/j.jssc.2019.121107, PubMed: 121107.

Ahmad, Z., A. Shah, M. Siddiq, and H.-B. Kraatz. "Polymeric Micelles as Drug Delivery Vehicles." *RSC Advances* 4, no. 33 (2014): 17028–38. doi:10.1039/C3RA47370H.

Ainbinder, D., and E. Touitou. "Testosterone Ethosomes for Enhanced Transdermal Delivery." *Drug Delivery* 12, no. 5 (2005): 297–303. doi:10.1080/10717540500176910.

Akbarzadeh, A., R. Rezaei-Sadabady, S. Davaran, S. W. Joo, N. Zarghami, Y. Hanifehpour, M. Samiei, M. Kouhi, and K. Nejati-Koshki. "Liposome: Classification, Preparation, and Applications." *Nanoscale Research Letters* 8, no. 1 (2013): 102. doi:10.1186/1556-276X-8-102.

Alarçin, Emine, Xiaofei Guan, Sara Saheb Kashaf, Khairat Elbaradie, Huazhe Yang, Hae Lin Jang, and Ali Khademhosseini. "Recreating Composition, Structure, Functionalities of Tissues at Nanoscale for Regenerative Medicine." *Regenerative Medicine* 11, no. 8 (2016): 849–58. doi:10.2217/rme-2016-0120.

Alonso, J., H. Khurshid, J. Devkota, Z. Nemati, N. K. Khadka, H. Srikanth, J. Pan, and M.-H. Phan. "Superparamagnetic Nanoparticles Encapsulated in Lipid Vesicles for Advanced Magnetic Hyperthermia and Biodetection." *Journal of Applied Physics* 119, no. 8 (2016). doi:10.1063/1.4942618, PubMed: 083904.

Alsulays, B. B., M. K. Anwer, G. A. Soliman, S. M. Alshehri, and E. S. Khafagy. "Impact of Penetratin Stereochemistry on the Oral Bioavailability of Insulin-Loaded Solid Lipid Nanoparticles." *International Journal of Nanomedicine* 14 (2019): 9127–38. doi:10.2147/ijn.s225086.

Alvarez-Berríos, M. P., and J. L. Vivero-Escoto. "In Vitro Evaluation of Folic Acid-Conjugated Redox-Responsive Mesoporous Silica Nanoparticles for the Delivery of Cisplatin." *International Journal of Nanomedicine* 11 (2016): 6251–65. doi:10.2147/ijn.s118196.

Amoozgar, Z., and Y. Yeo. "Recent Advances in Stealth Coating of Nanoparticle Drug Delivery Systems." *Wiley Interdisciplinary Reviews. Nanomedicine & Nanobiotechnology* 4, no. 2 (2012): 219–33. doi:10.1002/wnan.1157.

Anderson, S. D., V. V. Gwenin, and C. D. Gwenin. "Magnetic Functionalized Nanoparticles for Biomedical, Drug Delivery and Imaging Applications." *Nanoscale Research Letters* 14, no. 1 (2019): 188. doi:10.1186/s11671-019-3019-6.

Andreozzi, E., J. W. Seo, K. Ferrara, and A. Louie. "Novel Method to Label Solid Lipid Nanoparticles with 64cu for Positron Emission Tomography Imaging." *Bioconjugate Chemistry* 22, no. 4 (2011): 808–18. doi:10.1021/bc100478k.

Anselmo, A. C., and S. Mitragotri. "Nanoparticles in the Clinic: An Update." *Bioengineering & Translational Medicine* 4, no. 3 (2019): e10143. doi:10.1002/btm2.10143.

Arias, Jose L. *Nanotechnology and Drug Delivery, Volume Two: Nano-Engineering Strategies and Nanomedicines Against Severe Diseases*. 1st ed. Edited by J. L. Arias. Boca Raton, FL: CRC Press Press, 2016. doi:10.1201/b19976.

Arifin, D. R., and A. F. Palmer. "Polymersome Encapsulated Hemoglobin: A Novel Type of Oxygen Carrier." *Biomacromolecules* 6, no. 4 (2005): 2172–81. doi:10.1021/bm0501454.

Arts, Josje H. E., Mackenzie Hadi, Muhammad-Adeel Irfan, Athena M. Keene, Reinhard Kreiling, Delina Lyon, Monika Maier, Karin Michel, Thomas Petry, Ursula G. Sauer, David Warheit, Karin Wiench, Wendel

Wohlleben, and Robert Landsiedel. "A Decision-Making Framework for the Grouping and Testing of Nanomaterials (DF4nanoGrouping)." *Regulatory Toxicology & Pharmacology* 71, no. 2 (Suppl.) (2015): S1–SS27. doi:10.1016/j.yrtph.2015.03.007.

Ascenso, A., A. Salgado, C. Euletério, F. G. Praça, M. V. L. B. Bentley, H. C. Marques, H. Oliveira, C. Santos, and S. Simões. "In Vitro and In Vivo Topical Delivery Studies of Tretinoin-Loaded Ultradeformable Vesicles." *European Journal of Pharmaceutics & Biopharmaceutics* 88, no. 1 (2014): 48–55. doi:10.1016/j.ejpb.2014.05.002.

Attama, A. A. "SLN, NLC, LDC: State of the Art in Drug and Active Delivery." *Recent Pat Drug Deliv Formul* 5, no. 3 (2011): 178–87. doi:10.2174/187221111797200524.

Attia, M. F., N. Anton, J. Wallyn, Z. Omran, and T. F. Vandamme. "An Overview of Active and Passive Targeting Strategies to Improve the Nanocarriers Efficiency to Tumour Sites." *Journal of Pharmacy & Pharmacology* 71, no. 8 (2019): 1185–98. doi:10.1111/jphp.13098.

Avgoustakis, K. "Pegylated Poly(Lactide) and Poly(Lactide-Co-Glycolide) Nanoparticles: Preparation, Properties and Possible Applications in Drug Delivery." *Current Drug Delivery* 1, no. 4 (2004): 321–33. doi:10.2174/1567201043334605.

Bae, K. H., J. Y. Lee, S. H. Lee, T. G. Park, and Y. S. Nam. "Optically Traceable Solid Lipid Nanoparticles Loaded with siRNA and Paclitaxel for Synergistic Chemotherapy with In Situ Imaging." *Advanced Healthcare Materials* 2, no. 4 (2013): 576–84. doi:10.1002/adhm.201200338.

Bai, S., C. Thomas, and F. Ahsan. "Dendrimers as a Carrier for Pulmonary Delivery of Enoxaparin, a Low-Molecular Weight Heparin." *Journal of Pharmaceutical Sciences* 96, no. 8 (2007): 2090–106. doi:10.1002/jps.20849.

Ballou, B., B. C. Lagerholm, L. A. Ernst, M. P. Bruchez, and A. S. Waggoner. "Noninvasive Imaging of Quantum Dots in Mice." *Bioconjugate Chemistry* 15, no. 1 (2004): 79–86. doi:10.1021/bc034153y.

Bally, M., K. Bailey, K. Sugihara, D. Grieshaber, J. Vörös, and B. Städler. "Liposome and Lipid Bilayer Arrays Towards Biosensing Applications." *Small* 6, no. 22 (2010): 2481–97. doi:10.1002/smll.201000644.

Banga, R. J., B. Meckes, S. P. Narayan, A. J. Sprangers, S. T. Nguyen, and C. A. Mirkin. "Cross-Linked Micellar Spherical Nucleic Acids from Thermoresponsive Templates." *Journal of the American Chemical Society* 139, no. 12 (2017): 4278–81. doi:10.1021/jacs.6b13359.

BaoLin, G., and P. X. Ma. "Synthetic Biodegradable Functional Polymers for Tissue Engineering: A Brief Review." *Science in China (Chemistry)* 57, no. 4 (2014): 490–500. doi:10.1007/s11426-014-5086-y.

Barathmanikanth, S., K. Kalishwaralal, M. Sriram, S. R. K. Pandian, H.-S. Youn, S. Eom, and S. Gurunathan. "Anti-Oxidant Effect of Gold Nanoparticles Restrains Hyperglycemic Conditions in Diabetic Mice." *Journal of Nanobiotechnology* 8 (2010): 16. doi:10.1186/1477-3155-8-16.

Bárcena, C., A. K. Sra, and J. Gao. "Applications of Magnetic Nanoparticles in Biomedicine." In *Nanoscale Magnetic Materials and Applications*, edited by J. P. Liu, E. Fullerton, O. Gutfleisch, and D. J. Sellmyer, 591–626. Boston, MA: Springer, 2009.

Barone, A., M. Mendes, C. Cabral, R. Mare, D. Paolino, and C. Vitorino. "Hybrid Nanostructured Films for Topical Administration of Simvastatin as Coadjuvant Treatment of Melanoma." *Journal of Pharmaceutical Sciences* 108, no. 10 (2019): 3396–407. doi:10.1016/j.xphs.2019.06.002.

Bayda, S., M. Adeel, T. Tuccinardi, M. Cordani, and F. Rizzolio. "The History of Nanoscience and Nanotechnology: From Chemical–Physical Applications to Nanomedicine." *Molecules* 25, no. 1 (2019): 112. doi:10.3390/molecules25010112.

Beiranvand, S., and M. R. Moradkhani. "Bupivacaine Versus Liposomal Bupivacaine for Pain Control." *Drug Research* 68, no. 07 (2018): 365–9. doi:10.1055/s-0043-121142.

Beltrán-Gracia, E., A. López-Camacho, I. Higuera-Ciapara, J. B. Velázquez-Fernández, and A. A. Vallejo-Cardona. "Nanomedicine Review: Clinical Developments in Liposomal Applications." *Cancer Nanotechnology* 10, no. 1 (2019): 11. doi:10.1186/s12645-019-0055-y.

Bentolila, L. A. "5 - Photoluminescent Quantum Dots in Imaging, Diagnostics and Therapy." In *Applications of Nanoscience in Photomedicine*, edited by Michael R. Hamblin, and Pinar Avci, 77–104. Oxford: Chandos Publishing, 2015.

Bhalekar, M. R., A. R. Madgulkar, P. S. Desale, and G. Marium. "Formulation of Piperine Solid Lipid Nanoparticles (SLN) for Treatment of Rheumatoid Arthritis." *Drug Development & Industrial Pharmacy* 43, no. 6 (2017): 1003–10. doi:10.1080/03639045.2017.1291666.

Bharatwaj, B., A. K. Mohammad, R. Dimovski, F. L. Cassio, R. C. Bazito, D. Conti, Q. Fu, J. Reineke, and S. R. P. da Rocha. "Dendrimer Nanocarriers for Transport Modulation Across Models of the Pulmonary Epithelium." *Molecular Pharmaceutics* 12, no. 3 (2015): 826–38. doi:10.1021/mp500662z.

Bhardwaj, A., L. Kumar, S. Mehta, and A. Mehta. "Stimuli-Sensitive Systems-an Emerging Delivery System for Drugs." *Artificial Cells, Nanomedicine & Biotechnology* 43, no. 5 (2015): 299–310. doi:10.3109/21691401.2013.856016.

Bharti, C., U. Nagaich, A. K. Pal, and N. Gulati. "Mesoporous Silica Nanoparticles in Target Drug Delivery System: A Review." *International Journal of Pharmaceutical Investigation* 5, no. 3 (2015): 124–33. doi:10.4103/2230-973x.160844.

Boche, M., and V. Pokharkar. "Quetiapine Nanoemulsion for Intranasal Drug Delivery: Evaluation of Brain-Targeting Efficiency." *AAPS PharmSciTech* 18, no. 3 (2017): 686–96. doi:10.1208/s12249-016-0552-9.

Bock, N., A. Riminucci, C. Dionigi, A. Russo, A. Tampieri, E. Landi, V. A. Goranov, M. Marcacci, and V. Dediu. "A Novel Route in Bone Tissue Engineering: Magnetic Biomimetic Scaffolds." *Acta Biomaterialia* 6, no. 3 (2010): 786–96. doi:10.1016/j.actbio.2009.09.017.

Boduch-Lee, K. A., T. Chapman, S. E. Petricca, K. G. Marra, and P. Kumta. "Design and Synthesis of Hydroxyapatite Composites Containing an mPEG–dendritic Poly(l-lysine) Star Polycaprolactone." *Macromolecules* No. 37 (24)" (2004): 8959–66. doi:10.1021/ma0493630.

Bonoiu, A. C., S. D. Mahajan, H. Ding, I. Roy, K.-T. Yong, R. Kumar, R. Hu, E. J. Bergey, S. A. Schwartz, and P. N. Prasad. "Nanotechnology Approach for Drug Addiction Therapy: Gene Silencing Using Delivery of Gold Nanorod-siRNA Nanoplex in Dopaminergic Neurons." *Proceedings of the National Academy of Sciences of the United States of America* 106, no. 14 (2009): 5546–50. doi:10.1073/pnas.0901715106.

Bovier, P. A. "Epaxal®: A Virosomal Vaccine to Prevent Hepatitis A Infection." *Expert Review of Vaccines* 7, no. 8 (2008): 1141–50. doi:10.1586/14760584.7.8.1141.

Bragagni, M., N. Mennini, F. Maestrelli, M. Cirri, and P. Mura. "Comparative Study of Liposomes, Transfersomes and Ethosomes as Carriers for Improving Topical Delivery of Celecoxib." *Drug Delivery* 19, no. 7 (2012): 354–61. doi:10.3109/10717544.2012.724472.

Brown, S. D., P. Nativo, J.-A. Smith, D. Stirling, P. R. Edwards, B. Venugopal, D. J. Flint, J. A. Plumb, D. Graham, and N. J. Wheate. "Gold Nanoparticles for the Improved Anticancer Drug Delivery of the Active Component of Oxaliplatin." *Journal of the American Chemical Society* 132, no. 13 (2010): 4678–84. doi:10.1021/ja908117a.

Bursten, J. R., M. C. Roco, W. Yang, Y. Zhao, C. Chen, K. Savolainen, C. Gerber, K. Kataoka, Y. Krishnan, H. Bayley, L. Nazar, S. Milana, L. Vandersypen, P. S. Weiss, and J. Schummer. "Nano on Reflection." *Nature Nanotechnology* 11, no. 10 (2016): 828. doi:10.1038/nnano.2016.232.

Cabral, H., and K. Kataoka. "Progress of Drug-Loaded Polymeric Micelles into Clinical Studies." *Journal of Controlled Release* 190 (2014): 465–76. doi:10.1016/j.jconrel.2014.06.042.

Cai, X., Y. Luo, W. Zhang, D. Du, and Y. Lin. "pH-Sensitive ZnO Quantum Dots–Doxorubicin Nanoparticles for Lung Cancer Targeted Drug Delivery." *ACS Applied Materials & Interfaces* 8, no. 34 (2016): 22442–50. doi:10.1021/acsami.6b04933.

Castro, P. M., P. Baptista, A. R. Madureira, B. Sarmento, and M. E. Pintado. "Combination of PLGA Nanoparticles with Mucoadhesive Guar-Gum Films for Buccal Delivery of Antihypertensive Peptide." *International Journal of Pharmaceutics* 547, no. 1-2 (2018): 593–601. doi:10.1016/j.ijpharm.2018.05.051.

Cayero-Otero, M. D., M. J. Gomes, C. Martins, J. Álvarez-Fuentes, M. Fernández-Arévalo, and B. Sarmento. "In vivo Biodistribution of Venlafaxine-PLGA Nanoparticles for Brain Delivery: Plain vs. Functionalized Nanoparticles." *Expert Opinion on Drug Delivery* 16, no. 12 (2019):1413–1427. doi:10.1080/17425247.2019.16 90452.

Cha, B. G., and J. Kim. "Functional Mesoporous Silica Nanoparticles for Bio-Imaging Applications." *WIREs Nanomedicine & Nanobiotechnology* 11, no. 1 (2019): e1515. doi:10.1002/wnan.1515.

Chabra, S., M. Ranjan, R. Bhandari, T. Kaur, M. Aggrawal, V. Puri, N. Mahajan, I. P. Kaur, S. Puri, and R. C. Sobti. "Solid Lipid Nanoparticles Regulate Functional Assortment of Mouse Mesenchymal Stem Cells." *Journal of Stem Cells & Regenerative Medicine* 7, no. 2 (2011): 75–9. doi:10.46582/jsrm.0702012.

Chakraborty, I., and P. K. Mascharak. "Mesoporous Silica Materials and Nanoparticles as Carriers for Controlled and Site-Specific Delivery of Gaseous Signaling Molecules." *Microporous & Mesoporous Materials* 234 (2016): 409–19. doi:10.1016/j.micromeso.2016.07.028.

Chan, J. C., K. Burugapalli, H. Naik, J. L. Kelly, and A. Pandit. "Amine Functionalization of Cholecyst-derived Extracellular Matrix with Generation 1 PAMAM Dendrimer." *Biomacromolecules* 9, no. 2 (2008): 528–36. doi:10.1021/bm701055k.

Chan, J. M., P. M. Valencia, L. Zhang, R. Langer, and O. C. Farokhzad. "Polymeric Nanoparticles for Drug Delivery." *Methods in Molecular Biology* 624 (2010): 163–175. doi:10.1007/978-1-60761-609-2_11.

Charych, D. H., U. Hoch, J. L. Langowski, S. R. Lee, M. K. Addepalli, P. B. Kirk, D. Sheng, X. Liu, P. W. Sims, L. A. VanderVeen, C. F. Ali, T. K. Chang, M. Konakova, R. L. Pena, R. S. Kanhere, Y. M. Kirksey, C. Ji, Y. Wang, J. Huang, T. D. Sweeney, S. S. Kantak, and S. K. Doberstein. "NKTR-214, an Engineered Cytokine with Biased IL2 Receptor Binding, Increased Tumor Exposure, and Marked Efficacy in Mouse Tumor Models." *Clinical Cancer Research* 22, no. 3 (2016): 680–90. doi:10.1158/1078-0432.ccr-15-1631.

Charych, D., S. Khalili, V. Dixit, P. Kirk, T. Chang, J. Langowski, W. Rubas, S. K. Doberstein, M. Eldon, U. Hoch, and J. Zalevsky. "Modeling the Receptor Pharmacology, Pharmacokinetics, and Pharmacodynamics of

NKTR-214, a Kinetically-Controlled Interleukin-2 (IL2) Receptor Agonist for Cancer Immunotherapy." *PLOS ONE* 12, no. 7 (2017): e0179431. doi:10.1371/journal.pone.0179431.

Chatap, V., P. Patil, and S. D. Patil. "In-Vitro, Ex-Vivo Characterization of Furosemide Bounded Pharmacosomes for Improvement of Solubility and Permeability." *Advances in Pharmacological Sciences* 2, no. 5 (2014): 67–76. doi:10.13189/app.2014.020501.

Chato-Astrain, J., I. Chato-Astrain, D. Sánchez-Porras, Ó.-D. García-García, F. Bermejo-Casares, C. Vairo, M. Villar-Vidal, G. Gainza, S. Villullas, R.-I. Oruezabal, Á. Ponce-Polo, I. Garzón, V. Carriel, F. Campos, and M. Alaminos. "Generation of a Novel Human Dermal Substitute Functionalized with Antibiotic-Loaded Nanostructured Lipid Carriers (NLCs) with Antimicrobial Properties for Tissue Engineering." *Journal of Nanobiotechnology* 18, no. 1 (2020): 174. doi:10.1186/s12951-020-00732-0.

Chauhan, A. S. (2018). "Dendrimers for Drug Delivery." *Molecules* 23, no. 4: 938. doi:10.3390/molecules23040938.

Chen, C.-W., W.-J. Syu, T.-C. Huang, Y.-C. Lee, J.-K. Hsiao, K.-Y. Huang, H.-P. Yu, M.-Y. Liao, and P.-S. Lai. "Encapsulation of Au/Fe3O4 Nanoparticles into a Polymer Nanoarchitecture with Combined near Infrared-Triggered Chemo-Photothermal Therapy Based on Intracellular Secondary Protein Understanding." *Journal of Materials Chemistry B* 5, no. 29 (2017): 5774–82. doi:10.1039/C7TB00944E.

Chen, F., and D. Gerion. "Fluorescent CdSe/ZnS Nanocrystal–Peptide Conjugates for Long-Term, Nontoxic Imaging and Nuclear Targeting in Living Cells." *Nano Letters* 4, no. 10 (2004): 1827–32. doi:10.1021/nl049170q.

Chen, F., M. Ma, J. Wang, F. Wang, S.-X. Chern, E. R. Zhao, A. Jhunjhunwala, S. Darmadi, H. Chen, and J. V. Jokerst. "Exosome-like Silica Nanoparticles: A Novel Ultrasound Contrast Agent for Stem Cell Imaging." *Nanoscale* 9, no. 1 (2017): 402–11. doi:10.1039/C6NR08177K.

Chen, G.-J., Y.-Z. Su, C. Hsu, Y.-L. Lo, S.-J. Huang, J.-H. Ke, Y.-C. Kuo, and L.-F. Wang. "Angiopep-pluronic F127-Conjugated Superparamagnetic Iron Oxide Nanoparticles as Nanotheranostic Agents for BBB Targeting." *Journal of Materials Chemistry B* 2, no. 34 (2014): 5666–75. doi:10.1039/C4TB00543K.

Chen, L., X. Zhou, and C. He. "Mesoporous Silica Nanoparticles for Tissue-Engineering Applications." *Wiley Interdisciplinary Reviews. Nanomedicine & Nanobiotechnology* 11, no. 6 (2019): e1573. doi:10.1002/wnan.1573.

Chen, X., X. Ding, Z. Zheng, and Y. Peng. "Thermosensitive Cross-Linked Polymer Vesicles for Controlled Release System." *New Journal of Chemistry* 30, no. 4 (2006): 577–82. doi:10.1039/B516053G.

Chen, Y. H., C. Y. Tsai, P. Y. Huang, M. Y. Chang, P. C. Cheng, C. H. Chou, D. H. Chen, C. R. Wang, A. L. Shiau, and C. L. Wu. "Methotrexate Conjugated to Gold Nanoparticles Inhibits Tumor Growth in a Syngeneic Lung Tumor Model." *Molecular Pharmaceutics* 4, no. 5 (2007): 713–22. doi:10.1021/mp060132k.

Chertok, B., B. A. Moffat, A. E. David, F. Yu, C. Bergemann, B. D. Ross, and V. C. Yang. "Iron Oxide Nanoparticles as a Drug Delivery Vehicle for MRI Monitored Magnetic Targeting of Brain Tumors." *Biomaterials* 29, no. 4 (2008): 487–96. doi:10.1016/j.biomaterials.2007.08.050.

Chiappetta, D. A., C. Hocht, C. Taira, and A. Sosnik. "Oral Pharmacokinetics of the Anti-HIV Efavirenz Encapsulated Within Polymeric Micelles." *Biomaterials* 32, no. 9 (2011): 2379–87. doi:10.1016/j.biomaterials.2010.11.082.

Chorny, M., I. Fishbein, B. B. Yellen, I. S. Alferiev, M. Bakay, S. Ganta, R. Adamo, M. Amiji, G. Friedman, and R. J. Levy. "Targeting Stents with Local Delivery of Paclitaxel-Loaded Magnetic Nanoparticles Using Uniform Fields." *Proceedings of the National Academy of Sciences of the United States of America* 107, no. 18 (2010): 8346–51. doi:10.1073/pnas.0909506107.

Choudhary, S., L. Gupta, S. Rani, K. Dave, and U. Gupta. "Impact of Dendrimers on Solubility of Hydrophobic Drug Molecules." *Frontiers in Pharmacology* 8 (2017): 261. doi:10.3389/fphar.2017.00261.

Chu, C. H., S. H. Cheng, N. T. Chen, W. N. Liao, and L. W. Lo. "Microwave-Synthesized Platinum-Embedded Mesoporous Silica Nanoparticles as Dual-Modality Contrast Agents: Computed Tomography and Optical Imaging." *International Journal of Molecular Sciences* 20, no. 7 (2019): 1560. doi:10.3390/ijms20071560.

Collier, J. H., and P. B. Messersmith. "Phospholipid Strategies in Biomineralization and Biomaterials Research." *Annul Rev Mater Res* 31, no. 1 (2001): 237–63. doi:10.1146/annurev.matsci.31.1.237.

Comfort, C., G. Garrastazu, M. Pozzoli, and F. Sonvico. "Opportunities and Challenges for the Nasal Administration of Nanoemulsions." *Current Topics in Medicinal Chemistry* 15, no. 4 (2015): 356–68. doi:10.2174/1568026615666150108144655.

Conde, J., J. T. Dias, V. Grazu, M. Moros, P. V. Baptista, and J. M. de la Fuente. "Revisiting 30 Years of Biofunctionalization and Surface Chemistry of Inorganic Nanoparticles for Nanomedicine." *Frontiers in Chemistry* 2 (2014): 48. doi:10.3389/fchem.2014.00048.

Costa, A., B. Sarmento, and V. Seabra. "Mannose-Functionalized Solid Lipid Nanoparticles Are Effective in Targeting Alveolar Macrophages." *European Journal of Pharmaceutical Sciences* 114 (2018): 103–13. doi:10.1016/j.ejps.2017.12.006.

Couvreur, P. "Nanomedicine: From Where Are We Coming and Where Are We Going?" *Journal of Controlled Release* 311–312 (2019): 319–21. doi:10.1016/j.jconrel.2019.10.020.

Cozad, M. J., S. L. Bachman, and S. A. Grant. "Assessment of Decellularized Porcine Diaphragm Conjugated with Gold Nanomaterials as a Tissue Scaffold for Wound Healing." *Journal of Biomedical Materials Research: Part A* 99, no. 3 (2011): 426–34. doi:10.1002/jbm.a.33182.

Craparo, E. F., C. Sardo, R. Serio, M. G. Zizzo, M. L. Bondì, G. Giammona, and G. Cavallaro. "Galactosylated Polymeric Carriers for Liver Targeting of Sorafenib." *International Journal of Pharmacy* 466, no. 1–2 (2014): 172–80. doi:10.1016/j.ijpharm.2014.02.047.

Croy, S. R., and G. S. Kwon. "Polymeric Micelles for Drug Delivery." *Current Pharmaceutical Design* 12, no. 36 (2006): 4669–84. doi:10.2174/138161206779026245.

Crucho, C. I. C., and M. T. Barros. "Polymeric Nanoparticles: A Study on the Preparation Variables and Characterization Methods." *Materials Science & Engineering C – Materials for Biological Applications* 80 (2017): 771–84. doi:10.1016/j.msec.2017.06.004.

Cui, F., K. Shi, L. Zhang, A. Tao, and Y. Kawashima. "Biodegradable Nanoparticles Loaded with Insulin-Phospholipid Complex for Oral Delivery: Preparation, In Vitro Characterization and In Vivo Evaluation." *Journal of Controlled Release* 114, no. 2 (2006): 242–50. doi:10.1016/j.jconrel.2006.05.013.

Cui, W., Q. Liu, L. Yang, K. Wang, T. Sun, Y. Ji, L. Liu, W. Yu, Y. Qu, J. Wang, Z. Zhao, J. Zhu, and X. Guo. "Sustained Delivery of BMP-2-related Peptide from the True Bone Ceramics/Hollow Mesoporous Silica Nanoparticles Scaffold for Bone Tissue Regeneration." *ACS Biomaterials Science & Engineering* 4, no. 1 (2018): 211–21. doi:10.1021/acsbiomaterials.7b00506.

Curran, M. P., and P. L. McCormack. "Methoxy Polyethylene Glycol–Epoetin Beta: A Review of Its Use in the Management of Anaemia Associated with Chronic Kidney Disease." *Drugs* 68, no. 8 (2008): 1139–56. doi:10.2165/00003495-200868080-00009.

D'Emanuele, A., R. Jevprasesphant, J. Penny, and D. Attwood. "The Use of a Dendrimer-Propranolol Prodrug to Bypass Efflux Transporters and Enhance Oral Bioavailability." *Journal of Controlled Release* 95, no. 3 (2004): 447–53. doi:10.1016/j.jconrel.2003.12.006.

Dai, C., H. Guo, J. Lu, J. Shi, J. Wei, and C. Liu. "Osteogenic Evaluation of Calcium/Magnesium-doped Mesoporous Silica Scaffold with Incorporation of rhBMP-2 by Synchrotron Radiation-based μCT." *Biomaterials* 32, no. 33 (2011): 8506–17. doi:10.1016/j.biomaterials.2011.07.090.

Dal Magro, R., F. Ornaghi, I. Cambianica, S. Beretta, F. Re, C. Musicanti, R. Rigolio, E. Donzelli, A. Canta, E. Ballarini, G. Cavaletti, P. Gasco, and G. Sancini. "ApoE-Modified Solid Lipid Nanoparticles: A Feasible Strategy to Cross the Blood-Brain Barrier." *Journal of Controlled Release* 249 (2017): 103–10. doi:10.1016/j.jconrel.2017.01.039.

Daou, T. J., L. Li, P. Reiss, V. Josserand, and I. Texier. "Effect of Poly(Ethylene Glycol) Length on the in vivo Behavior of Coated Quantum Dots." *Langmuir* 25, no. 5 (2009): 3040–3044. doi:10.1021/la8035083.

Dapkute, D., S. Steponkiene, D. Bulotiene, L. Saulite, U. Riekstina, and R. Rotomskis. "Skin-Derived Mesenchymal Stem Cells as Quantum Dot Vehicles to Tumors." *International Journal of Nanomedicine* 12 (2017): 8129–42. doi:10.2147/ijn.s143367.

Das, S. C., M. Hatta, P. R. Wilker, A. Myc, T. Hamouda, G. Neumann, J. R. Baker, Jr., and Y. Kawaoka. "Nanoemulsion W805EC Improves Immune Responses upon Intranasal Delivery of an Inactivated Pandemic H1N1 Influenza Vaccine." *Vaccine* 30, no. 48 (2012): 6871–6877. doi:10.1016/j.vaccine.2012.09.007.

das Neves J., F. Araújo, F. Andrade, J. Michiels, K. K. Ariën, G. Vanham, M. Amiji, M. F. Bahia, and B. Sarmento. "In vitro and ex vivo Evaluation of Polymeric Nanoparticles for Vaginal and Rectal Delivery of the Anti-HIV Drug Dapivirine." *Molecular Pharmaceutics* 10, no. 7 (2013): 2793–2807. doi:10.1021/mp4002365.

Dave, K., and V. V. K. Venuganti. "Dendritic Polymers for Dermal Drug Delivery." *Therapeutic Delivery* 8, no. 12 (2017): 1077–96. doi:10.4155/tde-2017-0091.

Dayan, N., and E. Touitou. "Carriers for Skin Delivery of Trihexyphenidyl HCl: Ethosomes vs. Liposomes." *Biomaterials* 21, no. 18 (2000): 1879–85. doi:10.1016/s0142-9612(00)00063-6.

de Leeuw, J., H. C. de Vijlder, P. Bjerring, and H. A. Neumann. "Liposomes in Dermatology Today." *Journal of the European Academy of Dermatology & Venereology* 23, no. 5 (2009): 505–16. doi:10.1111/j.1468-3083.2009.03100.x.

de Vlieger, Jon S. B., Daan J. A. Crommelin, Katherine Tyner, Daryl C. Drummond, Wenlei Jiang, Scott E. McNeil, Sesha Neervannan, Rachael M. Crist, and Vinod P. Shah. "Report of the AAPS Guidance Forum on the FDA Draft Guidance for Industry: 'Drug Products, Including Biological Products, That Contain Nanomaterials'." *AAPS Journal* 21, no. 4 (2019): 56. doi:10.1208/s12248-019-0329-7.

Derfus, A. M., W. C. W. Chan, and S. N. Bhatia. "Intracellular Delivery of Quantum Dots for Live Cell Labeling and Organelle Tracking." *Advanced Materials* 16, no. 12 (2004): 961–6. doi:10.1002/adma.200306111.

Deyev, S., G. Proshkina, A. Ryabova, F. Tavanti, M. C. Menziani, G. Eidelshtein, G. Avishai, and A. Kotlyar. "Synthesis, Characterization, and Selective Delivery of DARPin-Gold Nanoparticle Conjugates to Cancer Cells." *Bioconjugate Chemistry* 28, no. 10 (2017): 2569–74. doi:10.1021/acs.bioconjchem.7b00410.

Dimitri, A., and M. Talamo. "The Use of Data Mining and Machine Learning in Nanomedicine: A Survey." *Front Nanosci Nanotech* 4, no. 3 (2018): 1–7. doi:10.15761/FNN.1000S1004.

Ding, Z., P. Liu, D. Hu, Z. Sheng, H. Yi, G. Gao, Y. Wu, P. Zhang, S. Ling, and L. Cai. "Redox-Responsive Dextran Based Theranostic Nanoparticles for Near-Infrared/Magnetic Resonance Imaging and Magnetically Targeted Photodynamic Therapy." *Biomaterials Science* 5, no. 4 (2017): 762–71. doi:10.1039/C6BM00846A.

Discher, B. M., Y.-Y. Won, D. S. Ege, J. C.-M. Lee, F. S. Bates, D. E. Discher, and D. A. Hammer. "Polymersomes: Tough Vesicles Made from Diblock Copolymers." *Science* 284, no. 5417 (1999): 1143–6. doi:10.1126/science.284.5417.1143.

Dixit, S., T. Novak, K. Miller, Y. Zhu, M. E. Kenney, and A. M. Broome. "Transferrin Receptor-targeted Theranostic Gold Nanoparticles for Photosensitizer Delivery in Brain Tumors." *Nanoscale* 7, no. 5 (2015): 1782–90. doi:10.1039/c4nr04853a.

Dowaidar, M., H. N. Abdelhamid, M. Hällbrink, K. Freimann, K. Kurrikoff, X. Zou, and Ü. Langel. "Magnetic Nanoparticle Assisted Self-Assembly of Cell Penetrating Peptides-Oligonucleotides Complexes for Gene Delivery." *Scientific Reports* 7, no. 1 (2017): 9159. doi:10.1038/s41598-017-09803-z.

Downing, M. A., and P. K. Jain. "Chapter 16: Mesoporous Silica Nanoparticles: Synthesis, Properties, and Biomedical Applications." In *Nanoparticles for Biomedical Applications*, edited by E. J. Chung, L. Leon, and C. Rinaldi, 267–81. Amsterdam: Elsevier, 2020.

Drexler, K. E., C. Peterson, and G. Pergamit. *Unbounding the Future: The Nanotechnology Revolution*. New York: Morrow, 1991.

Duan, Y., A. Dhar, C. Patel, M. Khimani, S. Neogi, P. Sharma, N. Siva Kumar, and R. L. Vekariya. "A Brief Review on Solid Lipid Nanoparticles: Part and Parcel of Contemporary Drug Delivery Systems." *RSC Advances* 10, no. 45 (2020): 26777–91. doi:10.1039/D0RA03491F.

Duangjit, S., P. Opanasopit, T. Rojanarata, and T. Ngawhirunpat. "Effect of Edge Activator on Characteristic and In Vitro Skin Permeation of Meloxicam Loaded in Elastic Liposomes." *Advances in Materials Research* 194–196 (2011): 537–40. doi:10.4028/www.scientific.net/AMR.194-196.537.

Dubey, V., D. Mishra, T. Dutta, M. Nahar, D. K. Saraf, and N. K. Jain. "Dermal and Transdermal Delivery of an Anti-Psoriatic Agent via Ethanolic Liposomes." *Journal of Controlled Release* 123, no. 2 (2007): 148–54. doi:10.1016/j.jconrel.2007.08.005.

Duncan, R., and L. Izzo. "Dendrimer Biocompatibility and Toxicity." *Advanced Drug Delivery Reviews* 57, no. 15 (2005): 2215–37. doi:10.1016/j.addr.2005.09.019.

EC. "Commission Recommendation: Commission Recommendation of 18 October 2011 on the Definition of Nanomaterial 2011/696/EU." 2011. Accessed 30/12/2020. https://ec.europa.eu/research/industrial_technologies/pdf/policy/commission-recommendation-on-the-definition-of-nanomater-18102011_en.pdf.

Edgar, J. Y. C., and H. Wang. "Introduction for Design of Nanoparticle Based Drug Delivery Systems." *Current Pharmaceutical Design* 23, no. 14 (2017): 2108–12. doi:10.2174/1381612822666161025154003.

Editorial. "Nanomedicine and the COVID-19 Vaccines." *Nature Nanotechnology* 15, no. 12 (2020): 963–. doi:10.1038/s41565-020-00820-0.

Ekladious, I., Y. L. Colson, and M. W. Grinstaff. "Polymer–Drug Conjugate Therapeutics: Advances, Insights and Prospects." *Nature Reviews. Drug Discovery* 18, no. 4 (2019): 273–94. doi:10.1038/s41573-018-0005-0.

Ellison, P. A., F. Chen, S. Goel, T. E. Barnhart, R. J. Nickles, O. T. DeJesus, and W. Cai. "Intrinsic and Stable Conjugation of Thiolated Mesoporous Silica Nanoparticles with Radioarsenic." *ACS Applied Materials & Interfaces* 9, no. 8 (2017): 6772–81. doi:10.1021/acsami.6b14049.

El-Nahas, A. E., A. N. Allam, and A. H. El-Kamel. "Mucoadhesive Buccal Tablets Containing Silymarin Eudragit-loaded Nanoparticles: Formulation, Characterisation and ex vivo Permeation." *Journal of Microencapsulation* 34, no. 5 (2017): 463–474. doi:10.1080/02652048.2017.1345996.

Eroglu, Y. I. "A Comparative Review of Haute Autorité de Santé and National Institute for Health and Care Excellence Health Technology Assessments of Ikervis® to Treat Severe Keratitis in Adult Patients with Dry Eye Disease Which Has Not Improved Despite Treatment with Tear Substitutes." *Journal of Market Access & Health Policy* 5, no. 1 (2017):1336043–1336043. doi:10.1080/20016689.2017.1336043.

Esposito, E., E. Menegatti, and R. Cortesi. "Ethosomes and Liposomes as Topical Vehicles for Azelaic Acid: A Preformulation Study." *Journal of Cosmetic Science* 55, no. 3 (2004): 253–64. doi:10.1111/j.1467-2494.2004.00233_2.x.

Estelrich, J., E. Escribano, J. Queralt, and M. A. Busquets. "Iron Oxide Nanoparticles for Magnetically-Guided and Magnetically-Responsive Drug Delivery." *International Journal of Molecular Sciences* 16, no. 4 (2015): 8070–101. doi:10.3390/ijms16048070.

Etrych, T., V. Subr, J. Strohalm, M. Šírová, B. Ríhová, and K. Ulbrich. "HPMA Copolymer-Doxorubicin Conjugates: The Effects of Molecular Weight and Architecture on Biodistribution and In Vivo Activity." *Journal of Controlled Release* 164, no. 3 (2012): 346–54. doi:10.1016/j.jconrel.2012.06.029.

Fadeel, Bengt, and Christoph Alexiou. "Brave New World Revisited: Focus on Nanomedicine." *Biochemical & Biophysical Research Communications* 533, no. 1 (2020): 36–49. doi:10.1016/j.bbrc.2020.08.046.

Fam, S. Y., C. F. Chee, C. Y. Yong, K. L. Ho, A. R. Mariatulqabtiah, and W. S. Tan. "Stealth Coating of Nanoparticles in Drug-delivery Systems." *Nanomaterials* 10, no. 4 (2020): 787. doi:10.3390/nano10040787.

Faria, M. J., R. Machado, A. Ribeiro, H. Goncalves, M. E. C. D. Real Oliveira, T. Viseu, J. das Neves, and M. Lucio. "Rational Development of Liposomal Hydrogels: A Strategy for Topical Vaginal Antiretroviral Drug Delivery in the Context of HIV Prevention." *Pharmaceutics* 11, no. 9 (2019): 485. doi:10.3390/pharmaceutics11090485.

Farias, P. M., A. C. D. Andrade, R. Milani, Y. P. Ruiz, T. Tabosa, A. Galembeck, and A. Stingl. "Quantum Dots Pushing up In Vitro Diagnostics Limits." *Proceedings of the SPIE* 10077 (2017): 1007708.

Farjadian, F., S. Ghasemi, and S. Mohammadi-Samani. "Hydroxyl-Modified Magnetite Nanoparticles as Novel Carrier for Delivery of Methotrexate." *International Journal of Pharmacy* 504, no. 1–2 (2016): 110–6. doi:10.1016/j.ijpharm.2016.03.022.

Farjadian, F., S. Ghasemi, R. Heidari, and S. Mohammadi-Samani. "In vitro and in vivo Assessment of EDTA-modified Silica Nano-spheres with Supreme Capacity of Iron Capture as a Novel Antidote Agent." *Nanomedicine* 13, no. 2 (2017): 745–53. doi:10.1016/j.nano.2016.10.012.

Farjadian, F., A. Ghasemi, O. Gohari, A. Roointan, M. Karimi, and M. R. Hamblin. "Nanopharmaceuticals and Nanomedicines Currently on the Market: Challenges and Opportunities." *Nanomedicine* 14, no. 1 (2019): 93–126. doi:10.2217/nnm-2018-0120.

Fatima, S., Z. Iqbal, A. K. Panda, S. Samim, S. Talegaonkar, and F. J. Ahmad. "Polymeric Nanoparticles as a Platform for Permeability Enhancement of Class III Drug Amikacin." *Colloids Surf B Biointerfaces* 169 (2018): 206–213. doi:10.1016/j.colsurfb.2018.05.028.

FDA. "U.S. Food and Drug Administration CDER. Guidance for Industry: PAT–A Framework for Innovative Pharmaceutical Development, Manufacturing, and Quality Assurance." 2004. Accessed 10/02/2018. https://www.fda.gov/downloads/drugs/guidances/ucm070305.pdf.

FDA. "Considering Whether an FDA-Regulated Product Involves the Application of Nanotechnology, Guidance for Industry 2014." n.d. Accessed 31/12/2020. https://www.fda.gov/media/88423/download.

FDA. "Drug Products, Including Biological Products, That Contain Nanomaterials: Guidance for Industry 2017." Accessed 31/12/2020. https://www.fda.gov/files/drugs/published/Drug-Products--Including-Biological-Products--that-Contain-Nanomaterials---Guidance-for-Industry.pdf.

Fernandes, E., T. B. Soares, H. Gonçalves, and M. Lúcio. "Spectroscopic Studies as a Toolbox for Biophysical and Chemical Characterization of Lipid-Based Nanotherapeutics." *Frontiers in Chemistry* 6, no. 323 (2018). doi:10.3389/fchem.2018.00323.

Fernández-García, R., A. Lalatsa, L. Statts, F. Bolás-Fernández, M. P. Ballesteros, and D. R. Serrano. "Transferosomes as Nanocarriers for Drugs Across the Skin: Quality by Design from Lab to Industrial Scale." *International Journal of Pharmacy* 573 (2020): 118817. doi:10.1016/j.ijpharm.2019.118817.

Ferreira, C., S. Goel, D. Jiang, E. Ehlerding, E. Aluicio-Sarduy, J. Engle, and W. Cai. "86/90Y-Labeled Ultrasmall Mesoporous Silica Nanoparticles for Cancer Theranostics." *Journal of Nuclear Medicine* 59, no. 3 (Suppl. 1) (2018): 468–.

Feynman, R. P. "There's Plenty of Room at the Bottom." *Journal of Engineering Sciences* 4, no. 2 (1960): 23–36.

Fleischer, S., M. Shevach, R. Feiner, and T. Dvir. "Coiled Fiber Scaffolds Embedded with Gold Nanoparticles Improve the Performance of Engineered Cardiac Tissues." *Nanoscale* 6, no. 16 (2014): 9410–9414. doi:10.1039/c4nr00300d.

Forni, G., A. Mantovani, L. Moretta, R. Rappuoli, G. Rezza, A. Bagnasco, G. Barsacchi, G. Bussolati, M. Cacciari, P. Cappuccinelli, E. Cheli, R. Guarini, M. L. Bacci, M. Mancini, C. Marcuzzo, M. C. Morrone, G. Parisi, C. Patrono, A. Q. Curzio, G. Remuzzi, A. Roncaglia, S. Schiaffino, P. Vineis, and Rome on behalf of the Covid-19 Commission of Accademia Nazionale dei Lincei. "COVID-19 Vaccines: Where We Stand and Challenges Ahead." *Cell Death & Disease* 28, no. 2 (2021): 626–39. doi:10.1038/s41418-020-00720-9.

Foster, C. S., R. Davanzo, T. E. Flynn, K. McLeod, R. Vogel, and R. S. Crockett. "Durezol (Difluprednate Ophthalmic Emulsion 0.05%) Compared with Pred Forte 1% Ophthalmic Suspension in the Treatment of Endogenous Anterior Uveitis." *Journal of Ocular Pharmacology & Therapeutics* 26, no. 5 (2010): 475–83. doi:10.1089/jop.2010.0059.

Foulkes, Rachel, Ernest Man, Jasmine Thind, Suet Yeung, Abigail Joy, and Clare Hoskins. "The Regulation of Nanomaterials and Nanomedicines for Clinical Application: Current and Future Perspectives." *Biomaterials Science* 8, no. 17 (2020): 4653–64. doi:10.1039/D0BM00558D.

Frank, L. A., G. Sandri, F. D'Autilia, R. V. Contri, M. C. Bonferoni, C. Caramella, A. G. Frank, A. R. Pohlmann, and S. S. Guterres. "Chitosan Gel Containing Polymeric Nanocapsules: A New Formulation for Vaginal Drug Delivery." *International Journal of Nanomedicine* 9 (2014): 3151–3161. doi:10.2147/ijn.s62599.

Freestone, I., N. Meeks, M. Sax, and C. Higgitt. "The Lycurgus Cup: A Roman Nanotechnology." *Gold Bulletin* 40, no. 4 (2007): 270–7. doi:10.1007/BF03215599.

Fu, X., Y. Shi, T. Qi, S. Qiu, Y. Huang, X. Zhao, Q. Sun, and G. Lin. "Precise Design Strategies of Nanomedicine for Improving Cancer Therapeutic Efficacy Using Subcellular Targeting." *Signal Transduction & Targeted Therapy* 5, no. 1 (2020): 262. doi:10.1038/s41392-020-00342-0.

Gainza, G., M. Pastor, J. J. Aguirre, S. Villullas, J. L. Pedraz, R. M. Hernandez, and M. Igartua. "A Novel Strategy for the Treatment of Chronic Wounds Based on the Topical Administration of rhEGF-Loaded Lipid Nanoparticles: In Vitro Bioactivity and In Vivo Effectiveness in Healing-Impaired Db/Db Mice." *Journal of Controlled Release* 185 (2014): 51–61. doi:10.1016/j.jconrel.2014.04.032.

Ganesan, P., and D. Narayanasamy. "Lipid Nanoparticles: Different Preparation Techniques, Characterization, Hurdles, and Strategies for the Production of Solid Lipid Nanoparticles and Nanostructured Lipid Carriers for Oral Drug Delivery." *Sustainable Chemistry & Pharmacy* 6 (2017): 37–56. doi:10.1016/j.scp.2017.07.002.

Ganta, S., A. Singh, P. Kulkarni, A. W. Keeler, A. Piroyan, R. R. Sawant, N. R. Patel, B. Davis, C. Ferris, S. O'Neal, W. Zamboni, M. M. Amiji, and T. P. Coleman. "EGFR Targeted Theranostic Nanoemulsion for Image-Guided Ovarian Cancer Therapy." *Pharmaceutical Research* 32, no. 8 (2015): 2753–63. doi:10.1007/s11095-015-1660-z.

Gao, F., P. Botella, A. Corma, J. Blesa, and L. Dong. "Monodispersed Mesoporous Silica Nanoparticles with Very Large Pores for Enhanced Adsorption and Release of DNA." *Journal of Physical Chemistry. Part B* 113, no. 6 (2009): 1796–804. doi:10.1021/jp807956r.

Gaspar, Rogério. "Nanomedicine: Nanomedicine: Current View, Present and Future Main Regulatory Current View, Present and Future Main Regulatory Challenges Challenges." 2009. Accessed 22/01/2021. https://www.ema.europa.eu/en/documents/presentation/nanomedicine-current-view-present-future-main-regulatory-challenges-rogacrio-gaspar_en.pdf.

Gaspar, R. "Therapeutic Products: Regulating Drugs and Medical Devices." In *International Handbook on Regulating Nanotechnologies*, edited by G. A. Hodge, D. M. Bowman, and A. D. Maynard, 291–320. Cheltenham: Edward Elgar Publishing, 2010.

Gaspar, Rogério S., Helena F. Florindo, Liana C. Silva, Mafalda A. Videira, M. Luísa Corvo, Bárbara F. Martins, and Beatriz Silva-Lima. "Regulatory Aspects of Oncologicals: Nanosystems Main Challenges." In *Nano-Oncologicals: New Targeting and Delivery Approaches*, edited by Maria José Alonso, and Marcos Garcia-Fuentes, 425–52. Cham: Springer, 2014.

Geng, J., M. Li, L. Wu, C. Chen, and X. Qu. "Mesoporous Silica Nanoparticle-Based H2O2 Responsive Controlled-Release System Used for Alzheimer's Disease Treatment." *Advanced Healthcare Materials* 1, no. 3 (2012): 332–6. doi:10.1002/adhm.201200067.

Gholipourmalekabadi, M., M. Mobaraki, M. Ghaffari, A. Zarebkohan, V. F. Omrani, A. M. Urbanska, and A. Seifalian. "Targeted Drug Delivery Based on Gold Nanoparticle Derivatives." *Current Pharmaceutical Design* 23, no. 20 (2017): 2918–29. doi:10.2174/1381612823666170419105413.

Giubilato, E., V. Cazzagon, M. J. B. Amorim, M. Blosi, J. Bouillard, H. Bouwmeester, A. L. Costa, B. Fadeel, T. F. Fernandes, C. Fito, M. Hauser, A. Marcomini, B. Nowack, L. Pizzol, L. Powell, A. Prina-Mello, H. Sarimveis, J. J. Scott-Fordsmand, E. Semenzin, B. Stahlmecke, V. Stone, A. Vignes, T. Wilkins, A. Zabeo, L. Tran, and D. Hristozov. "Risk Management Framework for Nano-Biomaterials Used in Medical Devices and Advanced Therapy Medicinal Products." *Materials* 13, no. 20 (2020). doi:10.3390/ma13204532.

Goel, S., F. Chen, S. Luan, H. F. Valdovinos, S. Shi, S. A. Graves, F. Ai, T. E. Barnhart, C. P. Theuer, and W. Cai. "Engineering Intrinsically Zirconium-89 Radiolabeled Self-Destructing Mesoporous Silica Nanostructures for In Vivo Biodistribution and Tumor Targeting Studies." *Advancement of Science* 3, no. 11 (2016): 1600122. doi:10.1002/advs.201600122.

Gong, H., Z. Xie, M. Liu, H. Sun, H. Zhu, and H. Guo. "Research on Redox-Responsive Mesoporous Silica Nanoparticles Functionalized with PEG via a Disulfide Bond Linker as Drug Carrier Materials." *Colloid & Polymer Science* 293, no. 7 (2015): 2121–8. doi:10.1007/s00396-015-3595-7.

González-Paredes, A., L. Sitia, A. Ruyra, C. J. Morris, G. N. Wheeler, M. McArthur, and P. Gasco. "Solid Lipid Nanoparticles for the Delivery of Anti-Microbial Oligonucleotides." *European Journal of Pharmaceutics & Biopharmaceutics* 134 (2019): 166–77. doi:10.1016/j.ejpb.2018.11.017.

Gorain, B., M. Tekade, P. Kesharwani, A. K. Iyer, K. Kalia, and R. K. Tekade. "The Use of Nanoscaffolds and Dendrimers in Tissue Engineering." *Drug Discovery Today* 22, no. 4 (2017): 652–64. doi:10.1016/j.drudis.2016.12.007.

Goreham, R. V., A. Mierczynska, L. E. Smith, R. Sedev, and K. Vasilev. "Small Surface Nanotopography Encourages Fibroblast and Osteoblast Cell Adhesion." *RSC Advances* 3, no. 26 (2013): 10309–17. doi:10.1039/C3RA23193C.

Gote, V., S. Sikder, J. Sicotte, and D. Pal. "Ocular Drug Delivery: Present Innovations and Future Challenges." *Journal of Pharmacology & Experimental Therapeutics* 370, no. 3 (2019): 602–24. doi:10.1124/jpet.119.256933.

Graham, M. L. "Pegaspargase: A Review of Clinical Studies." *Advanced Drug Delivery Reviews* 55, no. 10 (2003): 1293–302. doi:10.1016/s0169-409x(03)00110-8.

Greish, K., A. Mathur, M. Bakhiet, and S. Taurin. "Nanomedicine: Is it Lost in Translation?" *Therapeutic Delivery* 9, no. 4 (2018): 269–85. doi:10.4155/tde-2017-0118.

Grillo, R., J. Gallo, D. G. Stroppa, E. Carbó-Argibay, R. Lima, L. F. Fraceto, and M. Bañobre-López. "Sub-Micrometer Magnetic Nanocomposites: Insights into the Effect of Magnetic Nanoparticles Interactions on the Optimization of SAR and MRI Performance." *ACS Applied Materials & Interfaces* 8, no. 39 (2016): 25777–87. doi:10.1021/acsami.6b08663.

Gu, L., D. J. Hall, Z. Qin, E. Anglin, J. Joo, D. J. Mooney, S. B. Howell, and M. J. Sailor. "In Vivo Time-Gated Fluorescence Imaging with Biodegradable Luminescent Porous Silicon Nanoparticles." *Nature Communications* 4, no. 1 (2013): 2326. doi:10.1038/ncomms3326.

Guibert, C., V. Dupuis, V. Peyre, and J. Fresnais. "Hyperthermia of Magnetic Nanoparticles: Experimental Study of the Role of Aggregation." *Journal of Physical Chemistry C* 119, no. 50 (2015): 28148–54. doi:10.1021/acs.jpcc.5b07796.

Guo, X., J. Zhu, H. Zhang, Z. You, Y. Morsi, X. Mo, and T. Zhu. "Facile Preparation of a Controlled-Release Tubular Scaffold for Blood Vessel Implantation." *Journal of Colloid & Interface Science* 539 (2019): 351–60. doi:10.1016/j.jcis.2018.12.086.

Guo, Y., S. Li, J. Liu, G. Yang, Z. Sun, and J. Wan. "Double Functional Aptamer Switch Probes Based on Gold Nanorods for Intracellular ATP Detection and Targeted Drugs Transportation." *Sensors & Actuators. Part B* 235 (2016): 655–62. doi:10.1016/j.snb.2016.05.131.

Gupta, N., D. B. Rai, A. K. Jangid, and D. Pooja, and H. Kulhari. "Nanomaterials-based siRNA Delivery: Routes of Administration, Hurdles and Role of Nanocarriers." In *Nanotechnology in Modern Animal Biotechnology: Recent Trends and Future Perspectives*, edited by S. Singh, and P. K. Maurya, 67–114. Singapore: Springer, 2019.

Hagigit, T., M. Abdulrazik, F. Valamanesh, F. Behar-Cohen, and S. Benita. "Ocular Antisense Oligonucleotide Delivery by Cationic Nanoemulsion for Improved Treatment of Ocular Neovascularization: An In-Vivo Study in Rats and Mice." *Journal of Controlled Release* 160, no. 2 (2012): 225–31. doi:10.1016/j.jconrel.2011.11.022.

Ha-Lien Tran, P., T. Wang, C. Yang, T. T. D. Tran, and W. Duan. "Development of Conjugate-by-Conjugate Structured Nanoparticles for Oral Delivery of Docetaxel." *Materials Science and Engineering C: Materials for Biological Applications* 107 (2020): 110346. doi:10.1016/j.msec.2019.110346.

Hamaguchi, T., Y. Matsumura, M. Suzuki, K. Shimizu, R. Goda, I. Nakamura, I. Nakatomi, M. Yokoyama, K. Kataoka, and T. Kakizoe. "NK105, a Paclitaxel-Incorporating Micellar Nanoparticle Formulation, Can Extend In Vivo Antitumour Activity and Reduce the Neurotoxicity of Paclitaxel." *British Journal of Cancer* 92, no. 7 (2005): 1240–6. doi:10.1038/sj.bjc.6602479.

Has, C., and P. Sunthar. "A Comprehensive Review on Recent Preparation Techniques of Liposomes." *Journal of Liposome Research* 30, no. 4 (2019): 336–65. doi:10.1080/08982104.2019.1668010.

Hayashi, K., K. Ono, H. Suzuki, M. Sawada, M. Moriya, W. Sakamoto, and T. Yogo. "High-Frequency, Magnetic-Field-Responsive Drug Release from Magnetic Nanoparticle/Organic Hybrid Based on Hyperthermic Effect." *ACS Applied Materials & Interfaces* 2, no. 7 (2010): 1903–11. doi:10.1021/am100237p.

Hayek, S. S. "Synthesis and Characterization of CeGdZn-Ferrite Nanoparticles as Magnetic Hyperthermia Application Agents." *Advances in Materials Science & Engineering* 2019 (2019): 4868506 doi:10.1155/2019/4868506.

Hearnden, V., H. Lomas, S. Macneil, M. Thornhill, C. Murdoch, A. Lewis, J. Madsen, A. Blanazs, S. Armes, and G. Battaglia. "Diffusion Studies of Nanometer Polymersomes Across Tissue Engineered Human Oral Mucosa." *Pharmaceutical Research* 26, no. 7 (2009): 1718–28. doi:10.1007/s11095-009-9882-6.

Henriques, João, João Sousa, Francisco Veiga, Catarina Cardoso, and Carla Vitorino. "Process Analytical Technologies and Injectable Drug Products: Is There a Future?" *International Journal of Pharmaceutics* 554 (2019): 21–35. doi:10.1016/j.ijpharm.2018.10.070.

Heo, D. N., W.-K. Ko, M. S. Bae, J. B. Lee, D.-W. Lee, W. Byun, C. H. Lee, E.-C. Kim, B.-Y. Jung, and I. K. Kwon. "Enhanced Bone Regeneration with a Gold Nanoparticle–Hydrogel Complex." *Journal of Materials Chemistry B* 2, no. 11 (2014): 1584–93. doi:10.1039/C3TB21246G.

Hild, W. A., M. Breunig, and A. Goepferich. "Quantum Dots – Nano-Sized Probes for the Exploration of Cellular and Intracellular Targeting." *European Journal of Pharmaceutics & Biopharmaceutics* 68, no. 2 (2008): 153–68. doi:10.1016/j.ejpb.2007.06.009.

Ho, Dean, Peter Wang, and Theodore Kee. "Artificial Intelligence in Nanomedicine." *Nanoscale Horizons* 4, no. 2 (2019): 365–77. doi:10.1039/C8NH00233A.

Hoch, U., C. M. Staschen, R. K. Johnson, and M. A. Eldon. "Nonclinical Pharmacokinetics and Activity of Etirinotecan Pegol (NKTR-102), a Long-Acting Topoisomerase 1 Inhibitor, in Multiple Cancer Models." *Cancer Chemotherapy & Pharmacology* 74, no. 6 (2014): 1125–37. doi:10.1007/s00280-014-2577-7.

Hong, S.-P., S. H. Kang, D. K. Kim, and B. S. Kang. "Paramagnetic Gd_2O_3 Nanoparticle-Based Targeting Theranostic Agent for C6 Rat Glioma Cell." *Journal of Nanomaterials* 2016 (2016). doi:10.1155/2016/7617894, PubMed: 7617894.

Hörmann, K., and A. Zimmer. "Drug Delivery and Drug Targeting with Parenteral Lipid Nanoemulsions: A Review." *Journal of Controlled Release* 223 (2016): 85–98. doi:10.1016/j.jconrel.2015.12.016.

Houshmand, M., F. Garello, P. Circosta, R. Stefania, S. Aime, G. Saglio, and C. Giachino. "Nanocarriers as Magic Bullets in the Treatment of Leukemia." *Nanomaterials* 10, no. 2 (2020): 276. doi:10.3390/nano10020276.

Hsieh, S. C., F. F. Wang, C. S. Lin, Y. J. Chen, S. C. Hung, and Y. J. Wang. "The Inhibition of Osteogenesis with Human Bone Marrow Mesenchymal Stem Cells by CdSe/ZnS Quantum Dot Labels." *Biomaterials* 27, no. 8 (2006): 1656–64. doi:10.1016/j.biomaterials.2005.09.004.

Hu, Q., C. J. Rijcken, R. Bansal, W. E. Hennink, G. Storm, and J. Prakash. "Complete Regression of Breast Tumour with a Single Dose of Docetaxel-entrapped Core-cross-linked Polymeric Micelles." *Biomaterials* 53 (2015): 370–378. doi:10.1016/j.biomaterials.2015.02.085.

Huang, S. L., P. X. Ling, and T. M. Zhang. "Oral Absorption of Hyaluronic Acid and Phospholipids Complexes in Rats." *World Journal of Gastroenterology* 13, no. 6 (2007): 945–9. doi:10.3748/wjg.v13.i6.945.

Huefner, A., D. Septiadi, B. D. Wilts, I. I. Patel, W.-L. Kuan, A. Fragniere, R. A. Barker, and S. Mahajan. "Gold Nanoparticles Explore Cells: Cellular Uptake and Their Use as Intracellular Probes." *Methods* 68, no. 2 (2014): 354–63. doi:10.1016/j.ymeth.2014.02.006.

Hussain, M., M. Shchepinov, M. Sohail, I. F. Benter, A. J. Hollins, E. M. Southern, and S. Akhtar. "A Novel Anionic Dendrimer for Improved Cellular Delivery of Antisense Oligonucleotides." *Journal of Controlled Release* 99, no. 1 (2004): 139–55. doi:10.1016/j.jconrel.2004.06.009.

"ICHQ8." *Q8: Pharmaceutical Development.* 2017. Accessed 22/01/2021. https://www.ema.europa.eu/en/documents/scientific-guideline/international-conference-harmonisation-technical-requirements-registration-pharmaceuticals-human-use_en-11.pdf.

"ICHQ9." *ICH Guideline Q9 on Quality Risk Management.* 2015. Accessed 22/01/2021. https://www.ema.europa.eu/en/documents/scientific-guideline/international-conference-harmonisation-technical-requirements-registration-pharmaceuticals-human-use_en-3.pdf.

"ICHQ10." *ICH Guideline Q10 on Pharmaceutical Quality System.* 2017. Accessed 22/01/2021. https://www.ema.europa.eu/en/documents/scientific-guideline/international-conference-harmonisation-technical-requirements-registration-pharmaceuticals-human_en.pdf.

"ICHQ12." *ICH Guideline Q12 on Technical and Regulatory Considerations for Pharmaceutical Product Lifecycle Management.* 2020. Accessed 22/01/2021. https://www.ema.europa.eu/en/documents/scientific-guideline/ich-guideline-q12-technical-regulatory-considerations-pharmaceutical-product-lifecycle-management_en.pdf.

Iezzi, R., B. R. Guru, I. V. Glybina, M. K. Mishra, A. Kennedy, and R. M. Kannan. "Dendrimer-based Targeted Intravitreal Therapy for Sustained Attenuation of Neuroinflammation in Retinal Degeneration." *Biomaterials* 33, no. 3 (2012): 979–88. doi:10.1016/j.biomaterials.2011.10.010.

Indrasekara, A. S., B. J. Paladini, D. J. Naczynski, V. Starovoytov, P. V. Moghe, and L. Fabris. "Dimeric Gold Nanoparticle Assemblies as Tags for SERS-Based Cancer Detection." *Advanced Healthcare Materials* 2, no. 10 (2013): 1370–6. doi:10.1002/adhm.201200370.

Iqbal, N., C. Vitorino, and K. M. G. Taylor. "How Can Lipid Nanocarriers Improve Transdermal Delivery of Olanzapine?. " *Pharmaceutical Development & Technology* 22, no. 4 (2017): 587–96. doi:10.1080/10837450.2016.1200615.

Ishii, M., R. Shibata, Y. Numaguchi, T. Kito, H. Suzuki, H. Shimizu, A. Ito, H. Honda, and T. Murohara. "Enhanced Angiogenesis by Transplantation of Mesenchymal Stem Cell Sheet Created by a Novel Magnetic Tissue Engineering Method." *Arteriosclerosis, Thrombosis, & Vascular Biology* 31, no. 10 (2011): 2210–5. doi:doi. doi:10.1161/ATVBAHA.111.231100.

Ito, A., Y. Takizawa, H. Honda, K. Hata, H. Kagami, M. Ueda, and T. Kobayashi. "Tissue Engineering Using Magnetite Nanoparticles and Magnetic Force: Heterotypic Layers of Cocultured Hepatocytes and Endothelial Cells." *Tissue Engineering* 10, no. 5–6 (2004): 833–40. doi:10.1089/1076327041348301.

Ito, A., E. Hibino, C. Kobayashi, H. Terasaki, H. Kagami, M. Ueda, T. Kobayashi, and H. Honda. "Construction and Delivery of Tissue-Engineered Human Retinal Pigment Epithelial Cell Sheets, Using Magnetite Nanoparticles and Magnetic Force." *Tissue Engineering* 11, no. 3–4 (2005a): 489–96. doi:10.1089/ten.2005.11.489.

Ito, A., K. Ino, T. Kobayashi, and H. Honda. "The effect of RGD peptide-conjugated magnetite cationic liposomes on cell growth and cell sheet harvesting." *Biomaterials* 26, no. 31 (2005b): 6185–93. doi:10.1016/j.biomaterials.2005.03.039.

Ito, A., K. Ino, K. Shimizu, H. Honda, and M. Kamihira. "Fabrication of 3D Tissue-like Structure Using Magnetite Nanoparticles and Magnetic Force." Paper Read at 2006 IEEE International Symposium on MicroNanoMechanical and Human Science. Nagoya, Japan, 5–8 Nov. 2006, 2006.

Ito, A., H. Jitsunobu, Y. Kawabe, and M. Kamihira. "Construction of Heterotypic Cell Sheets by Magnetic Force-Based 3-D Coculture of HepG2 and NIH3T3 Cells." *Journal of Bioscience & Bioengineering* 104, no. 5 (2007): 371–8. doi:10.1263/jbb.104.371.

Izadifar, M., M. E. Kelly, and X. Chen. "Regulation of Sequential Release of Growth Factors Using Bilayer Polymeric Nanoparticles for Cardiac Tissue Engineering." *Nanomedicine* 11, no. 24 (2016): 3237–59. doi:10.2217/nnm-2016-0220.

Jackman, J. A., J. Lee, and N. J. Cho. "Nanomedicine for Infectious Disease Applications: Innovation Towards Broad-spectrum Treatment of Viral Infections." *Small* 12, no. 9 (2016): 1133–9. doi:10.1002/smll.201500854.

Jahed, V., E. Vasheghani-Farahani, F. Bagheri, A. Zarrabi, H. H. Jensen, and K. L. Larsen. "Quantum Dots-βcyclodextrin-histidine Labeled Human Adipose Stem Cells-laden Chitosan Hydrogel for Bone Tissue Engineering." *Nanomedicine* 27: (2020): 102217. doi:10.1016/j.nano.2020.102217.

Jameson, G. S., J. T. Hamm, G. J. Weiss, C. Alemany, S. Anthony, M. Basche, R. K. Ramanathan, M. J. Borad, R. Tibes, A. Cohn, I. Hinshaw, R. Jotte, L. S. Rosen, U. Hoch, M. A. Eldon, R. Medve, K. Schroeder, E. White, and D. D. Von Hoff. "A Multicenter, Phase I, Dose-Escalation Study to Assess the Safety, Tolerability, and Pharmacokinetics of Etirinotecan Pegol in Patients with Refractory Solid Tumors." *Clinical Cancer Research* 19, no. 1 (2013): 268–78. doi:10.1158/1078-0432.ccr-12-1201.

Jangdey, M. S., A. Gupta, S. Saraf, and S. Saraf. "Development and Optimization of Apigenin-Loaded Transfersomal System for Skin Cancer Delivery: In Vitro Evaluation." *Artificial Cells, Nanomedicine & Biotechnology* 45, no. 7 (2017): 1452–62. doi:10.1080/21691401.2016.1247850.

Jeong, H. J., R. J. Yoo, J. K. Kim, M. H. Kim, S. H. Park, H. Kim, J. W. Lim, S. H. Do, K. C. Lee, Y. J. Lee, and D. W. Kim. "Macrophage Cell Tracking PET Imaging Using Mesoporous Silica Nanoparticles via in vivo Bioorthogonal F-18 Labeling." *Biomaterials* 199: 32–39 (2019). doi:10.1016/j.biomaterials.2019.01.043.

Jhaveri, A. M., and V. P. Torchilin. "Multifunctional Polymeric Micelles for Delivery of Drugs and siRNA." *Frontiers in Pharmacology* 5, no. 77 (2014). doi:10.3389/fphar.2014.00077.

Jiang G., H. Jia, J. Qiu, Z. Mo, Y. Wen, Y. Zhang, Y. Wen, Q. Xie, and J. Ban. "PLGA Nanoparticle Platform for Trans-Ocular Barrier to Enhance Drug Delivery: A Comparative Study Based on the Application of Oligosaccharides in the Outer Membrane of Carriers." *International Journal of Nanomedicine* 15 (2020): 9373–9387. doi:10.2147/ijn.s272750.

Joshi, N., and M. Grinstaff. "Applications of Dendrimers in Tissue Engineering." *Current Topics in Medicinal Chemistry* 8, no. 14 (2008): 1225–36. doi:10.2174/156802608785849067.

Juillerat-Jeanneret, L., M. Dusinska, L. M. Fjellsbo, A. R. Collins, R. D. Handy, and M. Riediker. "Biological Impact Assessment of Nanomaterial Used in Nanomedicine. Introduction to the NanoTEST Project." *Nanotoxicology* 9, no. (Suppl.: 1) (2015): 5–12. doi:10.3109/17435390.2013.826743.

Kalam, M. A., and A. Alshamsan. "Poly (d, l-lactide-co-glycolide) Nanoparticles for Sustained Release of Tacrolimus in Rabbit Eyes." *Biomedicine & Pharmacotherapy* 94 (2017): 402–411. doi:10.1016/j.biopha.2017.07.110.

Kamalesh, M., B. Diraj, B. Kiran, and Wagh Kalpesh. "Formulation and Evaluation of Pharmacosomes of Ketoprofen." *Indo American Journal of Pharmaceutical Research* 4 (2014): 1363–8.

Kambhampati, S. P., I. A. Bhutto, A. J. Clunies-Ross, M. K. Mishra, S. D. McLeod, G. A. Lutty, and R. Kannan. "Dendrimer Based Targeted Intravenous Therapy for Choroidal and Retinal Neovascularization." *Investigative Ophthalmology & Visual Science* 55, no. 13 (2014): 4630–.

Kamkaew, A., L. Cheng, S. Goel, H. F. Valdovinos, T. E. Barnhart, Z. Liu, and W. Cai. "Cerenkov Radiation Induced Photodynamic Therapy Using Chlorin e6-Loaded Hollow Mesoporous Silica Nanoparticles." *ACS Applied Materials & Interfaces* 8, no. 40 (2016): 26630–7. doi:10.1021/acsami.6b10255.

Kannan, S., H. Dai, R. S. Navath, B. Balakrishnan, A. Jyoti, J. Janisse, R. Romero, and R. M. Kannan. "Dendrimer-Based Postnatal Therapy for Neuroinflammation and Cerebral Palsy in a Rabbit Model." *Science Translational Medicine* 4, no. 130 (2012): 130ra46. doi:10.1126/scitranslmed.3003162.

Kataoka, K., K. Itaka, N. Nishiyama, Y. Yamasaki, M. Oishi, and Y. Nagasaki. "Smart Polymeric Micelles as Nanocarriers for Oligonucleotides and siRNA Delivery." *Nucleic Acids Symposium Series* 49, no. 49 (2005): 17–8. doi:10.1093/nass/49.1.17.

Katare, Y. K., R. P. Daya, C. Sookram Gray, R. E. Luckham, J. Bhandari, A. S. Chauhan, and R. K. Mishra. "Brain Targeting of a Water Insoluble Antipsychotic Drug Haloperidol via the Intranasal Route Using PAMAM Dendrimer." *Molecular Pharmaceutics* 12, no. 9 (2015): 3380–8. doi:10.1021/acs.molpharmaceut.5b00402.

Kempen, P. J., S. Greasley, K. A. Parker, J. L. Campbell, H. Y. Chang, J. R. Jones, R. Sinclair, S. S. Gambhir, and J. V. Jokerst. "Theranostic Mesoporous Silica Nanoparticles Biodegrade after Pro-survival Drug Delivery and Ultrasound/Magnetic Resonance Imaging of Stem Cells." *Theranostics* 5, no. 6 (2015): 631–42. doi:10.7150/thno.11389.

Kesharwani, P., K. Jain, and N. K. Jain. "Dendrimer as Nanocarrier for Drug Delivery." *Progress in Polymer Science* 39, no. 2 (2014): 268–307. doi:10.1016/j.progpolymsci.2013.07.005.

Khandavilli, S., and R. Panchagnula. "Nanoemulsions as Versatile Formulations for Paclitaxel Delivery: Peroral and Dermal Delivery Studies in Rats." *Journal of Investigative Dermatology* 127, no. 1 (2007): 154–62. doi:10.1038/sj.jid.5700485.

Khang, Dongwoo, Joseph Carpenter, Young Wook Chun, Rajesh Pareta, and Thomas J. Webster. "Nanotechnology for Regenerative Medicine." *Biomedical Microdevices* 12, no. 4 (2010): 575–87. doi:10.1007/s10544-008-9264-6.

Khazaeinia, T., and F. Jamali. "A Comparison of Gastrointestinal Permeability Induced by Diclofenac-Phospholipid Complex with Diclofenac Acid and Its Sodium Salt." *Journal of Pharmacy & Pharmaceutical Sciences* 6, no. 3 (2003): 352–9.

Khong, Jeffrey, Peter Wang, Tiffany R. X. Gan, Jiansheng Ng, Truong Thanh Lan Anh, Agata Blasiak, Theodore Kee, and Dean Ho. "Chapter 22: The Role of Artificial Intelligence in Scaling Nanomedicine Toward Broad Clinical Impact." In *Nanoparticles for Biomedical Applications*, edited by Eun Ji Chung, Lorraine Leon, and Carlos Rinaldi, 385–407. Amsterdam: Elsevier, 2020.

Kim, E. Y., R. Schulz, P. Swantek, K. Kunstman, M. H. Malim, and S. M. Wolinsky. "Gold Nanoparticle-Mediated Gene Delivery Induces Widespread Changes in the Expression of Innate Immunity Genes." *Gene Therapy* 19, no. 3 (2012): 347–53. doi:10.1038/gt.2011.95.

Kim, M. W., H. Y. Jeong, S. J. Kang, M. J. Choi, Y. M. You, C. S. Im, T. S. Lee, I. H. Song, C. G. Lee, K.-J. Rhee, Y. K. Lee, and Y. S. Park. "Cancer-Targeted Nucleic Acid Delivery and Quantum Dot Imaging Using EGF Receptor Aptamer-Conjugated Lipid Nanoparticles." *Scientific Reports* 7, no. 1 (2017): 9474. doi:10.1038/s41598-017-09555-w.

Kim, Tae Hyung, Seulki Lee, and Xiaoyuan Chen. "Nanotheranostics for Personalized Medicine." *Expert Review of Molecular Diagnostics* 13, no. 3 (2013): 257–69. doi:10.1586/erm.13.15.

Kim, T.-H., M. Eltohamy, M. Kim, R. A. Perez, J.-H. Kim, Y.-R. Yun, J.-H. Jang, E.-J. Lee, J. C. Knowles, and H.-W. Kim. "Therapeutic Foam Scaffolds Incorporating Biopolymer-Shelled Mesoporous Nanospheres with Growth Factors." *Acta Biomaterialia* 10, no. 6 (2014): 2612–21. doi:10.1016/j.actbio.2014.02.005.

Kim, Y., M. Tewari, J. D. Pajerowski, S. Cai, S. Sen, J. H. Williams, S. R. Sirsi, G. J. Lutz, and D. E. Discher. "Polymersome Delivery of siRNA and Antisense Oligonucleotides." *Journal of Controlled Release* 134, no. 2 (2009): 132–40. doi:10.1016/j.jconrel.2008.10.020.

Kislukhin, A. A., H. Xu, S. R. Adams, K. H. Narsinh, R. Y. Tsien, and E. T. Ahrens. "Paramagnetic Fluorinated Nanoemulsions for Sensitive Cellular Fluorine-19 Magnetic Resonance Imaging." *Nature Materials* 15, no. 6 (2016): 662–8. doi:10.1038/nmat4585.

Kneer, W., M. Rother, S. Mazgareanu, E. J. Seidel, and European IDEA-033 study group. "A 12-Week Randomized Study of Topical Therapy with Three Dosages of Ketoprofen in Transfersome® Gel (IDEA-033) Compared with the Ketoprofen-Free Vehicle (TDT 064), in Patients with Osteoarthritis of the Knee." *Journal of Pain Research* 6 (2013): 743–53. doi:10.2147/jpr.s51054.

Kobayashi, H., S. Kawamoto, S. K. Jo, H. L. Bryant, Jr., M. W. Brechbiel, and R. A. Star. "Macromolecular MRI Contrast Agents with Small Dendrimers: Pharmacokinetic Differences Between Sizes and Cores." *Bioconjugate Chemistry* 14, no. 2 (2003): 388–94. doi:10.1021/bc025633c.

Kojima, C., S. Tsumura, A. Harada, and K. Kono. "A Collagen-Mimic Dendrimer Capable of Controlled Release." *Journal of the American Chemical Society* 131, no. 17 (2009): 6052–3. doi:10.1021/ja809639c.

Koli, J. R. *Development of Anti-Oxidant Ethosomes for Topical Delivery Utilizing the Synergistic Properties of Vitamin A Palmitate, Vitamin E and Vitamin C.* New York: St. John's University, 2010.

Kong, F. Y., M. T. Xu, J. J. Xu, and H. Y. Chen. "A Novel Lable-free Electrochemical Immunosensor for Carcinoembryonic Antigen based on Gold Nanoparticles-Thionine-reduced Graphene Oxide Nanocomposite Film Modified Glassy Carbon Electrode." *Talanta* 85, no. 5 (2011): 2620–5. doi:10.1016/j.talanta.2011.08.028.

Kong, F. Y., J. W. Zhang, R. F. Li, Z. X. Wang, W. J. Wang, and W. Wang. "Unique roles of gold nanoparticles in drug delivery, targeting and imaging applications." *Molecules* 22, no. 9 (2017): 1445. doi:10.3390/molecules22091445.

Krishnaswamy, K., and V. Orsat. "Chapter 2: Sustainable Delivery Systems Through Green Nanotechnology." In *Nano- and Microscale Drug Delivery Systems*, edited by A. M. Grumezescu, 17–32. Amsterdam: Elsevier, 2017.

Kundrotas, G., V. Karabanovas, M. Pleckaitis, M. Juraleviciute, S. Steponkiene, Z. Gudleviciene, and R. Rotomskis. "Uptake and Distribution of Carboxylated Quantum Dots in Human Mesenchymal Stem Cells: Cell Growing Density Matters." *Journal of Nanobiotechnology* 17, no. 1 (2019): 39. doi:10.1186/s12951-019-0470-6.

Kwon, E. J., M. Skalak, A. Bertucci, G. Braun, F. Ricci, E. Ruoslahti, M. J. Sailor, and S. N. Bhatia. "Porous Silicon Nanoparticle Delivery of Tandem Peptide Anti-Infectives for the Treatment of Pseudomonas aeruginosa Lung Infections." *Advanced Materials* 29, no. 35 (2017). doi:10.1002/adma.201701527.

Lalu, L., V. Tambe, D. Pradhan, K. Nayak, S. Bagchi, R. Maheshwari, K. Kalia, and R. K. Tekade. "Novel Nanosystems for the Treatment of Ocular Inflammation: Current Paradigms and Future Research Directions." *Journal of Controlled Release* 268 (2017): 19–39. doi:10.1016/j.jconrel.2017.07.035.

Landsiedel, Robert, Lan Ma-Hock, Karin Wiench, Wendel Wohlleben, and Ursula G. Sauer. "Safety Assessment of Nanomaterials Using an Advanced Decision-Making Framework, the DF4nanoGrouping." *Journal of Nanoparticle Research* 19, no. 5 (2017): 171. doi:10.1007/s11051-017-3850-6.

Lee, E. A., H. Yim, J. Heo, H. Kim, G. Jung, and N. S. Hwang. "Application of Magnetic Nanoparticle for Controlled Tissue Assembly and Tissue Engineering." *Archives of Pharmacal Research* 37, no. 1 (2014): 120–8. doi:10.1007/s12272-013-0303-3.

Lee, S. H., S. Y. Back, J. G. Song, and H. K. Han. "Enhanced Oral Delivery of Insulin via the Colon-targeted Nanocomposite System of Organoclay/Glycol Chitosan/Eudragit(®)S100." *Journal of Nanobiotechnology* 18, no. 1 (2020):104. doi:10.1186/s12951-020-00662-x.

Lefley, J., C. Waldron, and C. R. Becer. "Macromolecular Design and Preparation of Polymersomes." *Polymer Chemistry* 11, no. 45 (2020): 7124–36. doi:10.1039/D0PY01247E.

Leonavičienė, L., G. Kirdaitė, R. Bradūnaitė, D. Vaitkienė, A. Vasiliauskas, D. Zabulytė, A. Ramanavičienė, A. Ramanavičius, T. Ašmenavičius, and Z. Mackiewicz. "Effect of Gold Nanoparticles in the Treatment of Established Collagen Arthritis in Rats." *Medicina* 48, no. 2 (2012): 91–101.

Leong, J., J. Y. Teo, V. K. Aakalu, Y. Y. Yang, and H. Kong. "Engineering Polymersomes for Diagnostics and Therapy." *Advanced Healthcare Materials* 7, no. 8 (2018): e1701276. doi:10.1002/adhm.201701276.

Li, Fangyuan, Yu Qin, Jiyoung Lee, Hongwei Liao, Nan Wang, Thomas P. Davis, Ruirui Qiao, and Daishun Ling. "Stimuli-Responsive Nano-Assemblies for Remotely Controlled Drug Delivery." *Journal of Controlled Release* 322 (2020a): 566–92. doi:10.1016/j.jconrel.2020.03.051.

Li, G., Z. Rong, S. Wang, H. Zhao, D. Piao, X. Yang, G. Tian, and H. Jiang. "Rapid Detection of Brucellosis Using a Quantum Dot-Based Immunochromatographic Test Strip." *PLOS Neglected Tropical Diseases* 14, no. 9 (2020b): e0008557. doi:10.1371/journal.pntd.0008557.

Li, J., W. Y. Lee, T. Wu, J. Xu, K. Zhang, G. Li, J. Xia, and L. Bian. "Multifunctional Quantum Dot Nanoparticles for Effective Differentiation and Long-Term Tracking of Human Mesenchymal Stem Cells In Vitro and In Vivo." *Advanced Healthcare Materials* 5, no. 9 (2016): 1049–57. doi:10.1002/adhm.201500879.

Li, L. L., and H. Wang. "Enzyme-Coated Mesoporous Silica Nanoparticles as Efficient Antibacterial Agents In Vivo." *Advanced Healthcare Materials* 2, no. 10 (2013): 1351–60. doi:10.1002/adhm.201300051.

Li, S., B. Byrne, J. Welsh, and A. F. Palmer. "Self-Assembled Poly(Butadiene)-b-Poly(Ethylene Oxide) Polymersomes as Paclitaxel Carriers." *Biotechnology Progress* 23, no. 1 (2007): 278–85. doi:10.1021/bp060208+.

Liao, Y. H., Y. J. Chang, Y. Yoshiike, Y. C. Chang, and Y. R. Chen. "Negatively Charged Gold Nanoparticles Inhibit Alzheimer's Amyloid-β Fibrillization, Induce Fibril Dissociation, and Mitigate Neurotoxicity." *Small* 8, no. 23 (2012): 3631–9. doi:10.1002/smll.201201068.

Lim, C., D.-w. Kim, T. Sim, N. H. Hoang, J. W. Lee, E. S. Lee, Y. S. Youn, and K. T. Oh. "Preparation and Characterization of a Lutein Loading Nanoemulsion System for Ophthalmic Eye Drops." *Journal of Drug Delivery Science & Technology* 36 (2016): 168–74. doi:10.1016/j.jddst.2016.10.009.

Lin, G., H. Zhang, and L. Huang. "Smart Polymeric Nanoparticles for Cancer Gene Delivery." *Molecular Pharmaceutics* 12, no. 2 (2015): 314–321. doi:10.1021/mp500656v.

Lin, G., T. Chen, J. Zou, Y. Wang, X. Wang, J. Li, Q. Huang, Z. Fu, Y. Zhao, M. C. Lin, G. Xu, and K. T. Yong. "Quantum Dots-siRNA Nanoplexes for Gene Silencing in Central Nervous System Tumor Cells." *Frontiers in Pharmacology* 8 (2017): 182. doi:10.3389/fphar.2017.00182.

Lin, J. J., P. P. Ghoroghchian, Y. Zhang, and D. A. Hammer. "Adhesion of Antibody-functionalized Polymersomes." *Langmuir* 22, no. 9 (2006): 3975–3979. doi:10.1021/la052445c.

Lin, P. C., S. Lin, P. C. Wang, and R. Sridhar. "Techniques for Physicochemical Characterization of Nanomaterials." *Biotechnology Advances* 32, no. 4 (2014): 711–26. doi:10.1016/j.biotechadv.2013.11.006.

Lin, X., F. Xie, X. Ma, Y. Hao, H. Qin, and J. Long. "Fabrication and Characterization of Dendrimer-Functionalized Nano-Hydroxyapatite and Its Application in Dentin Tubule Occlusion." *Journal of Biomaterials Science: Polymer Edition* 28, no. 9 (2017): 846–63. doi:10.1080/09205063.2017.1308654.

Liu, G., N. M. K. Tse, M. R. Hill, D. F. Kennedy, and C. J. Drummond. "Disordered Mesoporous Gadolinosilicate Nanoparticles Prepared Using Gadolinium Based Ionic Liquid Emulsions: Potential as Magnetic Resonance Imaging Contrast Agents." *Australian Journal of Chemistry* 64, no. 5 (2011): 617–24. doi:10.1071/CH11064.

Liu, P. Y., W. Tong, K. Liu, S. H. Han, X. T. Wang, E. Badiavas, K. Rieger-Christ, and I. Summerhayes. "Liposome-Mediated Transfer of Vascular Endothelial Growth Factor cDNA Augments Survival of Random-Pattern Skin Flaps in the Rat." *Wound Repair & Regeneration* 12, no. 1 (2004): 80–5. doi:10.1111/j.1067-1927.2004.012114.x.

Liu, Q., L. Song, S. Chen, J. Gao, P. Zhao, and J. Du. "A Superparamagnetic Polymersome with Extremely High T(2) Relaxivity for MRI and Cancer-targeted Drug Delivery." *Biomaterials* 114 (2017): 23–33. doi:10.1016/j.biomaterials.2016.10.027.

Liu, X., M. J. Yaszemski, and L. Lu. "Expansile Crosslinked Polymersomes for pH Sensitive Delivery of Doxorubicin." *Biomaterials Science* 4, no. 2 (2016): 245–9. doi:10.1039/C5BM00269A.

Liu, Y., J. K. Tee, and G. N. Chiu. "Dendrimers in Oral Drug Delivery Application: Current Explorations, Toxicity Issues and Strategies for Improvement." *Current Pharmaceutical Design* 21, no. 19 (2015): 2629–42. doi:10.2174/1381612821666150416102058.

Lomas, H., I. Canton, S. MacNeil, J. Du, S. P. Armes, A. J. Ryan, A. L. Lewis, and G. Battaglia. "Biomimetic pH Sensitive Polymersomes for Efficient DNA Encapsulation and Delivery." *Advanced Materials* 19, no. 23 (2007): 4238–43. doi:10.1002/adma.200700941.

Lomas, H., M. Massignani, K. A. Abdullah, I. Canton, C. Lo Presti, S. MacNeil, J. Du, A. Blanazs, J. Madsen, S. P. Armes, A. L. Lewis, and G. Battaglia. "Non-Cytotoxic Polymer Vesicles for Rapid and Efficient Intracellular Delivery." *Faraday Discussions* 139, no. 0 (2008): 143–59. doi:10.1039/B717431D.

Lomas, H., J. Du, I. Canton, J. Madsen, N. Warren, S. P. Armes, A. L. Lewis, and G. Battaglia. "Efficient Encapsulation of Plasmid DNA in pH-Sensitive PMPC-PDPA Polymersomes: Study of the Effect of PDPA Block Length on Copolymer-DNA Binding Affinity." *Macromolecular Bioscience* 10, no. 5 (2010): 513–30. doi:10.1002/mabi.201000083.

Lombardo, D., M. A. Kiselev, and M. T. Caccamo. "Smart Nanoparticles for Drug Delivery Application: Development of Versatile Nanocarrier Platforms in Biotechnology and Nanomedicine." *Journal of Nanomaterials* 2019 (2019). doi:10.1155/2019/3702518, PubMed: 3702518.

Lopes, C. M., J. Silva, M. E. C. D. Real Oliveira, and M. Lúcio. "Chapter 14: Lipid-Based Colloidal Carriers for Topical Application of Antiviral Drugs." In *Design of Nanostructures for Versatile Therapeutic Applications*, edited by A. M. Grumezescu, 565–622. Oxford: William Andrew Publishing, 2018.

Lu, Y., S. Zhao, and X. Zhang. "Fabrication of Mn^{2+}-Doped Hollow Mesoporous Aluminosilica Nanoparticles for Magnetic Resonance Imaging and Drug Delivery for Therapy of Colorectal Cancer." *Journal of Nanomaterials* 2019 (2019). doi:10.1155/2019/3525143, PubMed: 3525143.

Lúcio, M., C. M. Lopes, E. Fernandes, H. Gonçalves, and M. E. C. D. Real Oliveira. "Organic Nanocarriers for Brain Drug Delivery." In *Nanoparticles for Brain Drug Delivery*, edited by C. Vitorino, A. Jorge, and A. A. C. C. Pais. Singapore: Jenny Stanford Publishing Pte. Ltd, 2021. "Chapter 4.

Luk, B. T., and L. Zhang. "Current Advances in Polymer-Based Nanotheranostics for Cancer Treatment and Diagnosis." *ACS Applied Materials & Interfaces* 6, no. 24 (2014): 21859–73. doi:10.1021/am5036225.

Luo, X., D. Niu, Y. Wang, Y. Zhai, J. Chen, J. Gu, J. Shi, and Y. Li. "One-Pot Synthesis of Magnetite-Loaded Dual-Mesoporous Silica Spheres for T2-Weighted Magnetic Resonance Imaging and Drug Delivery." *RSC Advances* 5, no. 50 (2015): 39719–25. doi:10.1039/C5RA04970A.

Lv, Y., R. Wu, K. Feng, J. Li, Q. Mao, H. Yuan, H. Shen, X. Chai, and L. S. Li. "Highly Sensitive and Accurate Detection of C-Reactive Protein by CdSe/ZnS Quantum Dot-Based Fluorescence-Linked Immunosorbent Assay." *Journal of Nanobiotechnology* 15, no. 1 (2017): 35. doi:10.1186/s12951-017-0267-4.

Lynch, Iseult, Carsten Weiss, and Eugenia Valsami-Jones. "A Strategy for Grouping of Nanomaterials Based on Key Physico-Chemical Descriptors as a Basis for Safer-by-Design NMs." *Nano Today* 9, no. 3 (2014): 266–70. doi:10.1016/j.nantod.2014.05.001.

Madni, A., M. A. Rahem, N. Tahir, M. Sarfraz, A. Jabar, M. Rehman, P. M. Kashif, S. F. Badshah, K. U. Khan, and H. A. Santos. "Non-Invasive Strategies for Targeting the Posterior Segment of Eye." *International Journal of Pharmacy* 530, no. 1 (2017): 326–45. doi:10.1016/j.ijpharm.2017.07.065.

Mahmoodi, N. O., A. Ghavidast, and N. Amirmahani. "A Comparative Study on the Nanoparticles for Improved Drug Delivery Systems." *Journal of Photochemistry & Photobiology, Part B* 162 (2016): 681–93. doi:10.1016/j.jphotobiol.2016.07.037.

Majidi, S., F. Zeinali Sehrig, M. Samiei, M. Milani, E. Abbasi, K. Dadashzadeh, and A. Akbarzadeh. "Magnetic Nanoparticles: Applications in Gene Delivery and Gene Therapy." *Artificial Cells, Nanomedicine & Biotechnology* 44, no. 4 (2016): 1186–93. doi:10.3109/21691401.2015.1014093.

Makino, A., S. Kizaka-Kondoh, R. Yamahara, I. Hara, T. Kanzaki, E. Ozeki, M. Hiraoka, and S. Kimura. "Near-infrared Fluorescence Tumor Imaging Using Nanocarrier Composed of Poly(l-Lactic Acid)-Block-Poly(Sarcosine) Amphiphilic Polydepsipeptide." *Biomaterials* 30, no. 28 (2009): 5156–5160. doi:10.1016/j.biomaterials.2009.05.046.

Manikkath, J., A. R. Hegde, G. Kalthur, H. S. Parekh, and S. Mutalik. "Influence of Peptide Dendrimers and Sonophoresis on the Transdermal Delivery of Ketoprofen." *International Journal of Pharmacy* 521, no. 1–2 (2017): 110–9. doi:10.1016/j.ijpharm.2017.02.002.

Martínez-Carmona, M., D. Lozano, M. Colilla, and M. Vallet-Regí. "Lectin-Conjugated pH-Responsive Mesoporous Silica Nanoparticles for Targeted Bone Cancer Treatment." *Acta Biomaterialia* 65 (2018): 393–404. doi:10.1016/j.actbio.2017.11.007.

Marwah, H., T. Garg, G. Rath, and A. K. Goyal. "Development of Transferosomal Gel for Trans-Dermal Delivery of Insulin Using Iodine Complex." *Drug Delivery* 23, no. 5 (2016): 1636–44. doi:10.3109/10717 544.2016.1155243.

Matsumura, Y., T. Hamaguchi, T. Ura, K. Muro, Y. Yamada, Y. Shimada, K. Shirao, T. Okusaka, H. Ueno, M. Ikeda, and N. Watanabe. "Phase I Clinical Trial and Pharmacokinetic Evaluation of NK911, a Micelle-Encapsulated Doxorubicin." *British Journal of Cancer* 91, no. 10 (2004): 1775–81. doi:10.1038/sj.bjc.6602204.

McBain, S. C., U. Griesenbach, S. Xenariou, A. Keramane, C. D. Batich, E. W. F. W. Alton, and J. Dobson. "Magnetic Nanoparticles as Gene Delivery Agents: Enhanced Transfection in the Presence of Oscillating Magnet Arrays." *Nanotechnology* 19, no. 40 (2008): 405102. doi:10.1088/0957-4484/19/40/405102.

Mclaughlin, S., J. Podrebarac, M. Ruel, E. J. Suuronen, B. McNeill, and E. I. Alarcon. "Nano-Engineered Biomaterials for Tissue Regeneration: What Has Been Achieved so Far?" *Frontiers in Materials* 3, no. 27 (2016). doi:10.3389/fmats.2016.00027.

Meerovich, I., and A. K. Dash. "Chapter 8: Polymersomes for Drug Delivery and Other Biomedical Applications." In *Materials for Biomedical Engineering*, edited by A.-M. Holban, and A. M. Grumezescu, 269–309. Amsterdam: Elsevier, 2019.

Mendes, A. I., A. C. Silva, J. A. Catita, F. Cerqueira, C. Gabriel, and C. M. Lopes. "Miconazole-Loaded Nanostructured Lipid Carriers (NLC) for Local Delivery to the Oral Mucosa: Improving Antifungal Activity." *Colloids & Surfaces, Part B: Biointerfaces* 111 (2013): 755–63. doi:10.1016/j.colsurfb.2013.05.041.

Mendes, M., J. J. Sousa, A. Pais, and C. Vitorino (2018). "Targeted Theranostic Nanoparticles for Brain Tumor Treatment." *Pharmaceutics* 10, no. 4: 181. doi:10.3390/pharmaceutics10040181.

Michalet, X., F. F. Pinaud, L. A. Bentolila, J. M. Tsay, S. Doose, J. J. Li, G. Sundaresan, A. M. Wu, S. S. Gambhir, and S. Weiss. "Quantum Dots for Live Cells, in vivo Imaging, and Diagnostics." *Science* 307, no. 5709 (2005): 538–44. doi:10.1126/science.1104274.

Mikhaylov, G., U. Mikac, A. A. Magaeva, V. I. Itin, E. P. Naiden, I. Psakhye, L. Babes, T. Reinheckel, C. Peters, R. Zeiser, M. Bogyo, V. Turk, S. G. Psakhye, B. Turk, and O. Vasiljeva. "Ferri-Liposomes as an MRI-Visible Drug-Delivery System for Targeting Tumours and Their Microenvironment." *Nature Nanotechnology* 6, no. 9 (2011): 594–602. doi:10.1038/nnano.2011.112.

Mishra, D., P. K. Mishra, V. Dubey, M. Nahar, S. Dabadghao, and N. K. Jain. "Systemic and Mucosal Immune Response Induced by Transcutaneous Immunization Using Hepatitis B Surface Antigen-Loaded Modified Liposomes." *European Journal of Pharmaceutical Sciences* 33, no. 4–5 (2008): 424–33. doi:10.1016/j. ejps.2008.01.015.

Mishra, M. K., C. A. Beaty, W. G. Lesniak, S. P. Kambhampati, F. Zhang, M. A. Wilson, M. E. Blue, J. C. Troncoso, S. Kannan, M. V. Johnston, W. A. Baumgartner, and R. M. Kannan. "Dendrimer Brain Uptake and Targeted Therapy for Brain Injury in a Large Animal Model of Hypothermic Circulatory Arrest." *ACS Nano* 8, no. 3 (2014): 2134–47. doi:10.1021/nn404872e.

Mochida, Y., H. Cabral, Y. Miura, F. Albertini, S. Fukushima, K. Osada, N. Nishiyama, and K. Kataoka. "Bundled Assembly of Helical Nanostructures in Polymeric Micelles Loaded with Platinum Drugs Enhancing Therapeutic Efficiency Against Pancreatic Tumor." *ACS Nano* 8, no. 7 (2014): 6724–38. doi:10.1021/nn500498t.

Molina, G., S. Murcia, J. Molera, C. Roldán, D. Crespo, and T. Pradell. "Color and Dichroism of Silver-Stained Glasses." *Journal of Nanoparticle Research* 15, no. 9 (2013): 1932. doi:10.1007/s11051-013-1932-7.

Möller, K., K. Müller, H. Engelke, C. Bräuchle, E. Wagner, and T. Bein. "Highly Efficient siRNA Delivery from Core–shell Mesoporous Silica Nanoparticles with Multifunctional Polymer Caps." *Nanoscale* 8, no. 7 (2016): 4007–19. doi:10.1039/C5NR06246B.

Monteiro, N., A. Martins, R. L. Reis, and N. M. Neves. "Liposomes in Tissue Engineering and Regenerative Medicine." *Journal of the Royal Society. Interface / the Royal Society* 11, no. 101 (2014):20140459. doi:10.1098/ rsif.2014.0459.

Monteiro, N., A. Martins, D. Ribeiro, S. Faria, N. A. Fonseca, J. N. Moreira, R. L. Reis, and N. M. Neves. "On the Use of Dexamethasone-Loaded Liposomes to Induce the Osteogenic Differentiation of Human Mesenchymal Stem Cells." *Journal of Tissue Engineering & Regenerative Medicine* 9, no. 9 (2015): 1056–66. doi:10.1002/ term.1817.

Montoya Mira, J., L. Wu, S. Sabuncu, A. Sapre, F. Civitci, S. Ibsen, S. Esener, and A. Yildirim. "Gas-Stabilizing sub-100 Nm Mesoporous Silica Nanoparticles for Ultrasound Theranostics." *ACS Omega* 5, no. 38 (2020): 24762–72. doi:10.1021/acsomega.0c03377.

Movassaghian, S., O. M. Merkel, and V. P. Torchilin. "Applications of Polymer Micelles for Imaging and Drug Delivery." *Wiley Interdisciplinary Reviews. Nanomedicine & Nanobiotechnology* 7, no. 5 (2015): 691–707. doi:10.1002/wnan.1332.

Müller, Laura K., and Katharina Landfester. "Natural Liposomes and Synthetic Polymeric Structures for Biomedical Applications." *Biochemical & Biophysical Research Communications* 468, no. 3 (2015): 411–8. doi:10.1016/j. bbrc.2015.08.088.

Müller, R. H., M. Radtke, and S. A. Wissing. "Solid Lipid Nanoparticles (SLN) and Nanostructured Lipid Carriers (NLC) in Cosmetic and Dermatological Preparations." *Advanced Drug Delivery Reviews* 54 (Suppl. 1) (2002): S131–S55. doi:10.1016/s0169-409x(02)00118-7.

Murdoch, C., K. J. Reeves, V. Hearnden, H. Colley, M. Massignani, I. Canton, J. Madsen, A. Blanazs, S. P. Armes, A. L. Lewis, S. Macneil, N. J. Brown, M. H. Thornhill, and G. Battaglia. "Internalization and Biodistribution of Polymersomes into Oral Squamous Cell Carcinoma Cells in vitro and in vivo." *Nanomedicine* 5, no. 7 (2010): 1025–36. doi:10.2217/nnm.10.97.

Mussi, S. V., and V. P. Torchilin. "Recent Trends in the Use of Lipidic Nanoparticles as Pharmaceutical Carriers for Cancer Therapy and Diagnostics." *Journal of Materials Chemistry B* 1, no. 39 (2013): 5201–9. doi:10.1039/ C3TB20990C.

Mutalik, S., P. K. Shetty, A. Kumar, R. Kalra, and H. S. Parekh. "Enhancement in Deposition and Permeation of 5-Fluorouracil Through Human Epidermis Assisted by Peptide Dendrimers." *Drug Delivery* 21, no. 1 (2014): 44–54. doi:10.3109/10717544.2013.845861.

Na, M., C. Yiyun, X. Tongwen, D. Yang, W. Xiaomin, L. Zhenwei, C. Zhichao, H. Guanyi, S. Yunyu, and W. Longping. "Dendrimers as Potential Drug Carriers. Part II. Prolonged Delivery of Ketoprofen by In Vitro and In Vivo Studies." *European Journal of Medicinal Chemistry* 41, no. 5 (2006): 670–4. doi:10.1016/j. ejmech.2006.01.001.

Naing, A., J. R. Infante, K. P. Papadopoulos, K. A. Autio, D. J. Wong, G. S. Falchook, M. R. Patel, S. Pant, M. Whiteside, J. Bendell, T. M. Bauer, F. Janku, M. Javle, R. Colen, N. Tannir, and M. Oft. "CD8+ T Cell Stimulation with Pegylated Recombinant Human IL-10 in the Patient with Advanced Solid Tumors: A Phase I Study." *Journal for ImmunoTherapy of Cancer* 3, no. Suppl 2 (2015): 204–P204, doi:10.1186/2051-1426-3-S2-P204.

Namdeo, M., S. Saxena, R. Tankhiwale, M. Bajpai, Y. M. Mohan, and S. K. Bajpai. "Magnetic Nanoparticles for Drug Delivery Applications." *Journal of Nanoscience & Nanotechnology* 8, no. 7 (2008): 3247–71. doi:10.1166/ jnn.2008.399.

NANoREG. "NANoREG Framework for the Safety Assessment of Nanomaterials." 2017. Accessed 14/12/2018. http://publications.jrc.ec.europa.eu/repository/bitstream/JRC105651/kjna28550enn.pdf.

Naseri, N., H. Valizadeh, and P. Zakeri-Milani. "Solid Lipid Nanoparticles and Nanostructured Lipid Carriers: Structure, Preparation and Application." *Advanced Pharmaceutical Bulletin* 5, no. 3 (2015): 305–13. doi:10.15171/apb.2015.043.

Nasr, M., S. Nawaz, and A. Elhissi. "Amphotericin B Lipid Nanoemulsion Aerosols for Targeting Peripheral Respiratory Airways via Nebulization." *International Journal of Pharmacy* 436, no. 1–2 (2012): 611–6. doi:10.1016/j.ijpharm.2012.07.028.

Nehoff, H., N. N. Parayath, L. Domanovitch, S. Taurin, and K. Greish. "Nanomedicine for Drug Targeting: Strategies Beyond the Enhanced Permeability and Retention Effect." *International Journal of Nanomedicine* 9 (2014): 2539–55. doi:10.2147/IJN.S47129.

Nie, W., X. Dai, D. Li, D. McCoul, G. J. Gillispie, Y. Zhang, B. Yu, and C. He. "One-Pot Synthesis of Silver Nanoparticle Incorporated Mesoporous Silica Granules for Hemorrhage Control and Antibacterial Treatment." *ACS Biomaterials Science & Engineering* 4, no. 10 (2018): 3588–99. doi:10.1021/ acsbiomaterials.8b00527.

Nisini, R., N. Poerio, S. Mariotti, F. De Santis, and M. Fraziano. "The Multirole of Liposomes in Therapy and Prevention of Infectious Diseases." *Frontiers in Immunology* 9 (2018) : 155. doi:10.3389/fimmu.2018.00155.

O'Konek, J. J., P. E. Makidon, J. J. Landers, Z. Cao, C. A. Malinczak, J. Pannu, J. Sun, V. Bitko, S. Ciotti, T. Hamouda, Z. W. Wojcinski, N. W. Lukacs, A. Fattom, and J. R. Baker, Jr. "Intranasal Nanoemulsion-Based Inactivated Respiratory Syncytial Virus Vaccines Protect Against Viral Challenge in Cotton Rats." *Human Vaccines & Immunotherapeutics* 11, no. 12 (2015): 2904–12. doi:10.1080/21645515.2015.1075680.

Obaid, G., I. Chambrier, M. J. Cook, and D. A. Russell. "Cancer Targeting with Biomolecules: A Comparative Study of Photodynamic Therapy Efficacy Using Antibody or Lectin Conjugated Phthalocyanine-PEG Gold Nanoparticles." *Photochemistry & Photobiological Sciences* 14, no. 4 (2015): 737–47. doi:10.1039/c4pp00312h.

Ogawa, M., I. O. Umeda, M. Kosugi, A. Kawai, Y. Hamaya, M. Takashima, H. Yin, T. Kudoh, M. Seno, and Y. Magata. "Development of 111In-Labeled Liposomes for Vulnerable Atherosclerotic Plaque Imaging." *Journal of Nuclear Medicine* 55, no. 1 (2014): 115–20. doi:10.2967/jnumed.113.123158.

Olerile, L. D., Y. Liu, B. Zhang, T. Wang, S. Mu, J. Zhang, L. Selotlegeng, and N. Zhang. "Near-Infrared Mediated Quantum Dots and Paclitaxel Co-Loaded Nanostructured Lipid Carriers for Cancer Theragnostic." *Colloids & Surfaces, Part B: Biointerfaces* 150 (2017): 121–30. doi:10.1016/j.colsurfb.2016.11.032.

Oliveira, H., E. Pérez-Andrés, J. Thevenot, O. Sandre, E. Berra, and S. Lecommandoux. "Magnetic Field Triggered Drug Release from Polymersomes for Cancer Therapeutics." *Journal of Controlled Release* 169, no. 3 (2013): 165–70. doi:10.1016/j.jconrel.2013.01.013.

Oliveira, J. M., N. Kotobuki, M. Tadokoro, M. Hirose, J. F. Mano, R. L. Reis, and H. Ohgushi. "Ex vivo Culturing of Stromal Cells with Dexamethasone-loaded Carboxymethylchitosan/poly(amidoamine) Dendrimer Nanoparticles Promotes Ectopic Bone Formation." *Bone* 46, no. 5 (2010): 1424–35. doi:10.1016/j.bone.2010.02.007.

Oomen, Agnes G., Klaus Günter Steinhäuser, Eric A. J. Bleeker, Fleur van Broekhuizen, Adriënne Sips, Susan Dekkers, Susan W. P. Wijnhoven, and Philip G. Sayre. "Risk Assessment Frameworks for Nanomaterials: Scope, Link to Regulations, Applicability, and Outline for Future Directions in View of Needed Increase in Efficiency." *NanoImpact* 9: 1–13 (2018). doi:10.1016/j.impact.2017.09.001.

Ooya, T., J. Lee, and K. Park. "Hydrotropic Dendrimers of generations 4 and 5: Synthesis, Characterization, and Hydrotropic Solubilization of Paclitaxel." *Bioconjugate Chemistry* 15, no. 6 (2004): 1221–9. doi:10.1021/bc049814l.

Ossa, Dolores. "Hernán Pérez de la". *Quality Aspects of Nano-based Medicines SME Workshop: Focus on Quality for Medicines Containing Chemical Entities.* 2014. Accessed 15/12/2020. https://www.ema.europa.eu/en/documents/presentation/presentation-quality-aspects-nano-based-medicines-dolores-hernan-pacrez-de-la-ossa_en.pdf.

Pandey, G., N. Mittapelly, G. R. Valicherla, R. P. Shukla, S. Sharma, V. T. Banala, S. Urandur, A. K. Jajoriya, K. Mitra, D. P. Mishra, J. R. Gayen, and P. R. Mishra. "P-gp Modulatory acetyl-11-keto-β-boswellic Acid Based Nanoemulsified Carrier System for Augmented Oral Chemotherapy of Docetaxel." *Colloids & Surfaces, Part B: Biointerfaces* 155 (2017): 276–86. doi:10.1016/j.colsurfb.2017.04.028.

Pandey, Y. R., S. Kumar, B. K. Gupta, J. Ali, and S. Baboota. "Intranasal Delivery of Paroxetine Nanoemulsion via the Olfactory Region for the Management of Depression: Formulation, Behavioural and Biochemical Estimation." *Nanotechnology* 27, no. 2 (2016): 025102. doi:10.1088/0957-4484/27/2/025102.

Pandita, A., and P. Sharma. "Pharmacosomes: An Emerging Novel Vesicular Drug Delivery System for Poorly Soluble Synthetic and Herbal Drugs." *ISRN Pharmacology* 2013 (2013): 348186. doi:10.1155/2013/348186.

Pankhurst, Q. A., J. Connolly, S. K. Jones, and J. Dobson. "Applications of Magnetic Nanoparticles in Biomedicine." *Journal of Physics. Part D* 36, no. 13 (2003): R167–R81. doi:10.1088/0022-3727/36/13/201.

Park, J., J. Park, E. J. Ju, S. S. Park, J. Choi, J. H. Lee, K. J. Lee, S. H. Shin, E. J. Ko, I. Park, C. Kim, J. J. Hwang, J. S. Lee, S. Y. Song, S. Y. Jeong, and E. K. Choi. "Multifunctional Hollow Gold Nanoparticles Designed for Triple Combination Therapy and CT Imaging." *Journal of Controlled Release* 207 (2015): 77–85. doi:10.1016/j.jconrel.2015.04.007.

Patel, Nimitt G., Ajeet Kumar, Veroni N. Jayawardana, Craig D. Woodworth, and Philip A. Yuya. "Fabrication, Nanomechanical Characterization, and Cytocompatibility of Gold-Reinforced Chitosan Bio-Nanocomposites." *Materials Science & Engineering. Part C* 44 (2014): 336–44. doi:10.1016/j.msec.2014.08.042.

Patel, S. K., W. Beaino, C. J. Anderson, and J. M. Janjic. "Theranostic Nanoemulsions for Macrophage COX-2 Inhibition in a Murine Inflammation Model." *Clinical Immunology* 160, no. 1 (2015): 59–70. doi:10.1016/j.clim.2015.04.019.

Patel, V., C. Rajani, D. Paul, P. Borisa, K. Rajpoot, S. R. Youngren-Ortiz, and R. K. Tekade. "Chapter 8: Dendrimers as Novel Drug-Delivery System and Its Applications." In *Drug Delivery Systems*, edited by R. K. Tekade, 333–92. London: Academic Press, 2020.

Patra, J. K., G. Das, L. F. Fraceto, E. V. R. Campos, M. D. P. Rodriguez-Torres, L. S. Acosta-Torres, L. A. Diaz-Torres, R. Grillo, M. K. Swamy, S. Sharma, S. Habtemariam, and H. S. Shin. "Nano Based Drug Delivery Systems: Recent Developments and Future Prospects." *Journal of Nanobiotechnology* 16, no. 1 (2018): 71. doi:10.1186/s12951-018-0392-8.

Patravale, V. B., P. G. Upadhaya, and R. D. Jain. "Preparation and Characterization of Micelles." In *Pharmaceutical Nanotechnology: Basic Protocols*, edited by Volkmar Weissig, and Tamer Elbayoumi, 19–29. New York: Springer, 2019.

Pederson, A. W., J. W. Ruberti, and P. B. Messersmith (2003). "Thermal Assembly of a Biomimetic Mineral/Collagen Composite." *Biomaterials* 24, no. 26: 4881–90. doi:10.1016/S0142-9612(03)00369-7.

Peira, E., P. Marzola, V. Podio, S. Aime, A. Sbarbati, and M. R. Gasco. "In Vitro and In Vivo Study of Solid Lipid Nanoparticles Loaded with Superparamagnetic Iron Oxide." *Journal of Drug Targeting* 11, no. 1 (2003): 19–24. doi:10.1080/1061186031000086108.

Pelegri-O'Day, E. M., E.-W. Lin, and H. D. Maynard. "Therapeutic Protein–Polymer Conjugates: Advancing Beyond Pegylation." *Journal of the American Chemical Society* 136, no. 41 (2014): 14323–32. doi:10.1021/ja504390x.

Perea, H., J. Aigner, U. Hopfner, and E. Wintermantel. "Direct Magnetic Tubular Cell Seeding: A Novel Approach for Vascular Tissue Engineering." *Cells, Tissues, Organs* 183, no. 3 (2006): 156–65. doi:10.1159/000095989.

Pinese, C., J. Lin, U. Milbreta, M. Li, Y. Wang, K. W. Leong, and S. Y. Chew. "Sustained Delivery of siRNA/ Mesoporous Silica Nanoparticle Complexes from Nanofiber Scaffolds for Long-Term Gene Silencing." *Acta Biomaterialia* 76 (2018): 164–77. doi:10.1016/j.actbio.2018.05.054.

Pinto, M., C. Fernandes, E. Martins, R. Silva, S. Benfeito, F. Cagide, R. F. Mendes, F. A. Almeida Paz, J. Garrido, F. Remião, and F. Borges. "Boosting Drug Discovery for Parkinson's: Enhancement of the Delivery of a Monoamine Oxidase-B Inhibitor by Brain-Targeted PEGylated Polycaprolactone-Based Nanoparticles." *Pharmaceutics* 11, no. 7 (2019): 331. doi:10.3390/pharmaceutics11070331.

Pirzada, M., and Z. Altintas. "Nanomaterials for Healthcare Biosensing Applications." *Sensors* 19, no. 23 (2019). doi:10.3390/s19235311.

Polyak, B., I. Fishbein, M. Chorny, I. Alferiev, D. Williams, B. Yellen, G. Friedman, and R. J. Levy. "High Field Gradient Targeting of Magnetic Nanoparticle-Loaded Endothelial Cells to the Surfaces of Steel Stents." *Proceedings of the National Academy of Sciences of the United States of America* 105, no. 2 (2008): 698–703. doi:10.1073/pnas.0708338105.

Pramanik, N., and T. Imae. "Fabrication and Characterization of Dendrimer-functionalized Mesoporous Hydroxyapatite." *Langmuir* 28, no. 39 (2012): 14018–27. doi:10.1021/la302066e.

Pujol-Autonell, I., M. J. Mansilla, S. Rodriguez-Fernandez, M. Cano-Sarabia, J. Navarro-Barriuso, R. M. Ampudia, A. Rius, S. Garcia-Jimeno, D. Perna-Barrull, E. Martinez-Caceres, D. Maspoch, and M. Vives-Pi. "Liposome-based Immunotherapy Against Autoimmune Diseases: Therapeutic Effect on Multiple Sclerosis." *Nanomedicine* 12, no. 11 (2017): 1231–42. doi:10.2217/nnm-2016-0410.

Qi, Jianping, Jie Zhuang, Yi Lu, Xiaochun Dong, Weili Zhao, and Wei Wu. "In Vivo Fate of Lipid-Based Nanoparticles." *Drug Discovery Today* 22, no. 1 (2017): 166–72. doi:10.1016/j.drudis.2016.09.024.

Qi, L., and X. Gao. "Emerging Application of Quantum Dots for Drug Delivery and Therapy." *Expert Opinion on Drug Delivery* 5, no. 3 (2008): 263–7. doi:10.1517/17425247.5.3.263.

Qiu, K., B. Chen, W. Nie, X. Zhou, W. Feng, W. Wang, L. Chen, X. Mo, Y. Wei, and C. He. "Electrophoretic Deposition of Dexamethasone-Loaded Mesoporous Silica Nanoparticles onto Poly(l-Lactic Acid)/Poly(ε-Caprolactone) Composite Scaffold for Bone Tissue Rngineering." *ACS Applied Materials & Interfaces* 8, no. 6 (2016): 4137–48. doi:10.1021/acsami.5b11879.

Quan, L., Y. Zhang, B. J. Crielaard, A. Dusad, S. M. Lele, C. J. F. Rijcken, J. M. Metselaar, H. Kostková, T. Etrych, K. Ulbrich, F. Kiessling, T. R. Mikuls, W. E. Hennink, G. Storm, T. Lammers, and D. Wang. "Nanomedicines for Inflammatory Arthritis: Head-to-Head Comparison of Glucocorticoid-Containing Polymers, Micelles, and Liposomes." *ACS Nano* 8, no. 1 (2014): 458–66. doi:10.1021/nn4048205.

Rafieerad, A., W. Yan, G. L. Sequiera, N. Sareen, E. Abu-El-Rub, M. Moudgil, and S. Dhingra. "Application of Ti3C2 mXene Quantum Dots for Immunomodulation and Regenerative Medicine." *Advanced Healthcare Materials* 8, no. 16 (2019). doi:10.1002/adhm.201900569, PubMed: 1900569.

Rahimpour, Y., and H. Hamishehkar. "Liposomes in Cosmeceutics." *Expert Opinion on Drug Delivery* 9, no. 4 (2012): 443–55. doi:10.1517/17425247.2012.666968.

Rai, D. B., N. Gupta, and D. Pooja, and H. Kulhari. "13: Dendrimers for Diagnostic Applications." In *Pharmaceutical Applications of Dendrimers*, edited by A. Chauhan, and H. Kulhari, 291–324. Amsterdam: Elsevier, 2020.

Rajan, R., S. Jose, V. P. B. Mukund, and D. T. Vasudevan. "Transferosomes: A Vesicular Transdermal Delivery System for Enhanced Drug Permeation." *Journal of Advanced Pharmaceutical Technology & Research* 2, no. 3 (2011): 138–43. doi:10.4103/2231-4040.85524.

Rajpoot, K., and S. K. Jain. "Oral Delivery of pH-Responsive Alginate Microbeads Incorporating Folic Acid-Grafted Solid Lipid Nanoparticles Exhibits Enhanced Targeting Effect Against Colorectal Cancer: A Dual-Targeted Approach." *International Journal of Biological Macromolecules* 151 (2020): 830–44. doi:10.1016/j.ijbiomac.2020.02.132.

Rameez, S., H. Alosta, and A. F. Palmer. "Biocompatible and Biodegradable Polymersome Encapsulated Hemoglobin: A Potential Oxygen Carrier." *Bioconjugate Chemistry* 19, no. 5 (2008): 1025–32. doi:10.1021/bc700465v.

Rameez, S., U. Banerjee, J. Fontes, A. Roth, and A. F. Palmer. "The Reactivity of Polymersome Encapsulated Hemoglobin with Physiologically Important Gaseous Ligands: Oxygen, Carbon Monoxide and Nitric Oxide." *Macromolecules* 45, no. 5 (2012): 2385–2389. doi:10.1021/ma202739f.

Ramyadevi, D., K. S. Rajan, B. N. Vedhahari, K. Ruckmani and N. Subramanian. "Heterogeneous Polymer Composite Nanoparticles Loaded in situ gel for Controlled Release Intra-Vaginal Therapy of Genital Herpes." *Colloids Surf B Biointerfaces* 146 (2016): 260–270. doi:10.1016/j.colsurfb.2016.06.022.

Rao, J. P., and K. E. Geckeler. "Polymer Nanoparticles: Preparation Techniques and Size-Control Parameters." *Progress in Polymer Science* 36, no. 7 (2011): 887–913. doi:10.1016/j.progpolymsci.2011.01.001.

Rata, D. M., A. N. Cadinoiu, L. I. Atanase, M. Popa, C. T. Mihai, C. Solcan, L. Ochiuz, and G. Vochita. "Topical Formulations Containing Aptamer-Functionalized Nanocapsules Loaded with 5-Fluorouracil: An Innovative Concept for the Skin Cancer Therapy." *Materials Science and Engineering C: Materials for Biological Applications* 119 (2021): 111591. doi:10.1016/j.msec.2020.111591.

Ravi, P. R., R. Vats, V. Dalal, and A. N. Murthy. "A Hybrid Design to Optimize Preparation of Lopinavir Loaded Solid Lipid Nanoparticles and Comparative Pharmacokinetic Evaluation with Marketed Lopinavir/Ritonavir Coformulation." *Journal of Pharmacy & Pharmacology* 66, no. 7 (2014): 912–26. doi:10.1111/jphp.12217.

Ravichandran, R., R. Sridhar, J. R. Venugopal, S. Sundarrajan, S. Mukherjee, and S. Ramakrishna. "Gold Nanoparticle Loaded Hybrid Nanofibers for Cardiogenic Differentiation of Stem Cells for Infarcted Myocardium Regeneration." *Macromolecular Bioscience* 14, no. 4 (2014): 515–25. doi:10.1002/mabi.201300407.

REFINE. "Anticipation of Regulatory Needs for Nanotechnology-Enabled Health Products: The REFINE White Paper." 2019. Accessed 01/01/2020. https://ec.europa.eu/jrc/en/publication/thematic-reports/anticipation-regulatory-needs-nanotechnology-enabled-health-products.

Ren, X., Y. Han, J. Wang, Y. Jiang, Z. Yi, H. Xu, and Q. Ke. "An Aligned Porous Electrospun Fibrous Membrane with Controlled Drug Delivery: An Efficient Strategy to Accelerate Diabetic Wound Healing with Improved Angiogenesis." *Acta Biomaterialia* 70 (2018): 140–53. doi:10.1016/j.actbio.2018.02.010.

Rezaei, G., M. Habibi-Anbouhi, M. Mahmoudi, K. Azadmanesh, S. Moradi-Kalbolandi, M. Behdani, L. Ghazizadeh, M. Abolhassani, and M. A. Shokrgozar. "Development of Anti-CD47 Single-chain Variable Fragment Targeted Magnetic Nanoparticles for Treatment of Human Bladder Cancer." *Nanomedicine* 12, no. 6 (2017): 597–613. doi:10.2217/nnm-2016-0302.

Richard, B. M., P. Newton, L. R. Ott, D. Haan, A. N. Brubaker, P. I. Cole, P. E. Ross, M. C. Rebelatto, and K. G. Nelson. "The Safety of EXPAREL ® (Bupivacaine Liposome Injectable Suspension) Administered by Peripheral Nerve Block in Rabbits and Dogs." *Journal of Drug Delivery* 2012 (2012): 962101. doi:10.1155/2012/962101.

Riehemann, K., S. W. Schneider, T. A. Luger, B. Godin, M. Ferrari, and H. Fuchs. "Nanomedicine--Challenge and Perspectives." *Angewandte Chemie International Edition in English* 48, no. 5 (2009): 872–97. doi:10.1002/anie.200802585.

Rogério, Gaspar, Helena Florindo, L. C. Silva, M. A. Videira, M. L. Corvo, B. F. Martins, and B. Silva-Lima. "Regulatory Aspects of Oncologicals: Nanosystems Main Challenges." In *Nano-Oncologicals. Advances in Delivery Science and Technology.* New York: Springer, 2014.

Rosenbrand, R., D. Barata, P. Sutthavas, R. Mohren, B. Cillero-Pastor, P. Habibovic, and S. van Rijt. "Lipid Surface Modifications Increase Mesoporous Silica Nanoparticle Labeling Properties in Mesenchymal Stem Cells." *International Journal of Nanomedicine* 13 (2018): 7711–25. doi:10.2147/IJN.S182428.

Rosi, N. L., D. A. Giljohann, C. S. Thaxton, A. K. Lytton-Jean, M. S. Han, and C. A. Mirkin. "Oligonucleotide-modified Gold Nanoparticles for Intracellular Gene Regulation." *Science* 312, no. 5776 (2006): 1027–30. doi:10.1126/science.1125559.

Rother, M., E. J. Seidel, P. M. Clarkson, S. Mazgareanu, U. Vierl, and I. Rother. "Efficacy of Epicutaneous Diractin (Ketoprofen in Transfersome Gel) for the Treatment of Pain Related to Eccentric Muscle Contractions." *Drug Design, Development & Therapy* 3 (2009): 143–9. doi:10.2147/dddt.s5501.

Rout, G. K., H.-S. Shin, S. Gouda, S. Sahoo, G. Das, L. F. Fraceto, and J. K. Patra. "Current Advances in Nanocarriers for Biomedical Research and Their Applications." *Artificial Cells, Nanomedicine & Biotechnology* 46, no. Suppl.2 (2018): 1053–62. doi:10.1080/21691401.2018.1478843.

Saha, B., J. Bhattacharya, A. Mukherjee, A. K. Ghosh, C. R. Santra, A. K. Dasgupta, and P. Karmakar. "In Vitro Structural and Functional Evaluation of Gold Nanoparticles Conjugated Antibiotics." *Nanoscale Research Letters* 2, no. 12 (2007): 614–22. doi:10.1007/s11671-007-9104-2.

Sainz, Vanessa, João Conniot, Ana I. Matos, Carina Peres, Eva Zupanǒiǒ, Liane Moura, Liana C. Silva, Helena F. Florindo, and Rogério S. Gaspar. "Regulatory Aspects on Nanomedicines." *Biochemical & Biophysical Research Communications* 468, no. 3 (2015): 504–10. doi:10.1016/j.bbrc.2015.08.023.

Salas, G., R. Costo, and M. del P. Morales. "Chapter 2: Synthesis of Inorganic Nanoparticles." In *Frontiers of Nanoscience*, edited by J. M. de la Fuente, and V. Grazu, 35–79. Amsterdam: Elsevier, 2012.

Saleh, Tawfik A. "Nanomaterials: Classification, Properties, and Environmental Toxicities." *Environmental Technology & Innovation* 20 (2020): 101067 doi:10.1016/j.eti.2020.101067.

Salim, N., N. Ahmad, S. H. Musa, R. Hashim, T. F. Tadros, and M. Basri. "Nanoemulsion as a Topical Delivery System of Antipsoriatic Drugs." *RSC Advances* 6, no. 8 (2016): 6234–50. doi:10.1039/C5RA14946K.

Salmaso, S., and P. Caliceti. "Stealth Properties to Improve Therapeutic Efficacy of Drug Nanocarriers." *Journal of Drug Delivery* 2013 (2013): 374252. doi:10.1155/2013/374252.

Salome Amarachi, C., F. Kenechukwu, and A. Attama. "Chapter 3: Nanoemulsions: Advances in Formulation, Characterization and Applications in Drug Delivery." In *Application of Nanotechnology in Drug Delivery*, 76–126. London: InTech, 2014.

Samia, A. C. S., X. Chen, and C. Burda. "Semiconductor Quantum Dots for Photodynamic Therapy." *Journal of the American Chemical Society* 125, no. 51 (2003): 15736–7. doi:10.1021/ja0386905.

Sang Yoo, H., and T. Gwan Park. "Biodegradable Nanoparticles Containing Protein-Fatty Acid Complexes for Oral Delivery of Salmon Calcitonin." *Journal of Pharmaceutical Sciences* 93, no. 2 (2004): 488–95. doi:10.1002/jps.10573.

Santo, V. E., J. Ratanavaraporn, K. Sato, M. E. Gomes, J. F. Mano, R. L. Reis, and Y. Tabata. "Cell Engineering by the Internalization of Bioinstructive Micelles for Enhanced Bone Regeneration." *Nanomedicine* 10, no. 11 (2015): 1707–21. doi:10.2217/nnm.15.11.

Santos, L. F., A. Sofia Silva, and J. F. Mano. "Complex-Shaped Magnetic 3D Cell-Based Structures for Tissue Engineering." *Acta Biomaterialia* 118 (2020): 18–31. doi:10.1016/j.actbio.2020.10.005.

Saraf, S., A. Jain, A. Tiwari, A. Verma, P. K. Panda, and S. K. Jain. "Advances in Liposomal Drug Delivery to Cancer: An Overview." *Journal of Drug Delivery Science & Technology* 56 (2020): 101549. doi:10.1016/j.jddst.2020.101549.

Saraiva, C., C. Praça, R. Ferreira, T. Santos, L. Ferreira, and L. Bernardino. "Nanoparticle-Mediated Brain Drug Delivery: Overcoming Blood–Brain Barrier to Treat Neurodegenerative Diseases." *Journal of Controlled Release* 235 (2016): 34–47. doi:10.1016/j.jconrel.2016.05.044.

Sato, M., A. Ito, H. Akiyama, Y. Kawabe, and M. Kamihira. "Effects of B-Cell lymphoma 2 Gene Transfer to Myoblast Cells on Skeletal Muscle Tissue Formation Using Magnetic Force-Based Tissue Engineering." *Tissue Engineering. Part A* 19, no. 1–2 (2013): 307–15. doi:10.1089/ten.tea.2011.0728.

Saulite, L., D. Dapkute, K. Pleiko, I. Popena, S. Steponkiene, R. Rotomskis, and U. Riekstina. "Nano-Engineered Skin Mesenchymal Stem Cells: Potential Vehicles for Tumour-Targeted Quantum-Dot Delivery." *Beilstein Journal of Nanotechnology* 8 (2017): 1218–30. doi:10.3762/bjnano.8.123.

Savić, R., A. Eisenberg, and D. Maysinger. "Block Copolymer Micelles as Delivery Vehicles of Hydrophobic Drugs: Micelle-Cell Interactions." *Journal of Drug Targeting* 14, no. 6 (2006): 343–55. doi:10.1080/10611860600874538.

Sawant, R. R., and V. P. Torchilin. "Multifunctionality of Lipid-Core Micelles for Drug Delivery and Tumour Targeting." *Molecular Membrane Biology* 27, no. 7 (2010): 232–46. doi:10.3109/09687688.2010.516276.

Sawant, R. R., A. M. Jhaveri, A. Koshkaryev, L. Zhu, F. Qureshi, and V. P. Torchilin. "Targeted Transferrin-Modified Polymeric Micelles: Enhanced Efficacy In Vitro and In Vivo in Ovarian Carcinoma." *Molecular Pharmaceutics* 11, no. 2 (2014): 375–81. doi:10.1021/mp300633f.

Schaffazick, S. R., A. R. Pohlmann, T. Dalla-Costa, and S. S. Guterres. "Freeze-Drying Polymeric Colloidal Suspensions: Nanocapsules, Nanospheres and Nanodispersion. A Comparative Study." *European Journal of Pharmaceutics & Biopharmaceutics* 56, no. 3 (2003): 501–5. doi:10.1016/s0939-6411(03)00139-5.

Schäffler, M., F. Sousa, A. Wenk, L. Sitia, S. Hirn, C. Schleh, N. Haberl, M. Violatto, M. Canovi, P. Andreozzi, M. Salmona, P. Bigini, W. G. Kreyling, and S. Krol. "Blood Protein Coating of Gold Nanoparticles as Potential Tool for Organ Targeting." *Biomaterials* 35, no. 10 (2014): 3455–66. doi:10.1016/j.biomaterials.2013.12.100.

Schipper, M. L., G. Iyer, A. L. Koh, Z. Cheng, Y. Ebenstein, A. Aharoni, S. Keren, L. A. Bentolila, J. Li, J. Rao, X. Chen, U. Banin, A. M. Wu, R. Sinclair, S. Weiss, and S. S. Gambhir. "Particle Size, Surface Coating, and PEGylation Influence the Biodistribution of Quantum Dots in Living Mice." *Small* 5, no. 1 (2009): 126–34. doi:10.1002/smll.200800003.

Scioli Montoto, S., G. Muraca, and M. E. Ruiz. "Solid Lipid Nanoparticles for Drug Delivery: Pharmacological and Biopharmaceutical Aspects." *Frontiers in Molecular Biosciences* 7, no. 319 (2020). doi:10.3389/fmolb.2020.587997.

Seigneuric, R., L. Markey, D. S. Nuyten, C. Dubernet, C. T. Evelo, E. Finot, and C. Garrido. "From Nanotechnology to Nanomedicine: Applications to Cancer Research." *Current Molecular Medicine* 10, no. 7 (2010): 640–52. doi:10.2174/156652410792630634.

Semalty, A., M. Semalty, B. S. Rawat, D. Singh, and M. S. Rawat. "Pharmacosomes: The Lipid-Based New Drug Delivery System." *Expert Opinion on Drug Delivery* 6, no. 6 (2009): 599–612. doi:10.1517/17425240902967607.

Sensenig, R., Y. Sapir, C. MacDonald, S. Cohen, and B. Polyak. "Magnetic Nanoparticle-based Approaches to Locally Target Therapy and Enhance Tissue Regeneration in vivo." *Nanomedicine* 7, no. 9 (2012): 1425–42. doi:10.2217/nnm.12.109.

Senthil Kumar, C., R. Thangam, S. A. Mary, P. R. Kannan, G. Arun, and B. Madhan. "Targeted Delivery and Apoptosis Induction of Trans-Resveratrol-Ferulic Acid Loaded Chitosan Coated Folic Acid Conjugate Solid Lipid Nanoparticles in Colon Cancer Cells." *Carbohydrate Polymers* 231 (2020):115682. doi:10.1016/j.carbpol.2019.115682.

Shah, B., D. Khunt, M. Misra, and H. Padh. "Application of Box-Behnken Design for Optimization and Development of Quetiapine Fumarate Loaded Chitosan Nanoparticles for Brain Delivery via Intranasal Route." *International Journal of Biological Macromolecules* 89 (2016): 206–218. doi:10.1016/j.ijbiomac.2016.04.076.

Shah, B. S., and J. J. Mao. "Labeling of Mesenchymal Stem Cells with Bioconjugated Quantum Dots." *Methods in Molecular Biology* 680 (2011): 61–75. doi:10.1007/978-1-60761-901-7_4.

Shen, B., Y. Ma, S. Yu, and C. Ji. "Smart Multifunctional Magnetic Nanoparticle-Based Drug Delivery System for Cancer Thermo-Chemotherapy and Intracellular Imaging." *ACS Applied Materials & Interfaces* 8, no. 37 (2016a): 24502–8. doi:10.1021/acsami.6b09772.

Shen, Z., M. P. Nieh, and Y. Li. "Decorating Nanoparticle Surface for Targeted Drug Delivery: Opportunities and Challenges." *Polymers* 8, no. 3 (2016b). doi:10.3390/polym8030083.

Shetab Boushehri, M. A., D. Dietrich, and A. Lamprecht. "Nanotechnology as a Platform for the Development of Injectable Parenteral Formulations: A Comprehensive Review of the Know-Hows and State of the Art." *Pharmaceutics* 12, no. 6 (2020): 510. doi:10.3390/pharmaceutics12060510.

Shevtsov, M. A., B. P. Nikolaev, L. Y. Yakovleva, A. V. Dobrodumov, A. V. Zhakhov, A. L. Mikhrina, E. Pitkin, M. A. Parr, V. I. Rolich, A. S. Simbircev, and A. M. Ischenko. "Recombinant Interleukin-1 Receptor Antagonist Conjugated to Superparamagnetic Iron Oxide Nanoparticles for Theranostic Targeting of Experimental Glioblastoma." *Neoplasia* 17, no. 1 (2015): 32–42. doi:10.1016/j.neo.2014.11.001.

Shi, Jinjun, Alexander R. Votruba, Omid C. Farokhzad, and Robert Langer. "Nanotechnology in Drug Delivery and Tissue Engineering: From Discovery to Applications." *Nano Letters* 10, no. 9 (2010): 3223–30. doi:10.1021/nl102184c.

Shi, M., Y. Zhou, J. Shao, Z. Chen, B. Song, J. Chang, C. Wu, and Y. Xiao. "Stimulation of Osteogenesis and Angiogenesis of hBMSCs by Delivering Si Ions and Functional Drug from Mesoporous Silica Nanospheres." *Acta Biomaterialia* 21 (2015): 178–89. doi:10.1016/j.actbio.2015.04.019.

Shi, M., Z. Chen, S. Farnaghi, T. Friis, X. Mao, Y. Xiao, and C. Wu. "Copper-Doped Mesoporous Silica Nanospheres, a Promising Immunomodulatory Agent for Inducing Osteogenesis." *Acta Biomaterialia* 30 (2016): 334–44. doi:10.1016/j.actbio.2015.11.033.

Shi, M., L. Xia, Z. Chen, F. Lv, H. Zhu, F. Wei, S. Han, J. Chang, Y. Xiao, and C. Wu. "Europium-doped Mesoporous Silica Nanosphere as an Immune-modulating Osteogenesis/Angiogenesis Agent." *Biomaterials* 144 (2017): 176–187. doi:10.1016/j.biomaterials.2017.08.027.

Shi, Y., R. van der Meel, X. Chen, and T. Lammers. "The EPR Effect and Beyond: Strategies to Improve Tumor Targeting and Cancer Nanomedicine Treatment Efficacy." *Theranostics* 10, no. 17 (2020): 7921–7924. doi:10.7150/thno.49577.

Shiang, Y.-C., C.-M. Ou, S.-J. Chen, T.-Y. Ou, H.-J. Lin, C.-C. Huang, and H.-T. Chang. "Highly Efficient Inhibition of Human Immunodeficiency Virus Type 1 Reverse Transcriptase By Aptamers Functionalized Gold Nanoparticles." *Nanoscale* 5, no. 7 (2013): 2756–64. doi:10.1039/C3NR33403A.

Shimizu, K., A. Ito, and H. Honda. "Enhanced Cell-Seeding into 3D Porous Scaffolds by Use of Magnetite Nanoparticles." *Journal of Biomedical Materials Research. Part B: Applied Biomaterials* 77, no. 2 (2006): 265–72. doi:10.1002/jbm.b.30443.

Shimizu, K., A. Ito, and H. Honda. "Mag-Seeding of Rat Bone Marrow Stromal Cells into Porous Hydroxyapatite Scaffolds for Bone Tissue Engineering." *Journal of Bioscience & Bioengineering* 104, no. 3 (2007a): 171–7. doi:10.1263/jbb.104.171.

Shimizu, K., A. Ito, T. Yoshida, Y. Yamada, M. Ueda, and H. Honda. "Bone Tissue Engineering with Human Mesenchymal Stem Cell Sheets Constructed Using Magnetite Nanoparticles and Magnetic Force." *Journal of Biomedical Materials Research. Part B: Applied Biomaterials* 82, no. 2 (2007b): 471–80. doi:10.1002/jbm.b.30752.

Shuhendler, A. J., P. Prasad, M. Leung, A. M. Rauth, R. S. DaCosta, and X. Y. Wu. "A Novel Solid Lipid Nanoparticle Formulation for Active Targeting to Tumor αvβ3 Integrin Receptors Reveals Cyclic RGD as a Double-Edged Sword." *Advanced Healthcare Materials* 1, no. 5 (2012): 600–8. doi:10.1002/adhm.201200006.

Silva, B., J. Marto, B. S. Braz, E. Delgado, A. J. Almeida and L. Gonçalves. "New Nanoparticles for Topical Ocular Delivery of Erythropoietin." *International Journal of Pharmaceutics* 576 (2020): 119020. doi:10.1016/j.ijpharm.2020.119020.

Simion, V., C. A. Constantinescu, D. Stan, M. Deleanu, M. M. Tucureanu, E. Butoi, I. Manduteanu, M. Simionescu, and M. Calin. "P-Selectin Targeted Dexamethasone-Loaded Lipid Nanoemulsions: A Novel Therapy to Reduce Vascular Inflammation." *Mediators of Inflammation* 2016 (2016):1625149. doi:10.1155/2016/1625149.

Singh, A., F. Dilnawaz, and S. K. Sahoo. "Long Circulating Lectin Conjugated Paclitaxel Loaded Magnetic Nanoparticles: A New Theranostic Avenue for Leukemia Therapy." *PLOS ONE* 6, no. 11 (2011): e26803. doi:10.1371/journal.pone.0026803.

Singh, Ajay Vikram, Mohammad Hasan Dad Ansari, Daniel Rosenkranz, Romi Singh Maharjan, Fabian L. Kriegel, Kaustubh Gandhi, Anurag Kanase, Rishabh Singh, Peter Laux, and Andreas Luch. "Artificial Intelligence and Machine Learning in Computational Nanotoxicology: Unlocking and Empowering Nanomedicine." *Advanced Healthcare Materials* 9, no. 17 (2020): 1901862. doi:10.1002/adhm.201901862.

Smith, A. M., and S. Nie. "Semiconductor Nanocrystals: Structure, Properties, and Band Gap Engineering." *Accounts of Chemical Research* 43, no. 2 (2010): 190–200. doi:10.1021/ar9001069.

Smith, A. M., H. Duan, A. M. Mohs, and S. Nie. "Bioconjugated Quantum Dots for In Vivo Molecular and Cellular Imaging." *Advanced Drug Delivery Reviews* 60, no. 11 (2008): 1226–40. doi:10.1016/j.addr.2008.03.015.

Smith, I. O., X. H. Liu, L. A. Smith, and P. X. Ma. "Nanostructured Polymer Scaffolds for Tissue Engineering and Regenerative Medicine." *Wiley Interdisciplinary Reviews. Nanomedicine & Nanobiotechnology* 1, no. 2 (2009): 226–36. doi:10.1002/wnan.26.

Soares, S., J. Sousa, A. Pais, and C. Vitorino. "Nanomedicine: Principles, Properties, and Regulatory Issues." *Frontiers in Chemistry* 6 (2018a): 360. doi:10.3389/fchem.2018.00360.

Soares, T. B., L. Loureiro, A. Carvalho, M. E. C. D. Real Oliveira, A. Dias, B. Sarmento, and M. Lúcio. "Lipid Nanocarriers Loaded with Natural Compounds: Potential New Therapies for Age Related Neurodegenerative Diseases?. " *Progress in Neurobiology* 168 (2018b): 21–41. doi:10.1016/j.pneurobio.2018.04.004.

Song, D., J. Cui, H. Sun, T.-H. Nguyen, S. Alcantara, R. De Rose, S. J. Kent, C. J. H. Porter, and F. Caruso. "Templated Polymer Replica Nanoparticles to Facilitate Assessment of Material-Dependent Pharmacokinetics and Biodistribution." *ACS Applied Materials & Interfaces* 9, no. 39 (2017): 33683–94. doi:10.1021/acsami.7b11579.

Souto, E. B., S. Doktorovova, J. R. Campos, P. Martins-Lopes, and A. M. Silva. "Surface-Tailored Anti-HER2/neu-Solid Lipid Nanoparticles for Site-Specific Targeting MCF-7 and BT-474 Breast Cancer Cells." *European Journal of Pharmaceutical Sciences* 128 (2019): 27–35. doi:10.1016/j.ejps.2018.11.022.

Spain, S. G., G. Yaşayan, M. Soliman, F. Heath, A. O. Saeed, and C. Alexander. "4.424: Nanoparticles for Nucleic Acid Delivery." In *Comprehensive Biomaterials*, edited by P. Ducheyne, 389–410. Oxford: Elsevier, 2011.

Spivak, M. Y., R. V. Bubnov, I. M. Yemets, L. M. Lazarenko, N. O. Tymoshok, and Z. R. Ulberg. "Development and Testing of Gold Nanoparticles for Drug Delivery and Treatment of Heart Failure: A Theranostic Potential for PPP Cardiology." *EPMA Journal* 4, no. 1 (2013): 20. doi:10.1186/1878-5085-4-20.

Sreejivungsa, K., N. Suchaichit, P. Moosophon, and A. Chompoosor. "Light-Regulated Release of Entrapped Drugs from Photoresponsive Gold Nanoparticles." *Journal of Nanomaterials* 2016 (2016): 4964693. doi:10.1155/2016/4964693.

Steinhäuser, Klaus Günter, and Philip G. Sayre. "Reliability of Methods and Data for Regulatory Assessment of Nanomaterial Risks." *NanoImpact* 7 (2017): 66–74. doi:10.1016/j.impact.2017.06.001.

Stirland, D. L., J. W. Nichols, S. Miura, and Y. H. Bae. "Mind the Gap: A Survey of How Cancer Drug Carriers Are Susceptible to the Gap Between Research and Practice." *Journal of Controlled Release* 172, no. 3 (2013): 1045–64. doi:10.1016/j.jconrel.2013.09.026.

Strebhardt, K., and A. Ullrich. "Paul Ehrlich's Magic Bullet Concept: 100 Years of Progress." *Nature Reviews. Cancer* 8, no. 6 (2008): 473–80. doi:10.1038/nrc2394.

Su, Shi, and Peter M. Kang. "Recent Advances in Nanocarrier-assisted Therapeutics Delivery Systems." *Pharmaceutics* 12, no. 9 (2020): 837. doi:10.3390/pharmaceutics12090837.

Sun, L., Z. Liu, L. Wang, D. Cun, H. H. Y. Tong, R. Yan, X. Chen, R. Wang and Y. Zheng. "Enhanced Topical Penetration, System Exposure and Anti-psoriasis Activity of Two Particle-sized, Curcumin-loaded PLGA Nanoparticles in Hydrogel." *Journal of Controlled Release* 254 (2017): 44–54. doi:10.1016/j.jconrel.2017.03.385.

Sun, W., Q. Hu, W. Ji, G. Wright, and Z. Gu. "Leveraging Physiology for Precision Drug Delivery." *Physiological Reviews* 97, no. 1 (2017): 189–225. doi:10.1152/physrev.00015.2016.

Sussman, E., A. Jayagopal, F. Haselton, and V. P. Shastri. "Engineering of Solid Lipid Nanoparticles for Biomedical Applications." In *New Delivery Systems for Controlled Drug Release from Naturally Occurring Materials*, edited by Nicholas Parris, LinShu Liu, Cunxian Song, and V. Prasad Shastri, 139–52. Washington DC: ACS, 2008.

Takeuchi, I., S. Kobayashi, Y. Hida and K. Makino. "Estradiol-loaded PLGA Nanoparticles for Improving Low Bone Mineral Density of Cancellous Bone Caused by Osteoporosis: Application of Enhanced Charged Nanoparticles with Iontophoresis." *Colloids and Surfaces B: Biointerfaces* 155 (2017): 35–40. doi:10.1016/j.colsurfb.2017.03.047.

Tan, J., Z. Deng, G. Liu, J. Hu, and S. Liu. "Anti-inflammatory Polymersomes of Redox-Responsive Polyprodrug Amphiphiles with Inflammation-triggered Indomethacin Release Characteristics." *Biomaterials* 178 (2018): 608–619. doi:10.1016/j.biomaterials.2018.03.035.

Taniguchi, N. "On the Basic Concept of Nanotechnology." In Proceeding of the ICPE, 18–23, Tokyo, 26–29 Aug., 1974.

Tanisaka, H., S. Kizaka-Kondoh, A. Makino, S. Tanaka, M. Hiraoka, and S. Kimura. "Near-Infrared Fluorescent Labeled Peptosome for Application to Cancer Imaging." *Bioconjugate Chemistry* 19, no. 1 (2008): 109–17. doi:10.1021/bc7001665.

Tao, Z. W., J. T. Favreau, J. P. Guyette, K. J. Hansen, J. Lessard, E. Burford, G. D. Pins, and G. R. Gaudette. "Delivering Stem Cells to the Healthy Heart on Biological Sutures: Effects on Regional Mechanical Function." *Journal of Tissue Engineering & Regenerative Medicine* 11, no. 1 (2017): 220–30. doi:10.1002/term.1904.

Taskintuna, I., A. S. Banker, M. Flores-Aguilar, G. Bergeron-Lynn, K. A. Aldern, K. Y. Hostetler, and W. R. Freeman. "Evaluation of a Novel Lipid Prodrug for Intraocular Drug Delivery: Effect of Acyclovir Diphosphate Dimyristoylglycerol in a Rabbit Model with Herpes Simplex Virus-1 Retinitis." *Retina* 17, no. 1 (1997): 57–64. doi:10.1097/00006982-199701000-00011.

Tayeb, H. H., and F. Sainsbury. "Nanoemulsions in Drug Delivery: Formulation to Medical Application." *Nanomedicine* 13, no. 19 (2018): 2507–25. doi:10.2217/nnm-2018-0088.

Teixeira, M. I., C. M. Lopes, M. H. Amaral, and P. C. Costa. "Current Insights on Lipid Nanocarrier-Assisted Drug Delivery in the Treatment of Neurodegenerative Diseases." *European Journal of Pharmaceutics & Biopharmaceutics* 149 (2020a): 192–217. doi:10.1016/j.ejpb.2020.01.005.

Teixeira, M. I., M. H. Amaral, P. C. Costa, C. M. Lopes, and Dimitrios A. Lamprou. "Recent Developments in Microfluidic Technologies for Central Nervous System Targeted Studies." *Pharmaceutics* 12, no. 6 (2020b): 542. doi:10.3390/pharmaceutics12060542.

Tekade, Rakesh K., Rahul Maheshwari, Namrata Soni, Muktika Tekade, and Mahavir B. Chougule. "Chapter 1: Nanotechnology for the Development of Nanomedicine." In *Nanotechnology-Based Approaches for Targeting and Delivery of Drugs and Genes*, edited by Vijay Mishra, and Prashant Kesharwani, Mohd Cairul Iqbal Mohd Amin and Arun Iyer, 3–61. London: Academic Press, 2017.

Teow, H. M., Z. Zhou, M. Najlah, S. R. Yusof, N. J. Abbott, and A. D'Emanuele. "Delivery of Paclitaxel Across Cellular Barriers Using a Dendrimer-Based Nanocarrier." *International Journal of Pharmacy* 441, no. 1–2 (2013): 701–11. doi:10.1016/j.ijpharm.2012.10.024.

Thevenot, P., S. Sohaebuddin, N. Poudyal, J. P. Liu, and L. Tang. "Magnetic Nanoparticles to Enhance Cell Seeding and Distribution in Tissue Engineering Scaffolds." *Proceedings of the IEEE* 2008 (2008): 646–9. doi:10.1109/NANO.2008.196.

Thomas, T. P., M. T. Myaing, J. Y. Ye, K. Candido, A. Kotlyar, J. Beals, P. Cao, B. Keszler, A. K. Patri, T. B. Norris, and J. R. Baker. "Detection and Analysis of Tumor Fluorescence Using a Two-Photon Optical Fiber Probe." *Biophysical Journal* 86, no. 6 (2004): 3959–65. doi:10.1529/biophysj.103.034462.

Tian, X., L. Zhang, M. Yang, L. Bai, Y. Dai, Z. Yu, and Y. Pan. "Functional Magnetic Hybrid Nanomaterials for Biomedical Diagnosis and Treatment." *Wiley Interdisciplinary Reviews. Nanomedicine & Nanobiotechnology* 10, no. 1 (2018). doi:10.1002/wnan.1476.

Tietze, R., R. Jurgons, S. Lyer, E. Schreiber, F. Wiekhorst, D. Eberbeck, H. Richter, U. Steinhoff, L. Trahms, and C. Alexiou. "Quantification of Drug-Loaded Magnetic Nanoparticles in Rabbit Liver and Tumor After In Vivo Administration." *Journal of Magnetism & Magnetic Materials* 321, no. 10 (2009): 1465–8. doi:10.1016/j.jmmm.2009.02.068.

Tinkle, S., S. E. McNeil, S. Mühlebach, R. Bawa, G. Borchard, Y. C. Barenholz, L. Tamarkin, and N. Desai. "Nanomedicines: Addressing the Scientific and Regulatory Gap." *Annals of the New York Academy of Sciences* 1313 (2014): 35–56. doi:10.1111/nyas.12403.

Torchilin, V. P. "Lipid-Core Micelles for Targeted Drug Delivery." *Current Drug Delivery* 2, no. 4 (2005): 319–27. doi:10.2174/156720105774370221.

Torchilin, V. P. "Chapter 1 Fundamentals of Stimuli-responsive Drug and Gene Delivery Systems." In *Stimuli-responsive Drug Delivery Systems*, edited by A. Singh, and M. M. Amiji, 1–32. Cambridge: The Royal Society of Chemistry, 2018.

Torchilin, V. P., M. D. Frank-Kamenetsky, and G. L. Wolf. "CT Visualization of Blood Pool in Rats by Using Long-Circulating, Iodine-Containing Micelles." *Academic Radiology* 6, no. 1 (1999): 61–5. doi:10.1016/S1076-6332(99)80063-4.

Torres-Ortega, P. V., L. Saludas, J. E. Idoyaga, C. Rodríguez-Nogales, E. Garbayo, and M. J. Blanco-Prieto. "Chapter 6: Hybrid Nanosystems." In *Nanoparticles for Brain Drug Delivery*, edited by C. Vitorino, A. Jorge, and A. A. C. C. Pais. Singapore: Jenny Stanford Publishing Pte. Ltd, 2021.

Tsai, F.-T., Y. Wang, and D. J. Darensbourg. "Environmentally Benign CO2-Based Copolymers: Degradable Polycarbonates Derived from Dihydroxybutyric Acid and Their Platinum–Polymer Conjugates." *Journal of the American Chemical Society* 138, no. 13 (2016): 4626–33. doi:10.1021/jacs.6b01327.

Tuguntaev, R. G., C. I. Okeke, J. Xu, C. Li, P. C. Wang, and X. J. Liang. "Nanoscale Polymersomes as Anti-Cancer Drug Carriers Applied for Pharmaceutical Delivery." *Current Pharmaceutical Design* 22, no. 19 (2016): 2857–65. doi:10.2174/1381612822666160217142319.

Tupal, A., M. Sabzichi, F. Ramezani, M. Kouhsoltani, and H. Hamishehkar. "Dermal Delivery of Doxorubicin-Loaded Solid Lipid Nanoparticles for the Treatment of Skin Cancer." *Journal of Microencapsulation* 33, no. 4 (2016): 372–80. doi:10.1080/02652048.2016.1200150.

Venuganti, V. V., and O. P. Perumal. "Poly(Amidoamine) Dendrimers as Skin Penetration Enhancers: Influence of Charge, Generation, and Concentration." *Journal of Pharmaceutical Sciences* 98, no. 7 (2009): 2345–56. doi:10.1002/jps.21603.

Verma, P., and K. Pathak. "Therapeutic and Cosmeceutical Potential of Ethosomes: An Overview." *Journal of Advanced Pharmaceutical Technology & Research* 1, no. 3 (2010): 274–82. doi:10.4103/0110-5558.72415.

Veronese, F. M., and A. Mero (2008). "The impact of PEGylation on biological therapies." *BioDrugs* no. 22 (5): 315–29. doi:10.2165/00063030-200822050-00004.

Videira, M. A., M. F. Botelho, A. C. Santos, L. F. Gouveia, J. J. de Lima, and A. J. Almeida. "Lymphatic Uptake of Pulmonary Delivered Radiolabelled Solid Lipid Nanoparticles." *Journal of Drug Targeting* 10, no. 8 (2002): 607–13. doi:10.1080/1061186021000054933.

Vieira, D. B., and L. F. Gamarra. "Getting into the Brain: Liposome-Based Strategies for Effective Drug Delivery Across the Blood-Brain Barrier." *International Journal of Nanomedicine* 11 (2016): 5381–414. doi:10.2147/IJN.S117210.

Viseu, T., C. M. Lopes, E. Fernandes, M. E. C. D. Real Oliveira, and M. Lucio. "A Systematic Review and Critical Analysis of the Role of Graphene-based Nanomaterialsin Cancer Theranostics." *Pharmaceutics* 10, no. 282 (2018): 1–45. doi:10.3390/pharmaceutics10040282.

Vitorino, C., A. Almeida, J. Sousa, I. Lamarche, P. Gobin, S. Marchand, W. Couet, J.-C. Olivier, and A. Pais. "Passive and Active Strategies for Transdermal Delivery Using Co-Encapsulating Nanostructured Lipid Carriers: In Vitro vs. In Vivo Studies." *European Journal of Pharmaceutics & Biopharmaceutics* 86, no. 2 (2014): 133–44. doi:10.1016/j.ejpb.2013.12.004.

Vrana, N. E., O. Erdemli, G. Francius, A. Fahs, M. Rabineau, C. Debry, A. Tezcaner, D. Keskin, and P. Lavalle. "Double Entrapment of Growth Factors by Nanoparticles Loaded into Polyelectrolyte Multilayer Films." *Journal of Materials Chemistry B* 2, no. 8 (2014): 999–1008. doi:10.1039/C3TB21304H.

Wang, D., and T. Imae. "Fluorescence Emission from Dendrimers and Its pH Dependence." *Journal of the American Chemical Society* 126, no. 41 (2004): 13204–5. doi:10.1021/ja0454992.

Wang, J., Y. Wei, Y.-R. Fei, L. Fang, H.-S. Zheng, C.-F. Mu, F.-Z. Li, and Y.-S. Zhang. "Preparation of Mixed Monoterpenes Edge Activated Pegylated Transfersomes to Improve the In Vivo Transdermal Delivery Efficiency of Sinomenine Hydrochloride." *International Journal of Pharmacy* 533, no. 1 (2017a): 266–74. doi:10.1016/j.ijpharm.2017.09.059.

Wang, J., J. Yu, Y. Yan, D. Yang, P. Wang, Y. Xu, J. Zhu, G. Xu, D. He, and G. Huang. "Biodegradable Polyester/Modified Mesoporous Silica Composites for Effective Bone Repair with Self-Reinforced Properties." *Polymers for Advanced Technologies* 30, no. 6 (2019): 1461–72. doi:10.1002/pat.4578.

Wang, J., D. Li, C. Liang, C. Wang, X. Zhou, L. Ying, Y. Tao, H. Xu, J. Shu, X. Huang, Z. Gong, K. Xia, F. Li, Q. Chen, J. Tang, and Y. Shen. "Scar Tissue-targeting Polymer Micelle for Spinal Cord Injury Treatment." *Small* 16, no. 8 (2020): 1906415. doi:10.1002/smll.201906415.

Wang, Q., C. Chen, W. Liu, X. He, N. Zhou, D. Zhang, H. Gu, J. Li, J. Jiang, and W. Huang. "Levofloxacin Loaded Mesoporous Silica Microspheres/Nano-Hydroxyapatite/Polyurethane Composite Scaffold for the Treatment of Chronic Osteomyelitis with Bone Defects." *Scientific Reports* 7 (2017b): 41808–. doi:10.1038/srep41808.

Wang, T., Y. Liu, and C. Wu. "Effect of Paclitaxel-Mesoporous Silica Nanoparticles with a Core-Shell Structure on the Human Lung Cancer Cell Line A549." *Nanoscale Research Letters* 12, no. 1 (2017c): 66–. doi:10.1186/s11671-017-1826-1.

Wang, X., H. Chen, Y. Chen, M. Ma, K. Zhang, F. Li, Y. Zheng, D. Zeng, Q. Wang, and J. Shi. "Perfluorohexane-Encapsulated Mesoporous Silica Nanocapsules as Enhancement Agents for Highly Efficient High Intensity Focused Ultrasound (HIFU)." *Advanced Materials* 24, no. 6 (2012): 785–91. doi:10.1002/adma.201104033.

Wang, X. Q., and Q. Zhang. "pH-Sensitive Polymeric Nanoparticles to Improve Oral Bioavailability of Peptide/Protein Drugs and Poorly Water-soluble Drugs." *European Journal of Pharmaceutics and Biopharmaceutics* 82, no. 2 (2012): 219–229. doi:10.1016/j.ejpb.2012.07.014.

Wang, Y., A. G. Cheetham, G. Angacian, H. Su, L. Xie, and H. Cui. "Peptide-Drug Conjugates as Effective Prodrug Strategies for Targeted Delivery." *Advanced Drug Delivery Reviews* 110–111 (2017): 112–26. doi:10.1016/j.addr.2016.06.015.

Wang, Y., and D. S. Kohane. "External Triggering and Triggered Targeting Strategies for Drug Delivery." *Nature Reviews Materials* 2, no. 6 (2017): 17020. doi:10.1038/natrevmats.2017.20.

Wang, Y., H. Cui, K. Li, C. Sun, W. Du, J. Cui, X. Zhao, and W. Chen. "A Magnetic Nanoparticle-Based Multiple-Gene Delivery System for Transfection of Porcine Kidney Cells." *PLOS ONE* 9, no. 7 (2014): e102886. doi:10.1371/journal.pone.0102886.

Wang, Y., C. Yang, R. Hu, H. T. Toh, X. Liu, G. Lin, F. Yin, H. S. Yoon, and K.-T. Yong. "Assembling Mn:ZnSe Quantum Dots-siRNA Nanoplexes for Gene Silencing in Tumor Cells." *Biomaterials Science* 3, no. 1 (2015): 192–202. doi:10.1039/C4BM00306C.

Wang, Y. S., S. Youngster, M. Grace, J. Bausch, R. Bordens, and D. F. Wyss. "Structural and Biological Characterization of Pegylated Recombinant Interferon Alpha-2B and Its Therapeutic Implications." *Advanced Drug Delivery Reviews* 54, no. 4 (2002): 547–70. doi:10.1016/s0169-409x(02)00027-3.

Wang, Z., L. Dong, L. Han, K. Wang, X. Lu, L. Fang, S. Qu, and C. W. Chan. "Self-Assembled Biodegradable Nanoparticles and Polysaccharides as Biomimetic ECM Nanostructures for the Synergistic Effect of RGD and BMP-2 on Bone Formation." *Scientific Reports* 6, no. 1 (2016): 25090. doi:10.1038/srep25090.

Wang, Z., Z. Wang, W. W. Lu, W. Zhen, D. Yang, and S. Peng. "Novel Biomaterial Strategies for Controlled Growth Factor Delivery for Biomedical Applications." *NPG Asia Materials* 9, no. 10 (2017): e435–e. doi:10.1038/am.2017.171.

Wen, Y., J. Ban, Z. Mo, Y. Zhang, P. An, L. Liu, Q. Xie, Y. Du, B. Xie, X. Zhan, L. Tan, Y. Chen, and Z. Lu. "A Potential Nanoparticle-loaded in situ Gel for Enhanced and Sustained Ophthalmic Delivery of Dexamethasone." *Nanotechnology* 29, no. 42 (2018): 425101. doi:10.1088/1361-6528/aad7da.

Werner, K., R. Ilka, R. Matthias, S. Egbert, and IDEA-033-III-01 Study Group. "A Multiple-Dose, Open-Label, Safety, Compliance, and Usage Evaluation Study of Epicutaneously Applied Diractin; (Ketoprofen in Transfersome) in Joint/Musculoskeletal Pain or Soft Tissue Inflammation." *Current Drug Safety* 4, no. 1 (2009): 5–10. doi:10.2174/157488609787354468.

Whelove, O. E., M. J. Cozad, B. D. Lee, S. Sengupta, S. L. Bachman, B. J. Ramshaw, and S. A. Grant. "Development and In Vitro Studies of a Polyethylene Terephthalate-Gold Nanoparticle Scaffold for Improved Biocompatibility." *Journal of Biomedical Materials Research. Part B: Applied Biomaterials* 99, no. 1 (2011): 142–9. doi:10.1002/jbm.b.31881.

Wu, D., J. Yang, J. Li, L. Chen, B. Tang, X. Chen, W. Wu, and J. Li. "Hydroxyapatite-Anchored Dendrimer for in situ Remineralization of Human Tooth Enamel." *Biomaterials* 34, no. 21 (2013): 5036–47. doi:10.1016/j.biomaterials.2013.03.053.

Wu, F., T. Xu, G. Zhao, S. Meng, M. Wan, B. Chi, C. Mao, and J. Shen. "Mesoporous Silica Nanoparticles-encapsulated Agarose and Heparin as Anticoagulant and Resisting Bacterial Adhesion Coating for Biomedical Silicone." *Langmuir* 33, no. 21 (2017): 5245–52. doi:10.1021/acs.langmuir.7b00567.

Wu, H., F. Li, S. Wang, J. Lu, J. Li, Y. Du, X. Sun, X. Chen, J. Gao, and D. Ling. "Ceria Nanocrystals Decorated Mesoporous Silica Nanoparticle based ROS-scavenging Tissue Adhesive for Highly Efficient Regenerative Wound Healing." *Biomaterials* 151: 66–77 (2018). doi:10.1016/j.biomaterials.2017.10.018.

Wu, K., D. Su, J. Liu, R. Saha, and J.-P. Wang. "Magnetic Nanoparticles in Nanomedicine: A Review of Recent Advances." *Nanotechnology* 30, no. 50 (2019): 502003. doi:10.1088/1361-6528/ab4241.

Wu, X., H. Liu, J. Liu, K. N. Haley, J. A. Treadway, J. P. Larson, N. Ge, F. Peale, and M. P. Bruchez. "Immunofluorescent Labeling of Cancer Marker Her2 and Other Cellular Targets with Semiconductor Quantum Dots." *Nature Biotechnology* 21, no. 1 (2003): 41–6. doi:10.1038/nbt764.

Xie, H., L. Li, Y. Sun, Y. Wang, S. Gao, Y. Tian, X. Ma, C. Guo, F. Bo, and L. Zhang. "An Available Strategy for Nasal Brain Transport of Nanocomposite based on PAMAM Dendrimers via in situ Gel." *Nanomaterials* 9, no. 2 (2019): 147. doi:10.3390/nano9020147.

Xie, J., Y. Bi, H. Zhang, S. Dong, L. Teng, R. J. Lee, and Z. Yang. "Cell-Penetrating Peptides in Diagnosis and Treatment of Human Diseases: From Preclinical Research to Clinical Application." *Frontiers in Pharmacology* 11 (2020): 697. doi:10.3389/fphar.2020.00697.

Xie, W., L. Wang, Y. Zhang, L. Su, A. Shen, J. Tan, and J. Hu. "Nuclear Targeted Nanoprobe for Single Living Cell Detection by Surface-Enhanced Raman Scattering." *Bioconjugate Chemistry* 20, no. 4 (2009): 768–173. doi:10.1021/bc800469g.

Xie, Z., C. B. Paras, H. Weng, P. Punnakitikashem, L. C. Su, K. Vu, L. Tang, J. Yang, and K. T. Nguyen. "Dual Growth Factor Releasing Multi-Functional Nanofibers for Wound Healing." *Acta Biomaterialia* 9, no. 12 (2013): 9351–9. doi:10.1016/j.actbio.2013.07.030.

Xing, H., K. Hwang, and Y. Lu (2016). "Recent Developments of Liposomes as Aanocarriers for Theranostic Applications." *Theranostics* 6, no. 9: 1336–52. doi:10.7150/thno.15464.

Xu, C., Y. Sun, Y. Yu, M. Hu, C. Yang, and Z. Zhang. "A Sequentially Responsive and Structure-Transformable Nanoparticle with a Comprehensively Improved 'CAPIR Cascade' for Enhanced Antitumor Effect." *Nanoscale* 11, no. 3 (2019): 1177–94. doi:10.1039/c8nr08781d.

Yamamoto, Y., A. Ito, M. Kato, Y. Kawabe, K. Shimizu, H. Fujita, E. Nagamori, and M. Kamihira. "Preparation of Artificial Skeletal Muscle Tissues by a Magnetic Force-Based Tissue Engineering Technique." *Journal of Bioscience & Bioengineering* 108, no. 6 (2009): 538–43. doi:10.1016/j.jbiosc.2009.05.019.

Yan, Y., J. Gong, J. Chen, Z. Zeng, W. Huang, K. Pu, J. Liu, and P. Chen. "Recent Advances on Graphene Quantum Dots: From Chemistry and Physics to Applications." *Advanced Materials* 31, no. 21 (2019): e1808283. doi:10.1002/adma.201808283.

Yang, B. B., and A. Kido. "Pharmacokinetics and Pharmacodynamics of Pegfilgrastim." *Clinical Pharmacokinetics* 50, no. 5 (2011): 295–306. doi:10.2165/11586040-000000000-00000.

Yang, C., H. Chen, J. Zhao, X. Pang, Y. Xi, and G. Zhai. "Development of a Folate-Modified Curcumin Loaded Micelle Delivery System for Cancer Targeting." *Colloids & Surfaces, Part B: Biointerfaces* 121 (2014): 206–13. doi:10.1016/j.colsurfb.2014.05.005.

Yang, H., H. Mao, Z. Wan, A. Zhu, M. Guo, Y. Li, X. Li, J. Wan, X. Yang, X. Shuai, and H. Chen. "Micelles Assembled with Carbocyanine Dyes for Theranostic Near-infrared Fluorescent Cancer Imaging and Photothermal Therapy." *Biomaterials* 34, no. 36 (2013): 9124–33. doi:10.1016/j.biomaterials.2013.08.022.

Yang, X., D. Wang, Y. Ma, Q. Zhao, J. K. Fallon, D. Liu, X. E. Xu, Y. Wang, Z. He, and F. Liu. "Theranostic Nanoemulsions: Codelivery of Hydrophobic Drug and Hydrophilic Imaging Probe for Cancer Therapy and Imaging." *Nanomedicine* 9, no. 18 (2014): 2773–85. doi:10.2217/nnm.14.50.

Yang, Yafeng, Aditya Chawla, Jin Zhang, Adam Esa, Hae Lin Jang, and Ali Khademhosseini. "Chapter 29: Applications of Nanotechnology for Regenerative Medicine: Healing Tissues at the Nanoscale." In *Principles of Regenerative Medicine*. 3rd ed., edited by Anthony Atala, Robert Lanza, Antonios G. Mikos, and Robert Nerem, 485–504. Boston, MA: Academic Press, 2019.

Yao, J., P. Li, L. Li, and M. Yang. "Biochemistry and Biomedicine of Quantum Dots: From Biodetection to Bioimaging, Drug Discovery, Diagnostics, and Therapy." *Acta Biomaterialia* 74 (2018): 36–55. doi:10.1016/j.actbio.2018.05.004.

Ye, M., Y. Qian, J. Tang, H. Hu, M. Sui, and Y. Shen. "Targeted Biodegradable Dendritic MRI Contrast Agent for Enhanced Tumor Imaging." *Journal of Controlled Release* 169, no. 3 (2013): 239–45. doi:10.1016/j.jconrel.2013.01.034.

Yi, C., D. Liu, C. C. Fong, J. Zhang, and M. Yang. "Gold Nanoparticles Promote Osteogenic Differentiation of Mesenchymal Stem Cells Through p38 MAPK Pathway." *ACS Nano* 4, no. 11 (2010): 6439–48. doi:10.1021/nn101373r.

Yilgor, P., K. Tuzlakoglu, R. L. Reis, N. Hasirci, and V. Hasirci. "Incorporation of a Sequential BMP-2/BMP-7 Delivery System into Chitosan-based Scaffolds for Bone Tissue Engineering." *Biomaterials* 30, no. 21 (2009): 3551–9. doi:10.1016/j.biomaterials.2009.03.024.

Yoo, J., C. Park, G. Yi, D. Lee, and H. Koo. "Active Targeting Strategies Using Biological Ligands for Nanoparticle Drug Delivery Systems." *Cancers* 11, no. 5 (2019): 640. doi:10.3390/cancers11050640.

Young, S. H., and E. Rozengurt. "Qdot Nanocrystal Conjugates Conjugated to Bombesin or ANG II Label the Cognate G Protein-Coupled Receptor in Living Cells." *American Journal of Physiology. Cell Physiology* 290, no. 3 (2006): C728–C32. doi:10.1152/ajpcell.00310.2005.

Zakrewsky, M., S. Kumar, and S. Mitragotri. "Nucleic Acid Delivery into Skin for the Treatment of Skin Disease: Proofs-of-Concept, Potential Impact, and Remaining Challenges." *Journal of Controlled Release* 219 (2015): 445–56. doi:10.1016/j.jconrel.2015.09.017.

Zhang, H., J. Yang, K. Liang, J. Li, L. He, X. Yang, S. Peng, X. Chen, C. Ding, and J. Li. "Effective Dentin Restorative Material Based on Phosphate-Terminated Dendrimer as Artificial Protein." *Colloids & Surfaces, Part B: Biointerfaces* 128 (2015): 304–14. doi:10.1016/j.colsurfb.2015.01.058.

Zhang, H., S. Yu, X. Zhao, Z. Mao, and C. Gao. "Stromal Cell-Derived factor-1α-encapsulated Albumin/Heparin Nanoparticles for Induced Stem Cell Migration and Intervertebral Disc Regeneration In Vivo." *Acta Biomaterialia* 72 (2018): 217–27. doi:10.1016/j.actbio.2018.03.032.

Zhang, J., C. Li, X. Zhang, S. Huo, S. Jin, F.-F. An, X. Wang, X. Xue, C. I. Okeke, G. Duan, F. Guo, X. Zhang, J. Hao, P. C. Wang, J. Zhang, and X.-J. Liang. "In vivo tumor-targeted dual-modal fluorescence/CT imaging using a nanoprobe co-loaded with an aggregation-induced emission dye and gold nanoparticles." *Biomaterials* 42 (2015): 103–111. doi:10.1016/j.biomaterials.2014.11.053.

Zhang, P., A. G. Cheetham, L. L. Lock, and H. Cui. "Cellular Uptake and Cytotoxicity of Drug–Peptide Conjugates Regulated by Conjugation Site." *Bioconjugate Chemistry* 24, no. 4 (2013): 604–13. doi:10.1021/bc300585h.

Zhang, X.-Y., and P.-Y. Zhang. "Polymersomes in Nanomedicine: A Review." *Current Medicinal Chemistry* 13, no. 2 (2017): 124–9. doi:10.2174/1573413712666161018144519.

Zhao, Y.-Z., X. Li, C.-T. Lu, M. Lin, L.-J. Chen, Q. Xiang, M. Zhang, R.-R. Jin, X. Jiang, X.-T. Shen, X.-K. Li, and J. Cai. "Gelatin Nanostructured Lipid Carriers-mediated Intranasal Delivery of Basic Fibroblast Growth Factor Enhances Functional Recovery in Hemiparkinsonian Rats." *Nanomedicine* 10, no. 4 (2014): 755–64. doi:10.1016/j.nano.2013.10.009.

Zhao, Z., A. Ukidve, J. Kim, and S. Mitragotri. "Targeting Strategies for Tissue-specific Drug Delivery." *Cell* 181, no. 1 (2020): 151–67. doi:10.1016/j.cell.2020.02.001.

Zheng, F.-F., P.-H. Zhang, Y. Xi, J.-J. Chen, L.-L. Li, and J.-J. Zhu. "Aptamer/Graphene Quantum Dots Nanocomposite Capped Fluorescent Mesoporous Silica Nanoparticles for Intracellular Drug Delivery and Real-Time Monitoring of Drug Release." *Analytical Sciences* 87, no. 23 (2015): 11739–45. doi:10.1021/acs.analchem.5b03131.

Zhou, J., Q. X. Wang, and C. Y. Zhang. "Liposome-Quantum Dot Complexes Enable Multiplexed Detection of Attomolar DNAs Without Target Amplification." *Journal of the American Chemical Society* 135, no. 6 (2013): 2056–9. doi:10.1021/ja3110329.

Zhou, X., L. Chen, W. Nie, W. Wang, M. Qin, X. Mo, H. Wang, and C. He. "Dual-Responsive Mesoporous Silica Nanoparticles Mediated Codelivery of Doxorubicin and Bcl-2 SiRNA for Targeted Treatment of Breast Cancer." *Journal of Physical Chemistry C* 120, no. 39 (2016): 22375–87. doi:10.1021/acs.jpcc.6b06759.

Zhou, X., W. Weng, B. Chen, W. Feng, W. Wang, W. Nie, L. Chen, X. Mo, J. Su, and C. He. "Mesoporous Silica Nanoparticles/Gelatin Porous Composite Scaffolds with Localized and Sustained Release of Vancomycin for Treatment of Infected Bone Defects." *Journal of Materials Chemistry B* 6, no. 5 (2018): 740–52. doi:10.1039/C7TB01246B.

Zhu, S.-P., Z.-G. Wang, Y.-Z. Zhao, J. Wu, H.-X. Shi, L.-B. Ye, F.-Z. Wu, Y. Cheng, H.-Y. Zhang, S. He, X. Wei, X.-B. Fu, X.-K. Li, H.-Z. Xu, and J. Xiao. "Gelatin Nanostructured Lipid Carriers Incorporating Nerve Growth Factor Inhibit Endoplasmic Reticulum Stress-Induced Apoptosis and Improve Recovery in Spinal Cord Injury." *Molecular Neurobiology* 53, no. 7 (2016): 4375–86. doi:10.1007/s12035-015-9372-2.

Zhu, Y., C. Liu, and Z. Pang. "Dendrimer-based Drug Delivery Systems for Brain Targeting." *Biomolecules* 9, no. 12 (2019): 790. doi:10.3390/biom9120790.

Zielinska, A., F. Carreiro, A. M. Oliveira, A. Neves, B. Pires, D. N. Venkatesh, A. Durazzo, M. Lucarini, P. Eder, A. M. Silva, A. Santini, and E. B. Souto (2020). "Polymeric Nanoparticles: Production, Characterization, Toxicology and Ecotoxicology." *Molecules* 25, no. 16. doi:10.3390/molecules25163731.

Zylberberg, C., and S. Matosevic. "Pharmaceutical Liposomal Drug Delivery: A Review of New Delivery Systems and a Look at the Regulatory Landscape." *Drug Delivery* 23, no. 9 (2016): 3319–29. doi:10.1080/10717544.2016.1177136.

Escaping Immune Clearance

3

Esmael M. Alyami, Ammar Tarar, and Ching-An Peng

Contents

3.1 INTRODUCTION

The mononuclear phagocyte system (MPS) involves the identification of foreign particles that will be eliminated from the body. Markers such as CD47 and CD200 allow cells to be recognized by the immune system as self. Red blood cells can have their surface self-markers for four months before they are destroyed by the immune system. The MPS is a barrier that all intravenous drug carriers must overcome to reach targeted sites. For a therapeutic carrier to be effective it is required to have prolonged longevity in the circulation system as well as the ability to target its specific site of entry.[1] For the biodistribution of particles to be effective, their size, shape, and surface characteristics must fall between ideal parameters. When particles are non-biocompatible, they are easily recognized by the MPS, rendering them ineffective as drug delivery carriers. Ideal carriers are between 10 and 200 nm; however, carriers larger than 200 nm can be modified to improve drug delivery efficiency.[2] For example, tethering targeting molecule enables therapeutic carriers to aim at disease sites.[3] Altering the surface characteristics of a carrier can also reduce the rate of opsonization and avoid complement activation. In order to overcome the biochemical and immunological obstacles that therapeutic carriers face, the ability to attach polyethylene glycol (PEG) chains to a molecule or carrier was developed, a process called PEGylation. It has been demonstrated that PEG chains offer stealth-like properties when attached, and subsequently, several conjugation strategies have been developed for therapeutic use.[4] PEGylated dendrimers, liposomes, and micelles have shown to be viable therapeutic agents in cancer therapy. The PEGylation of other compounds such as protein molecules and monoclonal antibodies has demonstrated an increased circulation time and a reduction of immunogenicity without a decrease in effectiveness[5] PEGylation has indeed improved the pharmacokinetics of therapeutic carriers, but there are still immunological obstacles that need to be overcome. Several studies focused on issues such as hypersensitivity and non-biodegradability as drawbacks that open the consideration for other biochemical processes that can reduce opsonization. The complexity of natural particulates has set the standard for synthetic biomaterials to have functionality and diversity. The erythrocyte exhibits a complex biological functionality where it can last in the circulation for up to four months while performing complex biological tasks without being recognized as a foreign particle. Pathogens have evolved immune-evading mechanisms that allow them to infect hosts efficiently.

While therapeutic alternatives are rapidly developing, combining this with the delivery mechanisms is not keeping pace. On the surface, it simply appears like packaging and delivering cargo; in essence, it is a complex amalgamation of the physicochemical availability of the drug, its route of administration, and the stability and interaction of the delivery system with the drug and the host[6] The last decade has seen the rise of several nanoparticles (NPs)-based delivery systems such as liposomes and micelles, which have been used for the treatment of cancer and other diseases.

Typically, NPs are solid, colloidal particles in the range of 10–1,000 nm and for drug delivery systems the preferred size is less than 200 nm.[6] The small size of particles enhances their solubility, increases their bioavailability, and permits better absorption in the various organ systems. For systemically delivered engineered NPs overcoming the protective mechanisms of multiple-level organ responses such as those operative in the MPS poses a great challenge. Design challenges need to take care of overcoming the host defense mechanisms but also need to modify vectors to achieve tailored release of the drug. Sensor-based drug release and the degradation of drug carriers post-release are also desirable traits.[7]

The quest to rationalize the above expectations delved into biomimicry wherein delivery systems mimicked biological systems, allowing them to overcome the "natural" biological barriers of the host under consideration and accentuate drug delivery. The current chapter discusses the use of chemical and bio-inspired strategies in the development of drug delivery carriers that allow them to overcome the natural host defense mechanisms.

3.2 HOST DEFENSE MECHANISM

Before we delve into understanding the prolonged circulation of NPs in the human host, one has to understand how the "innate" host immune mechanism clears the NPs from circulation. The mammalian immune system is a multi-tiered security platform that has a checkpoint at every level. The MPS in systemically fixed tissues with the help of their heterogeneous population of phagocytic cells play a significant role in the identification and clearance of perceived antigenic threats (immune complexes, exogenous and endogenous antigens). The composition of MPS includes the liver Kupffer cells, the brain microglia, lung alveolar macrophages, and lymph nodes. The antigens may be internalized (phagocytosed) either through non-immune receptor-mediated phagocytosis or by immunophagic effects mediated by binding to Fc receptors or complement receptors.[8] It was also found that macrophage phenotype has a role in NP uptake. The M1 polarized phenotype was shown to have a higher NP uptake in an isolated culture system in comparison to the M2 phenotype.[9] The MPS does not encounter "bare" NPs. The contact of NPs with blood or other tissues allows its conditioning to the host MPS and produces protein adsorption to the NPs' surface. This protein adsorption, also known as "corona", serves as opsonins that prime the NPs for enhanced uptake and clearance. These opsonized particles enter the phagocytes through several receptors such as the Toll-like receptors, Fc receptors, and scavenger receptors[10]

3.3 STEALTH FUNCTIONALIZATION

3.3.1 Chemical Approach

Having realized the challenges faced by the NPs in the human host by the innate immune responses, the plan is to prolong the blood circulation of NPs in the host to ensure targeted drug delivery. One of the means of achieving this stealth functionality is through polymer grafting. It was preliminarily observed that hydrophobic or charged particles have a higher propensity to opsonization versus hydrophilic or uncharged particles. Some of the polymers used to confer stealth properties on NPs include PEG, poly (2-oxazoline), and poly(zwitterions) (Figure 3.1). These molecules are hydrophilic and flexible, and their presence on the NP sterically impedes the interaction of the NPs with the opsonin proteins, thus resulting in their increased circulation in the blood.

3.3.1.1 Polyethylene Glycol

Among these polymers, PEG has received the most attention. The process of PEGylation involves the attachment of repeat units of EG to the NPs or the drug. PEGylation prevents the binding of opsonin proteins to the NPs in part due to their molecular weight, surface chain density, and conformation of the polymer.[9] Pegaspargase for leukemia and pegademase for severe combined immunodeficiency disorder were among the first PEGylated drugs approved by the FDA[11] Currently close to 20 PEGylated products are under review or have been approved by the FDA. These include various classes of drug molecules from recombinant proteins (cytokines, growth factors, coagulation factors, antibodies, hormones, peptides). While the PEGylation of biological products is discussed more often, there is development for expanding its use for non-biologic products (small organic molecules, aptamers, and synthetic peptides)[12] PEGylated drugs find application in the treatment of cancers, hepatitis C, acromegaly, neutropenia, and wound healing among other disorders.[11] While PEG has been a natural choice for the surface coating of several nanoparticles, reports indicate the presence of anti-PEG immunity in a significant proportion of PEG-naïve and exposed individuals.[13] Anti-PEG antibodies of type IgG and IgM are reported. It is believed that the presence of these antibodies contributes to the phenomenon of accelerated blood clearance. This

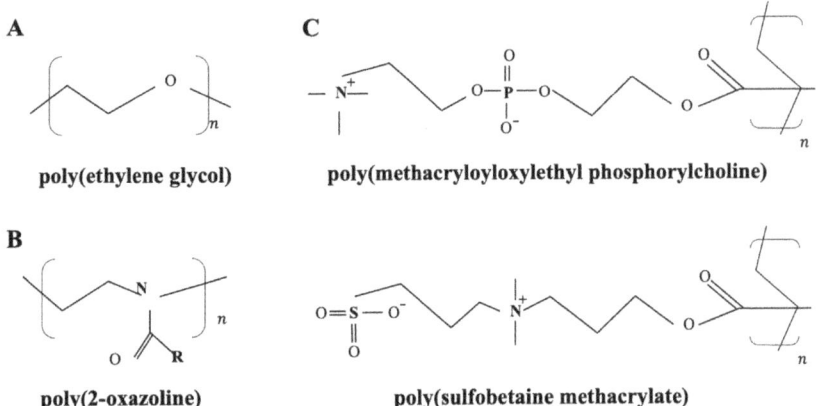

A poly(ethylene glycol)

B poly(2-oxazoline)

C poly(methacryloyloxylethyl phosphorylcholine)

poly(sulfobetaine methacrylate)

FIGURE 3.1 The chemical synthesis stealth approach. (A) polyethylene glycol, (B) poly (2-oxazoline), (C) examples of zwitterion polymers – poly (methacryloyloxylethyl phosphorylcholine) and poly(sulfobetaine methacrylate).

in turn may result in complications such as rapid clearance of drugs or non-effective therapeutic dose, and side effects to carriers, such as anaphylaxis.[14, 15]

3.3.1.2 Poly (2-Oxazoline)

Poly (2-oxazoline) (POX) polymers found rapid success, as a replacement for PEG in biomedicine. Their narrow molecular weight distribution, biocompatibility, low dispersity, thermo-responsiveness, low viscosity, and reduced synthesis time made them a desirable replacement. A series of POX polymers, poly(2-methyl-2-oxazoline) (PMeOx), poly(2-ethyl-2-oxazoline) (PEtOx), and poly(2-methyl-2-oxazine) (PMeOzi), have been tested for their biodistribution. They are reported to have low uptake in MPS. The particles were found to have low toxicity and maintained morphology *in vivo*. The high hydrophilicity of these molecules reduces their interaction with cells, microbes, and other biomolecules leading to the development of anti-fouling mechanisms.[16, 17]

The conjugation of POX and its derivatives with therapeutic proteins, drugs, amphiphilic molecules, and nucleic acids (genes, siRNA) has been explored for the treatment of cancer, metabolic diseases, and infections. Despite the desirable attributes of POX, its clinical use is still under consideration by the FDA. The only POX derivative approved by FDA is PEtox. The PEtox-rotigotine conjugate has cleared all the pre-clinical trials and is currently being tested in phase 1 of clinical trials as a treatment for Parkinson's disease. Preliminary results from the trials indicate that the drug is well-tolerated; the plasma levels of the drug increase gradually, plateau, and are then excreted[18] Despite the stealth functionality of POX polymers, they have been found to trigger complement activation through the C1q molecule. The C1q molecule further initiates the classical complement pathway resulting in the activation of C3 complement protein enhancing opsonization and clearance of the NPs.[19]

3.3.1.3 Zwitterions

Zwitterions contain equimolar cations and anions moieties thereby displaying an overall surface electroneutrality. Most zwitterions can be roughly classified as either betaine-like zwitterions or mixed-charge zwitterions. Most zwitterions belong to the former category. Some of the known betaine-like zwitterions include phosphorylcholine, sulfobetaine, carboxybetaine with phosphonate, sulfonates, and carboxylates. Whereas amino acids and some peptides serve as mixed-charge zwitterions[20] While zwitterions have most features comparable to other drug delivery systems – biocompatibility, long circulation time, negligible immunogenicity, and low cytotoxicity – one of their best properties is anti-fouling. The anti-fouling property is due to the dense hydration shells formed by zwitterions. A large number of cationic and anionic groups endow the zwitterions with super hydrophilicity and high hydration capability. Even under physiological conditions such as in the presence of saline solutions, zwitterions attract counterions resulting in a conformational change to a relatively stretched form, enhancing the anti-fouling effect. Overall, the electroneutrality of zwitterions reduces the chances of non-specific electrostatic bonding, resulting in better anti-fouling measures.[21-23] Zwitterions have been used as carriers of the drug in response to pH, redox changes, temperature, and targeted tissues. Both drugs and genetic material have been cargoed using zwitterions. *In-vitro* studies and *in-vivo* animal models of zwitterion-based drug delivery have proved to be of utility in cancer, diabetes, and genetic diseases.[24-26]

3.3.2 Bioinspired Approach

3.3.2.1 Bacterial Cells

The first line of defense against foreign pathogens is the immune system and its ability to distinguish between self and non-self. The innate immune system defends the host from the majority of infections and foreign particles including bacteria and viruses. If the foreign object cannot be neutralized by the innate immune system, then the burden of neutralizing this object lies with the adaptive immune system. Pathogens have evolved a mechanism to evade the scrutiny of the immune system, and it has been reported that these nano/microorganisms can interfere with macrophage signaling. Rosenberger et al. reported that pathogens possess genes and express proteins that function to interfere with macrophage signaling and result in phagocyte sabotage[27] To suppress the phagocytosis activation, interrupted signaling must occur between the immune cell and the pathogen. Phagocytic activity is downregulated upon virulence factor proteins delivery into a macrophage, which interferes with several cytoskeletal proteins to suppress phagocytosis signaling. The first strategy is displayed by Yad A proteins of *Yersinia enterocolitica* that bind to factor[28] and contribute to its pathogenicity.[29] In addition, *S. aureus* evolved a mechanism to captivate the opsonin and prevent it from binding to the bacteria. For instance, protein A, which is expressed in the bacterial cell wall, is capable of suppressing phagocytosis by specific binding to the Fc region of the IgG and blocking the antibody from interacting with Fcγ receptors.[30] Similarly, Sbi protein, expressed by most *S. aureus* strains, binds to the Fc region of the IgG and evades immunosurveillance.[31–33] Some *Staphylococcus* interacts with activator convertases and stabilizes surface-bound C3 convertase to inhibit its activation pathways, thus limiting enzymatic activity. Some other pathogens can evade phagocytosis by covering their surface with capsular polysaccharides, thus preventing the opsonization of antibodies and limiting elimination through phagocytosis[34] For example, a patient with cystic fibrosis presents with *Pseudomonas aureus* in their lungs, which is a pathogen that exhibits hydrophilic polyuronic polysaccharides, interfering with phagocytosis.

3.3.2.2 *Carrier Cells for Therapeutic Delivery*

The successful delivery of therapeutic agents to target sites in the presence of a hostile environment can be achieved by hiding them inside endogenous circulating cells, for example, erythrocyte-infused therapeutic delivery since these cells can travel through narrow capillaries networks escaping the spleen clearance.[35] T-lymphocytes use the circulatory system to move between lymphatic agents and sites of foreign antigen expressions, and these tumor-targeting T-cells can act as cell carriers for systematic delivery.[36] An attractive candidate as a cell carrier is the mesenchymal stem cell (MSC) which has the ability to differentiate into several lineages and also has the highest degree of plasticity.[37] These cells are isolated from a variety of human tissues and organs such as the brain, liver, kidneys, and lungs. MSC's ability to migrate to sites of injury and tumor microenvironments further supports their candidacy as ideal cell carriers. Furthermore, MSCs can be modified by gene vectors to release therapeutic agents.[38] For a cell carrier to be effective in releasing targeted therapeutics, it is necessary for these cells to travel across small spaces such as capillaries and the endothelium. MSCs migrate across the endothelium to targeted tissues by the physicochemical pairing of the respective cytokines and receptors (Figure 3.2).

3.3.2.2.1 *Erythrocyte*

Erythrocytes exhibit all the properties of an ideal drug carrier. They have a flexible structure, possess a unique shape, and are small in size. Erythrocytes' ability to pass through narrow capillary networks and avoid elimination makes them uniquely able to be employed as therapeutic carriers. To investigate their effective therapeutic carrier, researchers use the natural semi-permeable membrane to load with therapeutic agents (Figure 3.2). This offers a sustained release of small-molecule therapeutics and retention of larger proteins within the membrane. Advances in molecular biology and bioengineering have provided scientists with a greater understanding of the physicochemical and biological function of red blood cells. One major advancement was the discovery of CD47, the marker of self. Oldenburg et al. reported that CD47 functions as a marker of self and demonstrated the inverse relationship with increased phagocytosis and reduced marker levels.[39] This supports the role of CD47 expression in long-term erythrocytes in the bloodstream. CD47 regulates phagocytosis by its interaction with SIRP-alpha on macrophages. Through this ligation, tyrosine phosphatase is activated and myosin accumulation at the phagocytic synapse is suppressed. This leads to inhibition of Fcγ which mediates phagocytic signals.[39] Furthermore, by inhibiting Fcγ a reduction or inhibition of phagocytosis occurs.

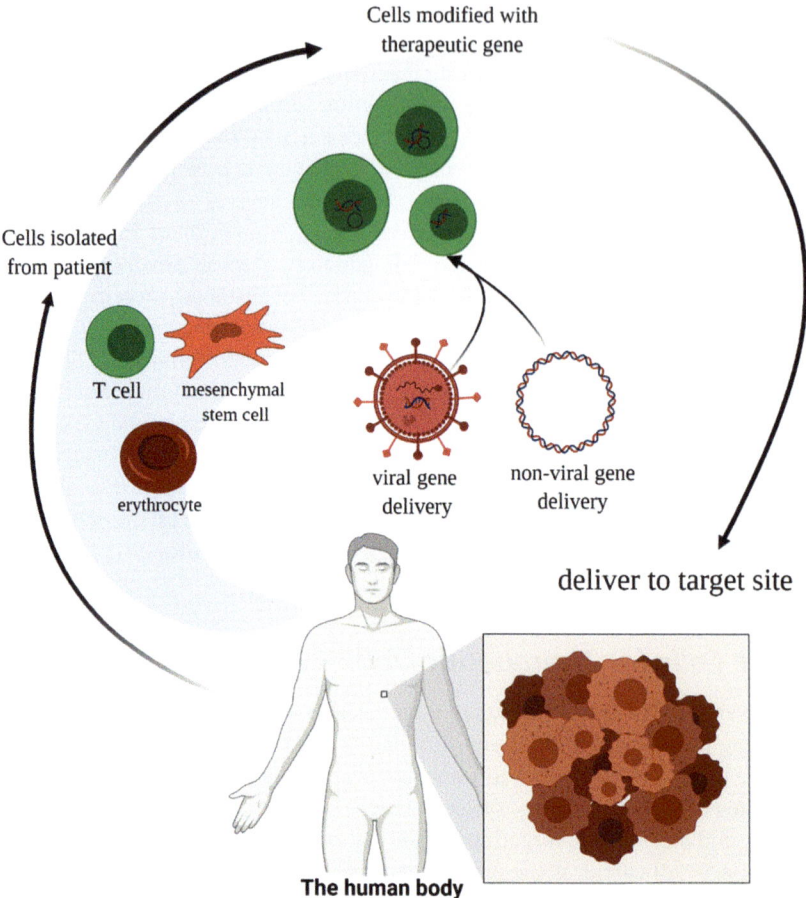

FIGURE 3.2 Native human cells such as T-cells, MSCs, and erythrocytes can be used as carriers for drug and gene delivery. Therapeutic genes are delivered through viral or non-viral methods to modify the cells which then home to target sites while escaping the immunity.

3.3.2.2.2 T-Lymphocytes

An advantage of using T-cells is the ability to exploit their tumor-homing capabilities. These cells can be used to deliver oncolytic viruses to the targeted tumor. The addition of therapeutic agents does not affect the integrity of these cells. Cytoine-induced killer cells have demonstrated the ability to localize into leukemia tissue and cause toxicity to the tissue.[40] These cells have been effective in the treatment of solid malignancies in ovaries. The success of this treatment *in vivo* has led to clinical studies with encouraging results. T-cell-based immunotherapies have been successful in tumor immunotherapy by increasing the numbers of endogenous NK and CD8 T-cells which are potent mediators of antitumor immunity. T-cells co-transcribed with prostate tumor antigens to target tumor cells were successfully used for tumor treatment by Kloss et al.[41] T-cells were rendered to be tumor-specific and demonstrated a result of tumor remission without sacrificing the reactivity of the cell. T-lymphocytes are attractive drug delivery systems as T-cells are specific and in response to antigenic stimuli can mediate lysis of the target (antigen-presenting) cell. Further, their ability to cross the blood–brain barrier makes them a potential agent of drug delivery for disorders of the nervous system[42] (Figure 3.2).

3.3.2.2.3 Mesenchymal Stem Cells

MSCs are also attractive for the targeted delivery of genes and viruses, which migrate to and incorporate within the connective tissue of tumors but actively seek out metastases far removed from the tumor site

(Figure 3.2). MSCs have been utilized as delivery vehicles of interactions to improve anti-cancer immune surveillance by activating cytotoxic lymphocytes and NK cells. Nakamua et al. delivered gene-modified MSCs by infection with an adenoviral vector encoding human IL-2 that enhanced antitumor effect and prolonged the survival of tumor-bearing rats.[43] MSCs are also delivery agents for gene-directed enzyme drug therapy. Results have shown that delivery of MSC transfected with cytosine deaminase (CD) resulted in a significant prolongation of survival of rats with glioma cells.[43] Transfected MSCs with antiviral vectors with CD demonstrated deceased tumor visibly.

3.3.2.3 Cell Membrane Components Coating

Membrane components have been used to coat NPs to enhance stealth functionalization. These components are different carbohydrates and proteins on human host cell surfaces. Since they are recognized as self by the host, they attract reduced immune attention and allow longer circulation of NPs.

3.3.2.3.1 Carbohydrates
Carbohydrates are a significant proportion of the eukaryotic and prokaryotic systems. Different classes of carbohydrates such as glycoproteins and glycolipids are on the cell membrane. Each of these molecules serves a specific function for the cell. Naturally occurring polysaccharides or synthetic derivatives that resemble natural polysaccharides in structure and function are being increasingly utilized for stealth functionalization, for instance, the use of glycosaminoglycans (GAGs). Sialic acid (SA) shows a high affinity towards siglecs. This property of sialic acid makes it a good coating choice to enhance cellular targeting[44] An increasing trend is also seen in the use of polysialic acid (PSA) as NPs coating. The utility of SA/PSA in delivering chemotherapeutic agents (DOX/epirubic) in cancer treatment is being explored, as well as its use in delivering proteins such as asparaginase. The proteins were found to remain active in comparison to PEG-asparaginase conjugation[45,46] The utility of other GAGs such as heparin has been explored in *in-vitro* studies and *in-vivo* mouse models for the delivery of exogenous proteins and siRNA and is proposed to be explored for the delivery of genome editing using CRISPR-Cas9 technology.[47] Heparin conjugated with other biomaterials such as chitosan has been used for siRNA delivery targeting vascular endothelial growth factor (VEGF) silencing in ARPE-19 cells *in vitro*. These particles were pH-sensitive and thus displayed 25% higher targeting.[48]

3.3.2.3.2 Dextran/Dextrin
The understanding of the immune evasion capabilities of pathogens has grown, and this natural mechanism has been investigated in therapeutic delivery. Technically, sucrose fermentation can be used for the production of bacterial dextran, followed by acid hydrolysis to decrease its molecular weight.[49] Dextran coating has also been recognized to stabilize micelle carriers[50] and prolong the blood circulation time of drug molecules,[51] including poly(methyl methacrylate) polymer carriers[52] and contrast agents.[53] One of the strategies is simply a coating of liposome with linear dextran which was one of the earliest attempts to use components of polysaccharides.[54] Moreover, poly(lactic acid) is another nanoparticle that was coated with dextran to reduce protein adsorption.[55] In another study investigating dextrin, which has an identical structure to dextran, it was found not to trigger an immune response,[56] but to prolong the blood circulation time.[57]

3.3.2.3.3 Hyaluronic Acid
Hyaluronic acid (HA) is another polysaccharide that has been explored for its stealth functionalization in NP-mediated drug delivery.[45,58] The non-immunogenic nature of the polysaccharides, their biocompatibility, biodegradability, size, conformation, and the ability to be coupled with other polymers make them desirable. However, the mixed molecular weights of the particles, low solubility in organic solvents, and slow enzymatic degradation limit their use as vehicles of delivery. However, surface modifications and the use of stimuli-responsive carriers help overcome these barriers to their use. HA is natural component of polysaccharide that can be obtained from *Streptococcus* bacteria. CD44 receptor is the cell membrane protein abundant on many tumor cell surfaces and is attracted to the HA ligand. HA bound on the surface

of lipid nanoparticles provides an increase in blood circulation time through interaction with CD44. For example, siRNA,[59] DOX,[60] and mitomycin C[61] are nanoparticles attached with HA that were employed to target tumor cells. This makes HA an excellent target for anti-cancer drug delivery.[62]

3.3.2.4 Membranes from Ghost Cells

The cell membrane is a lipid bilayer. Retrospectively, the cell does serve as a vehicle for intracellular components. Some of these vehicles are mobile whereas some are stationary. The use of lipids as NPs is discussed in the larger context of cell membrane-based NP. We will explore the use of four cell populations, *viz*, erythrocytes, MSCs, leukocytes, and platelets, which have been explored as NPs for drug delivery (Figure 3.3).

3.3.2.4.1 Ghost Erythrocytes
Their long half-life, availability, and motile nature make erythrocytes the most desirable drug delivery agents. The absence of a nucleus and genetic material makes them easy to manipulate. Additionally, their abundant numbers ease purification. The presence of a self-cell marker (CD47) on the RBC membrane shields them from phagocytosis. Two variants of erythrocytes, *viz*, erythrosomes and nanosponges, find application in drug delivery systems. While erythrosomes[63] are RBC membrane-derived liposomes, nanosponges[64] are erythrocyte membrane conjugated to polymers. To develop an RBC carrier, a multitude of techniques have been developed to load erythrocytes with therapeutic agents. Hypotonic treatment is the standard preparation that retains the physicochemical characteristics of the RBC membrane[65] Erythrocytes are placed in a hypotonic solution where osmotic pressure releases the intracellular contents within the RBC membrane. The therapeutic agent passively diffuses into RBCs and is retained via isotonic buffer resealing.[66] This technique has been done in using RBCs to deliver β-glucosidase and β-galactosidase for the treatment of Gaucher's disease[35] These specialized cells are called erythrocyte ghosts and have been harnessed for the delivery of oligonucleotide and plasma DNA. RBC carriers are also used to entrap small dry molecules which increases the biodistribution of therapeutics (Figure 3.3).

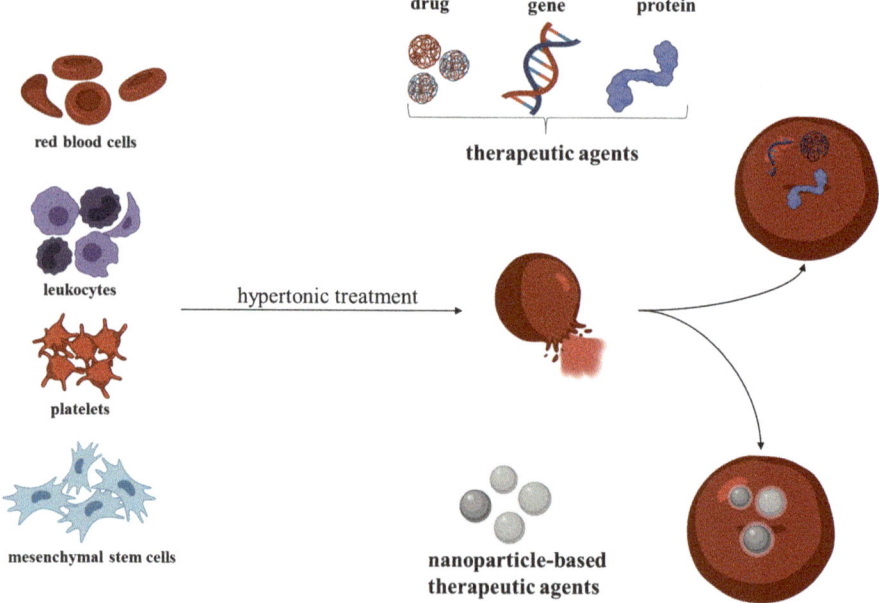

FIGURE 3.3 Ghost cell-derived nanocarriers using RBCs, leukocytes, platelets, and MSCs. These ghost-mediated therapeutic carriers are prepared using hypertonic treatment of cells and harbor various therapeutic agents.

Erythrocyte ghosts have been engineered to contain hemagglutinin fusion protein on lipid membranes which is the therapeutic design of the anti-cancer drug Decitabine.[67] Nano-erythrosomes were first reported and are RBC membrane-derived liposomes. Daunorubicin-conjugated nano-erythrosomes had a greater antineoplastic index than the free drug. The plasma membrane of erythrocyte ghosts is used to cloak biodegradable polymeric nanoparticles via membrane extension and demonstrate the extended blood circulation half-time of RBC membrane camouflaged polymeric nanoparticles. PEG-coated nanoparticles had an elimination half-life of 15.8 hours, while the RBC-coated nanoparticles had an elimination half-life of 39.6 hours. While this is a significant improvement in half-life circulation, risks include rejection of immunogenic species that are not removed and surface antigens of specific blood groups interfering with the drug optimization of the RBC carrier. Further research has used the properties of RBC cells by coupling therapeutic agents on the outer surface by covalent conjugation. Ligands on the RBC surface such as complement receptors, are sites for drug conjugation which would increase the circulation time. A hitchhiking strategy was employed to attach therapeutic polymeric nanoparticles to the surface to increase circulation time. Doshi et al. synthesized RBC-like particles that mimic the capabilities of RBCs such as the ability to carry oxygen and flow through smaller spaces than their diameter.[68] Merkel et al. synthesized hydrogel microparticles with tunable elasticity that resembled RBCs.[69] Both studies demonstrated that mechanobiological mimicry of RBCs was possible and has the capability of extended circulation times and increased particle deformability. One of the earliest such reported NPs was a polymer of poly(lactic-*co*-glycolic acid) (PLGA) coated with erythrocyte membrane. Some of the other polymers that are coated with erythrocyte membranes include polycaprolactone, polypyrrole, poly(lactic acid), Fe_3O_4, magnetic nanoclusters, mesoporous silica, gold, and gelatin. Erythrocyte membrane-coated nanoparticles have been used to deliver chemotherapeutic agents (doxorubicin, paclitaxel), proteins (β-glucosidase, β-galactosidase), and small molecules (folic acid, gambogic acid).[70]

3.3.2.4.2 Ghost MSC

The unique function and non-immunogenicity of MSC make it very popular in the field of medicine and drug/gene delivery. One study developed a natural gene delivery platform using nanoghosts derived from MSC (NG-MSC) with pDNA encoding cancer-toxic genes to target multiple cancers. Their results showed a significant suppression of prostate (80%) and metastatic orthotopic lung cancer growth as well as prolonged animal survival.[71,72] The same group also investigated the effect of NG-MSC obtained from MSC pretreated with cancer cells conditioned-media (CM-NGs) or proinflammatory cytokines (Cyto-NGs). Outcomes enhanced the targeting of cancer cells and immune cells, where Cyto-NGs revealed the more tumor-targeted ones while MC-NGs are more targeting immune cells[73] (Figure 3.3).

3.3.2.4.3 Ghost Leukocyte

Like erythrocytes, the utilization of white blood cells (leukocyte) membranes was explored for coating nanoparticles to achieve stability, the ability to cross immune barriers, targeting, and localization. Leukocytes comprise lymphocytes, monocytes, macrophages, and neutrophils (Figure 3.3). Leukocyte membrane-based NPs are either ghost leukocytes or leukocyte membranes coated onto other nanoparticles – termed leukolike NP. A study assessing the efficacy of leukolike NPs found that leukolike NP ligands could communicate with receptors on endothelial cells, were able to deliver payloads across an inflamed reconstructed endothelium, and could retain functionalization *in vivo*.[58] In addition, human cytotoxic T-lymphocytes serve as another membrane-based leukocyte that camouflaged PLGA nanoparticles, enabling the targeting of gastric cancer cells. As a result, T-lymphocytes ghost-membrane inhibit phagocytic activity by macrophages and therefore revealed more than 88% of the tumor growth suppression.[74] Monocyte/macrophages are among the most reviewed choice of leukocytes for developing leukolike particles. Drugs loaded in macrophages have a prolonged lifespan and are shielded from MPS elimination. The efficacy of macrophage biomimetic NPs has been assessed in artheroscelorsis,[75] cancers of varied origin,[76,77] and anti-HIV therapy.[76] Neutrophil membranes are preferred for neutrophil abundance, their ability to transmigrate, and the swelling of their numbers in response to inflammation. Kang et al. have shown that PLGA loaded with carfilzomib (a proteasome inhibitor) encapsulated in neutrophil membrane homed to premetastatic sites within the tumor.[78] In an independent study assessing *in-vivo* models of pancreatic tumors, treatment with celastrol loaded on naïve neutrophil membrane encapsulated PLGA or PEG was found to prolong survival and minimize liver metastases.[79]

3.3.2.4.4 Ghost Platelets

Platelet-derived nanoparticles (PNPs) are constructed by wrapping platelet membranes onto solid NP cores. PNPs target passively using natural markers on the cell surface or actively through engagement with specific markers such as CLEC-2, P-selectin, integrin α6β1, and integrin αIIbβ3. PNPs have been used to deliver drugs for the rebuilding of injured vasculature, tumors, and the inhibition of drug-resistant bacteria.[80] In addition to specific cell membrane particles being wrapped around a solid nanoparticle core, cancer cell membranes are also used for biomimicry. Either independently or as hybrids with macrophage or platelet membranes, these NPs are finding wide use in theranostics.[81-83]

3.3.2.5 Immunoglobulin Superfamily Proteins

Proteins serve a wide variety of functions in and for the cell such as recognition, transport, and metabolism. Proteins are also highly immunogenic and thus their use in stealth functionalization needs careful curation. The proteins are coated on to the solid NP core and thus used for drug delivery. Some of the commonly employed protein molecules for biomimetic drug delivery are discussed below.

3.3.2.5.1 CD47

CD47 is a self-cell marker that prevents the phagocytosis of self-cells through the CD172a phagocytic pathway. It has been reported that PEG NP, when coated with CD47, preferentially reduced phagocytic activity by the M1 phenotype.[84] Further higher accumulation of CD47-coated graphene oxide nanosheets was observed in tumor sites as compared to PEGylated graphene oxide nanosheets.[9] Another use of host protein for stealth functionalization is serum albumin (SA). SA is an abundant host protein. Studies with SA-coated tobacco mosaic virus were shown to exhibit reduced antibody recognition and longer circulation time.[85]

CD47 has been established as a marker of self on RBC surfaces. It is suggested that CD47 could represent a viable solution in the design of macrophage-evading therapeutics. CD47's N-terminal domain is a ligand for an immunoinhibitory receptor SIRPα that is abundant on macrophages and some non-phagocytic cells. Upon CD47 binding, SIRPα activates the phosphate SHP-1 which inhibits the cytoskeleton-intensive phagocytosis of cells and large particles that are opsonized by antibodies and complement factors.[86] By this pathway, it supports the discovery that CD47 acts as a marker of self. This was originally described when CD47-deficient red blood cells were injected into control mice and were rapidly cleared by splenic macrophages.

CD47 is less effective at inhibiting uptake for rigid targets, and viruses are much stiffer than red blood cells. Soluble CD47 protein's effect on phagocytosis activity was first demonstrated by Hsu et al. In the study, the extracellular domain of the CD47 gene was cloned into bacterial vector pre-constructed with streptavidin gene, expressed in a BL21 bacterial strain. After purifying the CD47-SA recombinant protein by a biotinylated agarose column, the antiphagocytic effect was evaluated by treated J774A.1 macrophages for 1 h, prior to adding perfluorocarbon-based oxygen carriers which successfully escape the immune clearance by macrophages[87] (Figure 3.4). Another study hypothesized that overexpression of full-length human CD47 on a standard virus-producing cell line would generate lentivirus with sufficient CD47 to signal against macrophage uptake.[86] During the structural studies of CD47-lentivirus, in-vitro assessment of the uptake by phagocytic cells and nonphagocytic cells was investigated. NOD SCID gamma (NSG) mice were then used to assess in vivo whether CD47-lentivirus showed enhanced circulation and gene delivery to lung cancer xenografts. NSG mice express a unique mouse variant of SIRPα that binds human CD47. It should be noted that NSG mice lack functional lymphocytes but have functional macrophages. Thus, the NSG model allows the focused study of macrophages in lentiviral vector clearance. It is suggested that this can be systemically delivered across multiple sites of disease. The marker of self-inhibition of liver clearance is less clear from past studies than splenic clearance, thus the

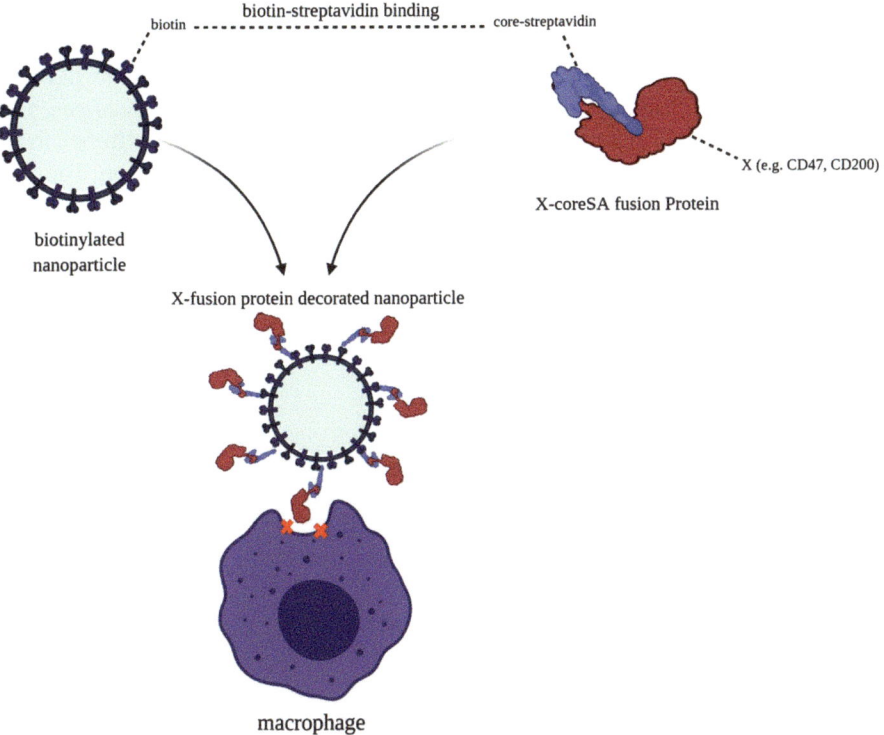

FIGURE 3.4 Biomimetic nanoparticles using fusion protein of streptavidin with immunoglobulin family proteins (e.g., CD47 and CD200) which helps the nanoparticle to escape immunosurveillance.

effects on Kupffer cells, which are the dominant liver macrophage, are still to be understood. It was found that splenic macrophages, as well as bone marrow-derived macrophages, are clearly inhibited by CD47 on cells. Findings suggest that lentivirus which buds through cell membranes rich in CD47 has the ability to inhibit the uptake of liver macrophages. This is a desirable target that warrants future investigation of the expression of transgenes in therapeutic drug delivery.

3.3.2.5.2 CD200

CD200 is known as an anti-inflammatory transmembrane glycoprotein in the immunoglobulin superfamily.[88] CD200 interacts with its receptor CD200R which is highly expressed on myeloid cells such as macrophages and neutrophils. This interaction has been known to reduce macrophage activation and chronic inflammation. To harness the immunomodulatory property of CD200 for surface modification, CD200-streptavidin fusion protein was expressed from bacteria transformed with PET20b plasmid-encoded with CD200 extracellular domain and core streptavidin.[88] The purified CD200-SA protein was bound to biotin-coated fluorescent polystyrene particles of various sizes ranging from 0.15 to 2 µm (Figure 3.4). In a culture with THP1 macrophages, these NPs showed reduced activation and phagocytic ability and significantly reduced amounts of pro-inflammatory cytokine TNF-alpha and Interleukin-6 (IL-6).[88]

3.4 CONCLUSION

Significant advancement has been made in the design of engineered nanoparticles in the past several decades. Despite these advancements, synthetic systems do not match the complexity of natural cells. The development of efficient therapeutic delivery vehicles requires evasion of the MPS localization to the target sites and sustained delivery. Inspired by the way innate biological cells from our body can accomplish everyday tasks in the body, the biomimetic approach to engineering delivery systems has expanded rapidly. RBCs, T-cells, and MSCs have all been exploited for the therapeutic delivery of genes, nucleotides, proteins, and drugs to tumor cells while maintaining the native cells' integrity. Delivery carriers based on pathogens' stealth mimicry have shown to offer a certain degree of immune evasion. The understanding of delivery mechanisms used by biological carriers is yet to be fully understood. Greater understanding will allow researchers to develop new and improved synthetic techniques based on innate biological cells. The field of nanobiotechnology continues to develop to accommodate the ever-expanding dynamism of therapeutic discovery. There are multiple combinations of chemical and bio-inspired molecules that aid better uptake and efficacy of NPs. The choice of the coating is dependent on the immune barrier that needs to be overcome, and the ease of synthesis.

REFERENCES

1. Müller, R. H., K. Mäder, and S. Gohla. "Solid Lipid Nanoparticles (SLN) for Controlled Drug Delivery: A Review of the State of the Art." *European Journal of Pharmaceutics & Biopharmaceutics* 50, no. 1 (2000): 161–77. doi:10.1016/S0939-6411(00)00087-4.
2. Kalachandra, S., T. Takamata, D. M. Lin, E. A. Snyder, and J. Webster-Cyriaque. "Stability and Release of Antiviral Drugs from Ethylene Vinyl Acetate (EVA) Copolymer." *Journal of Materials Science: Materials in Medicine* 17, no. 12 (2006): 1227–36. doi:10.1007/s10856-006-0596-6.
3. Farokhzad, O. C., and R. Langer. "Nanomedicine: Developing Smarter Therapeutic and Diagnostic Modalities." *Advanced Drug Delivery Reviews* 58, no. 14 (2006): 1456–9. doi:10.1016/j.addr.2006.09.011.
4. Duncan, R., and M. J. Vicent. "Polymer Therapeutics-Prospects for 21st Century: The End of the Beginning." *Advanced Drug Delivery Reviews* 65, no. 1 (2013): 60–70. doi:10.1016/j.addr.2012.08.012.
5. Plummer, R., R. H. Wilson, H. Calvert, A. V. Boddy, M. Griffin, J. Sludden, M. J. Tilby, M. Eatock, D. G. Pearson, C. J. Ottley, Y. Matsumura, K. Kataoka, and T. Nishiya. "A Phase I Clinical Study of Cisplatin-Incorporated Polymeric Micelles (NC-6004) in Patients with Solid Tumours." *British Journal of Cancer* 104, no. 4 (2011): 593–8. doi:10.1038/bjc.2011.6.
6. Rizvi, S. A. A., and A. M. Saleh. "Applications of Nanoparticle Systems in Drug Delivery Technology." *Saudi Pharmaceutical Journal* 26, no. 1 (2018): 64–70. doi:10.1016/j.jsps.2017.10.012.
7. Petros, R. A., and J. M. Desimone. "Strategies in the Design of Nanoparticles for Therapeutic Applications." *Nature Reviews. Drug Discovery* 9, no. 8 (2010): 615–27. doi:10.1038/nrd2591.
8. Yona, S., and S. Gordon. "From the Reticuloendothelial to Mononuclear Phagocyte System: The Unaccounted Years." *Frontiers in Immunology* 6, no. Jul (2015): 328. doi:10.3389/fimmu.2015.00328.
9. Fam, S. Y., C. F. Chee, C. Y. Yong, K. L. Ho, A. R. Mariatulqabtiah, and W. S. Tan. "Stealth Coating of Nanoparticles in Drug-Delivery Systems." *Nanomaterials* 10, no. 4 (2020): 1–18. doi:10.3390/nano10040787.
10. Gustafson, H. H., D. Holt-Casper, D. W. Grainger, and H. Ghandehari. "Nanoparticle Uptake: The Phagocyte Problem." *Nano Today* 10, no. 4 (2015): 487–510. doi:10.1016/j.nantod.2015.06.006.
11. Milton Harris, J., and R. B. Chess. "Effect of Pegylation on Pharmaceuticals." *Nature Reviews. Drug Discovery* 2, no. 3 (2003): 214–21. doi:10.1038/nrd1033.
12. Park, E. J., J. Choi, K. C. Lee, and D. H. Na. "Emerging Pegylated Non-Biologic Drugs." *Expert Opinion on Emerging Drugs* 24, no. 2 (2019): 107–19. doi:10.1080/14728214.2019.1604684.
13. Garay, R. P., R. El-Gewely, J. K. Armstrong, G. Garratty, and P. Richette. "Antibodies Against Polyethylene Glycol in Healthy Subjects and in Patients Treated with PEG-Conjugated Agents." *Expert Opinion on Drug Delivery* 9, no. 11 (2012): 1319–23. doi:10.1517/17425247.2012.720969.
14. Yang, Q., and S. K. Lai. "Anti-PEG Immunity: Emergence, Characteristics, and Unaddressed Questions." *Wiley Interdisciplinary Reviews. Nanomedicine & Nanobiotechnology* 7, no. 5 (2015): 655–77. doi:10.1002/wnan.1339.
15. Kozma, G. T., T. Shimizu, T. Ishida, and J. Szebeni. "Anti-PEG Antibodies: Properties, Formation, Testing and Role in Adverse Immune Reactions to Pegylated Nano-Biopharmaceuticals." *Advanced Drug Delivery Reviews* 154–155 (2020): 163–75. doi:10.1016/j.addr.2020.07.024.

16. Lorson, T., M. M. Lübtow, E. Wegener, M. S. Haider, S. Borova, D. Nahm, R. Jordan, M. Sokolski-Papkov, A. V. Kabanov, and R. Luxenhofer. "Poly(2-Oxazoline)s Based Biomaterials: A Comprehensive and Critical Update." *Biomaterials* 178 (2018): 204–80. doi:10.1016/j.biomaterials.2018.05.022.

17. De La Rosa, V. R. "Poly(2-Oxazoline)s as Materials for Biomedical Applications." *Journal of Materials Science: Materials in Medicine* 25, no. 5 (2014): 1211–25. doi:10.1007/s10856-013-5034-y.

18. Sedlacek, O., and R. Hoogenboom. "Drug Deliverys Systems Based on Poly(2-Oxazoline)s and Poly(2-Oxazine) s." *Advances in Therapy* 3, no. 1 (2020). doi:10.1002/adtp.201900168, PubMed: 1900168.

19. Tavano, R., L. Gabrielli, E. Lubian, C. Fedeli, S. Visentin, P. Polverino De Laureto, G. Arrigoni, A. Geffner-Smith, F. Chen, D. Simberg, G. Morgese, E. M. Benetti, L. Wu, S. M. Moghimi, F. Mancin, and E. Papini. "C1q-Mediated Complement Activation and C3 Opsonization Trigger Recognition of Stealth Poly(2-Methyl-2-Oxazoline)-Coated Silica Nanoparticles by Human Phagocytes." *ACS Nano* 12, no. 6 (2018): 5834–47. doi:10.1021/acsnano.8b01806.

20. Zhou, L. Y., Y. H. Zhu, X. Y. Wang, C. Shen, X. W. Wei, T. Xu, and Z. Y. He. "Novel Zwitterionic Vectors: Multi-Functional Delivery Systems for Therapeutic Genes and Drugs." *Computational & Structural Biotechnology Journal* 18 (2020): 1980–99. doi:10.1016/j.csbj.2020.07.015.

21. Zhang, Y., Y. Liu, B. Ren, D. Zhang, S. Xie, Y. Chang, J. Yang, J. Wu, L. Xu, and J. Zheng. "Fundamentals and Applications of Zwitterionic Antifouling Polymers." *Journal of Physics. Part D* 52, no. 40 (2019). doi:10.1088/1361-6463/ab2cbc, PubMed: 403001.

22. Van Andel, E., S. C. Lange, S. P. Pujari, E. J. Tijhaar, M. M. J. Smulders, H. F. J. Savelkoul, and H. Zuilhof. "Systematic Comparison of Zwitterionic and Non-Zwitterionic Antifouling Polymer Brushes on a Bead-Based Platform." *Langmuir* 35, no. 5 (2019): 1181–91. doi:10.1021/acs.langmuir.8b01832.

23. Liu, Y., D. Zhang, B. Ren, X. Gong, L. Xu, Z. Q. Feng, Y. Chang, Y. He, and J. Zheng. "Molecular Simulations and Understanding of Antifouling Zwitterionic Polymer Brushes." *Journal of Materials Chemistry B* 8, no. 17 (2020): 3814–28. doi:10.1039/d0tb00520g.

24. Sun, R., X. J. Du, C. Y. Sun, S. Shen, Y. Liu, X. Z. Yang, Y. Bao, Y. H. Zhu, and J. Wang. "A Block Copolymer of Zwitterionic Polyphosphoester and Polylactic Acid for Drug Delivery." *Biomaterials Science* 3, no. 7 (2015): 1105–13. doi:10.1039/c4bm00430b.

25. Wang, Y., D. Huang, X. Wang, F. Yang, H. Shen, and D. Wu. "Fabrication of Zwitterionic and pH-Responsive Polyacetal Dendrimers for Anticancer Drug Delivery." *Biomaterials Science* 7, no. 8 (2019): 3238–48. doi:10.1039/c9bm00606k.

26. Shan, W., X. Zhu, W. Tao, Y. Cui, M. Liu, L. Wu, L. Li, Y. Zheng, and Y. Huang. "Enhanced Oral Delivery of Protein Drugs Using Zwitterion-Functionalized Nanoparticles to Overcome Both the Diffusion and Absorption Barriers." *ACS Applied Materials & Interfaces* 8, no. 38 (2016): 25444–53. doi:10.1021/acsami.6b08183.

27. Rosenberger, C. M., and B. B. Finlay. "Phagocyte Sabotage: Disruption of Macrophage Signalling by Bacterial Pathogens." *Nature Reviews. Molecular Cell Biology* 4, no. 5 (2003): 385–96. doi:10.1038/nrm1104.

28. Shao, F., P. M. Merritt, Z. Bao, R. W. Innes, and J. E. Dixon. "A Yersinia Effector and a Pseudomonas Avirulence Protein Define a Family of Cysteine Proteases Functioning in Bacterial Pathogenesis." *Cell* 109, no. 5 (2002): 575–88. doi:10.1016/S0092-8674(02)00766-3.

29. Biedzka-Sarek, M., H. Jarva, H. Hyytiäinen, S. Meri, and M. Skurnik. "Characterization of Complement Factor H Binding to Yersinia enterocolitica serotype O:3." *Infection & Immunity* 76, no. 9 (2008): 4100–9. doi:10.1128/IAI.00313-08.

30. Sulica, A., C. Medesan, M. Laky, D. Onică, J. Sjöquist, and V. Ghetie. "Effect of Protein A of Staphylococcus aureus on the Binding of Monomeric and Polymeric IgG to Fc Receptor-Bearing Cells." *Immunology* 38, no. 1 (1979): 173–9.

31. Zhang, L., K. Jacobson, J. Vasi, M. Lindberg, and L. Frykberg. "A Second IgG-Binding Protein in Staphylococcus aureus." *Microbiology* 144, no. 4 (1998): 985–91. doi:10.1099/00221287.

32. Smith, E. J., L. Visai, S. W. Kerrigan, P. Speziale, and T. J. Foster. "The Sbi Protein Is a Multifunctional Immune Evasion Factor of Staphylococcus aureus." *Infection & Immunity* 79, no. 9 (2011): 3801–9. doi:10.1128/IAI.05075-11.

33. Smith, E. J., R. M. Corrigan, T. van der Sluis, A. Gründling, P. Speziale, J. A. Geoghegan, and T. J. Foster. "The Immune Evasion Protein Sbi of Staphylococcus aureus Occurs Both Extracellularly and Anchored to the Cell Envelope by Binding Lipoteichoic Acid." *Molecular Microbiology* 83, no. 4 (2012): 789–804. doi:10.1111/j.1365-2958.2011.07966.x.

34. Bomyea, T. A. W. B. "Pseudomonas aeruginosa Lipopolysaccharide: A Major Virulence Factor, Initiator of Inflammation and Target for Effective Immunity Gerald." *Bone* 23, no. 1 (2008): 1–7. https://www.ncbi.nlm.nih.gov/pmc/articles/PMC3624763/pdf/nihms412728.pdf.

35. Ihler, G. M., R. H. Glew, and F. W. Schnure. "Enzyme Loading of Erythrocytes." *Proceedings of the National Academy of Sciences of the United States of America* 70, no. 9 (1973): 2663–6. doi:10.1073/pnas.70.9.2663.

36. Jiang, Y., B. N. Jahagirdar, R. L. Reinhardt, R. E. Schwartz, C. D. Keene, X. R. Ortiz-Gonzalez, M. Reyes, T. Lenvik, T. Lund, M. Blackstad, J. Du, S. Aldrich, A. Lisberg, W. C. Low, D. A. Largaespada, and C. M. Verfaillie. "Erratum: Pluripotency of Mesenchymal Stem Cells Derived from Adult Marrow (Nature (2002) 418 (41–49) DOI: 10.1038/nature00870)." *Nature* 447, no. 7146 (2007): 879–80. doi:10.1038/nature05812.

37. Corsten, M. F., and K. Shah. "Therapeutic Stem-Cells for Cancer Treatment: Hopes and Hurdles in Tactical Warfare." *Lancet Oncology* 9, no. 4 (2008): 376–84. doi:10.1016/S1470-2045(08)70099-8.

38. Cihova M., V. Altanerova, and C. Altaner. "Stem Cell Based Cancer Gene Therapy." *Molecular Pharmacology* 8, no. 5 (2011): 1480–7. doi:10.1021/mp200151a l.

39. Oldenborg, P.-A. "CD47: A Cell Surface Glycoprotein Which Regulates Multiple Functions of Hematopoietic Cells in Health and Disease." *ISRN Hematology* 2013 (2013): 1–19. doi:10.1155/2013/614619.

40. Marin, V., E. Dander, E. Biagi, M. Introna, G. Fazio, A. Biondi, and G. D'Amico. "Characterization of In Vitro Migratory Properties of Anti-CD19 Chimeric Receptor-Redirected CIK Cells for Their Potential Use in B-ALL Immunotherapy." *Experimental Hematology* 34, no. 9 (2006): 1218–28. doi:10.1016/j.exphem.2006.05.004.

41. Kloss, C. C., M. Condomines, M. Cartellieri, M. Bachmann, and M. Sadelain. "Combinatorial Antigen Recognition with Balanced Signaling Promotes Selective Tumor Eradication by Engineered T Cells." *Nature Biotechnology* 31, no. 1 (2013): 71–5. doi:10.1038/nbt.2459.

42. Yu, H., Z. Yang, F. Li, L. Xu, and Y. Sun. "Cell-Mediated Targeting Drugs Delivery Systems." *Drug Delivery* 27, no. 1 (2020): 1425–37. doi:10.1080/10717544.2020.1831103.

43. Nakamura, K., Y. Ito, Y. Kawano, K. Kurozumi, M. Kobune, H. Tsuda, A. Bizen, O. Honmou, Y. Niitsu, and H. Hamada. "Antitumor Effect of Genetically Engineered Mesenchymal Stem Cells in a Rat Glioma Model." *Gene Therapy* 11, no. 14 (2004): 1155–64. doi:10.1038/sj.gt.3302276.

44. Ghosh, S. "Nanotechnology and Sialic Acid Biology." In *Sialic Acids & Sialoglycoconjugates in the Biology of Life, Health & Disease*, 297–325. Amsterdam: Elsevier, 2020. doi:10.1016/b978-0-12-816126-5.00011-1.

45. Gulati, N. M., P. L. Stewart, and N. F. Steinmetz. "Bioinspired Shielding Strategies for Nanoparticle Drug Delivery Applications." *Molecular Pharmaceutics* 15, no. 8 (2018): 2900–9. doi:10.1021/acs.molpharmaceut.8b00292.

46. Zhang, T., Z. She, Z. Huang, J. Li, X. Luo, and Y. Deng. "Application of Sialic Acid/Polysialic Acid in the Drug Delivery Systems." *Asian Journal of Pharmaceutical Sciences* 9, no. 2 (2014): 75–81. doi:10.1016/j.ajps.2014.03.001.

47. Nakamura, S., N. Ando, M. Ishihara, and M. Sato. "Development of Novel Heparin/Protamine Nanoparticles Useful for Delivery of Exogenous Proteins In Vitro and In Vivo." *Nanomaterials* 10, no. 8 (2020): 1–13. doi:10.3390/nano10081584.

48. Pilipenko, I., V. Korzhikov-Vlakh, V. Sharoyko, N. Zhang, M. Schäfer-Korting, C. Rühl, C. Zoschke, and T. Tennikova. "pH-Sensitive Chitosan–Heparin Nanoparticles for Effective Delivery of Genetic Drugs into Epithelial Cells." *Pharmaceutics* 11, no. 7 (2019). doi:10.3390/pharmaceutics11070317.

49. Sarwat, F., S. A. U. Qader, A. Aman, and N. Ahmed. "Production & Characterization of a Unique Dextran from an Indigenous Leuconostoc mesenteroides CMG713." *International Journal of Biological Sciences* 4, no. 6 (2008): 379–86. doi:10.7150/ijbs.4.379.

50. Houga, C., J. Giermanska, S. Lecommandoux, R. Borsali, D. Taton, Y. Gnanou, and J. F. Le Meins. "Micelles and Polymersomes Obtained by Self-Assembly of Dextran and Polystyrene Based Block Copolymers." *Biomacromolecules* 10, no. 1 (2009): 32–40. doi:10.1021/bm800778n.

51. Tu, J., S. Zhong, and P. Li. "Studies on Acyclovir–Dextran Conjugate: Synthesis and Pharmacokinetics." *Drug Development & Industrial Pharmacy* 30, no. 9 (2004): 959–65. doi:10.1081/DDC-200037232.

52. Passirani, C., G. Barratt, J. P. Devissaguet, and D. Labarre. "Long-Circulating Nanoparticles Bearing Heparin or Dextran Covalently Bound to Poly(Methyl Methacrylate)." *Pharmaceutical Research* 15, no. 7 (1998): 1046–50. doi:10.1023/a:1011930127562.

53. Chao, Y., M. Makale, P. P. Karmali, Y. Sharikov, I. Tsigelny, S. Merkulov, S. Kesari, W. Wrasidlo, E. Ruoslahti, and D. Simberg. "Recognition of Dextran–Superparamagnetic Iron Oxide Nanoparticle Conjugates (Feridex) via Macrophage Scavenger Receptor Charged Domains." *Bioconjugate Chemistry* 23, no. 5 (2012): 1003–9. doi:10.1021/bc200685a.

54. Pain, D., P. K. Das, P. Ghosh, and B. K. Bachhawat. "Increased Circulatory Half-Life of Liposomes After Conjunction with Dextran." *Journal of Bio-Science* 6, no. 6 (1984): 811–6. doi:10.1007/BF02716840.

55. Ma, W. J., X. B. Yuan, C. S. Kang, T. Su, X. Yuan, P. Pu, and J. Sheng. "Evaluation of Blood Circulation of Polysaccharide Surface-Decorated PLA Nanoparticles." *Carbohydrate Polymers* 72, no. 1 (2008): 75–81. doi:10.1016/j.carbpol.2007.07.033.

56. Gonçalves, C., J. A. Martins, and F. M. Gama. "Self-Assembled Nanoparticles of Dextrin Substituted with Hexadecanethiol. Technical." *Proceedings of the 2007 Nanotechnology Conference and Trade Show at Santa Clara. Cancer Nanotechnology* 2 (2007): 374–7.

57. Gonçalves, C., E. Torrado, T. Martins, P. Pereira, J. Pedrosa, and M. Gama. "Dextrin Nanoparticles: Studies on the Interaction with Murine Macrophages and Blood Clearance." *Colloids & Surfaces, Part B: Biointerfaces* 75, no. 2 (2010): 483–9. doi:10.1016/j.colsurfb.2009.09.024.

58. Barclay, T. G., C. M. Day, N. Petrovsky, and S. Garg. "Review of Polysaccharide Particle-Based Functional Drug Delivery." *Carbohydrate Polymers* 221 (2019): 94–112. doi:10.1016/j.carbpol.2019.05.067.

59. Liu, W. S., H. J. Yan, R. Y. Qin, R. Tian, M. Wang, J. X. Jiang, M. Shen, and C. J. Shi. "SiRNA Directed Against Survivin Enhances Pancreatic Cancer Cell Gemcitabine Chemosensitivity." *Digestive Diseases & Sciences* 54, no. 1 (2009): 89–96. doi:10.1007/s10620-008-0329-4.

60. Cai, S., S. Thati, T. R. Bagby, H. M. Diab, N. M. Davies, M. S. Cohen, and M. L. Forrest. "Localized Doxorubicin Chemotherapy with a Biopolymeric Nanocarrier Improves Survival and Reduces Toxicity in Xenografts of Human Breast Cancer." *Journal of Controlled Release* 146, no. 2 (2010): 212–8. doi:10.1016/j.jconrel.2010.04.006.

61. Gujrati, V., S. Kim, S.-H. Kim, J. J. Min, H. E. Choy, S. C. Kim, and S. Jon. "Bioengineered Bacterial Outer Membrane Vesicles as Cell-Specific Drug-Delivery Vehicles for Cancer Therapy." *ACS Nano* 8, no. 2 (2014): 1525–37. doi:10.1021/nn405724x.

62. Mattheolabakis, G., L. Milane, A. Singh, and M. M. Amiji. "Hyaluronic Acid Targeting of CD44 for Cancer Therapy: From Receptor Biology to Nanomedicine." *Journal of Drug Targeting* 23, no. 7–8 (2015): 605–18. doi:10.3109/1061186X.2015.1052072.

63. Paygude, S. R. "A Review Nanoerythrosomes: Milestone in Novel Drug Delivery System." *Asian Journal of Pharmaceutical Research & Development* 1, no. 4 (2013): 73–80.

64. Chhabria, V., and S. Beeton. "Development of Nanosponges from Erythrocyte Ghosts for Removal of Streptolysin-O from Mammalian Blood." *Nanomedicine* 11, no. 21 (2016): 2797–807. doi:10.2217/nnm-2016-0180.

65. Hu, C. M. J., R. H. Fang, and L. Zhang. "Erythrocyte-Inspired Delivery Systems." *Advanced Healthcare Materials* 1, no. 5 (2012): 537–47. doi:10.1002/adhm.201200138.

66. Bax, B. E., M. D. Bain, P. J. Talbot, E. J. Parker-Williams, and R. A. Chalmers. "Survival of Human Carrier Erythrocytes In Vivo." *Clinical Science* 96, no. 2 (1999): 171–8. doi:10.1042/cs0960171.

67. Byun, H. M., D. Suh, H. Yoon, J. M. Kim, H. G. Choi, W. K. Kim, J. J. Ko, and Y. K. Oh. "Erythrocyte Ghost-Mediated Gene Delivery for Prolonged and Blood-Targeted Expression." *Gene Therapy* 11, no. 5 (2004): 492–6. doi:10.1038/sj.gt.3302180.

68. Doshi, N., A. S. Zahr, S. Bhaskar, J. Lahann, and S. Mitragotri. "Red Blood Cell-Mimicking Synthetic Biomaterial Particles." *Proceedings of the National Academy of Sciences of the United States of America* 106, no. 51 (2009): 21495–9. doi:10.1073/pnas.0907127106.

69. Merkel, T. J., S. W. Jones, K. P. Herlihy, F. R. Kersey, A. R. Shields, M. Napier, J. C. Luft, H. Wu, W. C. Zamboni, A. Z. Wang, J. E. Bear, and J. M. DeSimone. "Using Mechanobiological Mimicry of Red Blood Cells to Extend Circulation Times of Hydrogel Microparticles." *Proceedings of the National Academy of Sciences of the United States of America* 108, no. 2 (2011): 586–91. doi:10.1073/pnas.1010013108.

70. Li, R., Y. He, S. Zhang, J. Qin, and J. Wang. "Cell Membrane-Based Nanoparticles: A New Biomimetic Platform for Tumor Diagnosis and Treatment." *Acta Pharmacologica Sinica B* 8, no. 1 (2018): 14–22. doi:10.1016/j.apsb.2017.11.009.

71. Toledano Furman, N. E., Y. Lupu-Haber, T. Bronshtein, L. Kaneti, N. Letko, E. Weinstein, L. Baruch, and M. Machluf. "Reconstructed Stem Cell Nanoghosts: A Natural Tumor Targeting Platform." *Nano Letters* 13, no. 7 (2013): 3248–55. doi:10.1021/nl401376w.

72. Kaneti, L., T. Bronshtein, N. Malkah Dayan, I. Kovregina, N. Letko Khait, Y. Lupu-Haber, M. Fliman, B. W. Schoen, G. Kaneti, and M. Machluf. "Nanoghosts as a Novel Natural Nonviral Gene Delivery Platform Safely Targeting Multiple Cancers." *Nano Letters* 16, no. 3 (2016): 1574–82. doi:10.1021/acs.nanolett.5b04237.

73. Lupu-Haber, Y., T. Bronshtein, H. Shalom-Luxenburg, D. D'Atri, J. Oieni, L. Kaneti, A. Shagan, S. Hamias, L. Amram, G. Kaneti, N. Cohen Anavy, and M. Machluf. "Pretreating Mesenchymal Stem Cells with Cancer Conditioned-Media or Proinflammatory Cytokines Changes the Tumor and Immune Targeting by Nanoghosts Derived from These Cells." *Advanced Healthcare Materials* 8, no. 10 (2019): 1–8. doi:10.1002/adhm.201801589.

74. Zhang, L., R. Li, H. Chen, J. Wei, H. Qian, S. Su, J. Shao, L. Wang, X. Qian, and B. Liu. "Human Cytotoxic T-Lymphocyte Membrane-Camouflaged Nanoparticles Combined with Low-Dose Irradiation: A New Approach to Enhance Drug Targeting in Gastric Cancer." *International Journal of Nanomedicine* 12 (2017): 2129–42. doi:10.2147/IJN.S126016.

75. Gao, C., Q. Huang, C. Liu, C. H. T. Kwong, L. Yue, J. B. Wan, S. M. Y. Lee, and R. Wang. "Treatment of Atherosclerosis by Macrophage-Biomimetic Nanoparticles via Targeted Pharmacotherapy and Sequestration of Proinflammatory Cytokines." *Nature Communications* 11, no. 1 (2020): 1–14. doi:10.1038/s41467-020-16439-7.

76. Huang, Y., X. Gao, and J. Chen. "Leukocyte-Derived Biomimetic Nanoparticulate Drug Delivery Systems for Cancer Therapy." *Acta Pharmacologica Sinica B* 8, no. 1 (2018): 4–13. doi:10.1016/j.apsb.2017.12.001.

77. Sun, K., W. Yu, B. Ji, C. Chen, H. Yang, Y. Du, M. Song, H. Cai, F. Yan, and R. Su. "Saikosaponin D Loaded Macrophage Membrane-Biomimetic Nanoparticles Target Angiogenic Signaling for Breast Cancer Therapy." *Applied Materials Today* 18 (2020). doi:10.1016/j.apmt.2019.100505, PubMed: 100505.

78. Kang, T., Q. Zhu, D. Wei, J. Feng, J. Yao, T. Jiang, Q. Song, X. Wei, H. Chen, X. Gao, and J. Chen. "Nanoparticles Coated with Neutrophil Membranes Can Effectively Treat Cancer Metastasis." *ACS Nano* 11, no. 2 (2017): 1397–411. doi:10.1021/acsnano.6b06477.

79. Jiménez-Jiménez, C., M. Manzano, and M. Vallet-Regí. "Nanoparticles Coated with Cell Membranes for Biomedical Applications." *Biology* 9, no. 11 (2020): 1–17. doi:10.3390/biology9110406.

80. Wang, S., Y. Duan, Q. Zhang, A. Komarla, H. Gong, W. Gao, and L. Zhang. "Drug Targeting via Platelet Membrane–Coated Nanoparticles." *Small Struct.* 1, no. 1 (2020). doi:10.1002/sstr.202000018, PubMed: 2000018.

81. Chen, H. Y., J. Deng, Y. Wang, C. Q. Wu, X. Li, and H. W. Dai. "Hybrid Cell Membrane-Coated Nanoparticles: A Multifunctional Biomimetic Platform for Cancer Diagnosis and Therapy." *Acta Biomaterialia* 112 (2020): 1–13. doi:10.1016/j.actbio.2020.05.028.

82. Gong, C., X. Yu, B. You, Y. Wu, R. Wang, L. Han, Y. Wang, S. Gao, and Y. Yuan. "Macrophage-Cancer Hybrid Membrane-Coated Nanoparticles for Targeting Lung Metastasis in Breast Cancer Therapy." *Journal of Nanobiotechnology* 18, no. 1 (2020): 92. doi:10.1186/s12951-020-00649-8.

83. Jin, J., and Z. M. Bhujwalla. "Biomimetic Nanoparticles Camouflaged in Cancer Cell Membranes and Their Applications in Cancer Theranostics." *Frontiers in Oncology* 9 (2020): 1560. doi:10.3389/fonc.2019.01560.

84. Qie, Y., H. Yuan, C. A. Von Roemeling, Y. Chen, X. Liu, K. D. Shih, J. A. Knight, H. W. Tun, R. E. Wharen, W. Jiang, and B. Y. Kim. "Surface Modification of Nanoparticles Enables Selective Evasion of Phagocytic Clearance by Distinct Macrophage Phenotypes." *Scientific Reports* 6, no. May (2016): 1–11. doi:10.1038/srep26269.

85. Mariam, J., S. Sivakami, and P. M. Dongre. "Albumin Corona on Nanoparticles: A Strategic Approach in Drug Delivery." *Drug Delivery* 23, no. 8 (2016): 2668–76. doi:10.3109/10717544.2015.1048488.

86. Discher, D. E., J. C. Andrechak, and L. J. Dooling. "The Macrophage Checkpoint CD47 : SIRPa for Recognition of "Self" Cells: From Clinical Trials of Blocking Antibodies to Mechanobiological Fundamentals." *Philosophical Transactions of the Royal Society of London Series B* 374, no. 1779 (2019). doi:10.1098/rstb.2018.0217, PubMed: 20180217.

87. Hsu, Y. C., M. Acuña, S. M. Tahara, and C. A. Peng. "Reduced Phagocytosis of Colloidal Carriers Using Soluble CD47." *Pharmaceutical Research* 20, no. 10 (2003): 1539–42. doi:10.1023/A:1026114713035.

88. Zhang, J., and C. A. Peng. "Diminution of Phagocytosed Micro/Nanoparticles by Tethering with Immunoregulatory CD200 Protein." *Scientific Reports* 10, no. 1 (2020): 8604. doi:10.1038/s41598-020-65559-z.

Passive Drug Delivery, Mechanisms of Uptake, and Intracellular Trafficking

4

Parisa Foroozandeh, Siti Asmaa Mat Jusoh, and Shaharum Shamsuddin

Contents

4.1 INTRODUCTION: BACKGROUND AND DRIVING FORCES

The cell membrane (CM), also known as the plasma membrane, is a phospholipid bilayer with hydrophilic heads and hydrophobic tails [1–3]. Cell membranes contain cholesterol in their phospholipid bilayer to maintain their fluidity at different temperatures [4, 5]. In addition, there are embedded proteins in cell membranes acting as membrane transporters [6]. Cell membranes separate cytoplasm and the contents of the cell from the extracellular environment. Protecting the cell and intracellular components from its surroundings is the key function of the plasma membrane [7–9]. Cell membranes also confer the shape of the cell by anchoring the cytoskeleton. In addition, cell membranes attach to the extracellular matrix and other cells to form tissues [10, 11]. Cellular membranes play a role in different cellular processes including cell signaling, ion conductivity, cell adhesion, and communication with the extracellular and extra-organelle space. Moreover, cell membranes maintain cell homeostasis, confer structural support,

DOI: 10.1201/9781003092773-5

and retain the composition of the cell [12, 13]. Cell membranes regulate the movement of nutrients into the cell and transport toxic substances outside of the cell [14].

A continuous flow of nutrients and the elimination of undesirable or used substances are needed for cells to survive [15–17]. In order to maintain the movement of proteins, lipids, and solutes, there are specialized pathways that work within the cells referred to as membrane trafficking pathways [18–20]. These pathways are vital to the process of maintaining the sustainability of the cell by delivering the nutrients and other solutes to all parts of the cellular system [21, 22]. These specialized pathways also deliver newly synthesized proteins to their desired locations inside the cells [23–25]. The membrane trafficking pathways control crucial cellular activities including cellular uptake, the transportation of nutrients for metabolism and pathogens for degradation, the trafficking of moieties to the desired location, the transportation of signaling molecules, and communication within or outside cells [26–28]. These trafficking processes which occur both at the cell membrane and subcellular levels have been employed directly, or otherwise, to mediate the localization of endogenous and exogenous substances [29–31]. Another aspect of membrane trafficking is the utilization of different receptors such as folate receptors, epidermal growth factor receptors, melanocortin receptor-1, and a-melanocyte stimulating hormone for targeted drug delivery to deliver therapeutic payloads [32–34]. The endosomal carriers assist in receptor binding, uptake, endosomal escape, and nuclear internalization [35, 36].

4.2 DIFFERENT TYPES OF UPTAKE PATHWAYS

The movement of substances across the cell membrane can be through passive transport which does not require energy or active transport which does employ energy. The cell membrane is a semi-permeable and highly selective barrier which means not all the substances can cross the cell membrane [37–39]. Some substances including small non-polar molecules, hydrophobic molecules such as benzene, uncharged molecules such as water and ethanol, and gases like oxygen and carbon dioxide can easily and rapidly pass through the membranes by diffusion, which is a passive transport process [40, 41]. This type of transport is along a concentration gradient which means it happens from higher concentration to lower concentration and, therefore, does not require energy [42, 43]. Highly charged molecules like ions, large molecules like carbohydrates and amino acids, and water-soluble materials like glucose need assistance to cross the membrane because they are repelled by the hydrophobic tails of the phospholipid bilayer [44, 45]. In fact, these molecules require transport proteins embedded in the membrane to cross the membrane which is a type of passive transport called facilitated diffusion [46–48].

In the case of moving substances against a concentration gradient, the substances cross the membrane through active transport processes which happen from lower concentration to higher concentration and, therefore, employ energy provided by adenosine triphosphate (ATP) [49–51]. One form of active transport is endocytosis in which cells internalize substances by enclosing them in vesicles generated from the cell plasma membrane. Endocytosis occurs in different steps; the first step is engulfing the substance by invagination of the cell membrane that forms membrane-bound vesicles referred to as endosomes [52–54]. Cells contain heterogeneous populations of endosomes equipped with distinct endocytic machinery, which originate at different sites of the cell membrane [55, 56]. In the second step, endosomes deliver the substances to various vesicles which take the substances to different destinations. Lastly, the substances are delivered to different intracellular compartments [57–59]. Endocytosis is classified into two broad categories including phagocytosis which is an uptake of bacteria and large particles and pinocytosis which is an uptake of fluids and solutes. Pinocytosis can be categorized into receptor-mediated endocytosis (RME) and macropinocytosis. Receptor-mediated endocytosis consists of clathrin-mediated endocytosis (CME), caveolin-mediated endocytosis (CVME), and clathrin/caveolae independent endocytosis [60, 61] (Figure 4.1).

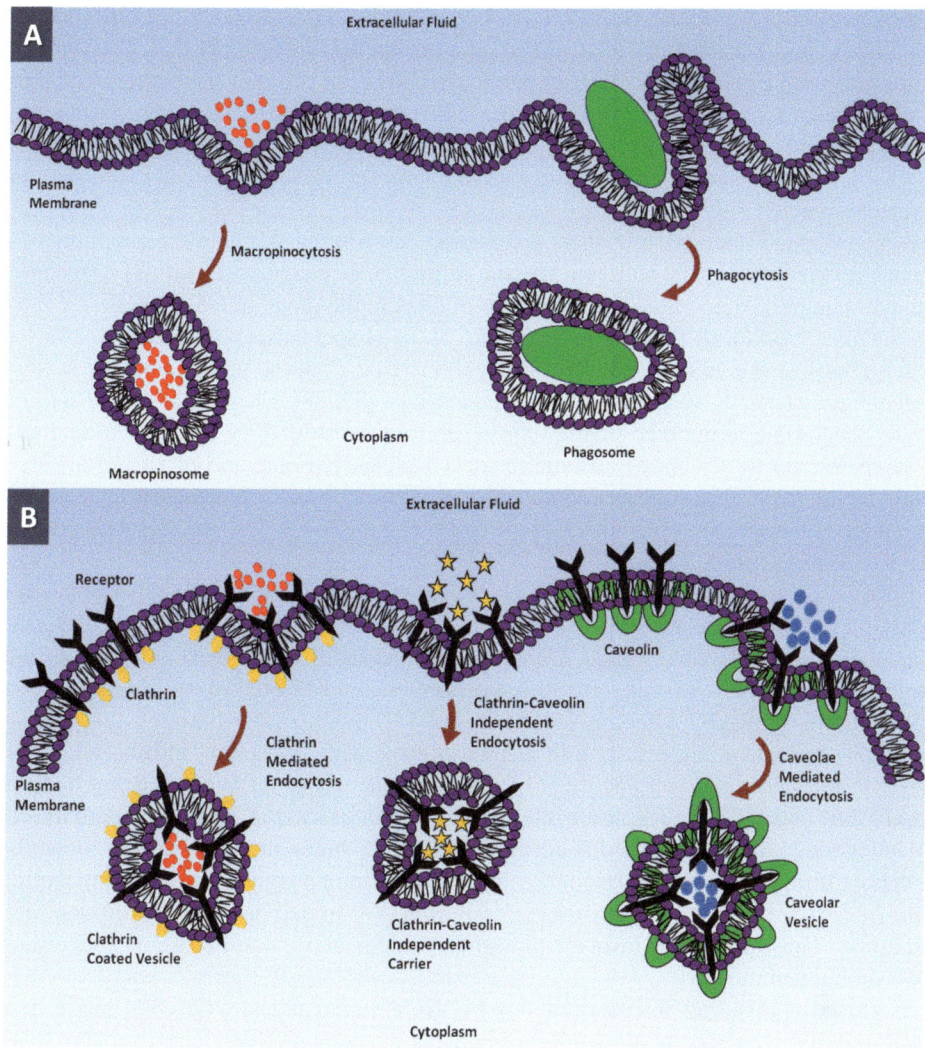

FIGURE 4.1   (A) Macropinocytosis and phagocytosis. (B) Clathrin-mediated endocytosis, clathrin- and caveolin-independent endocytosis, and caveolae-mediated endocytosis [39].

4.2.1 Phagocytosis

The phagocytosis process and phagocytic cells exist in all types of organisms ranging from unicellular organisms to complex, multicellular animals [62–64]. Phagocytosis occurs mainly in specialized cells called professional phagocytes such as macrophages, monocytes, neutrophils, and dendritic cells [65–67]. Other types of cells, called non-professional phagocytes, such as fibroblasts and epithelial and endothelial cells, may also show phagocytic activity, but to a lower extent [68, 69]. Phagocytosis plays a key role in the physiological processes including cell nutrition, immune defense, tissue remodeling, and autophagy. Phagocytosis is employed to engulf and degrade foreign substances, apoptotic cells, senescent cells, cell debris, and infectious microorganisms (bacteria and virus) as a response of innate and adaptive immunity [70, 71].

Phagocytosis occurs in three different steps of which the first step is the opsonization of particles and then the opsonized particles adhere to the cell membrane. In the last step, particles will be ingested by the cells [72, 73]. Particularly, the phagocytosis process usually initiates by opsonization whereby opsonins such as immunoglobulins (i.e., antibodies), complement proteins (C3, C4, C5), or other blood proteins (including laminin and fibronectin) are adsorbed onto the particle surface [74–76]. Then, the opsonized particles are detected by phagocytes resulting in the attachment of phagocytes to opsonized particles via specific ligand-receptor interactions. For instance, the Fc receptor (FcR) binds to the constant fragment of immunoglobulins and complement receptors (CR) bind to complement molecules adsorbed at the particle [77, 78]. Other receptors such as mannose/fructose receptors and scavenger receptors are also involved in the phagocytosis process [79, 80].

The receptor-ligand interaction triggers a signaling cascade that leads to the assembly of actin, an extension of the cell surface, and subsequently the formation of phagosome [81–83]. Depending on the size of the particle, phagosome may have a variety of sizes in the range of a few hundred nanometers to dozens of microns [84–86]. In fact, the main feature of the phagocytosis process is the ability to engulf large particles the size of a micron. As actin is depolymerized from the phagosome, the newly denuded vacuole membrane becomes accessible to early endosomes [87, 88]. Then, series of fusion and fission events cause phagosome to undergo maturation which results in the ferry of cargo to late endosomes. Finally, late endosome fuse with a lysosome to form a phagolysosome and the materials are digested at acidic pH by the hydrolytic enzymes contained within the lysosomal lumen. Ultimately particles are degraded, and the receptors are cycled back to the cell surface [89–92]. The phagocytosis process usually lasts from 30 minutes to several hours [93].

Levin-Konigsberg et al. studied the role of phosphoinositides in phagolysosome resolution. Phosphatidylinositol-4-phosphate (PtdIns(4)P), which is abundant in maturing phagolysosomes, was depleted as they tubulated and resorbed. Depletion was caused, in part, by the transfer of phagolysosomal PtdIns (4)P to the endoplasmic reticulum, a process mediated by oxysterol-binding protein-related protein 1L (ORP1L), a RAB7 effector. ORP1L formed discrete tethers between the phagolysosome and the endoplasmic reticulum, resulting in distinct regions with alternating PtdIns (4)P depletion and enrichment. Tubules emerged from PtdIns (4)P-rich regions, where ADP-ribosylation factor-like protein 8B (ARL8B) and SifA- and kinesin-interacting protein/pleckstrin homology domain-containing family M member 2 (SKIP/PLEKHM2) accumulated. SKIP binds preferentially to monophosphorylated phosphoinositides, of which PtdIns (4)P is most abundant in phagolysosomes, contributing to their tubulation. Accordingly, premature hydrolysis of PtdIns (4)P impaired SKIP recruitment and phagosome resolution. Thus, resolution involves phosphoinositides and the tethering of phagolysosomes to the endoplasmic reticulum [94].

Phagocytosis of invading microorganisms by professional phagocytic cells has a central role in innate immunity. However, several microorganisms developed strategies to subvert this process. Seixas et al. investigated the mechanism by which the malaria parasite *Plasmodium berghei* and the bacterium *Escherichia coli* subvert phagocytosis through the modulation of Rab14 or Rab9a expression, respectively. First, it was confirmed that the scavenger receptor CD36 and the Toll-like receptor (TLR) 4 are required for the phagocytosis of *P. berghei* and *E. coli*, respectively. Interestingly, it was observed that Rab14 silencing leads to an increase in the surface expression of CD36 in macrophages, which can explain the increase in the phagocytosis of *P. berghei* that was reported previously. Similar results were obtained for Rab9a and TLR4, i.e., Rab9a silencing causes an upregulation of TLR4 surface expression in macrophages. Furthermore, it was found that the decrease in the internalization of CD36 and TLR4, upon Rab14 or Rab9a silencing, respectively, can explain the increase in the surface levels of these receptors. Thus, this study provides evidence that the modulation of phagocytosis caused by changes in Rab expression is operated, at least partly, through changes in the surface levels of phagocytic receptors [95].

The role of the receptor tyrosine kinase (RTK) Mer and its ligands Protein S and Gas6 in the initial recognition and capture of apoptotic cells (ACs) by macrophages was investigated. Extremely rapid binding kinetics of both ligands to phosphatidylserine (PtdSer)-displaying ACs was demonstrated, and it was shown that ACs can be co-opsonized with multiple PtdSer opsonins. Furthermore, it was shown that macrophage phagocytosis of ACs opsonized with Mer ligands can occur independently of a requirement for αV integrins. Finally, a novel role for Mer in the tethering of ACs to the macrophage surface was demonstrated, showing that Mer-mediated tethering and subsequent AC engulfment can be distinguished by their requirement for Mer kinase activity. These findings identify Mer as a receptor uniquely capable of both tethering ACs to the macrophage surface and driving their subsequent internalization [96].

4.2.2 Pinocytosis

Non-phagocytic endocytosis generally called pinocytosis (i.e., cell drinking) is the internalization of fluids containing solutes and particles [97, 98]. This mode of endocytosis occurs by the formation of smaller size vesicles than those employed during phagocytosis [99]. In pinocytosis, small particles in the range of a few nanometers to several hundred nanometers are internalized [100, 101]. Unlike phago-cytosis that is limited to specialized cells, pinocytosis occurs in almost all cell types in a continuous manner and irrespective of the needs of the cell [102–104]. Phagocytosis and pinocytosis differ based on the size of endocytotic vesicles. In the phagocytosis process, large particles through large vesicles are engulfed whereas in the pinocytosis process fluids and solutes through small pinocytotic vesicles are internalized [105, 106]. Pinocytosis based on the size of the vesicle can be divided into macropino-cytosis and receptor-mediated endocytosis (RME). Receptor-mediated endocytosis in turn depends on the protein involved in vesicle formation and can be classified into three distinct mechanisms including clathrin-mediated endocytosis, caveolae-mediated endocytosis, and clathrin- and caveolin-independent endocytosis [107–109].

4.2.2.1 Macropinocytosis

Macropinocytosis is clathrin- and caveolin-independent endocytosis which happens in almost all cells with the exception of brain microvessel endothelial cells [110, 111]. This mode of endocytosis is a non-specific, actin-dependent process that takes up large particles in the micron range [112–114]. During macropinocytosis, all particles and substances in the extracellular fluid irrespective of specific receptors are internalized through large endocytic vesicles referred to as macropinosomes [115–117]. Due to the formation of large vesicles, micropinocytosis is a significant process for the internalization of large particles which would not be possible to take up via clathrin- or caveolae-dependent endocytosis [118, 119].

Macropinocytosis is a typical pathway for the uptake of apoptotic bodies, apoptosome, cell fragments, necrotic cells, viruses, bacteria, and nanosomes [120, 121]. Macropinocytosis also plays a role in antigen presentation in major histocompatibility complex II (MHCII) [122, 123]. Despite phagocytosis and receptor-mediated endocytosis, macropinocytosis is not regulated by the direct action of a receptor or the cargo molecules [124, 125]. This endocytosis pathway is originated by the activation of tyrosine kinases receptors such as the epidermal growth factor and the platelet-derived growth factor receptor which lead to an increase in actin polymerization and trigger the formation of membrane ruffles followed by macropinosome biogenesis. These formed ruffles engulf the surrounding substances in the extracellular fluid, and the formed macropinosomes undergo acidification and subsequent fusion with lysosome [126–129].

Recently, members of the Sorting Nexin (SNX) family have been localized to the cell surface and early macropinosomes and implicated in macropinosome formation. SNX-PX-BAR proteins form a subset of the SNX family and their lipid-binding (PX) and membrane-curvature sensing (BAR) domain architecture further implicate their functional involvement in macropinosome formation [130]. Li et al. used dynamic imaging to visualize membrane and cytoskeletal behavior in migrating neural crest cells in living tissue. It was found that forward movement of individual neural crest cells is accompanied by circular membrane flow, from anterior-to-posterior apically and posterior-to-anterior basally, coupled with the internalization of lipid vesicles via macropinocytosis in the soma. Macropinosomes become wrapped with actin, then undergo anterograde translocation via microtubules toward the lamellipodium, resulting in its expansion. It was elucidated how actin dynamics and membrane flow interact to drive the forward locomotion of individual cells [131].

4.2.2.2 Receptor-Mediated Endocytosis (RME)

Unlike macropinocytosis, receptor-mediated endocytosis (RME) is highly specific. In particular, RME relies on the binding of a ligand such as insulin or transferrin to its complementary receptor on the surface of a target cell [132–134]. Depending on the proteins involved in endocytic pathways, receptor-mediated endocytosis is categorized as clathrin-mediated endocytosis, caveolae-mediated endocytosis, or clathrin- and caveolae-independent endocytosis.

4.2.2.2.1 Clathrin-Mediated Endocytosis (CME)

Clathrin-mediated endocytosis is an important cellular entry pathway present in all mammalian cells. This pathway is employed to uptake a variety of ligand-receptor complexes. Therefore, clathrin-mediated endocytosis is of great importance not only for ligands but also for viruses such as influenza virus as well as for drug-loaded nanocarriers having targeting ligands on their surface [135–138]. This pathway is responsible for the internalization of vital nutrients such as cholesterol and iron which are carried into the cells by low-density lipoprotein (LDL) via the LDL receptor, and by transferrin (Tf) via the Tf receptor, respectively [139–141].

Clathrin-mediated endocytosis also plays a key role in the physiological process including membrane recycling, intracellular communication, down-regulation of cell signaling, and maintaining cellular homeostasis by trafficking ion pumps [142–144]. Furthermore, CME assists the internalization of lipoproteins, folic acid, transcobalamin, iron transport proteins, hormones, and growth factors into cells. Attaching these ligands to a nano-drug carrier facilitates their uptake by clathrin-mediated endocytosis into the targeted cells. The ligand-binding domain of RME has a negative charge; thus, CME is the primary path for the uptake of positively charged substances [145–147].

Clathrin-mediated endocytosis takes place in membrane regions enriched in clathrin proteins which are the main cytosolic coat protein and constitute 2% of the total area of the plasma membrane [148, 149]. The polymerization of clathrin protein leads to the formation of basket-like structures which in turn result in the development of a coated pit in the size range of 120 to 150 nm [150–152]. The clathrin protein assembly unit has a three-legged structure referred to as the triskelion which consists of three heavy and three light chains [153–155]. This protein, with the help of extensive protein machinery including accessory proteins (e.g., epsin, amphiphysin, SNX9, endophilin, and the FCHo2 F-BAR domain), adaptor protein complexes (e.g., the AP-2 heterotetrameric complex [a-b2-m2-s2], AP180), and clathrin assembly lymphoid myeloid leukemia [CALM] protein), generates and stabilizes curvature in the membrane. As the clathrin lattice formation continues, the pit becomes deeply invaginated [156–158].

In this process, the membranes invaginate inwards with the biogenesis of clathrin-coated vesicles. The vesicles are then released from the plasma membrane with the assistance of GTPases and dynamin that is assembled as a ring around the newly formed vesicle [159–161]. Actin supplies the energy and regulates the movement of clathrin-coated vesicles inside the cells. The destination of vesicles depends on the receptor that cargo ligands attach to [162–164]. After the internalization of vesicles, they lose the clathrin coating. At this stage, uncoated vesicles either traffic to early endosomes that are acidified by ATP-dependent proton pumps or some receptors and ligands such as LDL receptor, transferrin, and its receptor detached, recycled and transported back to plasma membrane for the next turn of delivery. Then, the early endosomes can also be targeted to late endosomes and later to compartments such as lysosomes and multivesicular bodies (MVBs) [165–167].

A three-dimensional mathematical model was used to study the contribution of clathrins during the process of cellular uptake of spherical nanoparticles under different membrane tensions. The clathrin-coated pit (CCP) that forms around the inward budding of the cell membrane was modeled as a vesicle with bending rigidity. An optimization algorithm was proposed for minimizing the total energy of the system; the model considers the deforming nanoparticle, receptor-ligand bonds, the cell membrane, and CCP. The results showed that the CCP enables full wrapping of the nanoparticles at various membrane tensions. When the cell membrane tension increases, the total deformation energy also increases, but the ratio of CCP bending to the minimum value of the total energy of the system decreases. The results also showed that the diameter of the endocytic vesicles (determined by the competition between the stretching of the cell membrane and confinement of the coated pits) is much larger than that of the nanoparticles, which is different from passive endocytosis that is not facilitated by the CCPs. These results indicate that variations of tension on cell membranes constitute a biophysical marker for understanding the size distribution of CCPs observed in experiments. These findings also suggest that the early initiation of endocytosis is related to the receptor-ligand bonds that cannot generate adequate force to wrap the nanoparticles into the cell membrane before clathrins respond to support the endocytic vesicles [169].

Simultaneous dual-color total-internal-reflection fluorescence microscopy (TIR-FM) was performed to analyze the internalization and distribution of markers for clathrin-mediated endocytosis (clathrin, dynamin1, dynamin2, and transferrin) in migrating cells. In MDCK cells, which endogenously express dynamin2, the dynamin2-EGFP fluorescence demonstrated identical spatial and temporal behavior as clathrin both prior to and during internalization. By contrast, in the same cells, the neuronal dynamin1 only localized with clathrin just prior to endocytosis. In migrating cells, each endocytic marker was polarized towards the leading edge, away from the lagging edge. These observations suggest a re-evaluation of the functional differences between dynamin1 and dynamin2, and of the role of clathrin-mediated endocytosis in cell migration [170].

The formation of clathrin-coated structures at the plasma membranes of BSC1 and HeLa cells depleted by RNAi of the clathrin adaptor, AP-2, was studied by using *in-vivo* imaging data obtained by spinning-disk confocal microscopy. Very few clathrin coats continue to assemble after AP-2 knockdown. Moreover, there is a total absence of clathrin-containing structures completely lacking AP-2 while all the remaining coats still contain a small amount of AP-2. These results suggest that AP-2 is essential for endocytic clathrin-coated-pit and coated-vesicle formation [171].

4.2.2.2.2 Caveolin-Mediated Endocytosis (CVME)

Caveolin-mediated endocytosis initiates at the level of caveolae which are flask-shaped membrane invaginations with the size range of 50–80 nm [172, 173]. Caveolae are abundant in muscle, endothelial cells, fibroblasts, and adipocytes and absent in neurons and leukocytes [174–176]. Caveolae consist of cholesterol, GPI-anchored proteins, sphingolipids, and the integral membrane proteins caveolin-1 and caveolin-2. Caveolin-1 promotes the binding of several molecules including fatty acids, glycosphingolipids, cholesterol, and membrane proteins [177–179]. Thus, caveolae sequester multiple ligands responsible for cellular signaling including heterotrimeric G proteins, non-receptor tyrosine kinases, insulin receptors, platelet-derived growth factor receptors, and endothelial nitric oxide synthase (eNOS) [180–182].

In caveolin-mediated endocytosis, cavin protein, a component of caveolae, is responsible for the induction of membrane curvature, dynamin enables vesicle detachment, and vesicle-associated membrane protein (VAMP2) and synaptosome-associated protein (SNAP) facilitate subsequent vesicle fusion [183–185]. Unlike CME, the protein involved in caveolae formation, caveolin-1, does not detach from the vesicle [186–188]. Caveolin vesicles fuse with other caveolin vesicles, forming multicaveolar structures referred to as caveosomes which then later fuse with early endosomes in a bidirectional way. Afterwards, based on the type of cell, vesicular structures may travel to the smooth endoplasmic reticulum or to the Golgi-trans network and from there they may enter the nucleus through the nuclear pore complex [189–191]. Similar to clathrin-dependent endocytosis, caveolar vesicles require actin to move and intact microtubules to traffic within the cell [192–194].

Caveolae-mediated endocytosis plays a significant role in many biological processes including transcytosis, cell signaling, and the regulation of lipids, fatty acids, membrane proteins, and membrane tension [195–197]. Moreover, caveolae-mediated endocytosis is involved in a variety of diseases, including cancer, diabetes, and viral infections [198–200]. In particular, many pathogens including simian virus 40 (SV40) viruses employ caveolae-mediated endocytosis to bypass lysosomes and escape degradation by lysosomal enzymes [201, 202]. For the same reason, this pathway is promising for targeting therapeutics to the intracellular organelles and cellular delivery of proteins and nucleic acids [203–205]. Moreover, cholera and Shiga toxins also exploit the caveolae-mediated endocytosis pathway to enter the cells [206, 207]. Hence, these molecules can be employed for drug delivery purposes. Particularly, cholera and Shiga toxins have a binding affinity for antigens on the surface of cancerous cells, making them an easy target. Therefore, the synthesis of drug carriers with these toxins makes them target specific [208–210]. In comparison with clathrin-mediated endocytosis, the uptake kinetics of caveolae-mediated endocytosis takes place at a slower rate and longer time. Moreover, caveolae-mediated endocytosis has smaller vesicles than clathrin-mediated endocytosis [211–213].

The endocytic pathway involved in the entry of *Leishmania donovani* into host macrophages, utilizing specific inhibitors against two major pathways of internalization, i.e., clathrin- and caveolin-mediated endocytosis, was explored. It was shown that pitstop 2, an inhibitor for clathrin-mediated endocytosis, does not affect the entry of *Leishmania donovani* promastigotes into host macrophages. Interestingly, a significant reduction in internalization was observed upon treatment with genistein, an inhibitor for caveolin-mediated endocytosis. These results are supported by a similar trend in intracellular amastigote load within host macrophages. These results suggest that *Leishmania donovani* utilizes caveolin-mediated endocytosis to internalize into the host cells [214].

While severe acute respiratory syndrome coronavirus (SARS-CoV) was initially thought to enter cells through direct fusion with the plasma membrane, more recent evidence suggests that virus entry may also involve endocytosis. It was found that SARS-CoV enters cells via pH- and receptor-dependent endocytosis. Treatment of cells with either SARS-CoV spike protein or spike-bearing pseudoviruses resulted in the translocation of angiotensin-converting enzyme 2 (ACE2), the functional receptor of SARS-CoV, from the cell surface to endosomes. In addition, the spike-bearing pseudoviruses and early endosome antigen 1 were found to colocalize in endosomes. Further analyses using specific endocytic pathway inhibitors and dominant-negative Eps15 as well as caveolin-1 colocalization study suggested that virus entry was mediated by a clathrin- and caveolae-independent mechanism. Moreover, cholesterol- and sphingolipid-rich lipid raft microdomains in the plasma membrane, which have been shown to act as platforms for many physiological signaling pathways, were shown to be involved in virus entry. Endocytic entry of SARS-CoV may expand the cellular range of SARS-CoV infection, and these findings here contribute to the understanding of SARS-CoV pathogenesis, providing new information for anti-viral drug research [215].

Wei et al. have demonstrated that porcine epidemic diarrhea virus (PEDV) enters cells via the clathrin- and caveolae-mediated endocytosis pathways, in which dynamin II, clathrin heavy chain, Eps15, cholesterol, and caveolin-1 were indispensably involved. In addition, lipid raft extraction assay showed that PEDV can also enter cells through lipid raft-mediated endocytosis. To investigate the trafficking of internalized PEDV, it was found that PEDV entry into cells relied on low pH and internalized virions reached lysosomes through the early endosome–late endosome–lysosome pathway. The results concretely revealed the entry mechanisms of PEDV and provided an insightful theoretical basis for the further understanding of PEDV pathogenesis and guidance for new targets of antiviral drugs [216].

4.2.2.2.3 Clathrin/Caveolae-Independent Endocytosis

In the cells deprived of clathrin and caveolin, cellular uptake occurs through clathrin- and caveolae-independent endocytosis which is a cholesterol-dependent pathway [217–219]. Vesicles in this mode of endocytosis internalize extracellular fluid, SV40, CTB, glycosylphosphatidylinositol (GPI)-linked proteins, interleukin-2, growth hormones, etc. [220–222]. Clathrin- and caveolae-independent endocytosis can be classified based on the protein involved in the endocytosis process, classified as Arf6-dependent, flotillin-dependent, Cdc42-dependent, and RhoA-dependent [223, 224].

One of the clathrin- and caveolae-independent endocytosis pathways is the ADP-ribosylation factor 6 (Arf6)-dependent pathway which involves endocytosis of the major histocompatibility complex (MHC) class I that is vital for antigen presentation and immune response, β-integrins, glucose transporter GLUT1, and other proteins that are involved in amino acid uptake and cell-extracellular matrix interactions [225–227]. Mukhamedova et al. have shown that the principal pathway responsible for the internalization of ATP-binding cassette transporter A1 (ABCA1) leading to its degradation in macrophages is the ARF6-dependent endocytic pathway. This pathway was predominant in the regulation of ABCA1 abundance and efflux of plasma membrane cholesterol. Conversely, the efflux of intracellular cholesterol was predominantly controlled by ARF6-independent pathways, and the inhibition of ARF6 shifted ABCA1 into recycling endosomes enhancing the efflux of intracellular cholesterol [228]. It was revealed that Arf6-mediated CD147 endocytic recycling is required for the malignant phenotypes of liver cancer. The Arf6-driven signaling machinery provides excellent biomarkers or therapeutic targets for the prevention of liver cancer [229].

It was found that siRNA-mediated depletion of clathrin or of adaptor protein 2 (AP-2)-complex subunits alters trafficking of Arf6 pathway cargo proteins, such as major histocompatibility complex class I (MHCI) and β1 integrin. Internalization of these cargoes from the plasma membrane was not affected in cells depleted of clathrin but was modestly delayed in cells lacking AP-2. Furthermore, the depletion of clathrin or AP-2 altered the intracellular distribution of MHCI and β1 integrin, inducing clustering in a perinuclear region. Despite this altered localization in both depleted populations, enhanced lysosomal targeting of MHCI was observed uniquely in cells that lack AP-2. Total levels of MHCI were modestly but consistently reduced in AP-2-depleted cells and restored by the lysosomal inhibitor bafilomycin A. Furthermore, the half-life of surface-derived MHCI was reduced in AP-2-depleted cells. Consistent with enhanced degradative sorting, colocalization of Arf6 cargo with the late endosome and lysosome markers CD63 and Lamp1 was increased in cells depleted of AP-2 but not clathrin. These studies indicate a role for AP-2 in maintaining normal post-endocytic trafficking through the Arf6-regulated, non-clathrin pathway, and reveal pervasive effects of clathrin and AP-2 depletion on the endosomal and lysosomal system [230].

Another subtype of the clathrin- and caveolae-independent endocytosis pathway is Cdc42 mediated which is a dynamin-independent pathway. This mode of endocytosis is the route for the internalization of cholera toxin B (CtxB) and the *Helicobacter pylori* vacuolating toxin (VacA) [231–234]. The interaction between the Rho GTPase Cdc42 and the GTPase-activating protein (GAP) GRAF1 (also known as ARHGAP26) was studied, and it was found that GRAF1 transiently assemble at discrete Cdc42-enriched punctae at the plasma membrane, resulting in a corresponding decrease in the microdomain association of Cdc42. However, Cdc42 captured in its active state was, through a GAP-domain-mediated interaction, localized together with GRAF1 on accumulated internal structures derived from the cell surface. Correlative fluorescence and electron tomography microscopy revealed that these structures were clusters of small membrane carriers with defective endosomal processing. It was concluded that a transient interaction between Cdc42 and GRAF1 drives endocytic turnover and controls the transition essential for endosomal maturation of plasma membrane internalized by this mechanism [235].

Garrett et al. found that endocytic downregulation reflects a decrease in endocytic activity controlled by Rho family GTPases, especially Cdc42. Blocking Cdc42 function by Toxin B treatment or the injection of dominant-negative inhibitors of Cdc42 abrogates endocytosis in immature dendritic cells (DCs). In mature DCs, the injection of constitutively active Cdc42 or microbial delivery of a Cdc42 nucleotide exchange factor reactivates endocytosis. DCs regulate endogenous levels of Cdc42-GTP with activated Cdc42 detectable only in immature cells. It was concluded that DCs developmentally regulate endocytosis at least in part by controlling levels of activated Cdc42 [236].

One clathrin- and caveolae-independent but dynamin-dependent pathway is mediated by small GTPase RhoA. RhoA-dependent endocytosis is employed in the uptake of the β-chain of the interleukin-2 receptor (IL-2R-β) and other proteins in both immune cells and fibroblasts [237–239]. Prosser et al. provide evidence for a clathrin-independent endocytic pathway in yeast. In cells lacking the clathrin-binding adaptor proteins Ent1, Ent2, Yap1801, and Yap1802, a second endocytic pathway that depends on the GTPase Rho1, the downstream formin Bni1, and the Bni1 cofactors Bud6 and Spa2 were identified. This second pathway does not require components of the better-studied endocytic pathway, including clathrin and Arp2/3 complex activators. These results revealed the existence of a second pathway for endocytosis in yeast, which suggests similarities with the RhoA-dependent endocytic pathways of mammalian cells [240].

It was observed that voiding-stimulated compensatory endocytosis (CE), which depended on β1 integrin-associated signaling pathways, occurred by a dynamin-, actin-, and RhoA-regulated mechanism and was independent of caveolins, clathrin, and flotillin. Internalized apical membrane and fluid were initially found in ZO-1-positive vesicles, which were distinct from discoidal/fusiform vesicles (DFV), classical early endosomes, or the Golgi, and subsequently in lysosomes. It was concluded that clathrin-independent CE in umbrella cells functions to recover membrane during voiding, is integrin regulated, occurs by a RhoA- and dynamin-dependent pathway, and terminates in degradation and not recapture of the membrane in DFV [241].

RhoA was reported that elicits suppression of Kv1.2 ionic current (a member of the Shaker family of voltage-sensitive potassium channels and contributes to the regulation of membrane excitability) by modulating channel endocytosis. This occurs through two distinct pathways, one clathrin-dependent and the other cholesterol-dependent. Activation of Rho kinase (ROCK) via the lysophosphatidic acid (LPA) receptor elicits clathrin-dependent Kv1.2 endocytosis and consequent attenuation of its ionic current. LPA-induced channel endocytosis is blocked by the ROCK inhibitor Y27632 or by clathrin RNA interference. In contrast, steady-state endocytosis of Kv1.2 in unstimulated cells is cholesterol-dependent. The inhibition of basal ROCK signaling with Y27632 increased surface Kv1.2, an effect that persists in the presence of clathrin small interfering RNA and that is not additive to the increase in surface channel levels elicited by the cholesterol sequestering drug filipin. Temperature block experiments show that ROCK affects cholesterol-dependent trafficking by modulating the recycling of the endocytosed channel back to the plasma membrane. Both receptor-stimulated and steady-state Kv1.2 trafficking modulated by RhoA/ROCK required the activation of dynamin as well as the ROCK effector Lim-kinase, indicating a key role for actin remodeling in RhoA-dependent Kv1.2 regulation [242].

CLIC/GEEC pathway is another clathrin- and caveolae-independent pathway that is utilized in the uptake of glycosylphosphatidylinositol-anchored proteins, transmembrane proteins including CD44 and dysferlin, extracellular fluids, toxins such as *Helicobacter pylori* vacuolating toxin A, cholera toxin, and viruses like adeno-associated virus 2 [243–246]. CLIC/GEEC pathway is regulated by the small GTPases, ADP-ribosylation factor 1 (ARF1), and cell division control protein 42 (CDC42) [247–249]. The CLIC/GEEC (CG) pathway occurs through uncoated tubulovesicular primary carriers referred to as clathrin-independent carriers (CLICs) which are invaginated from the plasma membrane [250, 251]. These carriers later mature into tubular early endocytic compartments termed glycosylphosphatidylinositol-anchored protein (GPI-AP) enriched compartments (GEECs). The GEECs subsequently fuse with the sorting endocytic vesicles in a Rab5 and PI3K dependent mechanism [252–255]. This pathway is a major contributor to membrane dynamics which enables rapid membrane turnover for key cellular processes like plasma membrane repair [256, 257]. Moreover, the CG pathway plays a significant role in regulating homoeostasis, the creation of a tubular vesicular endocytic network during cytokinesis as well as the repair of plasma membrane lesions induced by bacterial toxins [258–260].

Chadda et al. show that endocytosis via the GEECs pathway is inhibited by mild depletion of cholesterol, perturbation of actin polymerization, or overexpression of the Cdc42/Rac-interactive-binding (CRIB) motif of neural Wiskott2Aldrich syndrome protein (N-WASP). Consistent with the involvement of Cdc42-based actin nanomachinery, nascent endocytic vesicles containing cargo for the GEEC pathway co-localize with fluorescent protein-tagged isoforms of Cdc42, CRIB domain, N-WASP, and actin; high-resolution electron microscopy on plasma membrane sheets reveals Cdc42-labeled regions rich in green fluorescent protein–GPI. Using total internal reflection fluorescence microscopy at the single-molecule scale, it was found that mild cholesterol depletion alters the dynamics of actin polymerization at the cell surface by inhibiting Cdc42 activation and consequently its stabilization at the cell surface. These results suggest that endocytosis into GEECs occurs through cholesterol-sensitive, Cdc42-based recruitment of the actin polymerization machinery [261].

It was demonstrated that GRAF1 localizes to PtdIns(4,5)P2-enriched, tubular, and punctate lipid structures via N-terminal BAR and PH domains. These membrane carriers are relatively devoid of caveolin1 and flotillin1 but are associated with the activity of the small G protein Cdc42. This study provides the first specific non-cargo marker for CLIC/GEEC endocytic membranes and demonstrates how GRAF1 can coordinate small G protein signaling and membrane remodeling to facilitate internalization of CLIC/GEEC pathway cargoes [243].

Anupama and co-researchers have shown that Wingless signaling in *Drosophila* mainly occurs through a clathrin- and dynamin-independent endocytosis pathway with the aid of cell surface GPI-anchored proteins (CG pathway), mediated by Garz, Arf1, and Class I PI3 kinase. These Wingless carriers further fuse with endosomes derived from the CD pathway carrying the receptor, DFrizzled2. This culminates in a low pH-dependent transfer of Wingless to its signaling receptor resulting in effective signaling. The mediation of Wingless signaling by two distinct endocytosis pathways potentially allows cells to autonomously control Wingless uptake independent of the availability of DFrizzled2 [262].

Flotillins, also called Reggie protein comprised of flotillin 1 and flotillin 2 proteins, are membrane proteins that exist in certain microdomains or lipid rafts of the plasma membrane [263–265]. These proteins are highly homologous, conserved, and expressed ubiquitously [266, 267]. These proteins facilitate clathrin- and caveolae-independent endocytosis that is regulated by the Src family tyrosine kinase Fyn [268–270]. Currently, flotillins are employed as a marker protein for non-caveolar rafts [271–273]. The flotillin-dependent pathway is responsible for the uptake of cargos such as glycosylphosphatidylinositol (GPI)-linked proteins, cholera toxin B subunit, proteoglycans and their ligands, and Niemann-Pick C1-like1 (NPC1L1) [274–276]. Depending on the type of cell and the internalized cargo, flotillin-associated endocytosis can be either dependent or independent of dynamin [277–279].

In research conducted by Saslowsky et al., it was found that intoxication of cholera toxin in zebrafish embryos and mammals is flotillin dependent [280]. Pust et al. examined the importance of flotillin-1 and flotillin-2 for the uptake and transport of the bacterial Shiga toxin (Stx) and the plant toxin ricin and investigated whether toxin binding and uptake were associated with flotillin relocalization. A toxin-induced redistribution of the flotillins, which seemed to be regulated in a p38-dependent manner, was observed. These experiments provide no evidence for a changed endocytic uptake of Stx or ricin in cells silenced for flotillin-1 or -2. However, the Golgi-dependent sulfation of both toxins was significantly reduced in flotillin knockdown cells. Interestingly, when the transport of ricin to the ER was investigated, an increased mannosylation of ricin in flotillin-1 and flotillin-2 knockdown cells was obtained. The toxicity of both toxins was increased twofold in flotillin-depleted cells. Since Brefeldin A (BFA) inhibits the toxicity even in flotillin knockdown cells, the retrograde toxin transport is apparently still Golgi-dependent. Thus, flotillin proteins regulate and facilitate the retrograde transport of Stx and ricin [281].

It was found that the protein Flotillin-1 (Flot1) was required for stimuli including protein kinase C (PKC)-regulated internalization of members of two different NTT families, the DA transporter (DAT) and the glial glutamate transporter EAAT2, and a conserved serine residue in Flot1 that is essential for transporter internalization was identified. Further analysis revealed that Flot1 was also required to localize DAT within plasma membrane microdomains in stable cell lines and was essential for amphetamine-induced reverse transport of DA in neurons but not for DA uptake. In sum, these findings provide evidence for a critical role of Flot1-enriched membrane microdomains in PKC-triggered DAT endocytosis and the actions of amphetamine [282].

The function of plasma membrane microdomains defined by the proteins flotillin 1 and flotillin 2 in uropod formation and neutrophil chemotaxis was studied. Flotillins become concentrated in the uropod of neutrophils after exposure to chemoattractants such as N-formyl-Met-Leu-Phe (fMLP). It was shown that mice lacking flotillin 1 do not have flotillin microdomains, and that recruitment of neutrophils toward fMLP *in vivo* is reduced in these mice. *Ex vivo*, the migration of neutrophils through a resistive matrix is reduced in the absence of flotillin microdomains, but the machinery required for sensing chemoattractant functions normally. Flotillin microdomains specifically associate with myosin IIa and spectrin. Both uropod formation and myosin IIa activity are compromised in flotillin 1 knockout neutrophil. It was concluded that the association between flotillin microdomains and the cortical cytoskeleton has important functions during neutrophil migration, in uropod formation, and in the regulation of myosin IIa [283] (Figure 4.2).

4.3 INTRACELLULAR TRAFFICKING

After the internalization of substances into the cells, the next vital process is their intracellular location and translocation which is associated with the cytotoxicity, therapeutic efficacy, and the fate of internalized matter [284–286]. Generally, subsequent to the uptake of substances, they will first encounter

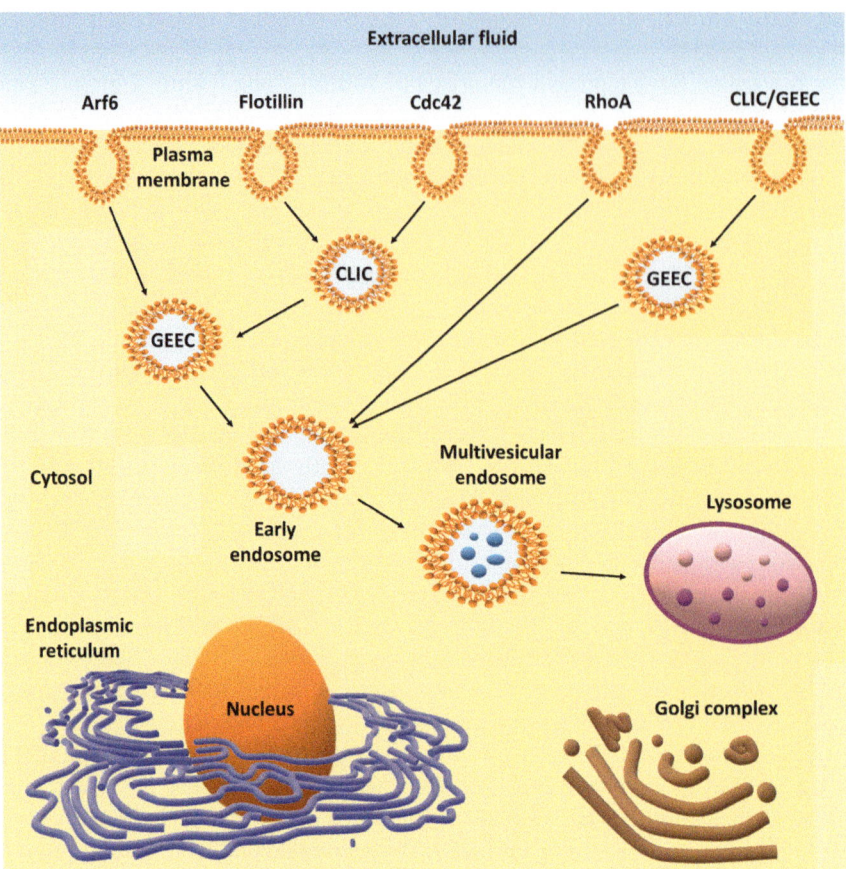

FIGURE 4.2   Clathrin- and caveolin-independent endocytosis pathways.

membrane-bound intracellular vesicles called early endosomes [287–289]. Endosomes are relatively large (up to 1 μm and even larger) intracellular membrane-bound compartments initially produced by the plasma membrane, and later they may fuse with Golgi-derived vesicles [290–293]. Endosomes are usually found in the cytoplasm of most human cells and can be categorized into three major forms including early endosomes, recycling endosomes, and late endosomes (also called multi-vesicular bodies – MVB). These three types of endosomes together compose the key part of the intracellular endocytic machinery [294–296].

Then, the early endosome delivers the cargo to the desired cellular destination. Part of the cargo is recycled to the plasma membrane in small vesicles, either directly or indirectly, by fusing with the recycling endosomes [297–299]. The rest of the cargo in early endosomes undergoes fission and fusion events which lead to maturation into late endosomes. Late endosomes can either fuse with the plasma membrane (releasing their cargo outside the cell in the form of exosomes) or fuse with lysosomes, forming endolysosomes [300–302]. Endolysosomes contain hydrolytic enzymes and hence lead to the degradation of the internalized substances. Occasionally, the internalized substance may not go through the mentioned endocytic pathway, and they are released into the cell cytoplasm [303–306]. If this incident occurs prior to the fusion with lysosomes the cargo can bypass lysosomal degradation and end up intact in the cytoplasm or in other intracellular compartments [307–309]. Another intracellular pathway that should be taken into consideration is the biological process called autophagy. Autophagy is an intracellular degradation pathway that is totally distinct from the endocytic pathway and ferries certain cytoplasmic constituents through autophagosome to lysosomal to be broken down and degraded [310–312]. This pathway plays a key role in the intracellular fate of substances as well as maintaining cellular homeostasis by the degradation of aggregated proteins and dysfunctional organelles [313, 314].

REFERENCES

1. Qian, S., V. K. Sharma, and L. A. Clifton. "Understanding the Structure and Dynamics of Complex Biomembrane Interactions by Neutron Scattering Techniques." *Langmuir* 2020, no. 36: 15189–211.
2. Lombardo, D. et al. "Interdisciplinary Approaches to the Study of Biological Membranes." 7 (2020): 267–90.
3. Berón, W., C. Alvarez-Dominguez, L. Mayorga, and P. D. Stahl. "Membrane Trafficking Along the Phagocytic Pathway." 5, no. 3 (1995): 100–4.
4. Kaddah, S., N. Khreich, F. Kaddah, C. Charcosset, and H. Greige-Gerges. "Cholesterol Modulates the Liposome Membrane Fluidity and Permeability for a Hydrophilic Molecule." 113 (2018): 40–8.
5. Ballweg, S., E. Sezgin, M. Doktorova, R. Covino, J. Reinhard, D. Wunnicke, I. Hänelt, I. Levental, G. Hummer, and R. Ernst. "Regulation of Lipid Saturation Without Sensing Membrane Fluidity." 11, no. 1 (2020): 1–13.
6. Edidin, M. "Lipids on the Frontier: A Century of Cell-Membrane Bilayers." 4, no. 5 (2003): 414–8.
7. Shi, Y., M. Cai, L. Zhou, and H. Wang. "The Structure and Function of Cell Membranes Studied by Atomic Force Microscopy." In *Seminars in Cell & Developmental Biology*. Amsterdam: Elsevier, 2018.
8. Shi, Y., and J. Massagué. "Mechanisms of TGF-β Signaling from Cell Membrane to the Nucleus." *Cell* 113, no. 6 (2003): 685–700.
9. Noack, J., and S. Mukherjee. "'Make way': Pathogen Exploitation of Membrane Traffic." *Current Opinion in Cell Biology* 65 (2020): 78–85.
10. Honigmann, A., and A. Pralle. "Compartmentalization of the Cell Membrane." *Journal of Molecular Biology* 428, no. 24 (2016): 4739–48.
11. Zalba, S., and T. L. Ten Hagen. "Cell Membrane Modulation as Adjuvant in Cancer Therapy." *Cancer Treatment Reviews* 52 (2017): 48–57.
12. McMahon, H. T., and J. L. Gallop. "Membrane Curvature and Mechanisms of Dynamic Cell Membrane Remodelling." *Nature* 438, no. 7068 (2005): 590–6.
13. García-Sánchez, T., A. Muscat, I. Leray, and L. M. Mir. "Pyroelectricity as a Possible Mechanism for Cell Membrane Permeabilization." 119 (2018): 227–33.
14. Lehman-McKeeman, L. D. "Biochemical and Molecular Basis of Toxicity." In *Haschek and Rousseaux's Handbook of Toxicologic Pathology*, 15–38. Amsterdam: Elsevier, 2013.
15. Broach, J. R. "Nutritional Control of Growth and Development in Yeast." *Genetics* 192, no. 1 (2012): 73–105.
16. Chen, Y., and J. L. Heazlewood. "Organellar Proteomic Profiling to Analyze Membrane Trafficking Pathways." *Trends in Plant Science* (2020).
17. Chambers, I. G., M. M. Willoughby, I. Hamza, and A. R. Reddi. "One Ring to Bring Them All and in the Darkness Bind Them: The Trafficking of Heme Without Deliverers." (2020): 118881.
18. Chen, X., and J. A. Williams. *Exocytosis*. 2004.
19. Stalder, D., and D. C. Gershlick. "Direct Trafficking Pathways from the Golgi Apparatus to the Plasma Membrane." In *Seminars in Cell & Developmental Biology*. Amsterdam: Elsevier (2020).
20. Mikuličić, S., and L. Florin. "The Endocytic Trafficking Pathway of Oncogenic Papillomaviruses." *Papillomavirus Research* 7 (2019): 135–7.
21. Martens, S., and H. T. McMahon. "Mechanisms of Membrane Fusion: Disparate Players and Common Principles." *Nature Reviews. Molecular Cell Biology* 9, no. 7 (2008): 543–56.
22. Harrison, M. J., and S. Ivanov. "Exocytosis for Endosymbiosis: Membrane Trafficking Pathways for Development of Symbiotic Membrane Compartments." *Current Opinion in Plant Biology* 38 (2017): 101–8.
23. Kumar, A., A. Ahmad, A. Vyawahare, and R. Khan. "Membrane Trafficking and Subcellular Drug Targeting Pathways." *Frontiers in Pharmacology* 11 (2020): 629.
24. Diaz-Rohrer, B., J. Lorent, I. Castello-Serrano, K. Levental, and I. Levental. "Pathways and Molecular Mechanisms of Microdomain-Dependent Membrane Trafficking." 116, no. 3 (2019): 218a–9a.
25. Makowski, S. L., R. S. Kuna, and S. J. Field. "Induction of Membrane Curvature by Proteins Involved in Golgi Trafficking." *Advances in Biological Regulation* 75 (2020): 100661.
26. Quinonez, R., and R. E. Sutton. "Lentiviral Vectors for Gene Delivery into Cells." *DNA & Cell Biology* 21, no. 12 (2002): 937–51.
27. Matsui, T., and M. Fukuda. "Methods of Analysis of the Membrane Trafficking Pathway from Recycling Endosomes to Lysosomes." In *Methods in Enzymology*, 195–206. Amsterdam: Elsevier, 2014.
28. Tan, J. Z. A., and P. A. Gleeson. "The Role of Membrane Trafficking in the Processing of Amyloid Precursor Protein and Production of Amyloid Peptides in Alzheimer's Disease." *Biochimica & Biophysica Acta* 1861, no. 4 (2019): 697–712.

29. Carter, C. J., S. Y. Bednarek, and N. V. Raikhel. "Membrane Trafficking in Plants: New Discoveries and Approaches." *Current Opinion in Plant Biology* 7, no. 6 (2004): 701–7.

30. Naslavsky, N., and S. Caplan. "Endocytic Membrane Trafficking in the Control of Centrosome Function." *Current Opinion in Plant Biology* (2020).

31. More, K., C. M. Klinger, L. D. Barlow, and J. B. Dacks. "Evolution and Natural History of Membrane Trafficking in Eukaryotes." 30, no. 10 (2020): R553–R64.

32. Scheffler, J. M., N. Schiefermeier, and L. A. Huber. "Mild Fixation and Permeabilization Protocol for Preserving Structures of Endosomes, Focal Adhesions, and Actin Filaments During Immunofluorescence Analysis." In *Methods in Enzymology*, 93–102. Amsterdam: Elsevier, 2014.

33. Blumenthal, R. et al. "Membrane Fusion." 103, no. 1 (2003): 53–70.

34. Jackson, C. L. "Membrane Trafficking: A Little Flexibility Helps Vesicles Get into Shape." *Current Biology* 28, no. 12 (2018): R706–R9.

35. Strickland, L. I., and D. R. Burgess. "Pathways for Membrane Trafficking During Cytokinesis." *Trends in Cell Biology* 14, no. 3 (2004): 115–8.

36. Ju, Y., H. Guo, M. Edman, and S. F. Hamm-Alvarez. "Application of Advances in Endocytosis and Membrane Trafficking to Drug Delivery." (2020).

37. Chen, R. R. "Permeability Issues in Whole-Cell Bioprocesses and Cellular Membrane Engineering." *Applied Microbiology & Biotechnology* 74, no. 4 (2007): 730–8.

38. Kotyk, A. *Cell Membrane Transport: Principles and Techniques*. Cham: Springer, 2012.

39. Foroozandeh, P., and A. A. Aziz. "Insight into Cellular Uptake and Intracellular Trafficking of Nanoparticles." *Nanoscale Research Letters* 13, no. 1 (2018): 339.

40. Douglas, R. G., R. Amino, P. Sinnis, and F. Frischknecht. "Active Migration and Passive Transport of Malaria Parasites." 31, no. 8 (2015): 357–62.

41. Di, L., P. Artursson, A. Avdeef, G. F. Ecker, B. Faller, H. Fischer, J. B. Houston, M. Kansy, E. H. Kerns, S. D. Krämer, H. Lennernäs, and K. Sugano. "Evidence-Based Approach to Assess Passive Diffusion and Carrier-Mediated Drug Transport." 17, no. 15–16 (2012): 905–12.

42. Backes, W. L. *Passive Diffusion of Drugs Across Membranes*. 2015.

43. Feher, J. J. *Quantitative Human Physiology: An Introduction*. Cambridge, MA: Academic Press, 2017.

44. Hooper, N. "Transport of Small Molecules." In *Instant Notes Biochemistry*, 145–50. Taylor & Francis, 2006.

45. Booth, L., R. Norman, and S. Pettigrew. "The Potential Implications of Autonomous Vehicles for Active Transport." 15 (2019): 100623.

46. Bauer, M., and R. Metzler. "In Vivo Facilitated Diffusion Model." *PLOS ONE* 8, no. 1 (2013): e53956.

47. Krepel, D., D. Gomez, S. Klumpp, and Y. Levy. "Mechanism of Facilitated Diffusion During a DNA Search in Crowded Environments." 120, no. 43 (2016): 11113–22.

48. Lévy, M., L. Resplandy, P. Klein, X. Capet, D. Iovino, and C. Ethé. "Grid Degradation of Submesoscale Resolving Ocean Models: Benefits for Offline Passive Tracer Transport." 48 (2012): 1–9.

49. Rubi, J., A. Lervik, D. Bedeaux, and S. Kjelstrup. "Entropy Facilitated Active Transport." 146, no. 18 (2017): 185101.

50. Dunn, J., and M. H. Grider. *Physiology, Adenosine Triphosphate (ATP)*. 2020.

51. Brown, V., M. Moodie, and R. Carter. "Evidence for Associations Between Traffic Calming and Safety and Active Transport or Obesity: A Scoping Review." 7 (2017): 23–37.

52. Kaźmierczak, Z., K. Szostak-Paluch, M. Przybyło, M. Langner, W. Witkiewicz, N. Jędruchniewicz, and K. Dąbrowska. "Endocytosis in Cellular Uptake of Drug Delivery Vectors: Molecular Aspects in Drug Development." 28, no. 18 (2020): 115556.

53. Deng, L., H. Liu, Y. Ma, Y. Miao, X. Fu, and Q. Deng. "Endocytosis Mechanism in Physiologically-Based Pharmacokinetic Modeling of Nanoparticles." 384 (2019): 114765.

54. Pasterkamp, R., and K. Burk. "Axon Guidance Receptors: Endocytosis, Trafficking and Downstream Signaling from Endosomes." *Progress in Neurobiology* (2020): 101916.

55. Zhang, X., Y. Cui, M. Yu, and J. Lin. "Single-Molecule Techniques for Imaging exo-Endocytosis Coupling in Cells." 24, no. 9 (2019): 879.

56. Hilgemann, D. W., M. J. Lin, M. Fine, and C. Deisl. "On the Existence of Endocytosis Driven by Membrane Phase Separations." 1862, no. 1 (2020): 183007.

57. Alberts, B. et al. "Transport into the Cell from the Plasma Membrane: Endocytosis." In *Molecular Biology of the Cell*. 4th ed. Garland Science, 2002.

58. Swanson, J. A. "Shaping Cups into Phagosomes and Macropinosomes." *Nature Reviews. Molecular Cell Biology* 9, no. 8 (2008): 639–49.

59. Nazario-Toole, A. E., and L. P. Wu. "Phagocytosis in Insect Immunity." In *Advances in Insect Physiology*. Amsterdam: Elsevier (2017): 35–82.

60. Rajendran, N. K., S. S. D. Kumar, N. N. Houreld, and H. Abrahamse. "A Review on Nanoparticle Based Treatment for Wound Healing." 44 (2018): 421–30.

61. Wang, H., W.-T. Lo, and V. Haucke. "Phosphoinositide Switches in Endocytosis and in the Endolysosomal System." *Current Opinion in Cell Biology* 59 (2019): 50–7.

62. Gallot-Lavallée, L., and J. M. Archibald. "Phagocytosis in a Shape-Shifting Bacterium." *Trends in Microbiology* (2020).

63. Ghose, P., and A. M. Wehman. "The Developmental and Physiological Roles of Phagocytosis in Caenorhabditis elegans." (2020).

64. Herb, M., A. Gluschko, and M. Schramm. "LC3-Associated Phagocytosis: The Highway to Hell for Phagocytosed Microbes." In *Seminars in Cell & Developmental Biology*. Amsterdam: Elsevier (2020).

65. Barger, S. R., N. C. Gauthier, and M. Krendel. "Squeezing in a Meal: Myosin Functions in Phagocytosis." *Trends in Cell Biology* 30, no. 2 (2020): 157–67.

66. Freeman, S. A., and S. Grinstein. "Phagocytosis: Mechanosensing, Traction Forces, and a Molecular Clutch." *Current Biology* 30, no. 1 (2020): R24–R6.

67. Hilu-Dadia, R., and E. Kurant. "Glial Phagocytosis in Developing and Mature Drosophila CNS: Tight Regulation for a Healthy Brain." *Current Opinion in Immunology* 62 (2020): 62–68.

68. Xiang, S., H. Tong, Q. Shi, J. C. Fernandes, T. Jin, K. Dai, and X. Zhang. "Uptake Mechanisms of Non-Viral Gene Delivery." 158, no. 3 (2012): 371–8.

69. Pleskova, S., R. N. Kriukov, E. N. Gorshkova, and A. V. Boryakov. "Characteristics of Quantum Dots Phagocytosis by Neutrophil Granulocytes." 5, no. 3 (2019): e01439.

70. Pauwels, A.-M., M. Trost, R. Beyaert, and E. Hoffmann. "Patterns, Receptors, and Signals: Regulation of Phagosome Maturation." 38, no. 6 (2017): 407–22.

71. Hillaireau, H., and P. Couvreur. "Nanocarriers' Entry into the Cell: Relevance to Drug Delivery." *Cellular & Molecular Life Sciences* 66, no. 17 (2009): 2873–96.

72. Liu, G., H. Zhai, T. Zhang, S. Li, N. Li, J. Chen, M. Gu, Z. Qin, and X. Liu. "New Therapeutic Strategies for IPF: Based on the Phagocytosis-Secretion-Immunization' Network Regulation Mechanism of Pulmonary Macrophages." 118 (2019): 109230.

73. Xin, C., H. Quan, J. M. Kim, Y. H. Hur, J. Y. Shin, H. B. Bae, and J. I. Choi. "Ginsenoside Rb1 Increases Macrophage Phagocytosis Through p38 Mitogen-Activated Protein Kinase/Akt Pathway." 43, no. 3 (2019): 394–401.

74. Yu, L., Y. Zheng, Y. Feng, and F. Ma. "Role of L-Selectin on Leukocytes in the Binding of Sialic Acids on Sperm Surface During the Phagocytosis of Sperm in Female Reproductive Tract." 120 (2018): 4–6.

75. Adolfsson, K., L. Abariute, A. P. Dabkowska, M. Schneider, U. Häcker, and C. N. Prinz. "Direct Comparison Between In Vivo and In Vitro Microsized Particle Phagocytosis Assays in Drosophila melanogaster." 46 (2018): 213–8.

76. Moussa, A.-T., A. Rabung, S. Reichrath, S. Wagenpfeil, T. Dinh, G. Krasteva-Christ, C. Meier, and T. Tschernig. "Modulation of Macrophage Phagocytosis In Vitro: A Role for Cholinergic Stimulation?" 214 (2017): 31–5.

77. Keller, S., S. Wieland, W. Gross, K. Berghoff, D. Gitschier, M. Eisentraut, and H. Kress. "Physical Determinants of Particle Uptake and Transport During Phagocytosis." 118, no. 3 (2020): 285a.

78. Ishidome, T., T. Yoshida, and R. Hanayama. "Induction of Live Cell Phagocytosis by a Specific Combination of Inflammatory Stimuli." *EBiomedicine* 22 (2017): 89–99.

79. Caviston, J. P., and E. L. Holzbaur. "Microtubule Motors at the Intersection of Trafficking and Transport." *Trends in Cell Biology* 16, no. 10 (2006): 530–7.

80. Jubrail, J., N. Kurian, and F. Niedergang. "Macrophage Phagocytosis Cracking the Defect Code in COPD." *Biomedical Journal* 40, no. 6 (2017): 305–12.

81. Martinez, J. "LAP It up, Fuzz Ball: A Short History of LC3-Associated Phagocytosis." *Current Opinion in Immunology* 55 (2018): 54–61.

82. Caisová, V., O. Uher, P. Nedbalová, I. Jochmanová, K. Kvardová, K. Masáková, G. Krejčová, L. Paďouková, J. Chmelař, J. Kopecký, and J. Ženka. "Effective Cancer Immunotherapy Based on Combination of TLR Agonists with Stimulation of Phagocytosis." 59 (2018): 86–96.

83. Cerrato, G., P. Liu, I. Martins, O. Kepp, and G. Kroemer. "Quantitative Determination of Phagocytosis by Bone Marrow-Derived Dendritic Cells via Imaging Flow Cytometry." In *Methods in Enzymology*. Amsterdam: Elsevier (2020): 27–37.

84. Kern, M. E., E. F. Nelsen, C. M. Hobson, J. Hsiao, E. T. E. O'Brien, M. R. Falvo, and R. Superfine. "Combined AFM and Vertical Light Sheet Microscopy to Correlate Actin Accumulation to Engulfment Forces During Phagocytosis." 118, no. 3 (2020): 33a.

85. Montironi, I. D., E. B. Reinoso, V. C. Paullier, M. I. Siri, M. J. Pianzzola, M. Moliva, N. Campra, G. Bagnis, I. Ferreira LaRocque-de-Freitas, D. Decote-Ricardo, C. G. Freire-de-Lima, J. M. Raviolo, and L. N. Cariddi. "Minthostachys verticillata Essential Oil Activates Macrophage Phagocytosis and Modulates the Innate Immune Response in a Murine Model of Enterococcus faecium Mastitis." 125 (2019): 333–44.

86. Valgardsdottir, R., I. Cattaneo, C. Klein, M. Introna, M. Figliuzzi, and J. Golay. "Human Neutrophils Mediate Trogocytosis Rather than Phagocytosis of CLL B Cells Opsonized with Anti-CD20 Antibodies." 129, no. 19 (2017): 2636–44.

87. Leigh, B. A. "Cooperation Among Conflict: Prophages Protect Bacteria from Phagocytosis." *Cell Host & Microbe* 26, no. 4 (2019): 450–2.

88. Baranov, M. V., R. A. Olea, and G. van den Bogaart. "Chasing Uptake: Super-Resolution Microscopy in Endocytosis and Phagocytosis." *Trends in Cell Biology* 29, no. 9 (2019): 727–39.

89. Bi, D., R. Zhou, N. Cai, Q. Lai, Q. Han, Y. Peng, Z. Jiang, Z. Tang, J. Lu, W. Bao, H. Xu, and X. Xu. "Alginate Enhances Toll-Like Receptor 4-Mediated Phagocytosis by Murine RAW264. 7 Macrophages." 105, no. 2 (2017): 1446–54.

90. Harik, V. M. "Geometry of Carbon Nanotubes and Mechanisms of Phagocytosis and Toxic Effects." *Toxicology Letters* 273 (2017): 69–85.

91. Ning, J., Y. Liu, and Z. J. A. Cui. "Identification and Functional Analysis of a Thioester-Containing Protein from Portunus Trituberculatus Reveals Its Involvement in the Prophenoloxidase System, Phagocytosis and AMP Synthesis." 510 (2019): 9–21.

92. Elguero, M. E., M. L. Sanchez Granel, M. G. Montes, N. G. Cid, N. O. Favale, C. B. Nudel, and A. D. Nusblat. "Uptake of Cholesterol by Tetrahymena thermophila Is Mainly Due to Phagocytosis." (2018).

93. Li, H., K. Tatematsu, M. Somiya, M. Iijima, and S. Kuroda. "Development of a Macrophage-Targeting and Phagocytosis-Inducing Bio-Nanocapsule-Based Nanocarrier for Drug Delivery." 73 (2018): 412–23.

94. Levin-Konigsberg, R., F. Montaño-Rendón, T. Keren-Kaplan, R. Li, B. Ego, S. Mylvaganam, J. E. DiCiccio, W. S. Trimble, M. C. Bassik, J. S. Bonifacino, G. D. Fairn, and S. Grinstein. "Phagolysosome Resolution Requires Contacts with the Endoplasmic Reticulum and Phosphatidylinositol-4-Phosphate Signalling." 21, no. 10 (2019): 1234–47.

95. Seixas, E., C. Escrevente, M. C. Seabra, and D. C. Barral. "Rab GTPase Regulation of Bacteria and Protozoa Phagocytosis Occurs Through the Modulation of Phagocytic Receptor Surface Expression." 8, no. 1 (2018): 1–10.

96. Dransfield, I., A. Zagórska, E. D. Lew, K. Michail, and G. Lemke. "Mer Receptor Tyrosine Kinase Mediates Both Tethering and Phagocytosis of Apoptotic Cells." 6, no. 2 (2015): e1646.

97. Lira, R. B., L. Benk, E. Ewins, J. P. Spatz, R. Lipowsky, I. Platzman, and R. Dimova. "Mimicking Cell Pinocytosis: Lipid Vesicles Engulfment of Oil-in-Water Droplets." 114, no. 3 (2018): 94a–5a.

98. Akinc, A., and G. Battaglia. "Exploiting Endocytosis for Nanomedicines." *Cold Spring Harbor Perspectives* 5, no. 11 (2013): a016980.

99. Zhao, F., Y. Zhao, Y. Liu, X. Chang, C. Chen, and Y. Zhao. "Cellular Uptake, Intracellular Trafficking, and Cytotoxicity of Nanomaterials." 7, no. 10 (2011): 1322–37.

100. Levin, E. R. "Plasma Membrane Estrogen Receptors." *Trends in Endocrinology & Metabolism* 20, no. 10 (2009): 477–82.

101. Rivero, F. "Endocytosis and the Actin Cytoskeleton in Dictyostelium discoideum." *International Review of Cell & Molecular Biology* 267 (2008): 343–97.

102. Panariti, A., G. Miserocchi, and I. Rivolta. "The Effect of Nanoparticle Uptake on Cellular Behavior: Disrupting or Enabling Functions?" 5 (2012): 87.

103. Sahay, G., D. Y. Alakhova, and A. V. Kabanov. "Endocytosis of Nanomedicines." *Journal of Controlled Release* 145, no. 3 (2010): 182–95.

104. Baldo, G., R. Giugliani, and U. Matte. "Lysosomal Enzymes May Cross the Blood–Brain-Barrier by Pinocytosis: Implications for Enzyme Replacement Therapy." *Medical Hypotheses* 82, no. 4 (2014): 478–80.

105. Hirota, K., and H. Terada. "Endocytosis of Particle Formulations by Macrophages and Its Application to Clinical Treatment." *Molecular Regulation of Endocytosis* 1 (2012).

106. Muley, H., R. Fadó, R. Rodríguez-Rodríguez, and N. Casals. "Drug Uptake-Based Chemoresistance in Breast Cancer Treatment." (2020): 113959.

107. Yu, Y. "Resolving Endosome Rotation in Intracellular Trafficking." *Biophysical Journal* 114, no. 3 (2018): 630a.

108. Brink, P. R., V. Valiunas, C. Gordon, M. R. Rosen, and I. S. Cohen. "Can Gap Junctions Deliver?" 1818, no. 8 (2012): 2076–81.

109. Danielsen, E. M., and G. H. Hansen. "Small Molecule Pinocytosis and Clathrin-Dependent Endocytosis at the Intestinal Brush Border: Two Separate Pathways into the Enterocyte." *Biochimica & Biophysica Acta* 1858, no. 2 (2016): 233–43.

110. Mercer, J., and A. Helenius. "Virus Entry by Macropinocytosis." *Nature Cell Biology* 11, no. 5 (2009): 510–20.

111. Li, Y.-X., and H.-B. Pang. "Macropinocytosis as a Cell Entry Route for Peptide-Functionalized and Bystander Nanoparticles." (2020).

112. Tekle, C., Bv Deurs, K. Sandvig, and T. G. Iversen. "Cellular Trafficking of Quantum Dot-Ligand Bioconjugates and Their Induction of Changes in Normal Routing of Unconjugated Ligands." 8, no. 7 (2008): 1858–65.

113. Stow, J. L., Y. Hung, and A. A. Wall. "Macropinocytosis: Insights from Immunology and Cancer." 65 (2020): 131–40.

114. Zhang, Y., and C. Commisso. "Macropinocytosis in Cancer: A Complex Signaling Network." 5, no. 6 (2019): 332–4.

115. Hobbs, G. A., and C. Der. "Binge Drinking: Macropinocytosis Promotes Tumorigenic Growth of RAS-Mutant Cancers." (2020).

116. Weerasekara, V. K., K. C. Patra, and N. Bardeesy. "EGFR Pathway Links Amino Acid Levels and Induction of Macropinocytosis." 50, no. 3 (2019): 261–3.

117. Ichimizu, S., H. Watanabe, H. Maeda, K. Hamasaki, K. Ikegami, V. T. G. Chuang, R. Kinoshita, K. Nishida, T. Shimizu, Y. Ishima, T. Ishida, T. Seki, H. Katsuki, S. Futaki, M. Otagiri, and T. Maruyama. "Cell-Penetrating Mechanism of Intracellular Targeting Albumin: Contribution of Macropinocytosis Induction and Endosomal Escape." 304 (2019): 156–63.

118. Lim, J. P., and P. A. J. I. Gleeson. "Macropinocytosis: An Endocytic Pathway for Internalising Large Gulps." 89, no. 8 (2011): 836–43.

119. Kuhn, D. A., D. Vanhecke, B. Michen, F. Blank, P. Gehr, A. Petri-Fink, and B. Rothen-Rutishauser. "Different Endocytotic Uptake Mechanisms for Nanoparticles in Epithelial Cells and Macrophages." 5, no. 1 (2014): 1625–36.

120. Torriani, G., J. Mayor, G. Zimmer, S. Kunz, S. Rothenberger, and O. Engler. "Macropinocytosis Contributes to Hantavirus Entry into Human Airway Epithelial Cells." 531 (2019): 57–68.

121. Hagiwara, M., and I. Nakase. "Epidermal Growth Factor Induced Macropinocytosis Directs Branch Formation of Lung Epithelial Cells." 507, no. 1–4 (2018): 297–303.

122. Kerr, M. C., and R. D. J. T. Teasdale. "Defining Macropinocytosis." 10, no. 4 (2009): 364–71.

123. Levin, R., S. Grinstein, and D. Schlam. "Phosphoinositides in Phagocytosis and Macropinocytosis." 1851, no. 6 (2015): 805–23.

124. Kühn, S., N. Lopez-Montero, Y. Y. Chang, A. Sartori-Rupp, and J. Enninga. "Imaging Macropinosomes During Shigella Infections." 127 (2017): 12–22.

125. Tomino, T., H. Tajiri, T. Tatsuguchi, T. Shirai, K. Oisaki, S. Matsunaga, F. Sanematsu, D. Sakata, T. Yoshizumi, Y. Maehara, M. Kanai, J. F. Cote, Y. Fukui, and T. Uruno. "DOCK1 Inhibition Suppresses Cancer Cell Invasion and Macropinocytosis Induced by Self-Activating Rac1P29S Mutation." 497, no. 1 (2018): 298–304.

126. Jones, A. T. "Macropinocytosis: Searching for an Endocytic Identity and Role in the Uptake of Cell Penetrating Peptides." 11, no. 4 (2007): 670–84.

127. Mao, M., L. Wang, C. C. Chang, K. E. Rothenberg, J. Huang, Y. Wang, B. D. Hoffman, P. B. Liton, and F. Yuan. "Involvement of a Rac1-Dependent Macropinocytosis Pathway in Plasmid DNA Delivery by Electrotransfection." 25, no. 3 (2017): 803–15.

128. Qian, Y., X. Wang, Y. Liu, Y. Li, R. A. Colvin, L. Tong, S. Wu, and X. Chen. "Extracellular ATP Is Internalized by Macropinocytosis and Induces Intracellular ATP Increase and Drug Resistance in Cancer Cells." 351, no. 2 (2014): 242–51.

129. Wang, J.-H., C. Wells, and L. J. V. Wu. "Macropinocytosis and Cytoskeleton Contribute to Dendritic Cell-Mediated HIV-1 Transmission to CD4+ T Cells." 381, no. 1 (2008): 143–54.

130. Wang, J. T., M. C. Kerr, S. Karunaratne, A. Jeanes, A. S. Yap, and R. D. Teasdale. "The SNX-PX-BAR Family in Macropinocytosis: The Regulation of Macropinosome Formation by SNX-PX-BAR Proteins." 5, no. 10 (2010): e13763.

131. Li, Y., W. G. Gonzalez, A. Andreev, W. Tang, S. Gandhi, A. Cunha, D. Prober, C. Lois, and M. E. Bronner. "Macropinocytosis-Mediated Membrane Recycling Drives Neural Crest Migration by Delivering F-Actin to the Lamellipodium." 117, no. 44 (2020): 27400–11.

132. Tashima, T. J. B. "Effective Cancer Therapy Based on Selective Drug Delivery into Cells Across Their Membrane Using Receptor-Mediated Endocytosis." 28, no. 18 (2018): 3015–24.

133. Alsford, S., M. C. Field, and D. Horn. "Receptor-Mediated Endocytosis for Drug Delivery in African Trypanosomes: Fulfilling Paul Ehrlich's Vision of Chemotherapy." 29, no. 5 (2013): 207–12.

134. Irannejad, R., N. G. Tsvetanova, B. T. Lobingier, and M. von Zastrow. "Effects of Endocytosis on Receptor-Mediated Signaling." 35 (2015): 137–43.

135. Lu, R., D. G. Drubin, and Y. Sun. "Clathrin-Mediated Endocytosis in Budding Yeast at a Glance." 129, no. 8 (2016): 1531–6.

136. Picco, A., and M. Kaksonen. "Quantitative Imaging of Clathrin-Mediated Endocytosis." 53 (2018): 105–10.

137. Chen, X., N. G. Irani, and J. Friml. "Clathrin-Mediated Endocytosis: The Gateway into Plant Cells." 14, no. 6 (2011): 674–82.

138. Wu, F., and P. Yao. "Clathrin-Mediated Endocytosis and Alzheimer's Disease: An Update." 8, no. 3 (2009): 147–9.

139. Ferguson, J. P., S. D. Huber, N. M. Willy, E. Aygün, S. Goker, T. Atabey, and C. Kural. "Mechanoregulation of Clathrin-Mediated Endocytosis." 130, no. 21 (2017): 3631–6.

140. Bhattacharyya, S., K. L. Warfield, G. Ruthel, S. Bavari, M. J. Aman, and T. J. Hope. "Ebola Virus Uses Clathrin-Mediated Endocytosis as an Entry Pathway." 401, no. 1 (2010): 18–28.

141. Rathnayake, S. S., K. Hristova, and M. E. Johnson. "Investigating How Membrane Localization Regulates Protein Assembly During Clathrin-Mediated Endocytosis." 116, no. 3 (2019): 369a.

142. Hassinger, J. E., G. Oster, D. G. Drubin, and P. Rangamani. "Design Principles for Robust Vesiculation in Clathrin-Mediated Endocytosis." 114, no. 7 (2017): E1118–E27.

143. Tacheva-Grigorova, S. K., A. J. Santos, E. Boucrot, and T. Kirchhausen. "Clathrin-Mediated Endocytosis Persists During Unperturbed Mitosis." 4, no. 4 (2013): 659–68.

144. Baisa, G. A., J. R. Mayers, and S. Y. Bednarek. "Budding and Braking News About Clathrin-Mediated Endocytosis." 16, no. 6 (2013): 718–25.

145. Doherty, G. J., and H. T. McMahon. "Mechanisms of Endocytosis." 78 (2009): 857–902.

146. Berro, J. "Uncovering the Mechanisms of Clathrin-Mediated Endocytosis Using Quantitative Biology Approaches." *Biophysical Journal* 116, no. 3 (2019): 150a.

147. Brach, T., C. Godlee, I. Moeller-Hansen, D. Boeke, and M. Kaksonen. "The Initiation of Clathrin-Mediated Endocytosis Is Mechanistically Highly Flexible." 24, no. 5 (2014): 548–54.

148. Conner, S. D., and S. L. Schmid. "Regulated Portals of Entry into the Cell." 422, no. 6927 (2003): 37–44.

149. Weinberg, J., and D. G. Drubin. "Clathrin-Mediated Endocytosis in Budding Yeast." *Trends in Cell Biology* 22, no. 1 (2012): 1–13.

150. Higgins, M. K., and H. T. McMahon. "Snap-Shots of Clathrin-Mediated Endocytosis." *Trends in Biochemical Sciences* 27, no. 5 (2002): 257–63.

151. Buss, F., J. P. Luzio, and J. Kendrick-Jones. "Myosin VI: A New Force in Clathrin Mediated Endocytosis." *FEBS Journal* 508, no. 3 (2001): 295–9.

152. Kaksonen, M., C. P. Toret, and D. G. Drubin. "A Modular Design for the Clathrin-and Actin-Mediated Endocytosis Machinery." *Cell* 123, no. 2 (2005): 305–20.

153. Cocucci, E., F. Aguet, S. Boulant, and T. Kirchhausen. "The First Five Seconds in the Life of a Clathrin-Coated Pit." 150, no. 3 (2012): 495–507.

154. Carvou, N., A. G. Norden, R. J. Unwin, and S. Cockcroft. "Signalling Through Phospholipase C Interferes with Clathrin-Mediated Endocytosis." 19, no. 1 (2007): 42–51.

155. Kural, C. "Mechanoregulation of Clathrin-Mediated Endocytosis in Isolated Cells and Developing Tissues." *Biophysical Journal* 112, no. 3 (2017): 91a.

156. Vanlandingham, P. A., M. P. Barmchi, S. Royer, R. Green, H. Bao, N. Reist, and B. Zhang. "AP180 Couples Protein Retrieval to Clathrin-Mediated Endocytosis of Synaptic Vesicles." 15, no. 4 (2014): 433–50.

157. Sorkin, A. "Cargo Recognition During Clathrin-Mediated Endocytosis: A Team Effort." *Current Opinion in Cell Biology* 16, no. 4 (2004): 392–9.

158. Takei, K., and V. Haucke. "Clathrin-Mediated Endocytosis: Membrane Factors Pull the Trigger." *Trends in Cell Biology* 11, no. 9 (2001): 385–91.

159. Rappoport, J. Z. "Focusing on Clathrin-Mediated Endocytosis." *Biochemical Journal* 412, no. 3 (2008): 415–23.

160. Ferguson, J. P., N. M. Willy, S. P. Heidotting, S. D. Huber, M. J. Webber, and C. Kural. "Dynamics of Clathrin-Mediated Endocytosis Within a Developing Organism." 112, no. 3 (2017): 473a.

161. Brodin, L., P. Löw, and O. Shupliakov. "Sequential Steps in Clathrin-Mediated Synaptic Vesicle Endocytosis." 10, no. 3 (2000): 312–20.

162. Soldati, T., and M. Schliwa. "Powering Membrane Traffic in Endocytosis and Recycling." *Nature Reviews. Molecular Cell Biology* 7, no. 12 (2006): 897–908.

163. Weinberg, J. S., and D. G. Drubin. "Regulation of Clathrin-Mediated Endocytosis by Dynamic Ubiquitination and Deubiquitination." *Current Biology* 24, no. 9 (2014): 951–9.

164. Owen, D. J., and J. P. Luzio. "Structural Insights into Clathrin-Mediated Endocytosis." *Current Opinion in Cell Biology* 12, no. 4 (2000): 467–74.

165. Capraro, B. R., Z. Shi, T. Wu, Z. Chen, J. M. Dunn, E. Rhoades, and T. Baumgart. "Kinetics of Endophilin N-BAR Domain Dimerization and Membrane Interactions." 288, no. 18 (2013): 12533–43.

166. Praefcke, G. J., and H. T. McMahon. "The Dynamin Superfamily: Universal Membrane Tubulation and Fission Molecules?." *Nature Reviews. Molecular Cell Biology* 5, no. 2 (2004): 133–47.

167. Ungewickell, E. J., and L. Hinrichsen. "Endocytosis: Clathrin-Mediated Membrane Budding." *Current Opinion in Cell Biology* 19, no. 4 (2007): 417–25.

168. Chen, F., L. Zhu, Y. Zhang, D. Kumar, G. Cao, X. Hu, Z. Liang, S. Kuang, R. Xue, and C. Gong. "Clathrin-Mediated Endocytosis Is a Candidate Entry Sorting Mechanism for Bombyx mori Cypovirus." 8, no. 1 (2018): 1–11.

169. Liu, X., H. Yang, Y. Liu, X. Gong, and H. Huang. "Numerical Study of Clathrin-Mediated Endocytosis of Nanoparticles by Cells Under Tension." 35, no. 3 (2019): 691–701.

170. Rappoport, J. Z., and S. M. Simon. "Real-Time Analysis of Clathrin-Mediated Endocytosis During Cell Migration." 116, no. 5 (2003): 847–55.

171. Boucrot, E., S. Saffarian, R. Zhang, and T. Kirchhausen. "Roles of AP-2 in Clathrin-Mediated Endocytosis." 5, no. 5 (2010): e10597.

172. Parton, R. G., and K. Simons. "The Multiple Faces of Caveolae." 8, no. 3 (2007): 185–94.

173. Del Pozo, M. A., F.-N. Lolo, and A. Echarri. "Caveolae: Mechanosensing and Mechanotransduction Devices Linking Membrane Trafficking to Mechanoadaptation." *Current Opinion in Cell Biology* 68 (2020): 113–23.

174. Thorn, H., K. G. Stenkula, M. Karlsson, U. Ortegren, F. H. Nystrom, J. Gustavsson, and P. Stralfors. "Cell Surface Orifices of Caveolae and Localization of Caveolin to the Necks of Caveolae in Adipocytes." 14, no. 10 (2003): 3967–76.

175. Yang, C., B. He, W. Dai, H. Zhang, Y. Zheng, X. Wang, and Q. Zhang. "The Role of caveolin-1 in the Biofate and Efficacy of Anti-Tumor Drugs and Their Nano-Drug Delivery Systems." (2020).

176. Yang, W., C. Geng, Z. Yang, B. Xu, W. Shi, Y. Yang, and Y. Tian. "Deciphering the Roles of Caveolin in Neurodegenerative Diseases: The Good, the Bad and the Importance of Context." (2020): 101116.

177. Wang, Z., C. Tiruppathi, J. Cho, R. D. Minshall, and A. B. Malik. "Delivery of Nanoparticle-Complexed Drugs Across the Vascular Endothelial Barrier via Caveolae." 63, no. 8 (2011): 659–67.

178. Pandit, R., W. K. Koh, R. K. P. Sullivan, T. Palliyaguru, R. G. Parton, and J. Götz. "Role for Caveolin-Mediated Transcytosis in Facilitating Transport of Large Cargoes into the Brain via Ultrasound." 327 (2020): 667–75.

179. Hagiwara, M., Y. Shirai, R. Nomura, M. Sasaki, K. Kobayashi, T. Tadokoro, and Y. Yamamoto. "Caveolin-1 Activates Rab5 and Enhances Endocytosis Through Direct Interaction." 378, no. 1 (2009): 73–8.

180. Pollard, T. D., Chapter 22-*Endocytosis and the Endosomal Membrane System*. 3rd ed, 377–92. Amsterdam: Elsevier, 2017.

181. Hou, K., S. Li, M. Zhang, and X. Qin. "Caveolin-1 in Autophagy: A Potential Therapeutic Target in Atherosclerosis." (2020).

182. Eom, H.-J., and J. Choi. "Clathrin-Mediated Endocytosis Is Involved in Uptake and Toxicity of Silica Nanoparticles in Caenohabditis elegans." *Chemico-Biological Interactions* 311 (2019): 108774.

183. Nabi, I. R. "Cavin Fever: Regulating Caveolae." *Nature Cell Biology* 11, no. 7 (2009): 789–91.

184. Zhang, F., H. Guo, J. Zhang, Q. Chen, and Q. Fang. "Identification of the Caveolae/Raft-Mediated Endocytosis as the Primary Entry Pathway for Aquareovirus." 513 (2018): 195–207.

185. Kulshrestha, R., H. Singh, A. Pandey, A. Mehta, S. Bhardwaj, and A. S. Jaggi. "Caveolin-1 as a Critical Component in the Pathogenesis of Lung Fibrosis of Different Etiology: Evidences and Mechanisms." 111 (2019): 104315.

186. Parton, R. G., and M. A. Del Pozo. "Caveolae as Plasma Membrane Sensors, Protectors and Organizers." *Nature Reviews. Molecular Cell Biology* 14, no. 2 (2013): 98–112.

187. Sakurai, Y., A. Kato, and H. Harashima. "Involvement of caveolin-1-mediated Transcytosis in the Intratumoral Accumulation of Liposomes." (2020).

188. Ning, P., L. Gao, Y. Zhou, C. Hu, Z. Lin, C. Gong, K. Guo, and X. Zhang. "Caveolin-1-mediated Endocytic Pathway Is Involved in Classical Swine Fever Virus Shimen Infection of Porcine Alveolar Macrophages." 195 (2016): 81–6.

189. Ray, A., and A. K. Mitra. "Nanotechnology in Intracellular Trafficking, Imaging, and Delivery of Therapeutic Agents." In *Emerging Nanotechnologies for Diagnostics, Drug Delivery & Medical Devices*, 169–88. Amsterdam: Elsevier, 2017.

190. Zhou, S., Y. Zu, F. Zhuang, and C. Yang. "Hypergravity-Induced Enrichment of β1 Integrin on the Cell Membranes of Osteoblast-Like Cells via Caveolae-Dependent Endocytosis." 463, no. 4 (2015): 928–33.

191. Vassilieva, E. V., A. I. Ivanov, and A. Nusrat. "Flotillin-1 Stabilizes caveolin-1 in Intestinal Epithelial Cells." 379, no. 2 (2009): 460–5.

192. Stillwell, W., ed. *Long-Range Membrane Properties*, 221–45. Amsterdam: Elsevier, 2016.

193. Gvaramia, D., M. E. Blaauboer, R. Hanemaaijer, and V. Everts. "Role of caveolin-1 in Fibrotic Diseases." 32, no. 6 (2013): 307–15.

194. Matveev, S., X. Li, W. Everson, and E. J. Smart. "The Role of Caveolae and Caveolin in Vesicle-Dependent and Vesicle-Independent Trafficking." 49, no. 3 (2001): 237–50.

195. Kruglikov, I. L., Z. Zhang, and P. E. Scherer. "Caveolin-1 in Skin Aging: From Innocent Bystander to Major Contributor." *Ageing Research Reviews* 55 (2019): 100959.
196. Gu, X., A. M. Reagan, M. E. McClellan, and M. H. Elliott. "Caveolins and Caveolae in Ocular Physiology and Pathophysiology." 56 (2017): 84–106.
197. Ferreira, A. P., and E. Boucrot. "Mechanisms of Carrier Formation During Clathrin-Independent Endocytosis." *Trends in Cell Biology* 28, no. 3 (2018): 188–200.
198. Sandvig, K., S. Pust, T. Skotland, and B. van Deurs. "Clathrin-Independent Endocytosis: Mechanisms and Function." 23, no. 4 (2011): 413–20.
199. Codenotti, S., M. Vezzoli, E. Monti, and A. Fanzani. "Focus on the Role of Caveolin and Cavin Protein Families in Liposarcoma." 94 (2017): 21–6.
200. Zielinski, J., A. M. Möller, M. Frenz, and M. Mevissen. "Evaluation of Endocytosis of Silica Particles Used in Biodegradable Implants in the Brain." 12, no. 6 (2016): 1603–13.
201. Tiwari, R., P. Jain, S. Asati, T. Haider, V. Soni, and V. Pandey. "State-of-Art Based Approaches for Anticancer Drug-Targeting to Nucleus." 48 (2018): 383–92.
202. Zhao, X., Y. Liu, Q. Ma, X. Wang, H. Jin, M. Mehrpour, and Q. Chen. "Caveolin-1 Negatively Regulates TRAIL-Induced Apoptosis in Human Hepatocarcinoma Cells." 378, no. 1 (2009): 21–6.
203. Rejman, J., M. Conese, and D. Hoekstra. "Gene Transfer by Means of Lipo-And Polyplexes: Role of Clathrin and Caveolae-Mediated Endocytosis." *Journal of Liposome Research* 16, no. 3 (2006): 237–47.
204. Smith, J. N., J. M. Edgar, J. M. Balk, M. Iftikhar, J. C. Fong, T. J. Olsen, D. A. Fishman, S. Majumdar, and G. A. Weiss. "Directed Evolution and Biophysical Characterization of a Full-Length, Soluble, Human caveolin-1 Variant." 1866, no. 9 (2018): 963–72.
205. Harris, J., D. Werling, J. C. Hope, G. Taylor, and C. J. Howard. "Caveolae and Caveolin in Immune Cells: Distribution and Functions." 23, no. 3 (2002): 158–64.
206. Singhal, S. S., R. Salgia, N. Verma, D. Horne, and S. Awasthi. "RLIP Controls Receptor-Ligand Signaling by Regulating Clathrin-Dependent Endocytosis." 1873, no. 1 (2020): 188337.
207. Fernandez-Rojo, M. A., and G. A. Ramm. "Filling the Gap on Caveolin-1 in Liver Carcinogenesis." *Trends in Cancer* 2, no. 12 (2016): 701–5.
208. Lu, Y., and P. S. Low. "Folate-Mediated Delivery of Macromolecular Anticancer Therapeutic Agents." *Advanced Drug Delivery Reviews* 54, no. 5 (2002): 675–93.
209. Kelemen, L. E. "The Role of Folate Receptor α in Cancer Development, Progression and Treatment: Cause, Consequence or Innocent Bystander?." *International Journal of Cancer* 119, no. 2 (2006): 243–50.
210. Gupta, R., C. Toufaily, and B. Annabi. "Caveolin and Cavin Family Members: Dual Roles in Cancer." *Biochimie* 107, no. B (2014): 188–202.
211. Oh, P., P. Borgström, H. Witkiewicz, Y. Li, B. J. Borgström, A. Chrastina, K. Iwata, K. R. Zinn, R. Baldwin, J. E. Testa, and J. E. Schnitzer. "Live Dynamic Imaging of Caveolae Pumping Targeted Antibody Rapidly and Specifically Across Endothelium in the Lung." 25, no. 3 (2007): 327–37.
212. El-Sayed, A., and H. Harashima. "Endocytosis of Gene Delivery Vectors: From Clathrin-Dependent to Lipid Raft-Mediated Endocytosis." *Molecular Therapy* 21, no. 6 (2013): 1118–30.
213. Lajoie, P., and I. R. Nabi. "Lipid Rafts, Caveolae, and Their Endocytosis." In *International Review of Cell & Molecular Biology*. Elsevier (2010): 135–63.
214. Kumar, G. A., J. Karmakar, C. Mandal, and A. Chattopadhyay. "Leishmania donovani Internalizes into Host Cells via Caveolin-Mediated Endocytosis." 9, no. 1 (2019): 1–11.
215. Wang, H., P. Yang, K. Liu, F. Guo, Y. Zhang, G. Zhang, and C. Jiang. "SARS Coronavirus Entry into Host Cells Through a Novel Clathrin-and Caveolae-Independent Endocytic Pathway." 18, no. 2 (2008): 290–301.
216. Wei, X., G. She, T. Wu, C. Xue, and Y. Cao. "PEDV Enters Cells Through Clathrin-, Caveolae-, and Lipid Raft-Mediated Endocytosis and Traffics via the Endo-/lysosome Pathway." 51, no. 1 (2020): 1–18.
217. Shafaq-Zadah, M., E. Dransart, and L. Johannes. "Clathrin-Independent Endocytosis, Retrograde Trafficking, and Cell Polarity." *Current Opinion in Cell Biology* 65 (2020): 112–21.
218. Orlando, M., D. Schmitz, C. Rosenmund, and M. A. Herman. "Calcium-Independent exo-Endocytosis Coupling at Small Central Synapses." 29, no. 12 (2019): 3767–74. e3.
219. Kirkham, M., and R. G. Parton. "Clathrin-Independent Endocytosis: New Insights into Caveolae and non-Caveolar Lipid Raft Carriers." *Biochimica & Biophysica Acta* 1745, no. 3 (2005): 273–86.
220. Kumari, S., M. Swetha, and S. Mayor. "Endocytosis Unplugged: Multiple Ways to Enter the Cell." *Cell Research* 20, no. 3 (2010): 256–75.
221. Kirkham, M., A. Fujita, R. Chadda, S. J. Nixon, T. V. Kurzchalia, D. K. Sharma, R. E. Pagano, J. F. Hancock, S. Mayor, and R. G. Parton. "Ultrastructural Identification of Uncoated Caveolin-Independent Early Endocytic Vehicles." 168, no. 3 (2005): 465–76.

222. Guo, S., X. Zhang, M. Zheng, X. Zhang, C. Min, Z. Wang, S. H. Cheon, M. H. Oak, S. Y. Nah, and K. M. Kim. "Selectivity of Commonly Used Inhibitors of Clathrin-Mediated and Caveolae-Dependent Endocytosis of G Protein–Coupled Receptors." 1848, no. 10 Pt A (2015): 2101–10.

223. Damm, E.-M. et al. "Clathrin-And caveolin-1–independent Endocytosis: Entry of Simian Virus 40 into Cells Devoid of Caveolae." 168, no. 3 (2005): 477–88.

224. Garaiova, Z., S. P. Strand, N. K. Reitan, S. Lélu, S. Ø Størset, K. Berg, J. Malmo, O. Folasire, A. Bjørkøy, and C. de L. Davies. "Cellular Uptake of DNA–Chitosan Nanoparticles: The Role of Clathrin-and Caveolae-Mediated Pathways." 51, no. 5 (2012): 1043–51.

225. Mellman, I., and W. J. Nelson. "Coordinated Protein Sorting, Targeting and Distribution in Polarized Cells." *Nature Reviews. Molecular Cell Biology* 9, no. 11 (2008): 833–45.

226. Bourmoum, M., and A. Claing. "Pase ARF6 Regulates Mitotic Exit and Cell Cycle Progression." *GT. Journal of Pharmacological & Toxicological Methods* 88 (2017): 169.

227. Pasternak, S. et al. "Arf6 Controls Rapid Lysosomal Transport of Cell Surface APP and Beta-Amyloid Production by Macropinocytosis." 4, no. 9 (2013): 532.

228. Mukhamedova, N., A. Hoang, H. L. Cui, I. Carmichael, Y. Fu, M. Bukrinsky, and D. Sviridov. "Small GTPase ARF6 Regulates Endocytic Pathway Leading to Degradation of ATP-Binding Cassette Transporter." A1 36, no. 12 (2016): 2292–303.

229. Qi, S., L. Su, J. Li, C. Zhang, Z. Ma, G. Liu, Q. Zhang, G. Jia, Y. Piao, and S. Zhang. "Arf6-Driven Endocytic Recycling of CD147 Determines HCC Malignant Phenotypes." 38, no. 1 (2019): 471.

230. Lau, A. W., and M. M. Chou. "The Adaptor Complex AP-2 Regulates Post-Endocytic Trafficking Through the Non-Clathrin Arf6-Dependent Endocytic Pathway." *Journal of Cell Science* 121, no. 24 (2008): 4008–17.

231. Haspel, N., H. Jang, and R. Nussinov. "Active and Inactive cdc42 Differ in Their Insert Region Conformational Dynamics." *Biophysical Journal* 120, no. 2 (2020): 306–18.

232. Liu, L., H. Jiang, W. Zhao, Y. Meng, J. Li, T. Huang, and J. Sun. "Cdc42-Mediated Supracellular Cytoskeleton Induced Cancer Cell Migration Under Low Shear Stress." 519, no. 1 (2019): 134–40.

233. Lv, J., J. Zeng, W. Zhao, Y. Cheng, L. Zhang, S. Cai, G. Hu, and Y. Chen. "Cdc42 Regulates LPS-Induced Proliferation of Primary Pulmonary Microvascular Endothelial Cells via ERK Pathway." 109 (2017): 45–53.

234. Aizawa, R., A. Yamada, T. Seki, J. Tanaka, R. Nagahama, M. Ikehata, T. Kato, A. Sakashita, H. Ogata, D. Chikazu, K. Maki, K. Mishima, M. Yamamoto, and R. Kamijo. "Cdc42 Regulates Cranial Suture Morphogenesis and Ossification." 512, no. 2 (2019): 145–9.

235. Francis, M. K. et al. "Endocytic Membrane Turnover at the Leading Edge Is Driven by a Transient Interaction Between Cdc42 and GRAF1." 128, no. 22 (2015): 4183–95.

236. Garrett, W. S., L. M. Chen, R. Kroschewski, M. Ebersold, S. Turley, S. Trombetta, J. E. Galán, and I. Mellman. "Developmental Control of Endocytosis in Dendritic Cells by Cdc42." 102, no. 3 (2000): 325–34.

237. Cavanaugh, K. E., M. F. Staddon, E. Munro, S. Banerjee, and M. L. Gardel. "RhoA Mediates Epithelial Cell Shape Changes via Mechanosensitive Endocytosis." 52, no. 2 (2020): 152–66. e5.

238. Iyer, M., M. D. Subramaniam, D. Venkatesan, S. G. Cho, M. Ryding, M. Meyer, and B. Vellingiri. "Role of RhoA-ROCK Signaling in Parkinson's Disease." (2020): 173815.

239. Jennings, R. T., M. Strengert, P. Hayes, J. El-Benna, C. Brakebusch, M. Kubica, and U. G. Knaus. "RhoA Determines Disease Progression by Controlling Neutrophil Motility and Restricting Hyperresponsiveness." 123, no. 23 (2014): 3635–45.

240. Prosser, D. C., T. G. Drivas, L. Maldonado-Báez, and B. Wendland. "Existence of a Novel Clathrin-Independent Endocytic Pathway in Yeast That Depends on Rho1 and Formin." 195, no. 4 (2011): 657–71.

241. Khandelwal, P., W. G. Ruiz, and G. Apodaca. "Compensatory Endocytosis in Bladder Umbrella Cells Occurs Through an Integrin-Regulated and RhoA-And Dynamin-Dependent Pathway." *EMBO Journal* 29, no. 12 (2010): 1961–75.

242. Stirling, L., M. R. Williams, and A. D. Morielli. "Dual Roles for RHOA/RHO-Kinase in the Regulated Trafficking of a Voltage-Sensitive Potassium Channel." *Molecular Biology of the Cell* 20, no. 12 (2009): 2991–3002.

243. Lundmark, R. et al. "Pase-Activating Protein." GRAF1 regulates the CLIC/GEEC endocytic pathway. *GT* 18, no. 22, 2008: 1802–8.

244. Nonnenmacher, M., and T. Weber. "Adeno-Associated Virus 2 Infection Requires Endocytosis Through the CLIC/GEEC Pathway." *Cell Host & Microbe* 10, no. 6 (2011): 563–76.

245. Surve, M. V. et al. "Streptococcus pneumoniae Utilizes a Novel Dynamin Independent Pathway for Entry and Persistence in Brain Endothelium." 1 (2020): 62–8.

246. Posor, Y., M. Eichhorn-Grünig, and V. Haucke. "Phosphoinositides in Endocytosis." 1851, no. 6 (2015): 794–804.

247. Howes, M. T., S. Mayor, and R. G. Parton. "Molecules, Mechanisms, and Cellular Roles of Clathrin-Independent Endocytosis." *Current Opinion in Cell Biology* 22, no. 4 (2010): 519–27.

248. Harper, C. B. et al. *Exploiting Endocytic Pathways to Prevent Bacterial Toxin Infection*, 1072, 2015.

249. Lundmark, R., and S. R. Carlsson. "Driving Membrane Curvature in Clathrin-Dependent and Clathrin-Independent Endocytosis." In *Seminars in Cell & Developmental Biology*. Amsterdam: Elsevier (2010).

250. Maeda, Y., and T. Kinoshita. "Structural Remodeling, Trafficking and Functions of Glycosylphosphatidylinositol-Anchored Proteins." *Progress in Lipid Research* 50, no. 4 (2011): 411–24.

251. Villaseñor, R., Y. Kalaidzidis, and M. Zerial. "Signal Processing by the Endosomal System." *Current Opinion in Cell Biology* 39 (2016): 53–60.

252. Maldonado-Báez, L., C. Williamson, and J. Donaldson. "Clathrin-Independent Endocytosis: A Cargo-Centric View." *Experimental Cell Research* 319, no. 18 (2013): 2759–69.

253. Diaz-Rohrer, B., K. R. Levental, and I. Levental. "Rafting Through Traffic: Membrane Domains in Cellular Logistics." *Biochimica & Biophysica Acta* 1838, no. 12 (2014): 3003–13.

254. Fujita, M., and T. Kinoshita. "GPI-Anchor Remodeling: Potential Functions of GPI-Anchors in Intracellular Trafficking and Membrane Dynamics." *Biochimica & Biophysica Acta* 1821, no. 8 (2012): 1050–8.

255. Józefowski, S., and M. Śróttek. "Lipid Raft-Dependent Endocytosis Negatively Regulates Responsiveness of J774 Macrophage-Like Cells to LPS by down Regulating the Cell Surface Expression of LPS Receptors." *Cellular Immunology* 312 (2017): 42–50.

256. Vercauteren, D., J. Rejman, T. F. Martens, J. Demeester, S. C. De Smedt, and K. Braeckmans. "On the Cellular Processing of Non-Viral Nanomedicines for Nucleic Acid Delivery: Mechanisms and Methods." 161, no. 2 (2012): 566–81.

257. Juliano, R., and K. Carver. "Cellular Uptake and Intracellular Trafficking of Oligonucleotides." *Advanced Drug Delivery Reviews* 87 (2015): 35–45.

258. Mercer, J., and U. F. Greber. "Virus Interactions with Endocytic Pathways in Macrophages and Dendritic Cells." *Trends in Microbiology* 21, no. 8 (2013): 380–8.

259. Suh, Y. H., K. Chang, and K. W. Roche. "Metabotropic Glutamate Receptor Trafficking." 91 (2018): 10–24.

260. Boquet, P., and V. Ricci. "Intoxication Strategy of Helicobacter pylori VacA Toxin." *Trends in Microbiology* 20, no. 4 (2012): 165–74.

261. Chadda, R., M. T. Howes, S. J. Plowman, J. F. Hancock, R. G. Parton, and S. Mayor. "Cholesterol-Sensitive Cdc42 Activation Regulates Actin Polymerization for Endocytosis via the GEEC Pathway." 8, no. 6 (2007): 702–17.

262. Anupama, H., C. Prabhakara, and S. Mayor. "Clathrin-Independent Endocytosis of Wingless via Clic/Geec Pathway Is Necessary for Effective Signalling in Drosophila Wing Discs." *Biophysical Journal* 110, no. 3 (2016): 595a.

263. Vercauteren, D., M. Piest, L. J. van der Aa, M. Al Soraj, A. T. Jones, J. F. Engbersen, S. C. De Smedt, and K. Braeckmans. "Flotillin-Dependent Endocytosis and a Phagocytosis-Like Mechanism for Cellular Internalization of Disulfide-Based Poly (Amido Amine)/DNA Polyplexes." 32, no. 11 (2011): 3072–84.

264. Dam, D., S. Jelsma, and A. Paller. "445 Discovery of an Alternate, Flotillin-Dependent, Clathrin-Mediated Endocytosis Pathway for IGF-1 Receptor Internalization and Signaling in Keratinocytes." *Journal of Investigative Dermatology* 136, no. 5 (2016): S79.

265. Xu, R., X. Song, P. Su, Y. Pang, and Q. Li. "Identification and Characterization of the Lamprey flotillin-1 Gene with a Role in Cell Adhesion." 71 (2017): 286–94.

266. Lalazar, G., A. Ben Ya'acov, D. M. Livovsky, M. El Haj, O. Pappo, S. Preston, L. Zolotarov, and Y. Ilan. "β-Glycoglycosphingolipid-Induced Alterations of the STAT Signaling Pathways Are Dependent on CD1d and the Lipid Raft Protein flotillin-2." 174, no. 4 (2009): 1390–9.

267. Biernatowska, A., K. Augoff, J. Podkalicka, S. Tabaczar, W. Gajdzik-Nowak, A. Czogalla, and A. F. Sikorski. "MPP1 Directly Interacts with Flotillins in Erythrocyte Membrane-Possible Mechanism of Raft Domain Formation." 1859, no. 11 (2017: 2203–12.

268. Schmidt, F., A. Thywißen, M. Goldmann, C. Cunha, Z. Cseresnyés, H. Schmidt, M. Rafiq, S. Galiani, M. H. Gräler, G. Chamilos, J. F. Lacerda, A. Campos, C. Eggeling, M. T. Figge, T. Heinekamp, S. G. Filler, A. Carvalho, and A. A. Brakhage. "Flotillin-Dependent Membrane Microdomains Are Required for Functional Phagolysosomes Against Fungal Infections." 32, no. 7 (2020): 108017.

269. Langhorst, M. F., A. Reuter, F. A. Jaeger, F. M. Wippich, G. Luxenhofer, H. Plattner, and C. A. Stuermer. "Trafficking of the Microdomain Scaffolding Protein reggie-1/flotillin-2." 87, no. 4 (2008): 211–26.

270. Langhorst, M. F., F. A. Jaeger, S. Mueller, L. Sven Hartmann, G. Luxenhofer, and C. A. Stuermer. "Reggies/flotillins Regulate Cytoskeletal Remodeling During Neuronal Differentiation via CAP/Ponsin and Rho GTPases." 87, no. 12 (2008): 921–31.

271. Lu, Z., Y. Liu, Y. Shi, X. Shi, X. Wang, C. Xu, H. Zhao, and Q. Dong. "Curcumin Protects Cortical Neurons Against Oxygen and Glucose Deprivation/Reoxygenation Injury Through flotillin-1 and Extracellular Signal-Regulated Kinase1/2 Pathway." 496, no. 2 (2018): 515–22.

272. Stuermer, C. A. "The Reggie/Flotillin Connection to Growth." *Trends in Cell Biology* 20, no. 1 (2010): 6–13.

273. Babuke, T., and R. Tikkanen. "Dissecting the Molecular Function of Reggie/Flotillin Proteins." *European Journal of Cell Biology* 86, no. 9 (2007): 525–32.

274. Dam, D. H. M., S. A. Jelsma, J. M. Yu, H. Liu, B. Kong, and A. S. Paller. "Flotillin and AP2A1/2 Promote IGF-1 Receptor Association with Clathrin and Internalization in Primary Human Keratinocytes." (2020).

275. Lu, Z., M. Cui, H. Zhao, T. Wang, Y. Shen, and Q. Dong. "Tissue Kallikrein Mediates Neurite Outgrowth Through Epidermal Growth Factor Receptor and flotillin-2 Pathway In Vitro." 26, no. 2 (2014): 220–32.

276. Sugawara, Y., H. Nishii, T. Takahashi, J. Yamauchi, N. Mizuno, K. Tago, and H. Itoh. "The Lipid Raft Proteins flotillins/reggies Interact with Gαq and Are Involved in Gq-Mediated p38 Mitogen-Activated Protein Kinase Activation Through Tyrosine Kinase." 19, no. 6 (2007): 1301–8.

277. Deng, Y., P. Ge, T. Tian, C. Dai, M. Wang, S. Lin, K. Liu, Y. Zheng, P. Xu, L. Zhou, Q. Hao, and Z. Dai. "Prognostic Value of Flotillins (flotillin-1 and flotillin-2) in Human Cancers: A Meta-Analysis." 481 (2018): 90–8.

278. Banning, A., C. R. Regenbrecht, and R. Tikkanen. "Increased Activity of Mitogen Activated Protein Kinase Pathway in flotillin-2 Knockout Mouse Model." *Cellular Signalling* 26, no. 2 (2014): 198–207.

279. Park, M.-Y., N. Kim, L. L. Wu, G. Y. Yu, and K. Park. "Role of Flotillins in the Endocytosis of GPCR in Salivary Gland Epithelial Cells." 476, no. 4 (2016): 237–44.

280. Saslowsky, D. E., J. A. Cho, H. Chinnapen, R. H. Massol, D. J. -F. Chinnapen, J. S. Wagner, H. E. De Luca, W. Kam, B. H. Paw, and W. I. Lencer. "Intoxication of Zebrafish and Mammalian Cells by Cholera Toxin Depends on the flotillin/reggie Proteins but Not Derlin-1 or -2." 120, no. 12 (2010).

281. Pust, S., A. B. Dyve, M. L. Torgersen, B. van Deurs, and K. Sandvig. "Interplay Between Toxin Transport and Flotillin Localization." 5, no. 1 (2010): e8844.

282. Cremona, M. L., H. J. Matthies, K. Pau, E. Bowton, N. Speed, B. J. Lute, M. Anderson, N. Sen, S. D. Robertson, R. A. Vaughan, J. E. Rothman, A. Galli, J. A. Javitch, and A. Yamamoto. "Flotillin-1 Is Essential for PKC-Triggered Endocytosis and Membrane Microdomain Localization of DAT." 14, no. 4 (2011): 469–77.

283. Ludwig, A., G. P. Otto, K. Riento, E. Hams, P. G. Fallon, and B. J. Nichols. "Flotillin Microdomains Interact with the Cortical Cytoskeleton to Control Uropod Formation and Neutrophil Recruitment." 191, no. 4 (2010): 771–81.

284. Jovic, M. et al. "The Early Endosome: A Busy Sorting Station for Proteins at the Crossroads." 25, no. 1 (2010): 99.

285. Lv, W., and J. A. Champion. "Demonstration of Intracellular Trafficking, Cytosolic Bioavailability, and Target Manipulation of an Antibody Delivery Platform." *Nanomedicine: Nanotechnology, Biology & Medicine* 32 (2020): 102315.

286. Guo, Y., M. Duan, X. Wang, J. Gao, Z. Guan, and M. Zhang. "Early Events in Rabies Virus Infection: Attachment, Entry, and Intracellular Trafficking." 263 (2019): 217–25.

287. Donahue, N. D., H. Acar, and S. Wilhelm. "Concepts of Nanoparticle Cellular Uptake, Intracellular Trafficking, and Kinetics in Nanomedicine." *Advanced Drug Delivery Reviews* 143 (2019): 68–96.

288. Nakamura, T., Y. Yamada, Y. Sato, I. A. Khalil, and H. Harashima. "Innovative Nanotechnologies for Enhancing Nucleic Acids/Gene Therapy: Controlling Intracellular Trafficking to Targeted Biodistribution." 218 (2019): 119329.

289. Martin, V., I. A. C. Ribeiro, M. M. Alves, L. Gonçalves, A. J. Almeida, L. Grenho, M. H. Fernandes, C. F. Santos, P. S. Gomes, and A. F. Bettencourt. "Understanding Intracellular Trafficking and Anti-Inflammatory Effects of Minocycline Chitosan-Nanoparticles in Human Gingival Fibroblasts for Periodontal Disease Treatment." 572 (2019): 118821.

290. Huotari, J., and A. Helenius. "Endosome Maturation." *EMBO Journal* 30, no. 17 (2011): 3481–500.

291. Simion, V., E. Henriet, V. Juric, R. Aquino, C. Loussouarn, Y. Laurent, F. Martin, P. Midoux, E. Garcion, C. Pichon, and P. Baril. "Intracellular Trafficking and Functional Monitoring of miRNA Delivery in Glioblastoma Using Lipopolyplexes and the miRNA-ON RILES Reporter System." 327 (2020): 429–43.

292. Zhang, L., T. Wang, M. Song, M. Jin, S. Liu, K. Guo, and Y. Zhang. "Rab1b-GBF1-ARFs Mediated Intracellular Trafficking Is Required for Classical Swine Fever Virus Replication in Swine Umbilical Vein Endothelial Cells." (2020): 108743.

293. Nyuzuki, H., S. Ito, K. Nagasaki, Y. Nitta, N. Matsui, A. Saitoh, and H. Matsui. "Degeneration of Dopaminergic Neurons and Impaired Intracellular Trafficking in Atp13a2 Deficient Zebrafish." (2020).

294. Grant, B. D., and J. G. Donaldson. "Pathways and Mechanisms of Endocytic Recycling." *Nature Reviews. Molecular Cell Biology* 10, no. 9 (2009): 597–608.

295. Ji, Y., Y. Wang, D. Shen, Q. Kang, and L. Chen. "Mucin Corona Delays Intracellular Trafficking and Alleviates Cytotoxicity of Nanoplastic-Benzopyrene Combined Contaminant." (2020): 124306.

296. Ono, D., K. Asada, D. Yui, F. Sakaue, K. Yoshioka, T. Nagata, and T. Yokota. "Separation-Related Rapid Nuclear Transport of DNA/RNA Heteroduplex Oligonucleotide: Unveiling Distinctive Intracellular Trafficking." (2020).

297. Gindhart, J., and K. Weber. *Lysosome and Endosome Organization and Transport in Neurons*, 2009.

298. Condon, K. H., and M. D. Ehlers. "Postsynaptic Machinery for Receptor Trafficking." In *Protein Trafficking in Neurons*, 143–74. Amsterdam: Elsevier, 2007.

299. de Pinho Favaro, M. T. et al. "Intracellular Trafficking of a Dynein-Based Nanoparticle Designed for Gene Delivery." 112 (2018): 71–8.

300. Park, M., J. M. Salgado, L. Ostroff, T. D. Helton, C. G. Robinson, K. M. Harris, and M. D. Ehlers. "Plasticity-Induced Growth of Dendritic Spines by Exocytic Trafficking from Recycling Endosomes." 52, no. 5 (2006): 817–30.

301. Martens, T. F., K. Remaut, J. Demeester, S. C. De Smedt, and K. Braeckmans. "Intracellular Delivery of Nanomaterials: How to Catch Endosomal Escape in the Act." 9, no. 3 (2014): 344–64.

302. Scott, C. C., F. Vacca, and J. Gruenberg. "Endosome Maturation, Transport and Functions." In *Seminars in Cell & Developmental Biology*. Amsterdam: Elsevier (2014).

303. Dominska, M., and D. M. Dykxhoorn. "Breaking down the Barriers: siRNA Delivery and Endosome Escape." *Journal of Cell Science* 123, no. 8 (2010): 1183–9.

304. Blower, M. D. "Molecular Insights into Intracellular RNA Localization." In *International Review of Cell & Molecular Biology*. Amsterdam: Elsevier (2013): 1–39.

305. Breusegem, S. Y., and M. N. Seaman. "Image-Based and Biochemical Assays to Investigate Endosomal Protein Sorting." In *Methods in Enzymology*. Amsterdam: Elsevier (2014): 155–78.

306. Shanmughapriya, S., D. Langford, and K. Natarajaseenivasan. "Inter and Intracellular Mitochondrial Trafficking in Health and Disease." *Ageing Research Reviews* (2020): 101128.

307. Ma, X., Y. Wu, S. Jin, Y. Tian, X. Zhang, Y. Zhao, L. Yu, and X. J. Liang. "Gold Nanoparticles Induce Autophagosome Accumulation Through Size-Dependent Nanoparticle Uptake and Lysosome Impairment." 5, no. 11 (2011): 8629–39.

308. Ulloa-Aguirre, A. et al. "Protein Homeostasis and Regulation of Intracellular Trafficking of G Protein-Coupled Receptors." In *Protein Homeostasis Diseases*, 247–77. Amsterdam: Elsevier, 2020.

309. Zhu, J., C. Schwartz, and I. Wheeldon. "Controlled Intracellular Trafficking Alleviates an Expression Bottleneck in S. cerevisiae Ester Biosynthesis." *Metabolic Engineering Communications* 8 (2019): e00085.

310. Mizushima, N. "Autophagy: Process and Function." *Genes & Development* 21, no. 22 (2007): 2861–73.

311. Stern, S. T., and D. N. Johnson. "Role for Nanomaterial-Autophagy Interaction in Neurodegenerative Disease." *Autophagy* 4, no. 8 (2008): 1097–100.

312. Bitoque, D. B., A. M. Rosa da Costa, and G. A. Silva. "Insights on the Intracellular Trafficking of PDMAEMA Gene Therapy Vectors." 93 (2018): 277–88.

313. Klionsky, D. J. "Autophagy: From Phenomenology to Molecular Understanding in Less than a Decade." *Nature Reviews. Molecular Cell Biology* 8, no. 11 (2007): 931–7.

314. Wang, J., Y. Yu, K. Lu, M. Yang, Y. Li, X. Zhou, and Z. Sun. "Silica Nanoparticles Induce Autophagy Dysfunction via Lysosomal Impairment and Inhibition of Autophagosome Degradation in Hepatocytes." 12 (2017): 809.

Tumor Targeting

5

Eva Y. Pan, Aubrey Johnson, and Jennifer Zhao

Contents

DOI: 10.1201/9781003092773-6

5.1 INTRODUCTION

Traditional cytotoxic chemotherapy has been the mainstay for treating cancer since its first clinical use in the mid-1900s (DeVita and Chu 2008). Although very effective in treating a multitude of cancer disease states, cytotoxic chemotherapy is notorious for causing a range of systemic side effects related to its non-specific action on rapidly dividing cells. Thus, the focus in recent decades has shifted to developing tumor-targeted therapy that has fewer off-target adverse events and potentially greater efficacy. Targeted therapy is specific for receptors, mutations, or proteins that regulate cellular functions and gene expression in tumor cells as opposed to eliminating all rapidly dividing cells.

There are three main types of targeted therapy drugs: small molecules, monoclonal antibodies (mAbs), and antibody–drug conjugates. Small molecule inhibitors are primarily oral drugs that can penetrate cells, allowing them to target intracellular signaling pathways in addition to cell surface receptors. The most common targets of small molecules are receptor tyrosine kinases (RTKs), which mediate a variety of cellular differentiation and proliferation pathways and are often overexpressed or hyperactive in cancers (Du and Lovly 2018). RTKs have a general structure consisting of an extracellular ligand binding domain, a transmembrane portion, and an intracellular region with the tyrosine kinase (TK) domain (see Figure 5.1). Small molecule inhibitors of TKs are typically ATP mimetics that block the ATP binding site. Other targets of small molecule inhibitors include proteasomes, apoptosis proteins, and Hedgehog signaling (Lavanya et al. 2014). The advantages of small molecule inhibitors include their ease of administration, their ability to target a molecule regardless of its cellular location, and their increased ability to penetrate the blood–brain barrier (Imai and Takaoka 2006).

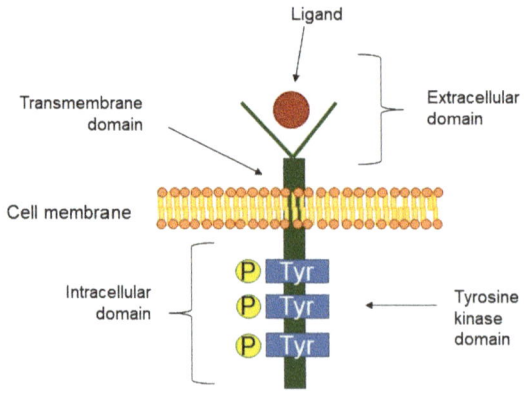

FIGURE 5.1   Receptor tyrosine kinase structure

Since the late 1990s, mAbs have been used in cancer treatment. The mAbs used in oncology are primarily IgG-based and consist of two functional units: the fragment of antigen binding (Fab) and the constant fragment (Fc). The Fab region is responsible for antigen binding and blockage of the receptor, whereas the Fc fragment is responsible for linkage to immune effector cells and stimulation of antibody-dependent cellular cytotoxicity. Due to their large molecular size and inability to penetrate cell membranes, mAbs most commonly target cell surface receptors or work in the tumor microenvironment (TME). Compared with small molecule inhibitors, mAbs have greater selectivity for antigens as well as longer half-lives. One unique concern with mAbs is their potential for immunogenicity, which could interfere with their efficacy. The risk of immunogenicity exists despite using humanized or even human mAbs (Imai and Takaoka 2006).

Antibody–drug conjugates (ADCs) are an emerging class of targeted anticancer therapy. ADCs utilize the antigen-targeting ability of mAbs and the cytotoxic properties of a second agent, which is most commonly a cytotoxic drug but in some cases, can be a radiopharmaceutical or immunotoxin (Chau, Steeg, and Figg 2019). As shown in Figure 5.2, the mAb and cytotoxic agent are connected through a chemical linker, which remains stable during administration and in systemic circulation. The linker either cleaves when exposed to cell conditions such as low pH or high glutathione concentrations or is degraded by lysosomal enzymes, allowing release of the cytotoxic component (see Figure 5.3) (Birrer et al. 2019).

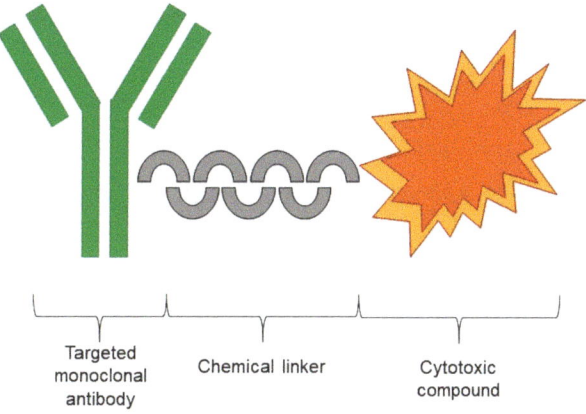

FIGURE 5.2   Antibody–drug conjugate (ADC) structure

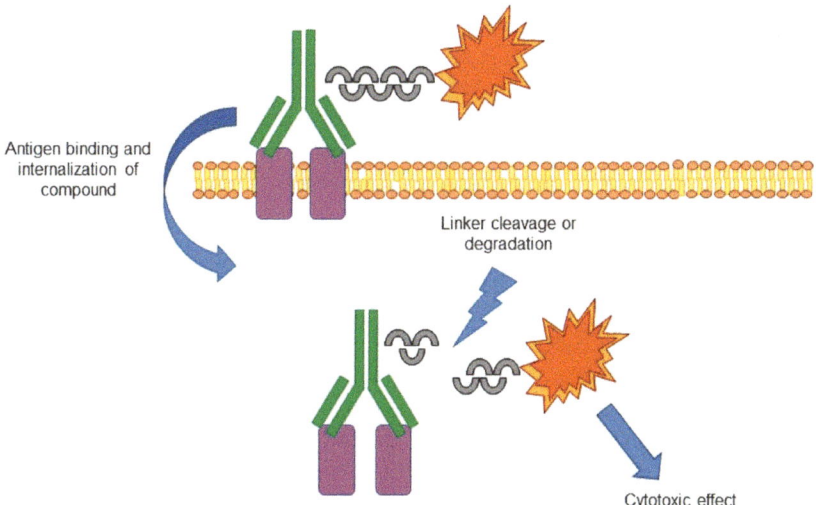

FIGURE 5.3   Mechanism of action of ADC

Targeted delivery with the ADC cytotoxic drug, also known as "payload," avoids some of the more pronounced challenges to conventional chemotherapy, including a narrow therapeutic window and off-target toxicities (Chau, Steeg, and Figg 2019). Current limitations of ADCs in anticancer therapy are related to adverse effects and antigen identification. On-target toxicities, such as skin rash with nectin-4 targeting, can occur in off-target cells that express the antigen (Rosenberg et al. 2019). Dose-limiting toxicities related to the payload are also a concern, such as ocular toxicities associated with cytotoxic tubulin inhibitors and veno-occlusive disease associated with calicheamicin cytotoxic mechanisms (Khongorzul et al. 2020). Future developments will focus both on personalization of therapy through antigen identification or stratification by measurement of antigen during phase II and III trials and on the development of new payload agents (Birrer et al. 2019; Khongorzul et al. 2020).

Overall, tumor targeting is an effective strategy for treating cancers, and the identification of suitable targets is key. Most importantly, tumor targets should be exclusively overexpressed on tumor cells compared with normal cells. Additionally, the number of available targets per cell and the distribution of positive/overexpressed cells within the tumor will impact the effectiveness of the targeted treatment (Boonstra et al. 2016). Depending on the treatment's mechanism of action, the stability of the receptor after the drug binds is also important. For example, receptor targets for ADCs should have a rapid rate of internalization, whereas receptors for drugs that do not need to be internalized should have good stability in the cell surface and negligible shedding into the tumor stroma or circulation. From a genetic standpoint, the gene coding for the receptor should not have a high rate of mutations, and there should be minimal to no variant forms of the receptor (Ghose 2002).

5.2 HORMONE THERAPIES

5.2.1 Estrogen Receptor

Estrogen receptor (ER) signaling modulates a variety of physiological functions, including reproductive maturation, bone modeling, cardiovascular health, and neuroprotection. There are two primary nuclear estrogen receptors, ERα and ERβ, and one estrogen membrane receptor known as the G protein–coupled estrogen receptor (GPER1). Estrogen signaling is categorized as genomic or non-genomic based on the mechanism of gene expression regulation (Fuentes and Silveyra 2019). Direct genomic signaling occurs when estrogen binds to ERα or ERβ in the cytoplasm, causing the receptor to dimerize and translocate to the nucleus. Once in the nucleus, the complex binds to DNA at estrogen response element sequences and recruits coregulator proteins that can activate or deactivate the receptor complex and impact gene expression (Patel and Bihani 2018). Non-genomic or indirect genomic signaling occurs when the estrogen receptor complex influences gene expression by interacting with other transcription factors, such as stimulating protein-1, activating transcription factor-2, and activator protein-1, instead of directly binding to DNA. Alternatively, estrogen binding to the membrane receptor GPER1 activates various protein kinase cascades such as the phospholipase C/protein kinase C (PLC/PKC) pathway, the Ras/Raf/ mitogen-activated protein kinase (MAPK) cascade, the PI3K/Akt cascade, and the cAMP/PKA signaling pathway (Fuentes and Silveyra 2019).

Approximately 75% of breast cancers express ER and are therefore subject to stimulation from circulating systemic estrogen and further cancer cell proliferation. The presence of ER in breast cancer cells offers a treatment target, as blocking the activity of estrogen from the receptors would reduce the downstream effects of cell cycle proliferation and growth. Since the late 1970s, antiestrogen agents have been used clinically to treat and reduce the risk of ER+ breast cancer. Antiestrogen agents consist of selective estrogen receptor modulators (SERMs), selective estrogen receptor degraders (SERDs), and aromatase inhibitors (AIs). SERMs compete with estrogen and prevent activation by inducing a conformational change of the receptor that impedes coactivator proteins from binding (Patel and Bihani 2018). They demonstrate selective estrogen agonist or antagonist effects based on the specific tissue. In breast tissue, SERMs act as antagonists to estrogen, whereas in uterine tissue, they agonize estrogen receptors (Riggs and Hartmann 2003).

The primary SERM used in breast cancer is tamoxifen, which is a non-steroidal triphenylethylene derivative that is metabolized by CYP2D6 to its primary active metabolite endoxifen (4-hydroxy-N-des-methyltamoxifen). Endoxifen binds to ER with high affinity to block estrogen from stimulating ER+ breast cancer cells. Clinically, tamoxifen reduced the risk of breast cancer recurrence by 47% after 5 years of treatment and reduced mortality by 26% after 10 years ("Early Breast Cancer Trialists' Collaborative Group" 1998). Although very effective, tamoxifen use increases the risk of endometrial cancer, since it stimulates estrogen receptors in uterine tissue. Other adverse events include hot flashes, arthralgias, mood swings, cataracts, bone loss in premenopausal women, and venous thromboembolism. In current clinical practice, tamoxifen is used primarily for breast cancer risk reduction and treatment in premenopausal women with ER+ breast tissue (Soltamox [package insert]). Based on findings that SERM-resistant breast cancers still utilize the ER signaling cascade, SERDs were designed to eradicate the ER pathway by inducing degradation of the estrogen receptor. Fulvestrant is a SERD that is used for metastatic ER+ breast cancer in postmenopausal women who have progressed on prior endocrine therapy or have not previously received endocrine therapy. It is well tolerated, with side effects consisting of postmenopausal symptoms and local injection site reactions.

In peripheral tissues such as adipose and bone, estrogen is generated from conversion of androstenedione and testosterone by aromatase enzymes to estrone and estradiol. After menopause, estrogen is largely produced by aromatase action in peripheral tissues rather than by the ovary. AIs suppress peripheral estrogen production by inhibiting aromatase enzyme function and are used in postmenopausal women with ER+ breast cancer. They can also be used in premenopausal women who undergo ovarian suppression with luteinizing hormone releasing hormone (LHRH) agonists or ovarian ablation with oophorectomy. Letrozole and anastrozole are non-steroidal AIs that reversibly bind to the aromatase enzyme, whereas exemestane is a steroidal AI that binds irreversibly to aromatase. All three of these agents inhibit aromatase activity by ≥97% and consequently, suppress plasma estrogen levels by >90% (Geisler 2011). Clinically, the agents are considered therapeutically equivalent and share similar toxicities of arthralgias, hot flashes, and bone loss.

5.2.2 Androgen Receptor

The androgen hormones (testosterone and dihydrotestosterone) exert their functions by binding to androgen receptors (ARs), which are expressed in a variety of tissues. Similar to estrogen receptors, ARs are nuclear transcription factors that act through genomic or non-genomic signaling (Davey and Grossmann 2016). In genomic signaling, androgen binds with the receptor, forming a complex that translocates to the nucleus and binds to androgen response elements. In non-genomic signaling, the androgen/AR complex can activate other pathways implicated in transcription, including ERK, Akt, and MAPK. Androgen receptor activation is critical for prostate cancer sustainability and is therefore an obvious target for inhibition. Blocking of androgen activity in prostate cancer is known as androgen deprivation therapy (ADT), which can be accomplished through chemical or surgical castration or with antiandrogens (Grossmann, Cheung, and Zajac 2013). Long-acting gonadotrophin-releasing hormone (GnRH) agonists stimulate the production of follicle stimulating hormone (FSH) and luteinizing hormone (LH), generating negative feedback in the hypothalamus and ultimately, suppressing androgen production. The initial surge of testosterone with GnRH agonists can cause tumor flare, especially in more advanced disease. The GnRH antagonist degarelix blocks GnRH receptors and directly reduces LH and FSH secretion and testosterone production, thereby avoiding a tumor flare.

Another approach to target androgen signaling in prostate cancer is competitive binding of the AR, thus inducing conformational changes that inhibit the transcriptional functions of the AR complex.

Non-steroidal antiandrogens were designed to act as pure antagonists to the AR and include the first-generation antiandrogens (bicalutamide, flutamide, nilutamide) and second-generation antiandrogens (enzalutamide, apalutamide, darolutamide). The first-generation antiandrogens are associated with development of drug resistance, conversion from antagonist to agonist activity in the presence of excess AR, and potential for antiandrogen withdrawal syndrome (Rice, Malhotra, and Stoyanova 2019). In light of these issues, second-generation antiandrogens were created to circumvent certain resistance mutations and to have greater selectivity and affinity for the AR.

Overall, the second-generation antiandrogens are more effective and better tolerated than the first-generation agents, although they are associated with an increased risk of seizure activity due to inhibition of gamma-aminobutyric acid (GABA)$_A$ (Rice, Malhotra, and Stoyanova 2019). The first-generation agents are now mainly used to prevent tumor flare during ADT initiation, whereas the second-generation agents are used for clinical treatment. Abiraterone acetate, a second-generation antiandrogen that differs mechanistically, inhibits the biosynthesis of androgens by irreversibly blocking CYP17-mediated production of testosterone precursors in the testes, adrenal glands, and prostatic tumor tissues (Rice, Malhotra, and Stoyanova 2019). The primary side effects of abiraterone, such as hypokalemia and hypertension, are due to low levels of mineralocorticoids; thus, it has become standard practice to administer abiraterone with a glucocorticoid such as prednisone (Rice, Malhotra, and Stoyanova 2019).

Clinically, ADT is used upfront in prostate cancer treatment with response rates up to 80%, but the cancer cells often develop resistance to androgen deprivation, which is known as castrate-resistant prostate cancer (CRPC) (Salonen et al. 2008). In CRPC, it is still necessary to continue ADT, since the tumor is heterogeneous, and some cells may still be responding to androgen suppression (Crawford et al. 2019). Current research is focused on determining the ideal sequence of treatment throughout the course of disease and how different combinations of androgen-targeted therapies can impact treatment outcomes.

5.3 SIGNAL TRANSDUCTION INHIBITORS

5.3.1 RAS/RAF/MEK/ERK Pathway

The MAPK signaling pathways are among the best-understood regulating pathways of human cell division, dissemination, and survival. One key MAPK pathway that contributes to cancer cell growth is the extracellular-signal-regulated kinase 1/2 (ERK) MAPK cascade. As shown in Figure 5.4, the pathway begins extracellularly, where ligands bind to RTKs, such as the transmembrane epidermal growth factor receptor (EGFR). Intracellularly, the RTK activates the signaling cascade, beginning with GTPase rat sarcoma protein (RAS and then extending to rapidly accelerated fibrosarcoma (RAF), MAPK/ERK kinase (MEK), and ERK. Once activated, ERK inserts into the nucleus, transmits the signal to transcription factors and effectors, and promotes cell proliferation (Sanchez, Wang, and Cohen 2018). The ERK/MAPK pathway also interacts with the AKT/ mammalian target of rapamycin (mTOR) and other pathways, which comprise a complex system of crosstalk and coordination (Lheureux et al. 2017). Under normal cellular conditions, this is a well-regulated pathway that is known to communicate with over 150 proteins to control cell division (Roberts and Der 2007).

Abnormalities in this pathway can instigate malignant growth by way of RTK overexpression or mutations (as in the case of EGFR) and RAS or RAF activating point mutations. RAS isoforms KRAS, NRAS, and HRAS are encoded by the RAS gene. Activating RAS driver mutations occur in approximately 90% of pancreatic cancers, 50% of colon cancers, 30% of lung cancers, and 30% of all cancers (Roberts and Der 2007). These mutations cause RAS to remain in an activated state, leading to excessive cell division and proliferation. Activations in RAS allow it to circumvent upstream targeted therapy, such as EGFR inhibition. Although RAS has been identified as a potential anticancer target for

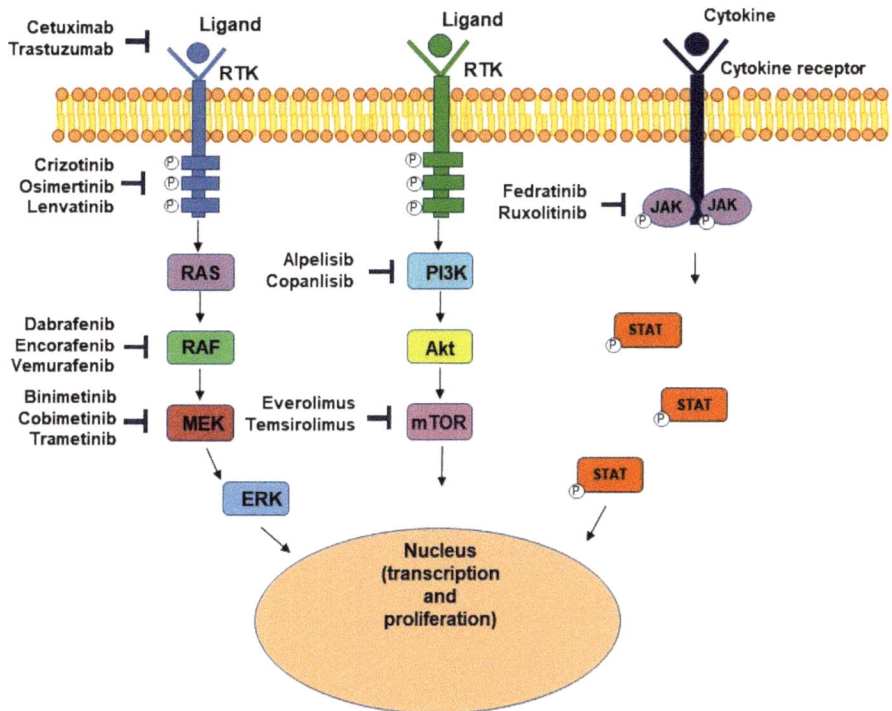

FIGURE 5.4   RAS/RAF/MEK/ERK, PI3K/Akt/m TOR, JAK/STAT pathways

decades, no specific RAS-targeted treatment has been deemed effective and safe by the Food and Drug Administration (FDA). However, recent progress has been made in the KRAS G12C point mutation, which has the highest amount of GTPase activity out of the common RAS mutations and is associated with smoking in lung adenocarcinoma (Moore et al. 2020). Additional targeted therapies are expected to target specific variant KRAS alleles, as wild-type RAS is essential for normal cell signaling. Indirect targeting through the nucleotide exchange cycle, RAS processing, or downstream mediators is also a potential therapeutic option.

RAF activating point mutations have been successfully targeted, and the inhibitors are currently standards of care in some cancer disease states. These mutations have been identified at RAF codon 600 in more than 50% of cases and more specifically, at V600E in close to 90% of cases (Sanchez, Wang, and Cohen 2018). BRAF V600E activating mutations are most commonly identified in melanoma, papillary thyroid cancer, colorectal cancer, hairy cell leukemia, and lung adenocarcinoma. Several oral BRAF inhibitors are FDA approved and work by inhibiting the RAF kinase activity, which prevents the activation of downstream effectors and inhibits unregulated cell growth. Vemurafenib was the first approved targeted BRAF inhibitor and showed a significant survival benefit compared with chemotherapy in patients with either V600E or V600K mutations, which set a new standard of care in patients with these mutations (McArthur et al. 2014). Following vemurafenib, dabrafenib was initially approved as monotherapy for advanced melanoma, although soon after approval, the BRAF inhibitors were found to have a greater effect in combination with MEK inhibition.

MEK inhibitors, such as trametinib, cobimetinib, and binimetinib, inhibit MEK1 and MEK2, thereby preventing downstream ERK signal transduction. Resistance to BRAF-targeted treatment can develop through reactivation of the MAPK signal transduction pathway. Therefore, dual BRAF and MEK inhibition provides greater efficacy by targeting the unregulated cascade at two steps in the signaling process, as clinically exemplified in the COMBI-d phase III trial in BRAF-mutated melanoma. Dabrafenib and trametinib demonstrated increased overall survival (OS) and progression-free survival (PFS) compared with dabrafenib monotherapy (Long et al. 2017). Combination therapy has also been shown to decrease specific RAF on-target adverse effects, such as skin lesions and skin squamous cell carcinoma due to compensatory ERK/MAPK pathway activation (Sanchez, Wang, and Cohen 2018; Kopetz et al. 2019). In colon cancer, BRAF monotherapy was not an option due to the rapid development of resistance. However, BRAF inhibition as part of a combination regimen, with an EGFR inhibitor and with or without a MEK inhibitor, recently demonstrated increased OS in the later-line setting for colon cancer (Kopetz et al. 2019). Combination therapy with vemurafenib/cobimetinib, dabrafenib/trametinib, and encorafenib/binimetinib is now recommended in the treatment of several cancers. As demonstrated by the aforementioned disease states, targeted therapy within the ERK/MAPK signaling pathway will need to be individualized by disease state.

5.3.2 PI3K/AKT/mTOR

The PI3K/Akt/mTOR pathway is one of the primary pathways regulating cell growth and survival. It is a complex network with many interconnected mediators. Phosphatidyl-inositol-3-kinases (PI3Ks) are a class of intracellular lipid kinases that phosphorylate inositol phospholipids. They are composed of three subunits: p85, p55, and p110, which is the catalytic subunit (Yang et al. 2019). In normal physiologic conditions, PI3K is activated by growth factors, cytokines, and hormones (see Figure 5.4) (Yang et al. 2019). PI3K activation catalyzes the production of phosphatidylinositol-3,4,5-triphosphate (PIP3), which is a second messenger that targets and phosphorylates Akt through the PDK1 enzyme (Yang et al. 2019). Activated Akt kinases then phosphorylate many downstream proteins that regulate cellular functions. One of the major downstream recipients of Akt signaling is mTOR (Porta, Paglino, and Mosca 2014). Akt phosphorylates a negative regulator of mTOR, TSC2, thus stimulating mTOR activity. mTOR consists of mTORC1 and mTORC2 complexes, and in general, it is responsible for carrying out many synthetic activities in promoting cell growth. One of the primary negative regulators of the PI3K pathway is PTEN, which dephosphorylates PIP3 to PIP2, blocking activation of downstream kinases. Loss or inactivation of PTEN is observed in many cancers, including glioblastoma; uterine, cervical, prostate, and breast cancer; melanoma; NSCLC; and others (Dillon and Miller 2014).

Many tumors exhibit alterations in the PI3K pathway that can lead to hyper-activation of the pathway and subsequent tumor proliferation. Therefore, several classes of drugs were developed to target various stages of the pathway. The mTOR inhibitors form a complex with the FK506 binding protein-12 that blocks mTOR activity and downstream signaling (Porta, Paglino, and Mosca 2014). The original mTOR inhibitor, rapamycin, had an unfavorable pharmacokinetic profile that precluded its use in cancer patients. Temsirolimus and everolimus are the currently available mTOR inhibitors; temsirolimus is used in endometrial and renal cell cancers, while everolimus is used in breast, renal cell, and neuroendocrine tumors (Porta, Paglino, and Mosca 2014). Toxicities of the mTOR inhibitors include stomatitis, skin rash, pneumonitis, metabolic abnormalities, and immunosuppression.

PI3K inhibitors are a newer class of agents that includes pan-inhibitors, isoform-specific inhibitors, or dual PI3K/mTOR inhibitors. Pan-inhibitors target multiple isoforms of p110 and include copanlisib and duvelisib. Copanlisib targets PI3Kα, β, γ, and δ, whereas duvelisib inhibits the δ and γ isoforms. PI3Kγ and PI3Kδ are expressed primarily in hematopoietic tissues; hence the use of copanlisib and duvelisib in hematologic malignancies (Mensah, Blaize, and Bryan 2018). PI3K isoform–specific inhibitors, such as idelalisib and alpelisib, were designed to have greater specificity for certain isoforms and thereby fewer toxicities compared with pan-inhibitors. Alpelisib targets PI3Kα, which is hyperactive in PIK3CA gene activating mutations. Alpelisib is used in metastatic ER+, HER2- breast cancer patients who have known mutations in PIK3CA (Yang et al. 2019). Idelalisib targets PI3Kδ and is used in chronic lymphocytic leukemia, small lymphocytic lymphoma, and follicular lymphoma (Yang et al. 2019). The PI3K inhibitors have a significant toxicity profile, including diarrhea, hyperglycemia, hypertension, cutaneous reactions, myelosuppression, infection, hepatic dysfunction, and pulmonary toxicity. Dual PI3K/mTOR inhibitors are currently still in clinical studies but have shown promising results in preclinical settings with improved efficacy compared with PI3K or mTOR inhibitors alone (Tarantelli et al. 2020).

5.3.3 EGFR

EGFRs are a family of transmembrane receptors consisting of ErbB1/HER1, ErbB2/HER2/Neu, ErbB3/HER3, and ErbB4/HER4. The EGFR receptor is composed of an extracellular ligand binding domain, transmembrane region, and intracellular domain with TK function (Wee and Wang 2017). The extracellular region consists of four domains: domains I and III partake in ligand binding; domain II forms homo- or hetero-dimers; and domain IV links to the transmembrane domain (Wee and Wang 2017). Epidermal growth factor (EGF) is considered the most important ligand for EGFR; other ligands that bind to the receptor include transforming growth factor-α, amphiregulin, heparin-binding EGF, and betacelulin. Ligand binding to EGFR results in receptor homo- or hetero-dimerization and autophosphorylation of the TK domain. Once the TK domain is phosphorylated, it serves as an anchor for various proteins that participate in downstream signal transduction. Two of the primary pathways activated by this phosphorylation are RAS/RAF/MEK and PI3K/AKT/mTOR (Herbst 2004). Since EGFR is implicated in several major pathways for cell proliferation and differentiation, it is a compelling target for treatment of associated cancers.

In normal cells, there are estimated to be 40,000–100,000 EGFR receptors per cell, whereas in cancerous cells, there can be more than 1,000,000 receptors per cell (Wee and Wang 2017). EGFR overexpression is observed in many cancers, such as head and neck, breast, non-small cell lung (NSCLC), colorectal, prostate, kidney, pancreas, ovary, and brain (Ayati et al. 2020). EGFR mutations can also lead to constitutive activation of the receptor by inducing ligand-independent receptor dimerization or rendering the TK overactive (Wee and Wang 2017). Two common activating kinase domain mutations are the L858R point mutation and various exon 19 in-frame deletions. These mutations are found in approximately 17% of patients with NSCLC (Morgensztern, Politi, and Herbst 2015). T790M is a kinase mutation that confers resistance to several EGFR TK inhibitors (TKIs) in the treatment of NSCLC and is present in about 50% of patients who acquire resistance.

Agents that inhibit EGFR activity include small molecule TKIs and mAbs targeting the extracellular receptor (Herbst 2004). mAbs demonstrate greater specificity for EGFR compared with small molecules, but they require intravenous administration and can induce immune-antibody responses that may inactivate the mAb (Herbst 2004). The currently approved EGFR mAbs are cetuximab and panitumumab. Both bind competitively to EGFR extracellular domain III, preventing ligand binding and receptor dimerization as well as promoting internalization of the receptor complex for degradation. Cetuximab is an IgG1 mAb, whereas panitumumab is IgG2, and this distinction is thought to result in an increase of immunostimulatory actions with cetuximab, theoretically increasing anticancer effect. Cetuximab is indicated for head and neck cancer and colorectal cancer (CRC), whereas panitumumab is only indicated for CRC. Mutations in the RAS gene can lead to constitutive activation of the RAS/RAF/MEK/ERK pathway in CRC, thus rendering upstream EGFR inhibition futile. Therefore, RAS mutation status is always checked prior to treatment with cetuximab or panitumumab in CRC and patients are only started on treatment if they have wild-type RAS.

Small molecule TKIs are classified by generations and include the following approved agents: gefitinib, erlotinib (first generation); afatinib, dacomitinib (second generation); and osimertinib (third generation) (Ayati et al. 2020). The TKIs bind to the ATP binding site in the mutated kinase domain and prevent intracellular phosphorylation and the subsequent downstream effects of cell proliferation. The first-generation agents bind reversibly to the TK domain, while the second- and third generation agents bind irreversibly. Afatinib and dacomitinib were designed to overcome resistance seen with erlotinib and gefitinib, and osimertinib was designed specifically to target the T790M mutation in addition to other common EGFR mutations. Osimertinib is now preferred for first-line treatment of NSCLC patients with sensitizing EGFR mutations due to superior efficacy compared with other agents.

The most common side effect of EGFR inhibitors is acneiform rash, occurring in 65–90% of patients. EGFR is expressed in the epidermis, where inhibition can lead to cell apoptosis and release of inflammatory chemokines, which manifests as acneiform rash (Fabbrocini et al. 2015). Studies have found that patients who develop a skin rash may respond better to EGFR inhibitors, so development of a rash is often used as a marker of clinical efficacy (Wacker et al. 2007). Other adverse events include diarrhea, nausea, and vomiting. Ongoing research is investigating mechanisms of resistance to current EGFR inhibitors and studying additional generations of EGFR TKIs.

5.3.4 HER2

HER2, a member of the EGFR receptor family, is overexpressed in a variety of tumors, most notably breast, gastric, and uterine cancers. Unlike the other ErbB receptors, HER2 is known as an orphan receptor because it does not bind to an identified ligand; rather, it heterodimerizes with other ErbB receptors. HER2 overexpression results in increased receptor homo- and heterodimerization, driving downstream signaling for cell differentiation and proliferation, and is associated with poor prognosis in breast cancer. Trastuzumab is a humanized mAb that binds to the extracellular domain IV and selectively exerts activity in HER2-positive cancer cells. A major mechanism of trastuzumab is antibody-dependent cell-mediated cytotoxicity, in which the Fc receptor on immune effector cells attaches to the Fc portion of trastuzumab, allowing the immune cell to attack the tumor cell (Nami, Maadi, and Wang 2018). Trastuzumab is used in HER2+ early-stage and metastatic breast cancer, gastric cancer, and uterine cancer. It is well tolerated, although the disruption of HER2 signaling in cardiomyocytes can cause suppression of autophagy and accumulation of reactive oxygen species, producing reversible cardiotoxicity.

Pertuzumab is another humanized HER2-targeting mAb, but it binds to domain II of the extracellular region and thus blocks receptor dimerization. Unlike trastuzumab, pertuzumab exhibits only modest activity when administered as a single agent, but it demonstrates clinical synergism when given in combination with trastuzumab. Since pertuzumab blocks HER2 from dimerizing with EGFR, it can cause diarrhea, as EGFR is expressed by epithelial cells throughout the gastrointestinal tract (Bines et al. 2020). Aside from diarrhea, there is a similar risk of cardiotoxicity as with trastuzumab.

There are three small molecule TKIs that target HER2: lapatinib, neratinib, and tucatinib. Lapatinib, a reversible inhibitor, was the first HER2 TKI to be approved for the treatment of metastatic HER2+ breast cancer in combination with capecitabine or letrozole and demonstrated a modest benefit in efficacy (Chien and Rugo 2017). Neratinib is an irreversible TKI that covalently binds to the ATP binding sites of several EGFR receptors. While potent, neratinib showed only a modest benefit in efficacy in the extended adjuvant and metastatic settings. Any benefit in efficacy would have to be weighed against the significant risk of diarrhea, which occurs in 95% of patients (Nerlynx [package insert]). Tucatinib is the newest TKI with greater selectivity for HER2 than EGFR. It was studied in combination with trastuzumab and capecitabine in metastatic HER2+ breast cancer patients and demonstrated a significant improvement in OS (Murthy et al. 2020). All three TKIs cross the blood–brain barrier and serve as viable choices for patients with brain metastases, who typically have limited treatment options.

5.3.5 MET

The mesenchymal epithelial transition factor (MET) receptor is a functioning transmembrane RTK that plays a role in trophoblast and hepatocyte development in the placenta. MET becomes activated through hepatocyte growth factor (HGF) binding, receptor homodimerization, phosphorylation of the TK domain, and subsequent activation of downstream signaling pathways, including cell proliferation pathways such as RAS/RAF/MEK/ERK, PI3K-AKT, Wnt/β-catenin, and JAK/STAT. In adults, the MET RTK is seen in a range of tissues and has an identified role in tissue injury response (Drilon et al. 2017). Similar to other RTKs, aberrations in the MET protein can result in oncogenesis. Constitutive activation of MET can be due to mutations, receptor or ligand overexpression, or rearrangements. These alterations are theoretically targetable through either mAb action on HGF or MET or TK inhibition of MET activation, with medications being studied for each of these targets (Wang et al. 2019). Unfortunately, MET inhibition has not shown significant clinical benefit so far (Reungwetwattana et al. 2017).

MET exon 14 alterations, however, have become an exception and have demonstrated recent benefit as a clinical target of MET inhibition. Exon 14 contributes to the MET juxtamembrane domain binding site function, and during normal MET protein synthesis, introns surrounding exon 14 are removed via RNA splicing. Alterations in exon 14 result in skipping, which leads to a non-function binding site and decreased degradation of the MET protein. The MET RTK then continues to activate the signal transduction proliferation pathways. These exon 14 alterations include a wide range of possible variations, including mutations and deletions, and they are estimated to be present in 3–4% of NSCLC adenocarcinomas (Drilon et al. 2017). Crizotinib, an oral TKI that is also used in ALK or ROS1 positive NSCLC, exhibits MET inhibition. Crizotinib demonstrated an objective response rate (ORR) of 32% when it was assessed in 69 patients with advanced MET exon 14 altered NSCLC (Drilon et al. 2020b). Capmatinib, another oral TKI with activity against MET exon 14 alterations, received FDA approval in 2020. This approval was based on a phase 2 trial of patients with advanced NSCLC with either MET exon 14 skipping mutation or MET amplification. In the patients with a MET exon 14 skipping alteration, 41% of patients who had previously received systemic treatment had a response compared with 68% of patients who had not received previous treatment. The responses were noted to have a quick onset of effect, and the median durations of response were 9.7 and 12.6 months, respectively, for the two groups. The MET amplification group had a less robust effect with capmatinib, with an ORR less than 20% (Wolf et al. 2020). Known adverse effects with MET inhibition include peripheral edema and nausea and vomiting, but the drugs have overall proved tolerable. Capmatinib also has the added benefit of crossing the blood–brain barrier, which is useful in brain metastases. Based on this data, capmatinib is the new standard of care as first-line therapy in MET exon 14 skipping NSCLC.

MET inhibition has also been suggested as a method to overcome resistance that develops during EGFR inhibitor treatment in NSCLC. The MET pathway demonstrates crosstalk with other RTK signal transduction pathways, such as the EGFR activation pathway, and can serve as a bypass pathway during EGFR inhibition (Drilon et al. 2017). Combination therapy with EGFR and MET inhibitors may help to potentially overcome one mechanism of resistance to EGFR inhibitors. Future development of MET inhibitor application may also involve identifying additional therapy targets, such as thresholds for protein or ligand amplification for clinical benefit, and identifying additional activating targets in addition to MET exon 14 skipping (Salgia 2017).

5.3.6 JAK/STAT

Myeloproliferative neoplasms (MPNs) are a group of diseases involving clonal proliferation of terminally differentiated cells of the myeloid lineage. These include essential thrombocytosis (ET), polycythemia vera (PV), and primary myelofibrosis (MF). The proliferation of these cells has been associated with Janus associated kinase 2 (JAK2) V617F mutation, which has been identified in 95% of patients with PV and in 50–60% of patients with ET and MF (Baxter et al. 2005; Kralovics et al. 2005).

The JAK/STAT signaling pathway regulates hematopoiesis and immune response. The JAK family includes four intracellular TKs bound to cytokine receptors. Once JAK is activated, it phosphorylates downstream signal transducer and activator of transcription (STAT) proteins to signal for gene transcription (see Figure 5.4). In MPNs, JAK2 mutation causes overactive signaling of the JAK/STAT pathway and aberrant downstream cell differentiation and proliferation (Bewersdorf et al. 2019). JAK/STAT modulates immune-cell activation and inflammation during acute graft-versus-host disease (GVHD), specifically neutrophil and dendritic cell activity.

Ruxolitinib inhibits JAK1 and JAK2 and is non-specific for the JAK2 V617F mutation. Its approval in MF is based on the COMFORT-I and COMFORT-II trials, which showed significant improvements in symptoms and spleen size when treated with ruxolitinib (Verstovsek et al. 2012; Harrison et al. 2012). However, 50–75% of patients experienced treatment failure or toxicities after 3–5 years. Ruxolitinib resistance has been postulated to be related to variable JAK2 V617F and other mutations, and possible JAK/STAT activation uninhibited by ruxolitinib. Fedratinib is a selective JAK2 inhibitor approved for primary or secondary MF. The JAKARTA-2 study showed significant improvements in symptoms and spleen size in patients with MF who were resistant or intolerant to ruxolitinib (Harrison et al. 2017). Lastly, ruxolitinib is also approved for steroid refractory acute GVHD based on the phase 3 REACH2 study showing improved overall response and OS (Zeiser et al. 2020).

5.3.7 ALK

Anaplastic lymphoma kinase (ALK) is a transmembrane RTK that has been identified as an oncogenic driver, currently most effectively targeted in NSCLC. The main function of the ALK protein, which is encoded by the ALK gene on chromosome 2, is neonatal nervous system development. In adults, only small amounts of the protein are produced and are limited to the nervous system, testes, and small intestine (Du et al. 2018; Lin, Riely, and Shaw 2017). Currently identified ligands include FAM150A (AUGβ) and FAM150B (AUGα), but additional ligands may be identified in the future (Hallberg and Palmer 2016). ALK activation by these ligands initiates the RAS/RAF/MEK/ERK, PI3K-AKT, JAK-STAT, and PLC-γ pathways, which produce the cell proliferation and survival necessary for oncogenesis (Du et al. 2018; Shaw and Engelman 2013). ALK-driven oncogenesis has also been identified as "oncogene addiction," which means that the cancers caused by receptor dimerization and stimulation are dependent on continued activation for survival and are susceptible to targeted inhibition (Shaw and Engelman 2013).

ALK rearrangements/fusions, point mutations, and amplifications have all been identified in cancer. The fusion between ALK and echinoderm microtubule-associated protein-like 4 (EML4) is created by a small inversion rearrangement in chromosome 2p and is the most commonly identified ALK fusion in NSCLC (Shaw and Engelman 2013; Du et al. 2018). Activating gene fusions cause continued activation of the ALK receptor and the downstream proliferation pathways, and they have also been identified in other cancers, including colorectal, breast, and anaplastic thyroid carcinoma (ATC), albeit at lower levels than in NSCLC (Lin, Riely, and Shaw 2017). Gene rearrangements within ALK occur in around 5% of NSCLC cases and are more common in non-smokers and younger patients (Du et al. 2018). ALK point mutations have been identified as oncogenic in neuroblastoma and ATC, but point mutations are also the most commonly identified cause of acquired resistance to ALK inhibitors in NSCLC, seen in approximately 30% of cases with an identified resistance mechanism (Du et al. 2018; Hallberg and Palmer 2016).

Several ALK-targeted TKIs have received approval from the FDA for metastatic ALK-positive NSCLC, including alectinib, brigatinib, ceritinib, crizotinib, and lorlatinib. Crizotinib was the first to receive approval in 2011 with evidence of improved PFS and response rate in comparison to cytotoxic chemotherapy, but it has since lost favor as first-line therapy in ALK-positive NSCLC due to increased rate of progression or death compared with alectinib in the phase 3 ALEX trial. Alectinib and several other later-generation ALK-targeted TKIs have greater penetration into the central nervous system (CNS), reducing brain metastasis development and progression. Additionally, they can overcome several point mutations that spur crizotinib resistance (Lin, Riely, and Shaw 2017). The identification of specific point mutations such as C1156Y (crizotinib resistance) or L11198F (lorlatinib resistance) can help guide targeted therapy for individual patients (Hallberg and Palmer 2016). Toxicities differ between the ALK-targeted TKIs, most likely due to off-target mechanisms. For example, ceritinib is associated with higher rates of diarrhea, nausea, and vomiting, while crizotinib has higher rates of QT prolongation (Costa et al. 2018). Selecting ALK-targeted therapy for specific patients requires consideration of both potential resistance mechanisms and adverse effects.

5.3.8 ROS1

ROS1 protein alterations have been successfully identified and targeted as an oncogenic driver mutation. Similar to other RTKs, ROS1 is a protein that affects cell proliferation pathways, including RAS/RAF/MEK/ERK, PI3K/AKT, JAK/STAT3, and SHP1/2, but less is known about the non-oncogenic role of

ROS1 in human cells. ROS1 has neither an identified function in human development nor an identified activating ligand. The oncogenic chromosomal rearrangement form of ROS1 was initially identified in glioblastoma cells. It has since been identified in several cancer types, including ovarian cancer, colorectal cancer, and cholangiocarcinoma. Moreover, 1–2% of NSCLC cases have an identified ROS1 gene fusion (Lin and Shaw 2017). This fusion occurs when the 3′ section of the ROS1 (the kinase domain) combines with the 5′ section of another gene. The CD74-ROS1 is the most commonly identified fusion in NSCLC, although numerous fusion partners are possible. It remains unclear how these fusion proteins are activated, as the typical RTK dimerization regions are not present (Bubendorf et al. 2016).

ROS1 possesses a similar binding site to the ALK protein, and several of the currently FDA-approved ALK inhibitors also target ROS1. The TKI crizotinib received approval as a ROS1 inhibitor in 2016 after a response rate of 72% was demonstrated in advanced NSCLC. Although the high response rate and PFS of 19.2 months show promising efficacy, the majority of patients with an initial response to treatment eventually develop acquired resistance, as with other TKIs (Shaw et al. 2014). The development of resistance can occur through acquired mutations, such as the G2032R mutation that limits medication binding, or through signaling pathways that bypass ROS1 inhibition (Lin and Shaw 2017). Ceritinib also inhibits ROS1 and has the added effect of penetrating the blood–brain barrier. Ceritinib demonstrated a response rate of 62%, although use in clinical practice has been limited by adverse effects, including diarrhea, nausea, and vomiting (Lin and Shaw 2017; Lim et al. 2017). Entrectinib has also demonstrated clinical activity in patients with ROS1 fusion–positive NSCLC who have not received another TKI, with a response rate of 77% and similar tolerability to crizotinib (Drilon et al. 2020c). As in ALK-positive NSCLC, lorlatinib is also active in the setting of ROS1 fusions but is currently recommended as a subsequent TKI therapy.

5.3.9 RET

Successful targeting of the RET proto-oncogene, which was named due to the fact that it was discovered "rearranged during transfection" in 1985, has led to improvements in the treatment of several types of cancers in recent years (Li et al. 2019a). The RET gene encodes the RET RTK, a protein most commonly expressed in humans during embryogenesis across tissue types, which decreases in prevalence after development (Mulligan 2014). The primary effects of RET occur in the kidneys and neural crest cells, where activation produces cell proliferation via the RAS/RAF/MEK/ERK, PI3K/AKT, and JNK pathways. RET is different from other RTKs in that it is not activated directly by ligands but instead, requires a separate receptor from the glial cell–derived neurotrophic factor (GDNF) family to bind and undergo dimerization (Subbiah et al. 2020). Pathogenic loss-of-function mutations in RET can produce Hirschsprung disease (lack of neuroblast migration and neuron development), kidney or urothelial abnormalities, and other developmental complications (Subbiah et al. 2020).

Abnormal RET expression and activation can also be oncogenic. RET protein expression is associated with cancer across several malignancies, and it can be activated through germline or somatic mutations. Germline RET mutations produce MEN2, a syndrome associated with multiple tumor types, most commonly early-onset medullary thyroid carcinoma (MTC) (Mulligan 2014). Somatic alterations include fusion gene production, which is the most commonly identified aberration, and activating mutations, of which more than 60 have been reported. Ionizing radiation and other genotoxic stress factors are well-known risk factors for RET alterations due to the formation of DNA double-strand breaks and inaccurate repair mechanisms (Subbiah et al. 2020; Romei, Ciampi, and Elisei 2016). The RET fusion gene is comprised of the RET 3′ sequence and the partner gene 5′ sequence, forming CCDC6-RET or NCOA-RET, most commonly seen in papillary thyroid cancer (PTC), and KIF5B-RET, most commonly in NSCLC (Subbiah et al. 2020; Romei, Ciampi, and Elisei 2016; Li et al. 2019a). These fusion proteins, which occur in 10–20% of PTC cases and 1–2% of NSCLC cases, cause constitutive activation of the receptor and decrease the degradation, thereby overstimulating cell proliferation (Subbiah et al. 2020).

Several multi-targeted TKIs include RET as a target, including cabozantinib, lenvatinib, sunitinib, sorafenib, alectinib, regorafenib, and vandetanib. Vandetanib is a standard of care option for systemic therapy of MTC, and it was compared with placebo in a randomized phase 3 trial. PFS was significantly improved in the vandetanib group (Wells et al. 2012). Two newly approved, more selective RET inhibitors are now available: selpercatinib, which has received approval in RET-mutant or RET fusion–positive thyroid cancer and NSCLC, and pralsetinib, which has been approved in NSCLC. Ideally, the more selective RET inhibitors would demonstrate higher potency with fewer adverse effects, and they have also demonstrated intracranial activity. Several "gatekeeper mutations" have been identified with previous RET inhibitors (such as vandetanib), including RET V804M and V804L, but inhibition of these specific mutations has been seen with the newer agents, which highlights the importance of identifying and targeting specific mutations (Subbiah et al. 2020; Li et al. 2019a). Both selpercatinib and pralsetinib were studied in later-line treatment of RET fusion–positive NSCLC, where they demonstrated response rates of 64% and 57%, respectively. Additionally, a response rate of 70% was seen in a small subset of patients who received pralsetinib as first-line therapy (Drilon et al. 2020a; Gainor, Curigliano, and Kim 2020). Overall, the more selective RET inhibitors have been considered well tolerated, with the most common adverse effects including hypertension, increased aspartate transaminase/alanine transaminase (ALT/AST) ratio, and constipation. Future directions for RET inhibitors may include implementation in combination therapy with other targeted drugs, as the RET fusion mutations have been identified as a mechanism of EGFR-targeted resistance (Subbiah et al. 2020).

5.3.10 FGFR

Fibroblast growth factor receptors (FGFRs) 1–4 are a group of transmembrane RTKs that play a role in cell migration, proliferation, and regulation. In normal cell function, the extracellular domain provides a space for 23 different fibroblast growth factor (FGF) ligands to bind, which leads to receptor dimerization and activation of the tyrosine residue. Once activated, the RTKs activate signaling through the PI3K-AKT, STAT, and RAS/MAPK pathways, inducing cell proliferation, angiogenesis, differentiation, and other functions depending on the specific cell (Mahipal et al. 2020; Pederzoli et al. 2020; Casadei et al. 2019). FGF and FGFRs regulate endocrine function, wound repair, bile acid and phosphate homeostasis, and embryogenesis (Mahipal et al. 2020; Babina and Turner 2017). FGFR overactivation can occur due to receptor amplification, activating mutations, overstimulation (FGF excess), or gene fusions.

Receptor amplification occurs most frequently in FGFR1 and is identified in around 17% of NSCLC cases with squamous histology (Babina and Turner 2017). FGFR receptor activating mutations occur more commonly with FGFR2 and FGFR3; FGFR2 mutations occur in approximately 10% of endometrial carcinomas, and FGFR3 mutations are identified in 75% of non-muscle-invasive urothelial carcinomas (Babina and Turner 2017). These activating mutations often produce dimerization of the receptor, which initiates the signaling cascade even without ligand present. Gene fusions, most commonly with TACC3, are currently the best-understood and most successfully targeted oncogenic processes relating to FGFR. The active fusion proteins may produce continual stimulation of the TK domain (Babina and Turner 2017; Pederzoli et al. 2020). FGFR2 fusions are known to play a role in intrahepatic cholangiocarcinoma, and FGFR3 fusions have been increasingly identified in urothelial carcinoma, especially the luminal I subtype (Babina and Turner 2017; Loriot et al. 2019).

Erdafitinib is an oral FGFR inhibitor that acts on FGFR1–4 and has received approval in advanced urothelial carcinoma. In a phase 2 study, patients with FGFR mutations experienced a numerically higher response rate of 49% than those with FGFR fusions with a rate of 16% (Loriot et al. 2019). Pemigatinib is another oral FGFR-targeted therapy that inhibits FGFR1–3. In patients with cholangiocarcinoma with FGFR2 alterations, 35.5% had a response to treatment with pemigatinib in the second-line setting (Abou-Alfa et al. 2020). Additional FGFR inhibitors currently in development include infigratinib, vofatamab, and ragaratinib; a few additional multi-targeted TKIs such as lenvatinib also inhibit FGFR1–4 (Pederzoli et al. 2020). Current limitations to anti-FGFR therapy include identifying patients with susceptible alterations and managing unacceptable adverse effects. On-target toxicity of FGFR-targeted therapy includes diarrhea, hyperphosphatemia, and retinal detachment (Babina and Turner 2017; Mahipal et al. 2020), which are due to the regulatory roles that FGFR1–4 have in normal cell function, such as phosphate and bile acid homeostasis.

5.3.11 KIT

c-Kit is a gene that encodes the KIT RTK, which is in the same family as platelet-derived growth factor receptor (PDGFR). The KIT receptor is found throughout many types of human tissue cells and plays a crucial role in hematopoiesis, mast cell growth, melanin development, and germ cell production (Liang et al. 2013; Pittoni et al. 2011). Stem cell factor (SCF) is an activation ligand for the transmembrane KIT protein; once SCF is bound, the KIT receptor undergoes dimerization, which leads to activation of the TK region. This activation can initiate activity in multiple pathways depending on the cell type, including SRC kinases, JAK/STAT, RAS/RAF/MEK/ERK, PI3K, and PLCγ (Pittoni et al. 2011; Sattler and Salgia 2004). KIT receptors play a role in cell proliferation through several pathways, and loss of function can lead to a range of consequences, including alterations in hair or skin pigmentation and loss of hearing (Sattler and Salgia 2004; Liang et al. 2013). c-KIT has been labeled as a proto-oncogene due to its role in cancer cell proliferation, and KIT has been targeted in the treatment of several tumor types.

KIT mutations are present in around 20% of core binding factor acute myeloid leukemia (AML) and were initially associated with decreased duration of response and survival (Liang et al. 2013). The data have since become increasingly unclear regarding the role of KIT mutations in differing prognostic genetic classifications, and there is currently no widely accepted strategy for targeting KIT in AML. KIT targeting in melanoma has proven slightly more successful. Acral, mucosal, and chronic sun-damage melanoma are associated with KIT mutations, but the mutations occur much less commonly in the population of melanoma with intermittent sun exposure or without sun damage (Curtin et al. 2006). KIT-targeted therapy is currently recommended as subsequent therapy in melanoma with activating KIT mutations. Gastrointestinal stromal tumors (GISTs) have been the most successful target of KIT inhibition. Activating KIT mutations are found in 80–90% of GISTs, with an estimated 50% occurring in exon 11 (Liang et al. 2013; Sattler and Salgia 2004). Exon 11 encodes the juxtamembrane region, which normally provides an inhibitory function by preventing independent activation. Additional KIT mutation sites include exon 9 (the extracellular domain) and exon 13 (the kinase domain) (Sattler and Salgia 2004).

Imatinib is a multi-targeted TKI that is the current standard of care in GIST, largely due to its inhibition of KIT as well as its effect on PDGFR. Imatinib competes with the ATP binding site of the TK domain, thus blocking the activation of cell proliferation pathways (Pittoni et al. 2011). Certain KIT mutations affect response to imatinib and may warrant higher baseline dosing of imatinib. Exon 11 mutations have been associated with better response and survival in GIST, and the typical 400 mg daily dose of imatinib is considered sufficient. Exon 9 mutations, however, have shown greater response and survival with high-dose imatinib at a total of 800 mg per day (von Mehren, Kane, and Bui 2020). Adverse effects of imatinib include nausea/vomiting, fluid retention, hemorrhage, and skin rash. Additional TKIs with KIT targeting activity include midostaurin, dasatinib, and sorafenib, although these agents primarily work through other mechanisms.

5.3.12 PDGFR

Platelet-derived growth factors (PDGFs) and platelet-derived growth factor receptors (PDGFRs) are a group of four ligands and two RTKs that are critical in organ development, bone formation, and wound healing (Raica and Cimpean 2010). PDGFs are secreted by endothelial and epithelial cells and are released during platelet degranulation, and they possess angiogenic properties through the increase in VEGF production and regulation of hematopoietic precursor differentiation (Kazlauskas 2017; Raica and Cimpean 2010). PDGF-C specifically has been shown to play a role in maintaining the blood–brain barrier (Papadopoulos and Lennartsson 2018). Once bound and activated, PDGFR initiates intracellular signaling pathways that result in cell proliferation. Abnormal PDGF expression or function has been identified in conditions including scleroderma, fibrosis, atherosclerosis, and cancer (Papadopoulos and Lennartsson 2018). Within tumor cell proliferation, activating point mutations, rearrangements, and amplification of the receptor can all lead to increased activation and function. PDGFR has been implicated in glioblastoma, lung cancer, melanoma, breast cancer, and sarcomas, both in cancerous cells and in the tumor stroma or microenvironment (Kazlauskas 2017; Papadopoulos and Lennartsson 2018).

Soft tissue sarcomas (STS) in particular have been identified as a therapeutic focus of PDGFR inhibition. Increased expression of both the ligand and the receptor has been identified in a wide range of STS and has been identified as a poor prognostic factor through *in vitro* analysis (Andrick and Gandhi 2017). In addition, 5–10% of GISTs express a mutation in the gene encoding PDGFR-alpha (PDGFRA) (Zobniw et al. 2019). Imatinib, an oral TKI, is the standard of care for GIST due to its activity against c-Kit and PDGFRA (including many exon 18 mutations). Imatinib is also used in hypereosinophilic syndrome with PDGFRA fusion kinase, myelodysplastic syndrome with PDGFR rearrangements, and PDGFR-expressing chordomas. Avapritinib is a recently approved TKI that targets PDGFRA exon 18 mutations, which commonly cause imatinib resistance in GIST, allowing therapy to be further individualized. Additional multi-targeted TKIs that partially exert action through PDGFR inhibition in multiple disease states include nilotinib, dasatinib, ponatinib, sunitinib, axitinib, midostaurin, pazopanib, regorafenib, sorafenib, nindetanib, lenvatinib, and ripretinib (Papadopoulos and Lennartsson 2018).

Olaratumab is a mAb that had been approved by the FDA but was later withdrawn from the market due to a lack of clinical benefit in survival outcomes in STS. Olaratumab is an IgG1 mAb that binds to PDGFRA, preventing binding and initiation of the cell growth and angiogenesis cascades (Andrick and Gandhi 2017). Olaratumab had initially shown a significant improvement in OS in STS in a phase 1b/2 study, but the phase 3 randomized trial did not confirm the effect. It is currently being reviewed in additional clinical trials for STS, pancreatic cancer, ovarian cancer, prostate cancer, and NSCLC. PDGFR-targeted TKIs and mAbs have been shown to have adverse effects including gastrointestinal toxicity, edema, and increased risk of hemorrhage or bleeding. Although PDGFR-specific targeting has not yet demonstrated significant efficacy in a broad population on its own, future research will continue to evaluate specific populations and combination therapy with other anticancer treatments.

5.3.13 Hedgehog Pathway

Hedgehog (HH) pathway signaling acts as a vital process during mammalian development and then becomes inactivated in adult tissue. Under typical circumstances, the cell surface receptor PTCH1 is a tumor suppressor gene that prevents the smoothened (SMO) protein pathway from initiating aberrant cell growth. During activation, the extracellular ligands sonic HH, Indian HH, and desert HH bind to the PTCH1 receptor, which reactivates SMO and initiates a cascade of signals through suppressor of fused (SUFU) and GlI1, GlI2, and GlI3 transcription factors (Epstein 2008). The reactivation of the pathway can produce unwanted cell division, which has been identified in cancer types including both hematologic malignancies and solid tumors, such as breast, lung, and prostate cancers (Cortes et al. 2019b). In addition, crosstalk between signaling pathways has also been noted with both the PI3K-Akt and Ras/Raf/MEK/ERK, both of which contribute to cancer development and growth (Epstein 2008; Cortes et al. 2019b).

Three drugs have been approved to directly target the HH pathway: sonidegib, vismodegib, and glasdegib. All three inhibit signal transduction through binding at SMO and were developed by targeting specific populations and disease states in which HH signaling was more pronounced, including basal cell carcinoma (BCC) and leukemia. BCC exhibits activating mutations in PTCH1 in 90% of cases and mutations in SMO in 10% of cases (Epstein 2008). Although most BCC can be surgically resected, sonidegib and vismodegib provide a targeted treatment option for locally advanced or metastatic cases. In the leukemia setting, glasdegib was shown to induce regression and reduce expression of stem-cell regulators in preclinical models. Clinically, glasdegib resulted in an increased OS in combination with low-dose cytarabine as compared with cytarabine alone in adults with AML who were not candidates for intensive chemotherapy (Cortes et al. 2019a). Adverse effects observed with these agents include muscle cramping, alopecia, dysgeusia, and weight loss, and these are thought to be on-target effects. HH signaling plays a role in hair growth and taste bud production, so alopecia and dysgeusia are expected when the SMO signaling is blocked (Sekulic et al. 2013). The HH pathway will continue to be an area of tumor targeting in clinical trials because of its known effect on cancer cell division in multiple tumor types.

5.3.14 BCR-ABL

From the 1960s to the 1990s, major discoveries were made in the understanding of chronic myeloid leukemia (CML), including the discovery of the Philadelphia (Ph) chromosome, the translocation involved with chromosomes 9 and 22, the resultant BCR/ABL oncoprotein, and their roles in CML (Goldman and Daley 2007). With these discoveries, tumor-targeted drugs such as TKIs were developed, drastically changing the CML treatment landscape. The Philadelphia chromosome is an oncogene that results from the reciprocal translocation t(9;22)(q34;q11.20): the fusion of the Abelson TK (ABL) gene at chromosome band 9q34 with the breakpoint cluster region (BCR) gene at chromosome band 22q11.2. This fusion gene encodes the oncoprotein BCR/ABL (Li et al. 1999). The juxtaposition of BCR activates ABL TK by dimerization or tetramerization of the fusion protein, encouraging autophosphorylation and subsequent increase in binding sites for SH2 domains of other proteins. With its many binding sites, BCR/ABL interacts with other cytoplasmic molecules in the oncogenic pathway, leading to abnormal multi-protein signaling processes that increase cell proliferation (Melo and Deininger 2004).

Imatinib was the first BCR/ABL TKI approved in 2001 for the treatment of CML. It is a 2-phenylaminopyrimidine TKI of ABL kinase, BCR-ABL fusion kinase, PDGFR, C-KIT, and *Abelson-related genes*. Imatinib binds to the BCR/ABL ATP binding site and stabilizes the inactive form of the oncoprotein, preventing autophosphorylation and phosphorylation of other molecules. This stops the downstream signaling in the oncogenic pathway. The IRIS trial compared imatinib with interferon-alfa in the treatment of CML and found imatinib to have a significantly higher OS rate. Imatinib also induced deeper cytogenetic and molecular responses that translated to reduced risk of relapse, progression, and death (Fava and Saglio 2010).

Despite the success observed with imatinib, some patients develop resistance after attaining initial response. Several newer generations of BCR/ABL TKIs have been developed to overcome imatinib resistance. These include second-generation agents (dasatinib, nilotinib, bosutinib) and a third-generation agent (ponatinib) (Bitencourt, Zalcberg, and Louro 2011). Nevertheless, resistance to these newer TKIs has also been identified. Several mechanisms of resistance have been proposed. These include BCR/ABL gene amplification, point mutations in the BCR/ABL kinase domain, and overexpression of multi-drug resistance genes (P-glycoprotein) (Milojkovic and Apperley 2009). The most common mutation identified is T315I (the gate keeper mutation), which is a point mutation in the BCR/ABL protein ATP binding site. This mutation confers resistance to not only imatinib but also dasatinib and nilotinib. Ponatinib is the only TKI that can effectively bind to BCR/ABL with T315I mutations. Other mutations identified include V299L (confers resistance to bosutinib and dasatinib) and E255K/V (confers resistance to nilotinib) (Bitencourt, Zalcberg, and Louro 2011). Due to possible drug resistance stemming from genetic aberrations, part of tumor-targeted treatment involves the identification of the aforementioned mutations and selecting a TKI based on resistance patterns.

5.3.15 BCL2

Dysregulation of apoptosis, evident in certain cancers, can lead to uncontrolled cell proliferation, eventually resulting in an accumulation of malignant cells. Hematologic malignancies are especially prone to consequences from dysregulated apoptosis due to their high cell turnover. B-cell lymphoma-2 (BCL-2) is one anti-apoptotic protein that has been found to be upregulated in hematologic malignancies such as

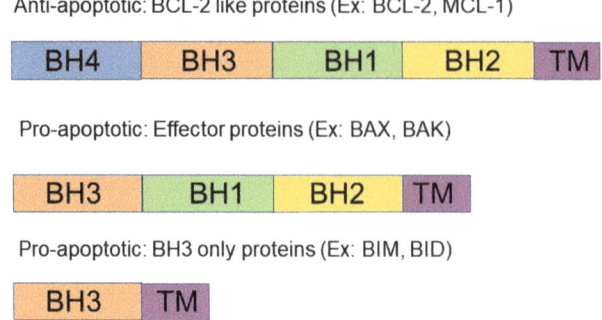

FIGURE 5.5   BCL2 protein family

chronic lymphocytic lymphoma (CLL) and AML. High levels of BCL-2 gene expression were initially observed in follicular lymphoma, which prompted the development of BCL-2 inhibitors such as venetoclax (Campbell and Tait 2018).

The intrinsic apoptosis pathway is regulated by BCL-2 family proteins, which include both pro- and anti-apoptotic proteins. Anti-apoptotic BCL-2 protein inhibits pro-apoptotic BAX and BAK proteins from initiating the apoptotic cascade. By inhibition of BCL-2, BAX and BAK proteins are activated, creating oligomeric pore formations on the mitochondrial membrane. This causes mitochondrial outer membrane permeability (MOMP) and the subsequent release of cytochrome C complex. Cytochrome C binds to APAF-1 to form apoptosomes, eventually resulting in cell death (Lachowiez, DiNardo, and Konopleva 2020; Zaman, Wang, and Gandhi 2014).

The BCL-2 protein family is classified by four amino acid domains: BCL-2 homology (BH) 1 to 4 (see Figure 5.5). BH3-only proteins are pro-apoptotic and inhibit the anti-apoptotic actions of BCL-2 by binding to the BH3 region of BCL-2. The understanding of this interaction between BH3-only proteins and BCL-2 led to the discovery of BCL-2-dependent malignancies through BH3 profiling, as well as the development of BH3 mimetic drugs. BH3 profiling is a mitochondrial assay that uses BH3 peptides to examine the dependence of cell survival on anti-apoptotic proteins such as BCL-2. Several hematologic malignancies have been shown to be dependent on BCL-2, including CLL/SLL, AML, and MM (Del Gaizo Moore et al. 2007; Pollyea et al. 2019; Touzeau et al. 2016).

Venetoclax is an oral BH3 mimetic small molecule co-crystal that confers high selectivity for BCL-2. It binds to the BH3-domain of the BCL-2 protein to initiate the pro-apoptotic cascade. It is approved for the treatment of adult patients with CLL/small lymphocytic lymphoma (SLL), and in combination with azacitidine, decitabine, or low-dose cytarabine (LDAC), for newly diagnosed AML patients who are 75 years or older, or who have comorbidities that preclude use of intensive induction chemotherapy (Venetoclax [package insert]). In CLL, venetoclax was studied in the CLL14 phase 3 trial in combination with obinutuzumab versus chlorambucil with obinutuzumab in previously untreated CLL patients with significant comorbidities. Results showed that venetoclax with obinutuzumab improved PFS and had a better overall response rate, including complete response, and better undetected minimal residual disease (MRD) at 3 and 12 months (Fischer et al. 2019). Venetoclax was also studied in the MURANO phase 3 study in combination with rituximab versus bendamustine with rituximab in CLL patients who had received at least one prior line of therapy. The results showed that venetoclax with rituximab improved ORR and PFS (Seymour et al. 2018).

In AML, venetoclax was initially granted accelerated approval in combination with azacitidine (aza/ven), decitabine (dec/ven), or low-dose cytarabine (LDAC-ven) in newly diagnosed AML patients who are 75 years or older based on phase 2 trials showing impressive response rates and OS (DiNardo et al. 2019; Wei et al. 2019). The phase 3 VIALE-A trial confirmed phase 2 findings with 34% reduction in the risk of death and much improved OS with aza/ven versus azacitidine alone in the same patient population (DiNardo et al. 2020). Similarly, the phase 3 VIALE-C trial showed a trend towards improved survival with LDAC/ven and offered a treatment option for patients previously exposed to azacitidine (Wei et al. 2020). With the introduction of targeted therapy in AML and its evident clinical efficacy, aza/ven has become the new standard of care for older patients who are not eligible for inductive chemotherapy.

5.3.16 FLT3

FMS-related tyrosine kinase 3 (FLT3) is an RTK expressed by progenitor cells that are lineage-restricted. FLT3-internal tandem duplication (ITD) mutation in AML blast cells constitutively activates the TK function and is associated with increased disease relapse and lower OS (Kiyoi et al. 1999; Kottaridis et al. 2002; Pratz and Levis 2017). Another identified mutation is the FLT3-tyrosine kinase domain (TKD), which does not carry the same prognostic risk as the ITD mutation (Abu-Duhier et al. 2001).

With several FLT3-targeted drugs available, the use of these agents exerts the most benefit in different settings depending on their spectrum and potency of inhibitory activity. Five FLT3 TKIs (midostaurin, sorafenib, quizartinib, gilteritinib, and crenolanib) have been investigated in early-phase or phase 3 trials with promising results (Pratz and Levis 2017). The first-generation FLT3 inhibitors, including sorafenib and midostaurin, were broad-spectrum multi-kinase inhibitors that did not exclusively target FLT3. Midostaurin was originally developed as a protein kinase C (PKC) inhibitor but was found to inhibit multiple other kinases, including FLT3, VEGFR2, c-KIT, and PDGFR-α (Propper et al. 2001). Initial studies of midostaurin monotherapy in AML patients showed significant blast reduction but failed to induce durable responses (Fischer et al. 2010). This led to midostaurin combination therapy with cytarabine and anthracycline, as studied in the phase 3 RATIFY trial in newly diagnosed FLT3-mutated AML. Significantly prolonged OS and event-free survival (EFS) shown in the RATIFY trial led to the FDA approval of midostaurin as the first FLT3 inhibitor, indicated in combination with cytarabine and anthracycline for newly diagnosed AML (Stone et al. 2017). It has been hypothesized that multi-kinase FLT3 inhibitors would be more effective than selective FLT3 inhibitors in the front-line setting due to the polyclonal nature of newly diagnosed AML. Similarly, sorafenib, another multi-kinase inhibitor, has also shown improved EFS in the phase 2 SORAML trial when used with induction therapy in newly diagnosed AML patients (Röllig et al. 2015).

Second-generation FLT3 inhibitors, including gilteritinib, quizartinib, and crenolanib, were developed to target FLT3 specifically and thus are more selective and potent. Gilteritinib is the second FDA-approved FLT3 inhibitor, indicated as monotherapy for the treatment of relapsed or refractory FLT3 mutated AML. The phase 3 ADMIRAL trial showed significantly improved OS compared with salvage chemotherapy (Perl et al. 2019). It is hypothesized that monotherapy with highly potent and selective FLT3 inhibitors may be more beneficial in patients with relapsed or refractory FLT3 mutated AML due to its likely oligoclonal nature.

5.3.17 BTK Inhibitors

Bruton tyrosine kinase (BTK) is a part of the B-cell receptor signaling pathway. B-cell receptor signaling is a very important regulator of cell proliferation and survival in a number of B-cell malignancies. Upregulated BTK expression is seen in malignant B-cell disorders such as CLL, mantle cell lymphoma (MCL), and Waldenstrom's microglobulinemia (WM). This upregulation results in BTK-dependent B-cell receptor activation for aberrant cellular proliferation, which makes BTK ideal for targeted treatment (Akinleye et al. 2013; Niemann et al. 2016). Several BTK inhibitors have been FDA approved for the treatment of B-cell malignancies (Morabito et al. 2020).

Ibrutinib is a first-generation BTK inhibitor approved for CLL/SLL, WM, MCL, and marginal zone lymphoma (MZL). It binds to the ATP binding site, inactivating the protein and inhibiting subsequent cell proliferation. Aside from BTK, ibrutinib also inhibits many other TKs, including EGFR, interleukin 2–inducible T-cell kinase (ITK), and protein tyrosine kinase (TEC) (Akinleye et al. 2013). This off-target inhibition leads to ibrutinib's many side effects, such as bleeding, atrial fibrillation, hypertension, diarrhea, cytopenias, and serious infections. Due to its side effect profile, ibrutinib use has been limited to certain patients, and other BTK inhibitors or treatments may be preferred. The second-generation BTK inhibitors acalabrutinib and zanubrutinib have greater BTK specificity with minimal off-target inhibition and fewer side effects compared with ibrutinib. Acalabrutinib is approved for CLL/SLL and MCL, and zanubrutinib is approved for MCL (Morabito et al. 2020).

In CLL, ibrutinib, acalabrutinib, and venetoclax with a CD20 mAb are all category 1 recommended treatment options for both treatment-naive and relapsed/refractory disease. However, ibrutinib is rarely used as front-line therapy, and acalabrutinib is often preferred in the relapsed/refractory (R/R) setting. Acalabrutinib showed impressive clinical efficacy and safety in the phase III trials ELEVATE-TN and ASCEND. ELEVATE-TN compared acalabrutinib monotherapy, or acalabrutinib with obinutuzumab, against chlorambucil with obinutuzumab in untreated CLL patients. Patients treated with acalabrutinib and obinutuzumab achieved a 90% reduction in risk of disease progression or death relative to chlorambucil with obinutuzumab (Sharman et al. 2020). The ASCEND trial evaluated acalabrutinib monotherapy compared with rituximab in combination with idelalisib or bendamustine in patients with R/R CLL. The results showed a significantly better PFS with acalabrutinib and a 69% risk reduction of disease progression or death (Ghia et al. 2020).

In MCL, the introduction of BTK inhibitors drastically changed the treatment landscape. Ibrutinib showed impressive PFS results in the phase 3 study. Later, acalabrutinib and zanubrutinib also showed improved response rates and PFS in the ACE-LY-004 and the BGB-3111-206 phase 2 studies, respectively, in patients with R/R MCL (Wang et al. 2018; Song et al. 2018). Furthermore, both showed better toxicity profiles and tolerance than ibrutinib.

5.3.18 NTRK Gene Fusions

The tropomyosin receptor kinase family (TRKA, TRKB, and TRKC) is present in tissues of the human nervous system and activates neurotrophins (NTs) during normal development and embryonal neuronal differentiation. These TRK receptors are transmembrane proteins that are encoded by neurotrophic receptor tyrosine kinase genes NTRK1, NTRK2, and NTRK3, and they bind preferentially to NGF, brain-derived neurotrophic factor (BDNF), neurotrophin 4 (NT-4), and neurotrophin 3 (NT-3) (Amatu, Sartore-Bianchi, and Siena 2016; Cocco, Scaltriti, and Drilon 2018). In more recent times, NTRK alterations have been identified as a targetable oncogenic pathway. Although overexpression, in-frame deletions, and alternative splicing of the NTRK genes are all possible, the most common activating NTRK alteration is gene fusion (Ricciuti et al. 2017). The NTRK gene 3′ segment is combined with a 5′ segment of a partner gene (of which over 60 possibilities have been pinpointed), forming a chimeric oncoprotein that leads to proliferation, differentiation, and survival of tumor cells (Amatu, Sartore-Bianchi, and Siena 2016; Scott 2019).

NTRK gene fusions have been identified in up to 1% of all solid tumors, which includes much higher percentages in some rare cancers such as secretory breast carcinoma, mammary analogue secretory carcinoma (MASC), congenital mesoblastic nephroma, and infantile fibrosarcomas. Expression is estimated to be in the range of 5–25% in papillary thyroid cancers and gastrointestinal stromal tumors (without the commonly identified KIT and PDGFRA mutations) and is considered to be <1% in NSCLC, squamous cell carcinoma (SCC) of the head and neck, breast cancer, colon cancer, renal cell carcinomas, non-GIST soft tissue sarcomas, and other solid tumors(Cocco, Scaltriti, and Drilon 2018; Ricciuti et al. 2017). Due to this expression across tumor types, there are currently two drugs with tumor-agnostic FDA-approved indications for NTRK gene fusion: larotrectinib and entrectinib.

Larotrectinib and entrectinib are both orally bioavailable TKIs, with larotrectinib being highly selective, whereas entrectinib also inhibits ROS1 and ALK oncogenic drivers. This inhibition of TRK induces cellular apoptosis and blocks signal transduction through the MAPK and PI3K pathways that would lead to tumor cell growth (Amatu, Sartore-Bianchi, and Siena 2016; Scott 2019). In two separate pooled analyses of phase 1 and 2 clinical trials of solid tumors with NTRK gene fusions, larotrectinib elicited an ORR of 79% and entrectinib an ORR of 57% (n = 159 and n = 54, respectively) (Hong et al. 2020; Doebele et al. 2020). Responses were seen across tumor types and in patients with brain metastases. The most common grade 3 or 4 adverse events were increased weight and anemia with entrectenib and increased ALT, anemia, and decreased neutrophil count with larotrectinib, all of which were reported at ≤10% incidence. Additional expected on-target side effects include paresthesias, dizziness, cognitive disturbance, and pain flares (with treatment discontinuation) due to the TRK receptor's role in the nervous system (Cocco, Scaltriti, and Drilon 2018).

5.4 ANGIOGENESIS INHIBITORS

5.4.1 VEGF

Angiogenesis is a vital process that is highly regulated in normal physiology by a balance of endogenous inducers and inhibitors, but this process can become overactive in pathologic conditions. Tumors need a reliable blood source to obtain oxygen and nutrients for growth; therefore, they create a pro-angiogenic environment. A variety of mediators are involved in promoting angiogenesis, including different growth factors, cytokines, bioactive lipids, matrix-degrading enzymes, and small molecules (El-Kenawi and El-Remessy 2013). Among the various pathways, vascular endothelial growth factor (VEGF) signaling is the rate-limiting step to angiogenesis. The VEGF family consists of five growth factors: VEGF-A, VEGF-B, VEGF-C, VEGF-D, and placenta growth factor (PLGF) (Koch and Claesson-Welsh 2012). Tumor cells and tumor-associated stroma can secrete VEGF, which then binds to tyrosine kinase receptors VEGFR1–R3. Of the growth factors, VEGF-A (known as VEGF) is the primary ligand, which acts mostly on VEGFR2 on endothelial cells (Simons, Gordon, and Claesson-Welsh 2016). The VEGFR is a cell surface receptor that has an extracellular domain for ligand binding, a transmembrane domain, and a cytoplasmic domain containing the TK portion (Shibuya 2011). When VEGF binds to VEGFR, the receptors homo- or heterodimerize and undergo conformational changes to allow auto- or trans-phosphorylation of tyrosine residues, stimulating a cascade of signaling pathways that initiates the process of forming new blood vessels (Koch and Claesson-Welsh 2012). Higher VEGF expression has been found in certain cancers, including colorectal cancer, breast cancer, NSCLC, renal cell cancer, and glioblastoma multiforme (Niu and Chen 2010).

Since tumors cannot survive without adequate vascularization, inhibition of angiogenesis has been an attractive target since the early 1970s. Bevacizumab was the first treatment developed to target the VEGF pathway, and it was approved in 2004 for its initial indication in metastatic CRC (Ferrara et al. 2004). Bevacizumab is a humanized mAb, but unlike most mAbs, it does not target the cell surface receptor. Rather, it binds to and neutralizes the VEGF-A ligand, thus preventing it from binding to the VEGF receptor (Ferrara et al. 2004). Since its initial approval in CRC, bevacizumab has been studied in many cancers and is now used in cervical cancer, endometrial cancer, glioblastoma, hepatocellular carcinoma (HCC), malignant mesothelioma, NSCLC, ovarian cancer, renal cell carcinoma, and soft tissue sarcoma. Due to its unique mechanism of action of targeting tumor angiogenesis, it is often used in combination with traditional cytotoxic chemotherapy, but it can also be used as a single agent. The major side effects of bevacizumab are related to the fact that platelets produce VEGF and absorb bevacizumab; therefore, blockage of platelet VEGF can lead to hypertension, impaired wound healing, bleeding, and gastrointestinal perforations (Kazazi-Hyseni, Beijnen, and Schellens 2010).

Ramucirumab differs from bevacizumab in that it binds to the VEGFR2 instead of the ligand. It is indicated for the treatment of gastric cancer, NSCLC, CRC, and HCC ("Cyramza [package insert]. Eli Lilly and Company. Indianapolis, IN. June 2020"). Ziv-aflibercept is a novel fusion protein that binds to VEGF-A, VEGF-B, and PLGF ligands. Although it binds to more ligands than bevacizumab, it demonstrated only a marginal benefit in efficacy when added to chemotherapy and plays a minimal role in current clinical practice (Van Cutsem et al. 2012). Aside from the large molecules, many small molecule TKIs were also developed to target VEGF signaling. These include axitinib, cabozantinib, lenvatinib, pazopanib, ponatinib, regorafenib, sorafenib, sunitinib, and vandetanib (Zirlik and Duyster 2018). All these agents also target other TKs such as PDGFR and FGFR, among others. They are used in a variety of cancers, such as renal cell carcinoma (RCC), hepatocellular carcinoma (HCC), thyroid cancer, GIST, soft tissue sarcoma, and endometrial cancer. Due to their multi-TKI functionality, these agents have significant toxicities, including the typical anti-VEGF side effects in addition to diarrhea, fatigue, hand-foot skin reaction, hepatotoxicity, and more.

5.5 IMMUNE SYSTEM TARGETS

5.5.1 PD-1, PDL-1, CTLA-4

The immune system is a key component in preventing cancer development and progression. Immunosuppressive medications, such as tacrolimus and azathioprine, and conditions like HIV are known to increase the risk of certain cancer types. In normal physiology, antigens (including those related to cancer cells) are presented to T-cells by antigen-presenting cells (APCs). When the T-cell receptor and the major histocompatibility complex on the APC bind at the same time as the CD28 receptor on the T-cell and the B7 receptor on the APC, a costimulatory response is generated. This stimulation produces trafficking and activation of the immune system against the antigen. Cytotoxic T lymphocyte antigen 4 (CTLA-4) is a counterpart to CD28 that also binds to B7 molecules but produces the opposite response (see Figure 5.6). CTLA-4 decreases T-cell function and induces T-cell apoptosis (Gibney, Weiner, and Atkins 2016; Postow, Callahan, and Wolchok 2015). Programmed cell death protein 1 (PD-1) also contributes to T-cell downregulation upon its binding to PD-L1 or PD-L2 on the tumor cell by suppressing T-cell proliferation, activity, and survival (Buchbinder and Desai 2016). These immune checkpoints maintain immune homeostasis but can also impact oncogenesis and evasion or overpowering of the immune system.

The immune checkpoints have been a major focus in anticancer therapy over the last decade. Immune checkpoint inhibitors (ICIs) transformed cancer care based on their novel mechanism and adverse effect profile compared with traditional chemotherapy. By inhibiting certain immune checkpoints such as CTLA-4 or PD-1, ICIs effectively stimulate the immune system to attack cancer cells. Ipilimumab, a CTLA-4 inhibitor, gained FDA approval in 2011 as monotherapy for the treatment of melanoma. Nivolumab and pembrolizumab, both PD-1 inhibitors, received approval in 2014 and have since been followed by additional PD-1 and PD-L1 inhibitors, including atezolizumab, avelumab, cemiplimab, and durvalumab. As a group, these agents have led to a new standard of care in the first-line setting in multiple cancer types, with notable benefits in NSCLC, melanoma, RCC, and small cell lung cancer (SCLC), among others. Since their initial approvals, additional benefit has been seen with concomitant CTLA-4 and PD-1 inhibition by combining ipilimumab and nivolumab, as CTLA-4 prevents T-cell activation at initial antigen presentation, while PD-1 affects multiple stages of the later immune response (Buchbinder and Desai 2016).

ICIs have demonstrated durable responses in subsets of patients across disease states, suggesting that there may be factors within individual immune systems or TMEs that prompt significant response, while other immune systems may not have the same robust response. Much research has concentrated on identifying a biomarker to predict which patients or specific cancer subsets will respond to ICI treatment, but no single predictor has yet been identified. PD-L1 expression on tumor and/or immune cells currently provides guidance in several disease states, including NSCLC and urothelial carcinoma, although it has

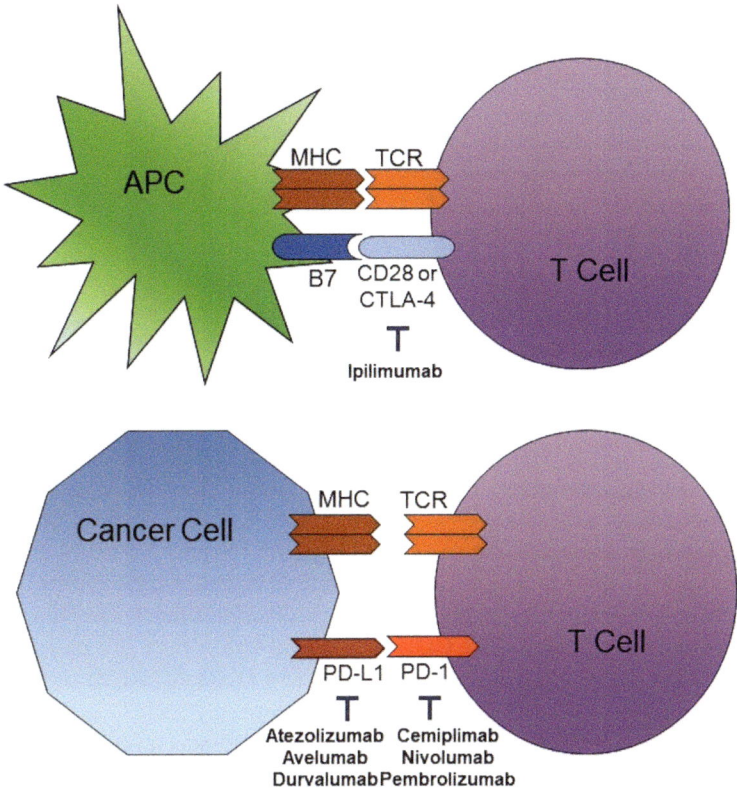

FIGURE 5.6   Immune targeting of cancer cells

not proved to be predictive of response in others. The presence of mutations or neoantigens within the tumor has also been identified as an indicator of ICI response. The number of mutations that occur in a specific tumor may correlate with how well the cancer cells will be recognized by the immune system, and this can be measured via tumor mutational burden (TMB). Similarly, cancers that possess mismatch repair deficiency (dMMR) express a higher amount of neoantigens due to errors in nucleotide matching, which can be identified by the immune system. Microsatellite instability (MSI) refers to the number of neoantigens present. Pembrolizumab has received FDA approval as a tumor non-specific treatment for TMB-high, dMMR, or MSI-high tumors. Although these developments in ICI targeting have led to more specific guidance, they are neither exclusive nor comprehensive (Gibney, Weiner, and Atkins 2016).

ICIs avoid the traditional cytotoxic chemotherapy effects like myelosuppression and alopecia, but they are not without serious side effects. Immune activation by ICIs can produce off-target autoimmune effects, such as rash, colitis, hepatitis, nephritis, hypophysitis, pneumonitis, myocarditis, endocrinopathies, and others. While most of these adverse effects can be managed with immunosuppressive treatments such as steroids, they can be fatal in certain cases. These toxicities are becoming more important to identify and manage as the use of ICIs continues to expand. Additionally, another area of research is treatment duration, as lasting immune responses can occur with shorter exposures to ICI in some patients.

5.5.2 CD19

CD19 is a surface protein expressed on B-cells during their life cycle. It is an important receptor in the PI3K/AKT pathway that is involved in B-cell differentiation and proliferation. Most non-Hodgkin B-cell lymphomas, such as diffuse large B-cell lymphoma (DLBCL), highly express CD19 and use it to

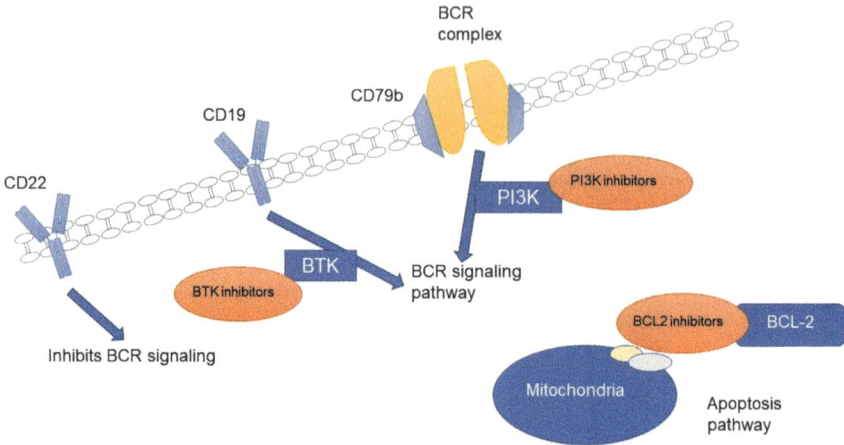

FIGURE 5.7   B-cell signaling pathways

enhance B-cell receptor signaling, leading to proliferation (see Figure 5.7) (Salles et al. 2020). Although CD19 surface expression is relatively lower than CD20 in B-cell malignancies, it is expressed early in the B-cell life cycle and persists longer throughout maturation (Tedder, Inaoki, and Sato 1997). Of note, it is not expressed on stem cells or plasma cells. CD19 is especially of interest as a targeted therapy in B-cell malignancies that cannot be treated with rituximab, such as CD20-negative tumors, or relapsed disease that has lost CD20 expression after previous rituximab exposure.

Tafasitamab-cxix is a CD19-targeted antibody with an Fc-enhanced region that increases the binding affinity to Fcγ receptors on effector cells such as macrophages and natural killer (NK) cells (Horton et al. 2008). Studies have shown that B-cell depletion by anti-CD19 antibodies depends on interactions with Fcγ receptors on immune effector cells (Horton et al. 2008). Thus, the Fc-enhanced region of tafasitamab increases the drug's cytotoxic activity, which is mediated through immune effector mechanisms, including antibody-dependent cell-mediated cytotoxicity (ADCC) with NK cells and antibody-dependent cellular phagocytosis (ADCP) with macrophages. In addition, tafasitamab-cxix also induces apoptosis by directly binding to CD19 receptors, halting the BCR signaling pathway for proliferation and leading to cell lysis (Tafasitamab [package insert]). Tafasitamab-cxix is approved in combination with lenalidomide for the treatment of R/R DLBCL not otherwise specified, including those transformed from indolent lymphomas and those ineligible for transplant (Tafasitamab [package insert]). *In vitro*, lenalidomide enhanced NK cell–mediated ADCC when used in combination with tafasitamab-cxix, demonstrating synergistic activity (Awan et al. 2010). The phase 2 L-MIND trial in R/R DLBCL patients who had CD20-directed antibody therapy and were ineligible for transplant showed an overall response rate of 55% and a median duration of response of 21.7 months (Salles et al. 2020). This led to its FDA approval in 2020.

5.5.3 CD20

CD20 is a nonglycosylated phosphoprotein expressed on the surface of B-cells throughout their life cycle, from pre-B-cells to mature B-cells. It is not expressed on early pre-B-cells or stem cells. More than 90% of B-cell non-Hodgkin lymphomas (NHL) express CD20. Upon antibody binding to CD20, the bound moiety is not immediately internalized. Therefore, CD20 cannot be used as a mAb–drug conjugate to deliver cytotoxic molecules; instead, CD20-targeted drugs elicit an immune response. Antitumor effects of CD20-targeted drugs have been shown in numerous preclinical and clinical studies (Zhou, Hu, and Qin 2008; Freeman and Sehn 2018). Rituximab is a type I chimeric CD20-targeted mAb that induces cell death mainly through ADCC and complement-dependent cytotoxicity (CDC). It has minimal direct cell death (DCD) mechanisms (Freeman and Sehn 2018). Rituximab was initially approved in 1997 for the treatment of R/R NHL. Since then, it has been studied in a variety of B-cell diseases as monotherapy, in combination with chemotherapy, and as maintenance therapy. It has also moved into the front-line setting in addition to the R/R setting.

Although its therapeutic benefit is undeniable, the development of resistance is a concern. The exact resistance mechanisms are unknown, but many have been postulated. Because rituximab relies heavily on the host immune response, resistance may stem from host- and tumor-related conditions. Rituximab's CDC activity may be decreased by complement consumption and complement resistance expression. Its ADCC activity may be reduced by exhausted effector cells, low-affinity Fc binding due to Fc receptor polymorphism, and lower CD20 expression. CLL and MCL express less CD20 compared with follicular lymphoma (FL) or DLBCL after exposure to rituximab (Freeman and Sehn 2018). Other proposed mechanisms of resistance include trogocytosis (phagocytosis of antibody–antigen complex while leaving malignant B-cell intact), resistance to caspase-dependent apoptosis, and decreased BAX/BAK pro-apoptotic proteins. Newer generations of CD20-targeted drugs such as obinutuzumab were developed to overcome these potential resistance mechanisms. Furthermore, augmenting the antibody's DCD abilities was also explored, as many B-cell malignancies have dysregulated apoptotic pathways (Freeman and Sehn 2018).

Obinutuzumab is a type II humanized CD20-targeted mAb. It was developed with glycoengineered type II properties, including an afucosylated Fc portion that increases binding to effector cells, translating to more potent ADCC and ADP activity compared with rituximab. It also induces caspase-independent DCD and increases levels of BAX/BAK, leading to apoptosis (Freeman and Sehn 2018). Obinutuzumab has been compared with rituximab in several head-to-head trials, showing an advantage in some but not all.

In the GALLIUM phase 3 study in treatment-naive patients with FL, chemotherapy plus obinutuzumab (G-chemo) was compared with chemotherapy plus rituximab (R-chemo) followed by the respective antibody maintenance for 2 years. Three-year PFS was improved with G-chemo compared with R-chemo (80% vs. 73.3%, p = 0.001), although ORR was similar, and no difference in OS was observed (Marcus et al. 2017). In the absence of a significant OS benefit, obinutuzumab is not currently recommended over rituximab for the treatment of newly diagnosed advanced stage FL. However, obinutuzumab may be considered in relapsed FL patients with resistance to rituximab, as it has shown a survival advantage in the GADOLIN trial comparing the combination of obinutuzumab and bendamustine with bendamustine alone in rituximab-refractory patients (Cheson et al. 2018). Obinutuzumab failed to show superiority compared with rituximab in DLBCL in the phase 3 GOYA trial (Vitolo et al. 2017). Currently, rituximab remains the CD20-targeted mAb of choice in the treatment of DLBCL. However, in CLL11, the obinutuzumab plus chlorambucil arm had better PFS, ORR, complete response (CR), and MRD negativity compared with rituximab plus chlorambucil, demonstrating a robust advantage over rituximab (Goede et al. 2014). Therefore, obinutuzumab is the CD20-targeted mAb of choice in the treatment of CLL.

A third CD20-targeted mAb, ofatumumab, was designed to improve complement-dependent cytotoxicity. Ofatumumab is theorized to be useful in patients with advanced disease who may have exhausted effector cells after extensive exposure to prior therapies. With a less robust host immune system and deficient effector cell function, patients with advanced disease may derive less benefit from mAbs that depend on ADCC activity. Thus, CDC-mediated cytotoxicity may be the preferred mechanism in this setting (Freeman and Sehn 2018). However, this theoretical advantage has not been clinically proven. A meta-analysis did not find ofatumumab to have an advantage over non-ofatumumab regimens when used in R/R CLL (Wu et al. 2017).

5.5.4 CD38

CD38 is a transmembrane glycoprotein that is highly and universally expressed on MM cells. CD38 is important in the functions of adhesion, proliferation, and activation of leukocytes, B-cell differentiation, and ecto-enzymatic activity such as calcium mobilization (van de Donk et al. 2016). Daratumumab is a human IgG1 kappa mAb that binds to a unique CD38 epitope. It causes cell death through multiple

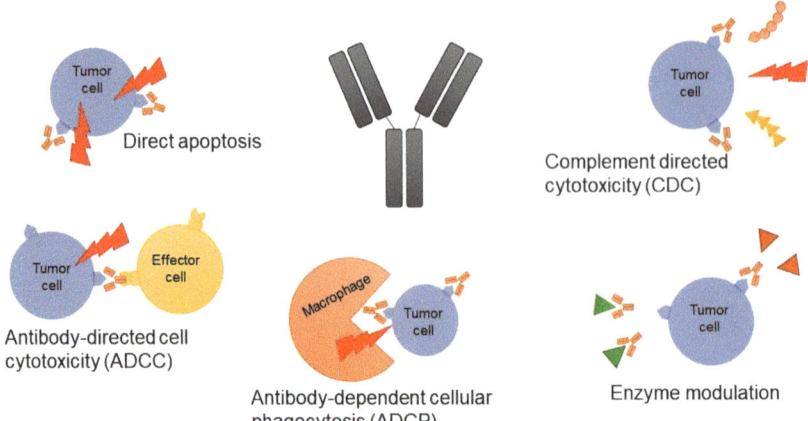

FIGURE 5.8   Antibody-mediated mechanisms of cytotoxicity

mechanisms, as shown in Figure 5.8, including ADCC, ADCP, CDC, direct apoptosis via crosslinking, and immunomodulatory effects via enzyme modulation (de Weers et al. 2011). Daratumumab was initially approved by the FDA in 2015 after showing promising single-agent efficacy in R/R MM in a phase 1/2 study (Lokhorst et al. 2015). It has since been approved both for front-line treatment and for R/R disease in various combinations with immunomodulators, proteasome inhibitors, melphalan, and steroids (Daratumumab [package insert]). In clinical trials, the addition of daratumumab to standard of care therapies has improved outcomes (Daratumumab [package insert]).

In 2020, a second CD38-targeted mAb, isatuximab, was FDA approved in combination with pomalidomide and dexamethasone for the treatment of R/R MM after at least two prior therapies, including lenalidomide and a proteasome inhibitor. Isatuximab also binds to a unique CD38 epitope. Similar to daratumumab, it causes cell death through multiple mechanisms including ADCC, CDC, ADCP, direct apoptosis, and immunomodulatory effects. Its approval was based on the ICARIA-MM trial, which showed that the addition of isatuximab to pomalidomide and dexamethasone significantly improved overall response rate and PFS (Attal et al. 2019).

5.5.5 SLAMF7

Signaling lymphocyte activation molecule-F7 (SLAMF7) is a glycoprotein that is highly expressed on NK cells, plasma cells, and MM cells. More than 95% of bone marrow myeloma cells express SLAMF7 (Lonial et al. 2015). Selective immune cells such as CD8+ T-cells, activated monocytes, and dendritic cells express SLAMF7 sparingly, while normal tissue cells have no expression (Hsi et al. 2008).

Elotuzumab is a humanized IgG1 mAb directed towards SLAMF7. Elotuzumab depletes MM cells through a dual mechanism of action. First, it activates NK cells directly through the SLAMF7 pathway by coupling with adapter protein EAT-2, leading to downstream signaling for cytotoxic granule synthesis and release. Second, elotuzumab tags MM cells by binding to SLAMF7 on the MM cell surface and activates NK cells via CD16 to facilitate NK cell–mediated ADCC. Because MM cells lack adapter protein EAT-2, elotuzumab can tag MM cells without triggering proliferation. This dual mechanism allows selective killing of MM cells (Lonial et al. 2015). Elotuzumab is FDA approved for the treatment of R/R MM in combination with lenalidomide and dexamethasone after one to three prior lines of therapy based on the ELOQUENT-2 study, or in combination with pomalidomide and dexamethasone after at least two prior lines of therapy based on the ELOQUENT-3 study.

The ELOQUENT-2 phase 3 trial compared the combination of elotuzumab plus lenalidomide and dexamethasone with lenalidomide and dexamethasone alone in R/R MM patients who progressed after one to three previous therapies. Results showed that the addition of elotuzumab improved PFS and OS. Patients had a 30% relative reduction in the risk of disease progression or death (Lonial et al. 2015). The ELOQUENT-3 phase 3 trial compared elotuzumab plus pomalidomide and dexamethasone with pomalidomide and dexamethasone alone in patients with R/R MM. Results showed that the addition of elotuzumab improved PFS and ORR. PFS benefit was consistent across subgroups, such as those who were refractory to both lenalidomide and a proteasome inhibitor and those with high-risk disease. Patients had a 46% reduction in the risk of disease progression or death (Dimopoulos et al. 2018).

5.5.6 CCR4

CC chemokine receptor 4 (CCR4) is a transmembrane G protein receptor expressed on certain types of T-cells, such as helper T-cells, regulatory T-cells, memory T-cells, and cutaneous lymphocyte-associated antigen (CLA)–positive T-cells. It plays an important role in trafficking lymphocytes to the skin. Adult T-cell leukemia/lymphoma (ATLL) tumor cells strongly express CCR4, while peripheral T-cell lymphoma (PTCL) and cutaneous T-cell lymphoma (CTCL) have variable expression based on disease subtype (Makita and Tobinai 2017; Wilcox 2015). CTCL subtypes such as mycosis fungoides (MF) and Sézary syndrome (SS) overexpress CCR4, and higher frequencies have been seen with more advanced disease (Kasamon et al. 2019).

Mogamulizumab is a humanized defucosylated antibody that binds to the B-terminal region of CCR4. Its antitumor effects on CCR4-positive cells are through NK cell–mediated ADCC. Mogamulizumab is the first glycol-engineered antibody to be FDA approved. Compared with traditional IgG mAbs, fucose residues are removed from the oligosaccharide structure of the Fc region, as shown in Figure 5.9. Defucosylation increases the binding affinity to the Fcγ receptor on effector cells, thus enhancing ADCC activity. Defucosylation permits ADCC to occur at lower antigen densities and effector-to-target-cell ratios. Studies have shown that removing the fucose residues increases ADCC 50-fold (Makita and Tobinai 2017). Potent cytotoxicity is demonstrated by mogamulizumab via ADCC activity alone, without any CDC or DCD mechanisms observed (Duvic, Evans, and Wang 2016; Afifi et al. 2019). Furthermore, mogamulizumab depletes regulatory T-cells that suppress host antitumor immunity. The depletion of regulatory T-cells increases the intrinsic immune response against tumor cells and enhances tumor killing (Wilcox 2015). Mogamulizumab is FDA approved for R/R CTCL, including both MF and SS, regardless of CCR4 expression. FDA approval is based on the phase 3 MAVORIC trial, which showed that mogamulizumab improved PFS compared with vorinostat (7.7 vs. 3.1 months). Mogamulizumab also improved response in all three compartments of the disease (skin, node, and blood) and had a significantly better overall response rate, and longer duration of response (Kim et al. 2018).

5.5.7 CD19-CD3

As aforementioned, CD19 is a surface protein expressed on B-cells during their life cycle that works through the PI3K/AKT pathway, which is involved in B-cell differentiation and proliferation. CD19 is

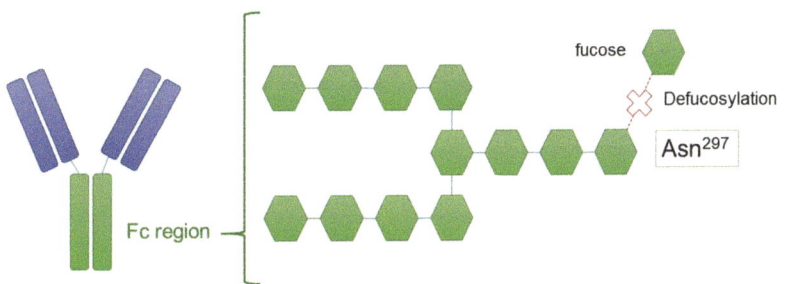

FIGURE 5.9 Mogamulizumab: Defucosylation of the Fc region

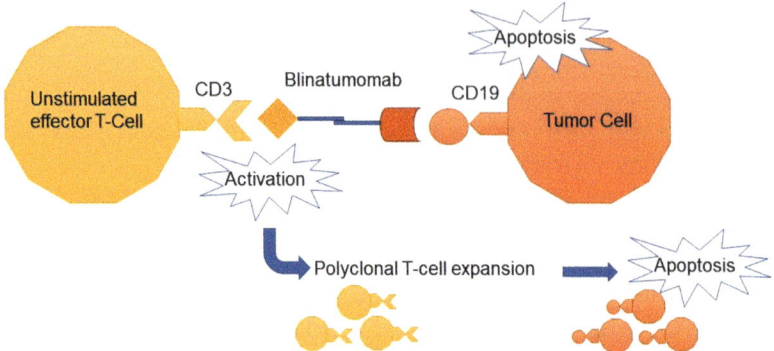

FIGURE 5.10 Blinatumomab: A bispecific T-cell engaging antibody (BiTE)

rarely expressed on plasma cells but is universally expressed on ALL of B-cell origin (Sanford 2015; Hoelzer 2011). Blinatumomab is a first-in-class bispecific T-cell-engaging antibody (BiTE). It contains two tandem single-chain variable fragments, of which one binds to CD19 antigens on malignant B-cells while the other binds to CD3 on T-cells. The single-chain antibody fragment BiTE structure lacks the constant region of traditional mAbs and thus, has a molecular weight one-third that of traditional mAbs. Blinatumomab physically links T-cells with malignant B-cells through simultaneous binding of CD19 and CD3, as shown in Figure 5.10. By binding to CD3, blinatumomab activates previously unstimulated effector T-cells and induces polyclonal T-cell expansion (Wu et al. 2015). Blinatumomab also increases cell adhesion molecules, cytolytic protein production, and inflammatory cytokine release to aid endogenous T-cells in the lysis of CD19-positive B-cells (Sanford 2015).

Blinatumomab was initially approved by the FDA in 2014 for Philadelphia chromosome (Ph)-negative R/R B-cell precursor acute lymphoblastic leukemia (BCP-ALL). Later, it also gained approval for MRD-positive BCP-ALL. The phase 3 TOWER study in heavily pretreated R/R BCP-ALL showed improved OS compared with standard of care chemotherapy (Kantarjian et al. 2017a). The phase 2 BLAST study in MRD-positive BCP-ALL showed undetectable MRD achieved by 70% of patients after blinatumomab (Goekbuget et al. 2014). Because blinatumomab activates T-cell proliferation and stimulates associated inflammatory cytokine release, including neurotoxic cytokines, cytokine release syndrome (CRS) and neurologic toxicities are commonly observed. Due to the risk of CRS and neurologic toxicities, premedication with dexamethasone is required, and the first cycle of treatment follows a step-up dosing scheme.

5.5.8 CSF-1R

The TME is an increasingly studied contributor to cancer development, growth, and response to treatment. Host immune response is a key defender against malignant growth, but several factors contribute to an immunosuppressive TME, allowing tumor cells to avoid targeting by the immune system. One factor in this process is the differentiation of macrophages between M1 (pro-inflammatory) and M2 (anti-inflammatory and tumor-promoting) (Zhu et al. 2019). In cancer, the M2 macrophages or "tumor-associated macrophages" (TAMs) predominate, supporting malignant cell growth, angiogenesis, and resistance to treatment. Colony-stimulating factor-1 receptor (CSF-1R) is an RTK that is activated by cytokines including CSF-1 and interleukin (IL)-34. CSF-1R mediates the differentiation of immune precursors, specifically TAMs, contributing to an immunosuppressive TME. The increased presence of TAMs has been identified as a negative prognostic factor in several cancer types (Kumari, Silakari, and Singh 2018; Cannarile et al. 2017), and CSF-R1 has been recognized as a target in inflammatory, autoimmune, and oncologic disorders. Suppressing activity mediated by CSF-1 and CSF-1R can promote a less immunosuppressive TME.

Several CSF-1 or CSF-R1 inhibitors are in development, including small molecule inhibitors and mAbs. Cabiralizumab, a CSF-1R-targeted mAb, is currently being studied in peripheral T-cell lymphoma, pancreatic cancer, breast cancer, and other cancer types. Pexidartinib, an oral TKI, was the first targeted CSF-1R inhibitor approved in 2019 and is used for tenosynovial giant cell tumor, which is associated with irregular expression of CSF1 (Lamb 2019). Thus far, side effects associated with this class include edema, pruritus, dry skin, and elevated liver enzymes (Cannarile et al. 2017; Lamb 2019). As CSF-R1-targeted therapy continues to advance, future areas of study will likely include the identification of which tumor types are the most amenable to inhibition and where these agents fit into current treatment schemes. Combination therapy with checkpoint inhibitors is a special area of interest, since reducing the immunosuppressive TME with CSF-1/CSF-R1 inhibitors may improve response to ICIs (Cannarile et al. 2017; Zhu et al. 2019).

5.6 ANTIBODY–DRUG CONJUGATES

5.6.1 CD33

CD33 is a surface antigen expressed on more than 90% of AML blast cells, early myeloid precursor cells, a few lymphoid cells, and hepatic sinusoidal endothelial cells. CD33 is not found on stem cells, thus making CD33 an attractive target for the treatment of AML while sparing stem cells (Ricart 2011). Gemtuzumab ozogamicin was the first antibody–drug conjugate approved by the FDA in 2000, indicated for the treatment of AML patients in first relapse who are 60 and older and not considered suitable for other cytotoxic chemotherapy. It is a humanized IgG4 antibody conjugated to ozogamicin, a semisynthetic derivative of the plant toxin calicheamicin. Calicheamicin is a natural antitumor antibiotic from *Micromonospora echinospora calichensis*, a soil bacterium (Zein et al. 1988). Gemtuzumab does not exert any clinically significant toxic effects as an unconjugated antibody (Hamann et al. 2002). Gemtuzumab is covalently bonded to ozogamicin with a hydrolysable 4-(4-acetylphenoxy) butanoic acid (AcBut) linker (see Figure 5.11). The AcBut linker is stable at the physiologic blood pH of 7.4 and is easily released via acid hydrolysis inside lysosomes. After gemtuzumab binds to cells expressing the CD33 antigen, the antibody–drug conjugate is quickly internalized, whereby ozogamicin is released to cause DNA strand break and ultimately, cell death (Ricart 2011).

Because of CD33 expression on myeloid progenitor cells and hepatic sinusoidal endothelial cells, gemtuzumab ozogamicin has side effects, including myelosuppression and sinusoidal obstruction syndrome (SOS), also previously known as veno-occlusive disease (VOD). The mechanism of SOS/VOD is hypothesized to be due to gemtuzumab's effect on CD33 positive hepatic sinusoid cells, causing ischemic hepatic necrosis or sinusoidal vasoconstriction. In 2010, gemtuzumab was voluntarily withdrawn from the U.S. market due to both lack of clinical benefit seen in the phase III SWOG S0106 study and safety concerns with increased rates of

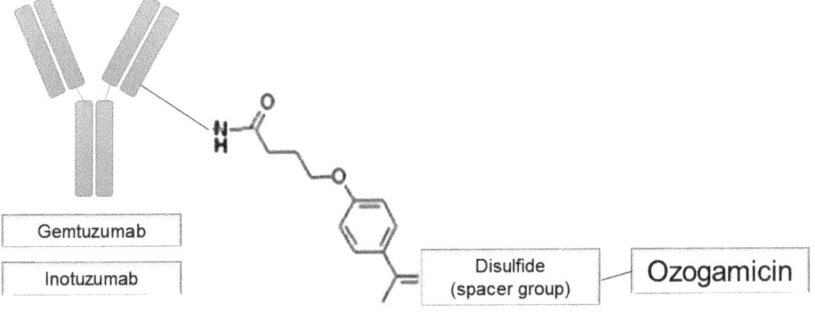

FIGURE 5.11   Antibody–drug conjugate cleavable 4-(4-acetylphenoxy) butanoic (AcBut) linkers

SOS/VOD seen during post-marketing surveillance (Petersdorf et al. 2013). In 2017, gemtuzumab ozogamicin returned to the market with FDA re-approval for the treatment of both relapsed/refractory and newly diagnosed CD33-positive AML with new fractionated and capped dosing based on clinical trials.

The phase 3 ALFA-0701 trial evaluated the addition of fractionated dose gemtuzumab ozogamicin to induction chemotherapy daunorubicin and cytarabine in younger, newly diagnosed AML patients. Two-year EFS was significantly better with the addition of gemtuzumab (40.8 vs. 17.1%, p = 0.0003) (Castaigne et al. 2012). The phase 3 AML-19 study compared gemtuzumab monotherapy with best supportive care in newly diagnosed older adults and showed improved OS (4.9 vs. 3.6 months, p = 0.005) (Amadori et al. 2016). The phase 2 MyloFrance-1 trial assessed gemtuzumab monotherapy in adult AML patients in first relapse and showed an overall response of 33.3% with complete response in 26% of patients, which is concluded to be beneficial (Taksin et al. 2007). VOD was reported in 5% of patients in the ALFA-0701 and the AML-19 studies and in zero patients in the MyloFrance-1 trial. Based on all trial experience taken together, gemtuzumab ozogamicin carries a black box warning for hepatotoxicity, including severe VOD/SOS (Castaigne et al. 2012; Amadori et al. 2016; Taksin et al. 2007).

5.6.2 CD22

CD22 surface antigen is expressed in virtually all BCP-ALL. It is an ideal target for antibody-based therapy because it is not expressed on memory B-cells, stem cells, T-cells, or non-lymphoid cells (Boué and LeBien 1988). Normally, CD22 functions as a receptor in the BCR signaling pathway (see Figure 5.7). It is one of the better-internalized molecules compared with other B-cell surface antigens, and it does not shed in the extracellular space (Ricart 2011). Inotuzumab ozogamicin is a CD22-directed IgG4 antibody conjugated to the cytotoxic molecule ozogamicin. The unconjugated antibody inotuzumab does not exert any antitumor effect. Once the ADC is bound to CD22-expressing B-cells, it is internalized, and ozogamicin is released to cause DNA strand breaking and apoptosis. Similarly to gemtuzumab, the ADC is linked via an AcBut linker that is stable at physiologic pH but easily cleaved via acid hydrolysis inside lysosomes (see Figure 5.11) (Aujla, Aujla, and Liu 2019).

Inotuzumab ozogamicin monotherapy is FDA approved for CD22-positive relapsed or refractory BCP-ALL based on the phase 3 INO-VATE trial. The trial compared inotuzumab monotherapy with standard chemotherapy including FLAG (fludarabine, cytarabine, and granulocyte stimulating factor), cytarabine with mitoxantrone, or cytarabine alone in patients with Ph-positive or Ph-negative relapsed or refractory B-cell ALL. Results showed that inotuzumab significantly improved complete remission rate compared with chemotherapy (73.8 vs. 30.9%, p < 0.0001) and had a better OS and longer duration of response (4.6 vs. 3.1 months, p = 0.03) (Kantarjian et al. 2019).

Unlike CD33-targeted gemtuzumab ozogamicin, inotuzumab ozogamicin's target CD22 is not expressed on hepatocytes. Nevertheless, inotuzumab ozogamicin carries a black box warning of VOD/SOS and a higher post-transplant non-relapse mortality. In the INO-VATE study, patients treated with inotuzumab had more SOS/VOD than those treated with chemotherapy (14% vs. 2.1%) (Kantarjian et al. 2019). Multivariate analysis also showed that transplant conditioning regimens with two alkylating agents and pre-transplant bilirubin greater than the upper limit of normal were associated with increased risk of SOS/VOD (Kantarjian et al. 2017b). Due to these findings, even though the mechanism of this toxicity is not clearly understood, inotuzumab ozogamicin increases the risk of hepatotoxicity and requires careful consideration in transplant patients and others at high risk for SOS.

5.6.3 CD30

CD30 cell surface receptor is a member of the tumor necrosis factor receptor (TNFR) family. It plays a role in TNFR-medicated apoptosis via factor 2 degradation. Specific tumor types such as classical Hodgkin lymphoma (cHL), systemic anaplastic large cell lymphoma (sALCL), and certain types of T-cell

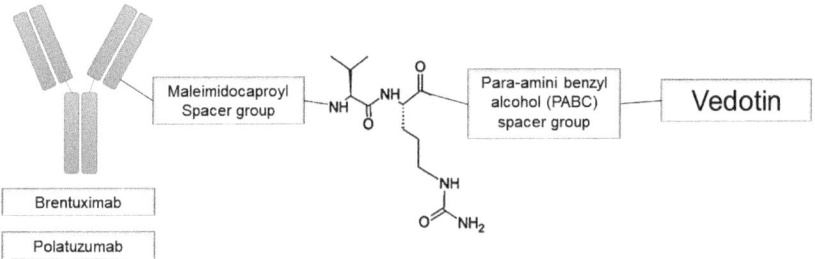

FIGURE 5.12 Antibody–drug conjugate cleavable valine-citrulline (ValCit) linker

lymphoma express high levels of CD30, while normal tissue cells have limited expression. Some T- and B-cells express CD30, but only in the activated form and not during resting conditions (Senter and Sievers 2012). Brentuximab vedotin is a CD30-directed human chimeric IgG1 antibody covalently linked to monomethyl auristatin E (MMAE), a microtubule-disrupting agent. The vedotin moiety is the structure of MMAE with the valine–citrulline (ValCit) dipeptide linker (see Figure 5.12). Each antibody molecule is bound to four MMAE molecules (Francisco et al. 2003). MMAE is a synthetic derivative of the naturally occurring antimitotic agent dolastatin 10, extracted from *Dolabella auricularia,* a marine shell-less mollusk (Senter and Sievers 2012). Dolastatin and its analogs are highly toxic and cannot be used as the plain drug, and the unconjugated CD30 antibody does not have any antitumor effect (Senter and Sievers 2012). However, as an ADC, brentuximab vedotin delivers effective targeted antitumor activity. It is currently FDA approved in HL, sALCL, and CD30-positive PTCL.

Once brentuximab is bound to CD30 positive cells, the ADC is engulfed by the cell, and the ValCit linker is cleaved by proteases within lysosomes (Scott 2017). The ADC and the ValCit linker are stable in physiologic conditions, and only 2% of MMAE was released during a 10-day incubation in human plasma *in vitro* (Hamblett et al. 2004) Free MMAE binds to tubulin, causing G2/M phase cell division arrest and eventually, apoptosis (Scott 2017). In addition to its intracellular activity, MMAE crosses the cell membrane and has a cytotoxic effect on nearby tumor cells *in vitro*, exerting an indirect "bystander" effect (Okeley et al. 2010). While the bystander effect provides an extra layer of tumor killing, it may also translate to toxicity, particularly neuropathy. Similarly to vinca alkaloids, neuropathy may present with brentuximab due to MMAE's tubulin-disrupting mechanism of cytotoxicity (Moskowitz et al. 2015).

5.6.4 CD79b

CD79b is a BCR signaling antigen receptor expressed on normal B-cells and most malignant B-cell lymphomas. CD79 is a crucial component in the BCR signaling complex and is required for BCR cell surface expression for downstream signaling (Polson et al. 2007). Virtually all DLBCL cells express CD79b. Importantly, CD79b is not expressed on hematopoietic stem cells (Shingleton and Dave 2020). These characteristics of CD79b are ideal for targeted drug therapy.

Polatuzumab vedotin is a CD79b-targeted antibody conjugated to MMAE. As with brentuximab vedotin, polatuzumab is covalently linked to MMAE via a ValCit bi-peptide linker that is very stable in plasma but easily cleavable intracellularly (see Figure 5.12). Each polatuzumab antibody is linked to two MMAE molecules (Shingleton and Dave 2020). Interestingly, unconjugated anti-CD79b antibody showed some activity in non-Hodgkin B-cell lymphoma (DOHH2) cells in *in vivo* xenograft models (Polson et al. 2007). This suggests some degree of ADCC or CDC leading to apoptosis in addition to MMAE-mediated cell killing.

Polatuzumab vedotin is FDA approved in combination with bendamustine and rituximab (P+BR) for the treatment of relapsed/refractory DLBCL after at least two prior therapies (Deeks 2019). FDA approval was based on the phase 1b/2 study GO29365 that compared P+BR with BR in patients with R/R DLBCL who were ineligible for transplant. P+BR showed higher complete remission (40% vs. 18%), better overall

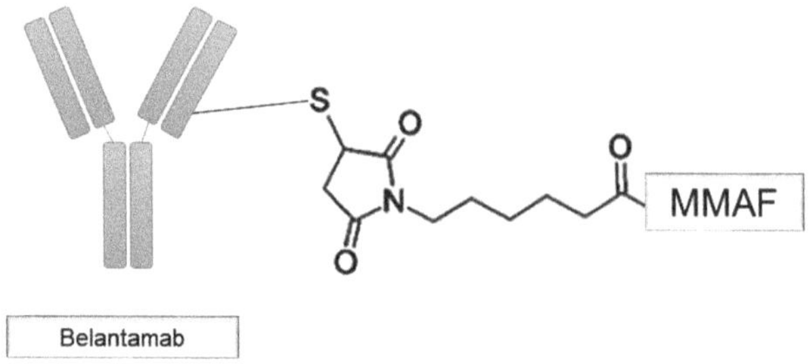

FIGURE 5.13   Antibody–drug conjugate non-cleavable maleimidocaproyl linker

response rate (CR + PR) (63% vs. 25%), and longer duration of response, PFS, and OS (Sehn et al. 2020). Similarly to brentuximab vedotin, peripheral neuropathy is also observed in patients receiving polatuzumab vedotin (Sehn et al. 2020).

5.6.5 BCMA

B-cell maturation antigen (BCMA) is a receptor in the TNFR superfamily that normally promotes plasma cell differentiation and growth. It is exclusively expressed by B-cells at later stages of maturation and absent on naive and memory B-cells. MM cells universally express BCMA at much higher levels than regular plasma cells and are dependent on BCMA for long-term survival (Tai et al. 2014). Belantamab mafodotin is a first-in-class afucosylated IgG1 BCMA-targeted mAb conjugated to monomethyl auristatin F (MMAF) via a protease-resistant maleimidocaproyl linker, as shown in Figure 5.13 (Trudel et al. 2019). Both the antibody and the ADC induce apoptosis through several mechanisms, including MMAF-induced cell toxicity, ADCC, and antibody-mediated phagocytosis. Afucosylation of the drug molecule increases the binding affinity of belantamab to FcγRIIIa (low-affinity Igγ Fc receptor III-A) receptors and enhances ADCC activity by recruiting and activating immune effector cells. Belantamab mafodotin also mediates antibody-dependent phagocytosis by recruiting macrophages. Lastly, antitubulin agent MMAF exerts cytotoxicity intracellularly by arresting G2/M phase cell division after release inside the cell. Unlike MMAE, MMAF is neither permeable nor cleaved from the ADC extracellularly to exert any "bystander" effect (Tai et al. 2014).

Belantamab mafodotin was approved as monotherapy in August 2020 for the treatment of R/R MM after at least four prior therapies, including an anti-CD38 mAb, a proteasome inhibitor, and an immunomodulatory agent. It was approved after the phase 2 DREAMM-2 study showed 31% overall response at the approved dose in the indicated patient population (Lonial et al. 2020). Common grade 3–4 adverse events include keratopathy, thrombocytopenia, and anemia. Of note, neuropathy was not observed (Lonial et al. 2020).

5.6.6 HER2

Ado-trastuzumab emtansine (T-DM1) was the first antibody–drug conjugate to target the HER2 receptor. Trastuzumab is linked to DM1, a derivative of maytansine, via non-reducible thioether linkers with a ratio of 3.5 DM1 molecules to 1 molecule of trastuzumab (Barok, Joensuu, and Isola 2014). The addition of DM1 neither alters the binding of trastuzumab to HER2 nor affects the natural antitumor effects of trastuzumab. Binding of T-DM1 onto HER2 receptors causes endocytosis of the antibody–receptor complex. Inside the cell, the antibody is degraded, and DM1 is released into the cell. DM1 inhibits microtubule assembly, which leads to mitotic arrest and cell apoptosis (Barok, Joensuu, and Isola 2014). T-DM1 is approved for use in HER2+ breast cancer in the early-stage adjuvant setting for residual disease as well as in the metastatic setting after initial treatment with trastuzumab and a taxane (von Minckwitz et al.

2019). For metastatic disease, T-DM1 significantly prolonged PFS and OS compared with lapatinib plus capecitabine (Verma et al. 2012). In terms of tolerability, T-DM1 has a considerable number of toxicities due to the combined effects of both trastuzumab and a cytotoxic agent. Adverse events that can be expected with T-DM1 include decreased left ejection fraction, myelosuppression, hepatic enzyme elevations, peripheral neuropathy, nausea, constipation, and arthralgias.

Trastuzumab deruxtecan (DS-8201a) is a newer ADC that targets HER2+ cancer cells. It consists of trastuzumab, a peptide linker, and exatecan methanesulfonate (Dxd), a topoisomerase I inhibitor. The trastuzumab component binds to the HER2 receptor on the cell, causing the ADC to be internalized, where the Dxd portion is released by lysosomal enzymes and exerts its cytotoxic effects. DS-8201a is a novel ADC in that it has a substantially higher drug-to-antibody ratio compared with other ADCs. While most ADCs have drug-to-antibody ratios around 2 to 4, DS-8201a has 8 Dxd molecules per antibody (Andrikopoulou et al. 2020). This allows for increased delivery of cytotoxic payload to tumor cells and more potent antitumor activity. In clinical studies for metastatic HER2+ breast cancer, 60.9% of patients responded to DS-8201a, which is even more impressive when considering that these patients had already received a median of six prior lines of therapy (Modi et al. 2020). Toxicities for DS-8201a include myelosuppression, nausea, vomiting, diarrhea, fatigue, alopecia, reduced ejection fraction, and interstitial lung disease.

5.6.7 Trop2

Trop2 is a type I transmembrane glycoprotein that is overexpressed in many cancers. It is coded by the *Tacstd2* (tumor-associated calcium signal transducer 2) gene and was initially discovered in trophoblast cells by Lipinski and colleagues (Lipinski et al. 1981). Trop2 expression activates downstream MAPK signaling and ERK phosphorylation, increases levels of cyclin D1 and cyclin E, induces mobilization of intracellular calcium, and increases expression of Ki-67. As a result, Trop2 plays a significant role in cell cycle progression and tumor proliferation. Regulated intramembrane proteolysis via TNF-α converting enzyme and γ-secretase cleaves Trop2 into an intracellular and an extracellular domain (Shvartsur and Bonavida 2015). The intracellular domain accumulates in the nucleus and is responsible for most of the functions of Trop2.

Although Trop2 mutations are associated with certain conditions, such as Gelatinous Drop-Like Corneal Dystrophy, no known Trop2 mutations have been linked to cancers. Instead, Trop2 overexpression has been found in many types of cancer, including breast, gastric, bladder, leukemia, and non-Hodgkin's lymphoma. Therapeutic targeting of Trop2 started with the design of anti-Trop2 antibodies and progressed with the development of Trop2-targeted ADCs. SN-38, a topoisomerase I inhibitor, is the water-insoluble active metabolite of irinotecan and is used as a drug conjugate with Trop2-targeted antibodies (Goldenberg et al. 2015). The ADC, known as IMMU-132, was constructed with several features in the crosslinker to optimize the use of SN-38 as a drug conjugate: a short polyethylene glycol moiety to enhance water solubility; a maleimide group for thiol–maleimide conjugation; a benzylcarbonate site for pH-mediated cleavage to release SN-38 from the linker; and attachment of the crosslinker in a position that prevents the transition of the lactone ring to the less active carboxylic acid form (Goldenberg et al. 2015). Compared with other ADCs, IMMU-132 is unique in that it utilizes a moderately toxic drug instead of an ultratoxic drug and conveys a bystander effect through local release of SN-38 at the tumor site in addition to ADC internalization. It also carries a high ratio of drug to mAb at approximately 8:1 (Goldenberg et al. 2015).

Positive Trop2 staining occurred in over 95% of tumors in a microarray with triple-negative breast cancer (TNBC) and hormone receptor- or HER2-positive breast cancer specimens. Based on strong preclinical data in TNBC, IMMU-132 was further pursued in clinical studies with metastatic TNBC patients and demonstrated a response rate of 33.3% and a median PFS of 5.5 months (Bardia et al. 2019). In April 2020, IMMU-132, otherwise known as sacituzumab govitecan-hziy, received FDA approval for adult patients with metastatic TNBC who had received at least two prior lines of treatment for metastatic disease. The most common adverse events (>5% incidence) of grade 3 or higher included neutropenia, anemia, diarrhea, fatigue, hypophosphatemia, nausea, and vomiting. Sacituzumab govitecan provides an effective and relatively well-tolerated treatment option for metastatic TNBC patients who otherwise would be limited to cytotoxic agents that are either more toxic or less effective. IMMU-132 is currently being studied in a variety of other cancers, including, but not limited to, endometrial cancer, prostate cancer, urothelial cancer, and SCLC (Syed 2020).

5.6.8 Nectin-4

Nectin-1, -2, -3, and -4 are cell adhesion molecules with varying expression and function in multicellular organism development processes. These proteins interact both within the nectin class and with other cell surface receptors. Nectin-4 specifically is a transmembrane protein that has been associated with viral adhesion, including serving as the epithelial receptor for the measles virus (Mandai et al. 2015). In recent years, nectin-4 has additionally been identified as an anticancer target based on its higher expression in urothelial, breast, lung, and pancreatic cancer tissues compared with non-malignant tissues; higher expression correlates with a poorer disease prognosis (Hanna 2020). Interactions with PDGFR, FGFR, VEGFR, and integrin and activation of the PI3K-AKT signaling pathway allow nectin-4 to impact cell proliferation, differentiation, and survival, although these proliferative effects are still being elucidated (Kedashiro et al. 2019). The difference in expression of nectin-4 between malignant and normal cells and the fact that nectin-4 does not play vital roles on normal cells have led to the development of nectin-4 as an effective ADC target.

Enfortumab vedotin is a fully humanized antibody connected to a linker and cytotoxic agent complex (vedotin). The conjugate exerts its action by selectively binding to nectin-4 on cell surfaces, internalizing into the cell, and releasing the cytotoxic monomethyl auristatin E (MMAE). Once MMAE is enzymatically cleaved from the enfortumab antibody, it acts as a microtubule-disrupting agent by preventing the polymerization of microtubules and inducing apoptosis through cell cycle arrest in the G2/M phase (Hanna 2020). In addition to the expected MMAE side effects such as neuropathy, enfortumab vedotin is also associated with a skin rash, which is thought to be an on-target effect due to epithelial nectin-4 antigen expression. Hyperglycemia can also occur, which has an unclear cause but is thought to be an on-target effect (Rosenberg et al. 2019).

Enfortumab vedotin first gained FDA approval in the United States for the treatment of locally advanced or metastatic urothelial carcinoma in patients whose disease has progressed after treatment with standard agents. In the major clinical trial, ORR at the time of data cutoff was 44%, which included 12% of patients experiencing a complete response. Previous clinical trials with antimicrotubule agents in this setting resulted in an ORR of 11–13%, which suggests that the targeting of nectin-4 provides substantial benefit to the cytotoxic mechanism (Rosenberg et al. 2019). Enfortumab vedotin is currently being further studied in urothelial carcinoma as monotherapy and as combination treatment with immunotherapy or chemotherapy, as well as in additional solid tumors with nectin-4 expression including breast cancer, NSCLC, and gastric cancer.

5.7 OTHER TARGETS

5.7.1 BRCA

The BRCA genes are a class of tumor suppressor genes that are highly involved in maintaining genomic stability through homologous recombination (HR) and DNA double-strand repair. The two genes in the BRCA family, BRCA1 and BRCA2, have different structures and functions. BRCA1 is involved in

DNA repair pathways, such as HR, non-homologous end joining (NHEJ), and single-strand annealing, as well as checkpoint activations in the cell cycle. BRCA2, on the other hand, functions mostly in HR. HR is a highly accurate method of repairing DNA double-strand breaks that would otherwise be lethal to cells. Mutations in the BRCA genes disrupt the normal DNA repair functions and are associated with an increased risk of ovarian, pancreatic, stomach, laryngeal, fallopian tube, and prostate cancers (Roy, Chun, and Powell 2011). These mutations can be either germline or somatic in origin; germline mutations occur in 5–7 % of all breast cancers and in 10–15% of ovarian cancers (Roy, Chun, and Powell 2011; Konstantinopoulos, Lacchetti, and Annunziata 2020).

The poly (ADP-ribose) polymerase (PARP) inhibitors are a class of drugs that are particularly effective in targeting BRCA-mutated tumors. PARP enzymes bind to DNA single-strand break (SSB) sites and add poly(ADP-ribose) (pADPr) units to various repair factors to activate the repair process. Inhibition of PARP enzymes thus leads to suppression of DNA single-strand repair. PARP inhibition in the context of BRCA-mutated cancer cells produces blockage of both single-strand and double-strand repair, making cell death nearly inevitable, as shown in Figure 5.14. This concept of exploiting more than one genetic defect to induce cell death is known as synthetic lethality (Javle and Curtin 2011).

The currently approved PARP inhibitors include olaparib, rucaparib, niraparib, and talazoparib. These small molecule agents prevent PARP enzymes from disassociating from the SSB sites, a mechanism known as "PARP trapping," which leads to accumulation of unrepaired SSBs (Pommier, O'Connor, and de Bono 2016). Talazoparib has the most potent PARP trapping activity, niraparib has the second most, and olaparib and rucaparib are the least potent. Niraparib, olaparib, and rucaparib are used in both BRCA-mutated and wild-type ovarian cancers. While these agents are most effective in BRCA-mutated tumors or tumors with HR deficiency, they have demonstrated efficacy in BRCA wild-type cancers as well. Talazoparib and olaparib are also approved for BRCA-mutated metastatic breast cancer (Lynparza [package insert]; Talzenna [package insert]). Most recently, olaparib has been approved for maintenance treatment in BRCA-mutated metastatic pancreatic cancer, and rucaparib has been approved for treatment of BRCA-mutated metastatic castration resistant pancreatic cancer (mCRPC) (Lynparza [package insert]; Rubraca [package insert]). The indications for PARP inhibitors continue to expand as they are studied in additional cancers associated with BRCA mutations. Due to their impact on DNA repair and cell cycle regulation, the PARP inhibitors can cause significant myelosuppression, especially in heavily pretreated patients. Other major toxicities include fatigue, nausea, diarrhea, increased serum creatinine, hepatic enzyme abnormalities, and the rare but serious side effect of AML or myelodysplastic syndrome (MDS) (Lynparza [package insert]; Talzenna [package insert]; Rubraca [package insert]; Zejula [package insert]).

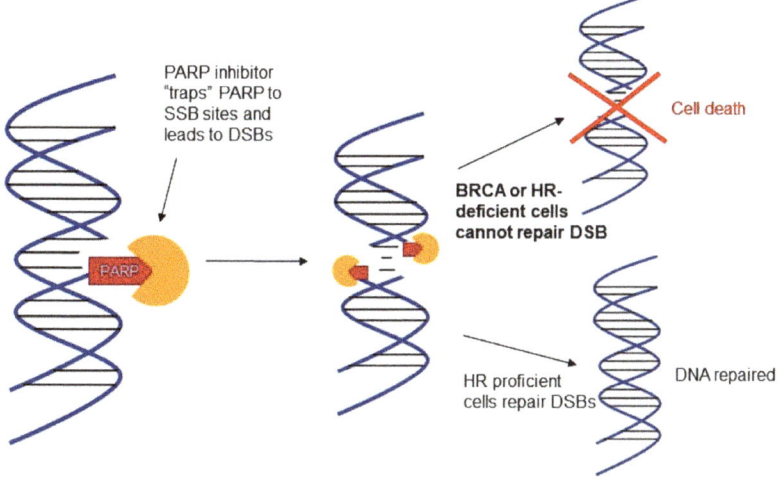

FIGURE 5.14   Mechanism of action of PARP inhibitors

5.7.2 CDK4/6

The cyclin D1-CDK4/6-Rb pathway helps regulate normal mammary tissue proliferation as a checkpoint in the cell cycle, but it can lead to breast cancer development when hyperactive. Cyclin D1 binds to cyclin-dependent kinase 4 and 6 (CDK4/6) to form a complex that phosphorylates retinoblastoma (Rb) protein. Rb then releases the E2F transcription factors, leading to gene expression that stimulates transition of the cell from G1 into S phase (Pernas et al. 2018). The EGFR/HER2, PI3K/AKT/mTOR, and ER pathways can also influence CDK4/6 activity by increasing cyclin D1 expression. Endogenous proteins known as INK4 proteins serve as natural inhibitors of CDK4/6 enzyme activity (Pernas et al. 2018). Small molecule CDK4/6 inhibitors were developed to mimic these proteins and target tumor cells early in the cell cycle to stop proliferation. By blocking CDK4/6 phosphorylation of Rb, these drugs effectively cause cell cycle arrest. ER+ breast cancer is optimal for targeting with CDK4/6 inhibitors because this tumor type typically retains function of Rb protein and overexpresses cyclin D1 (Finn et al. 2009).

Since the initial approval of palbociclib in 2016, the three CDK4/6 inhibitors (palbociclib, ribociclib, and abemaciclib) in combination with endocrine therapy have become the mainstay of treatment for metastatic ER+, HER2– breast cancer due to their impressive efficacy results of doubling PFS compared with AIs alone (Shah, Nunes, and Stearns 2018). Of the three CDK4/6 inhibitors, abemaciclib is the most potent and appears to have the most robust penetration into the CNS. Palbociclib and ribociclib cause more neutropenia and thrombocytopenia compared with abemaciclib, whereas abemaciclib is associated with a high rate of diarrhea (Pernas et al. 2018). Overall, the CDK4/6 inhibitors have changed the landscape of metastatic ER+, HER2– breast cancer. Ongoing studies of CDK4/6 inhibitors are investigating their role in early-stage breast cancer and HER2+ breast cancer (Pernas et al. 2018).

5.8 DRUG DELIVERY STRATEGIES

Distributing anticancer therapy to tumor cells has been a challenge since the introduction of systemic therapies. Tumors possess specific qualities that complicate medication delivery, including dense or compact tissue and abnormal tissue structure with undifferentiated cells. Additionally, tumor angiogenesis produces immature vasculature, so blood supply to the area is not consistent (Kutova et al. 2019). Chemotherapy and other systemic anticancer therapy cause undesired side effects when they act on healthy tissues in the body. Both efficacy and safety concerns emphasize the importance of targeted drug delivery directly to the site of the tumor.

One of the most developed strategies for optimizing chemotherapy delivery is the enhanced permeability and retention effect of liposomal and nano-dispersed albumin formulations of traditional medications. Because of this effect, the liposomal drugs leak from the immature vasculature and accumulate in the tumor site, creating more of a tumor-targeted effect. Examples of chemotherapy formulations utilizing these methods include liposomal doxorubicin, cytarabine, vincristine, and irinotecan and albumin-bound paclitaxel. In addition to enhancing drug delivery, these formulations also decrease some toxicities typically seen with individual agents, such as cardiotoxicity with doxorubicin and hypersensitivity associated with the Cremophor solubilizer in traditional paclitaxel. Encapsulation of chemotherapy can also increase the bioavailability and efficacy of the agents, although this method has not proved as promising as expected (Li et al. 2019b; Kutova et al. 2019). Additional nanomedicine carriers can include other organic carriers like dendrimers and carbon nanotubes and inorganic carriers like layered double hydroxides and superparamagnetic iron oxide nanoparticles, which are expected to develop further in coming years (Senapati et al. 2018).

Antibody treatments have been considered to be limited to extracellular targets in cancer therapy due to the large molecular size of antibodies. Several delivery methods are in use or in development to overcome this issue. One effective method to take advantage of antibody-targeted effects and the potential for intracellular delivery is the use of ADCs, which have been previously discussed. Another technique is the use of plasmid or viral vectors, delivered intracellularly via nanoparticles or liposomes, to induce the production of intracellular antibodies. Additional mechanisms to utilize antibody effects intracellularly are in development (Trenevska, Li, and Banham 2017).

Another focus of antibody–drug delivery has been on identifying more convenient routes of administration than the traditional intravenous option. Subcutaneous (SC) administration of several mAbs is now possible, which decreases treatment time, improves ease of preparation and administration for the healthcare provider, and reduces the risk of hypersensitivity reactions. Recombinant hyaluronidase increases the absorption of the mAb by breaking down hyaluronan in the skin, allowing a greater volume of administration and dispersion of drug than with typical SC delivery. Several SC-targeted mAb/hyaluronidase combinations are currently used in clinical practice with demonstrated clinical non-inferiority to the traditional formulations, including rituximab, trastuzumab with or without pertuzumab, and daratumumab (Locke, Maneval, and LaBarre 2019).

Stimuli-responsive medication release is an additional potential mechanism to target anticancer drug delivery in the future. Currently, intra-tumor stimuli for drug release include pH, reactive oxygen species, temperature, and the presence of certain enzymes. External factors that are in development for drug release include light, temperature, and electrical and magnetic triggers (Li et al. 2019b; Senapati et al. 2018). Research continues with these targeted drug delivery systems, which may translate into clinical applications that improve anticancer tolerability and efficacy.

5.9 CONCLUSION

Targeted therapy has ushered in a new era of cancer treatment that focuses on cancer cells with certain molecular alterations as opposed to any rapidly dividing cell. This shift in treatment focus has brought about the concept of precision medicine, which is the use of medicine tailored to an individual's genetic profile (White Al-Habeeb et al. 2016). While the origins of precision medicine are not entirely clear, this approach largely gained traction in 2015 when President Obama signed the Precision Medicine Initiative. Since then, scientists and clinicians have worked towards applying precision medicine to determining the diagnosis, prognosis, and treatment of cancers. One key way precision medicine is being utilized in treatment is by conducting basket trials in which patients with different tumor types but a common driver mutation are treated universally with a specific targeted therapy (Gambardella et al. 2020). In fact, several drugs have been approved under tumor-agnostic indications, such as the NTRK inhibitors for solid tumors with NTRK gene fusion or pembrolizumab for MSI-high, MMR-deficient, or TMB-high cancers.

While targeted therapy has drastically changed the landscape of cancer treatment, it is not without its own set of drawbacks. One of the primary concerns with targeted therapy is the development of drug resistance, which can occur through several major mechanisms. Cancer cells can directly reactivate the target that was blocked by the drug, such as in EGFR-hyperactivated NSCLC cells that develop the gate-keeper T790M mutation. This mutation arises when methionine is substituted for threonine at amino acid position 790 of the EGFR gene domain, rendering the receptor resistant to first-generation TKIs (Ma, Wei, and Song 2011). Alternatively, tumor cells can bypass the intended inhibition of a pathway by utilizing a parallel or downstream pathway to promote cell proliferation. For instance, one key method of resistance to endocrine therapies in ER+ breast cancer is signaling through the PI3K/AKT/mTOR pathway. AKT or S6K1, a downstream effector of mTOR, can directly phosphorylate ERα independently of estrogen, thereby triggering cell growth despite blockage of the estrogen receptor (Ciruelos Gil 2014). Cancer cells can also activate pro-survival signaling pathways in the setting of targeted therapy inhibition, such as recruitment of NFκB upon inhibition of EGFR (Neel and Bivona 2017). Ultimately, resistance to targeted therapy is a significant barrier to its use, and much of the current research is dedicated to understanding and overcoming resistance mechanisms.

Aside from drug resistance, another area of concern regarding targeted therapy is tumor heterogeneity. Receptor heterogeneity on the tumor cell has minimal impact on the efficacy of traditional cytotoxic chemotherapy. However, for targeted therapy, drug efficacy is highly associated with the quantity of available receptors or targets on or within a tumor cell. Tumor heterogeneity also significantly impacts the validity of data from tumor sampling and molecular profiling (Dagogo-Jack and Shaw 2018). For example, a biopsy from one site of the tumor may not capture the same molecular profile as a biopsy from another site. Likewise, treatment may not work in a portion of the tumor if the target is not present in all the tumor cells. As targeted therapy continues to evolve, it is crucial to expand our understanding of tumor heterogeneity and design treatment regimens that account for heterogeneity. Despite the shortcomings of targeted therapy, it is a very effective class of treatments that allows therapeutic tailoring to individual biomarkers and tumor profiling. Though cytotoxic chemotherapy will likely always have a role in cancer treatment, targeted therapy is undeniably becoming the mainstay of cancer therapy.

REFERENCES

Abou-Alfa, G. K., V. Sahai, A. Hollebecque, G. Vaccaro, D. Melisi, R. Al-Rajabi, A. S. Paulson, M. J. Borad, D. Gallinson, A. G. Murphy, D. Y. Oh, E. Dotan, D. V. Catenacci, E. Van Cutsem, T. Ji, C. F. Lihou, H. Zhen, L. Féliz, and A. Vogel. "Pemigatinib for Previously Treated, Locally Advanced or Metastatic Cholangiocarcinoma: A Multicentre, Open-Label, phase 2 Study." *Lancet Oncology* 21, no. 5 (2020): 671–84. doi:10.1016/S1470-2045(20)30109-1. https://www.ncbi.nlm.nih.gov/pubmed/32203698.

Abu-Duhier, F. M., A. C. Goodeve, G. A. Wilson, R. S. Care, I. R. Peake, and J. T. Reilly. "Identification of Novel FLT-3 Asp835 Mutations in Adult Acute Myeloid Leukaemia." *British Journal of Haematology* 113, no. 4 (2001): 983–8. doi:10.1046/j.1365-2141.2001.02850.x. https://www.ncbi.nlm.nih.gov/pubmed/11442493.

Afifi, S., S. Mohamed, J. Zhao, and F. Foss. "A Drug Safety Evaluation of Mogamulizumab for the Treatment of Cutaneous T-Cell Lymphoma." *Expert Opinion on Drug Safety* 18, no. 9 (2019): 769–76. doi:10.1080/1474033 8.2019.1643837. https://www.ncbi.nlm.nih.gov/pubmed/31303060.

Akinleye, A., Y. Chen, N. Mukhi, Y. Song, and D. Liu. "Ibrutinib and Novel BTK Inhibitors in Clinical Development." *Journal of Hematology & Oncology* 6 (2013): 59. doi:10.1186/1756-8722-6-59. https://www.ncbi.nlm.nih.gov/pubmed/23958373.

Amadori, S., S. Suciu, D. Selleslag, F. Aversa, G. Gaidano, M. Musso, L. Annino, A. Venditti, M. T. Voso, C. Mazzone, D. Magro, P. De Fabritiis, P. Muus, G. Alimena, M. Mancini, A. Hagemeijer, F. Paoloni, M. Vignetti, P. Fazi, L. Meert, S. M. Ramadan, R. Willemze, T. de Witte, and F. Baron. "Gemtuzumab Ozogamicin Versus Best Supportive Care in Older Patients with Newly Diagnosed Acute Myeloid Leukemia Unsuitable for Intensive Chemotherapy: Results of the Randomized phase III EORTC-GIMEMA AML-19 Trial." *Journal of Clinical Oncology* 34, no. 9 (2016): 972–9. doi:10.1200/JCO.2015.64.0060. https://www.ncbi.nlm.nih.gov/pubmed/26811524.

Amatu, A., A. Sartore-Bianchi, and S. Siena. "Gene Fusions as Novel Targets of Cancer Therapy Across Multiple Tumour Types." *ESMO Open* 1, no. 2 (2016): e000023. doi:10.1136/esmoopen-2015-000023. https://www.ncbi.nlm.nih.gov/pubmed/27843590.

Andrick, B. J., and A. Gandhi. "Olaratumab: A Novel Platelet-Derived Growth Factor Receptor α-Inhibitor for Advanced Soft Tissue Sarcoma." *Annals of Pharmacotherapy* 51, no. 12 (2017): 1090–8. doi:10.1177/1060028017723935. https://www.ncbi.nlm.nih.gov/pubmed/28778132.

Andrikopoulou, A., E. Zografos, M. Liontos, K. Koutsoukos, M. A. Dimopoulos, and F. Zagouri. "Trastuzumab Deruxtecan (DS-8201a): The Latest Research and Advances in Breast Cancer." *Clinical Breast Cancer* (2020). doi:10.1016/j.clbc.2020.08.006. https://www.ncbi.nlm.nih.gov/pubmed/32917537.

Attal, M., P. G. Richardson, S. V. Rajkumar, J. San-Miguel, M. Beksac, I. Spicka, X. Leleu, F. Schjesvold, P. Moreau, M. A. Dimopoulos, J. S. Huang, J. Minarik, M. Cavo, H. M. Prince, S. Macé, K. P. Corzo, F. Campana, S. Le-Guennec, F. Dubin, K. C. Anderson, and ICARIA-MM Study Group. "Isatuximab plus Pomalidomide and Low-Dose Dexamethasone Versus Pomalidomide and Low-Dose Dexamethasone in Patients with Relapsed and Refractory Multiple Myeloma (Icaria-MM): A Randomised, Multicentre, Open-Label, phase 3 Study." *Lancet* 394, no. 10214 (2019): 2096–107. doi:10.1016/S0140-6736(19)32556-5. https://www.ncbi.nlm.nih.gov/pubmed/31735560.

Aujla, A., R. Aujla, and D. Liu. "Inotuzumab Ozogamicin in Clinical Development for Acute Lymphoblastic Leukemia and Non-Hodgkin Lymphoma." *Biomarker Research* 7 (2019): 9. doi:10.1186/s40364-019-0160-4. https://www.ncbi.nlm.nih.gov/pubmed/31011424.

Awan, F. T., R. Lapalombella, R. Trotta, J. P. Butchar, B. Yu, D. M. Benson, J. M. Roda, J. Cheney, X. Mo, A. Lehman, J. Jones, J. Flynn, D. Jarjoura, J. R. Desjarlais, S. Tridandapani, M. A. Caligiuri, N. Muthusamy, and J. C. Byrd. "CD19 Targeting of Chronic Lymphocytic Leukemia with a Novel Fc-Domain-Engineered Monoclonal Antibody." *Blood* 115, no. 6 (2010): 1204–13. doi:10.1182/blood-2009-06-229039. https://www.ncbi.nlm.nih.gov/pubmed/19965644.

Ayati, A., S. Moghimi, S. Salarinejad, M. Safavi, B. Pouramiri, and A. Foroumadi. "A Review on Progression of Epidermal Growth Factor Receptor (EGFR) Inhibitors as an Efficient Approach in Cancer Targeted Therapy." *Bioorganic Chemistry* 99 (2020): 103811. doi:10.1016/j.bioorg.2020.103811. https://www.ncbi.nlm.nih.gov/pubmed/32278207.

Babina, I. S., and N. C. Turner. "Advances and Challenges in Targeting FGFR Signalling in Cancer." *Nature Reviews. Cancer* 17, no. 5 (2017): 318–32. doi:10.1038/nrc.2017.8. https://www.ncbi.nlm.nih.gov/pubmed/28303906.

Bardia, A., I. A. Mayer, L. T. Vahdat, S. M. Tolaney, S. J. Isakoff, J. R. Diamond, J. O'Shaughnessy, R. L. Moroose, A. D. Santin, V. G. Abramson, N. C. Shah, H. S. Rugo, D. M. Goldenberg, A. M. Sweidan, R. Iannone, S. Washkowitz, R. M. Sharkey, W. A. Wegener, and K. Kalinsky. "Sacituzumab govitecan-hziy in Refractory Metastatic Triple-Negative Breast Cancer." *New England Journal of Medicine* 380, no. 8 (2019): 741–51. doi:10.1056/NEJMoa1814213. https://www.ncbi.nlm.nih.gov/pubmed/30786188.

Barok, M., H. Joensuu, and J. Isola. "Trastuzumab Emtansine: Mechanisms of Action and Drug Resistance." *Breast Cancer Research* 16, no. 2 (2014): 209. doi:10.1186/bcr3621. https://www.ncbi.nlm.nih.gov/pubmed/24887180.

Baxter, E. J., L. M. Scott, P. J. Campbell, C. East, N. Fourouclas, S. Swanton, G. S. Vassiliou, A. J. Bench, E. M. Boyd, N. Curtin, M. A. Scott, W. N. Erber, A. R. Green, and Cancer Genome Project. "Acquired Mutation of the Tyrosine Kinase JAK2 in Human Myeloproliferative Disorders." *Lancet* 365, no. 9464 (2005): 1054–61. doi:10.1016/S0140-6736(05)71142-9. https://www.ncbi.nlm.nih.gov/pubmed/15781101.

Bewersdorf, J. P., S. M. Jaszczur, S. Afifi, J. C. Zhao, and A. M. Zeidan. "Beyond Ruxolitinib: Fedratinib and Other Emergent Treatment Options for Myelofibrosis." *Cancer Management & Research* 11 (2019): 10777–90. doi:10.2147/CMAR.S212559. https://www.ncbi.nlm.nih.gov/pubmed/31920387.

Bines, J., M. Procter, E. Restuccia, G. Viale, D. Zardavas, T. Suter, A. Arahmani, V. Van Dooren, J. Baselga, E. Clark, J. Eng-Wong, R. D. Gelber, M. Piccart, V. Mobus, E. de Azambuja, and APHINITY Steering Committee and Investigators. "Incidence and Management of Diarrhea with Adjuvant Pertuzumab and Trastuzumab in Patients with Human Epidermal Growth Factor receptor 2-Positive Breast Cancer." *Clinical Breast Cancer* 20, no. 2 (2020): 174-181.e3. doi:10.1016/j.clbc.2019.06.016. https://www.ncbi.nlm.nih.gov/pubmed/31924513.

Birrer, M. J., K. N. Moore, I. Betella, and R. C. Bates. "Antibody-Drug Conjugate-Based Therapeutics: State of the Science." *Journal of the National Cancer Institute* 111, no. 6 (2019): 538–49. doi:10.1093/jnci/djz035. https://www.ncbi.nlm.nih.gov/pubmed/30859213.

Bitencourt, R., I. Zalcberg, and I. D. Louro. "Imatinib Resistance: A Review of Alternative Inhibitors in Chronic Myeloid Leukemia." *Revista Brasileira de Hematologia e Hemoterapia* 33, no. 6 (2011): 470–5. doi:10.5581/1516-8484.20110124. https://www.ncbi.nlm.nih.gov/pubmed/23049365.

Boonstra, M. C., S. W. de Geus, H. A. Prevoo, L. J. Hawinkels, C. J. van de Velde, P. J. Kuppen, A. L. Vahrmeijer, and C. F. Sier. "Selecting Targets for Tumor Imaging: An Overview of Cancer-Associated Membrane Proteins." *Biomarkers in Cancer* 8 (2016): 119–33. doi:10.4137/BIC.S38542. https://www.ncbi.nlm.nih.gov/pubmed/27721658.

Boué, D. R., and T. W. LeBien. "Expression and Structure of CD22 in Acute Leukemia." *Blood* 71, no. 5 (1988): 1480–6. https://www.ncbi.nlm.nih.gov/pubmed/3258772.

Bubendorf, L., R. Büttner, F. Al-Dayel, M. Dietel, G. Elmberger, K. Kerr, F. López-Ríos, A. Marchetti, B. Öz, P. Pauwels, F. Penault-Llorca, G. Rossi, A. Ryška, and E. Thunnissen. "Testing for ROS1 in Non-Small Cell Lung Cancer: A Review with Recommendations." *Virchows Archiv* 469, no. 5 (2016): 489–503. doi:10.1007/s00428-016-2000-3. https://www.ncbi.nlm.nih.gov/pubmed/27535289.

Buchbinder, E. I., and A. Desai. "CTLA-4 and PD-1 Pathways: Similarities, Differences, and Implications of Their Inhibition." *American Journal of Clinical Oncology* 39, no. 1 (2016): 98–106. doi:10.1097/COC.0000000000000239. https://www.ncbi.nlm.nih.gov/pubmed/26558876.

Campbell, K. J., and S. W. G. Tait. "Targeting BCL-2 Regulated Apoptosis in Cancer." *Open Biology* 8, no. 5 (2018). doi:10.1098/rsob.180002. https://www.ncbi.nlm.nih.gov/pubmed/29769323.

Cannarile, M. A., M. Weisser, W. Jacob, A. M. Jegg, C. H. Ries, and D. Rüttinger. "Colony-Stimulating factor 1 Receptor (CSF1R) Inhibitors in Cancer Therapy." *Journal for ImmunoTherapy of Cancer* 5, no. 1 (2017): 53. doi:10.1186/s40425-017-0257-y. https://www.ncbi.nlm.nih.gov/pubmed/28716061.

Casadei, C., N. Dizman, G. Schepisi, M. C. Cursano, U. Basso, D. Santini, S. K. Pal, and U. De Giorgi. "Targeted Therapies for Advanced Bladder Cancer: New Strategies with FGFR Inhibitors." *Therapeutic Advances in Medical Oncology* 11 (2019): 1758835919890285. doi:10.1177/1758835919890285. https://www.ncbi.nlm.nih.gov/pubmed/31803255.

Castaigne, S., C. Pautas, C. Terré, E. Raffoux, D. Bordessoule, J. N. Bastie, O. Legrand, X. Thomas, P. Turlure, O. Reman, T. de Revel, L. Gastaud, N. de Gunzburg, N. Contentin, E. Henry, J. P. Marolleau, A. Aljijakli, P. Rousselot, P. Fenaux, C. Preudhomme, S. Chevret, H. Dombret, and Acute Leukemia French Association. "Effect of Gemtuzumab Ozogamicin on Survival of Adult Patients with De-Novo Acute Myeloid Leukaemia (ALFA-0701): A Randomised, Open-Label, phase 3 Study." *Lancet* 379, no. 9825 (2012): 1508–16. doi:10.1016/S0140-6736(12)60485-1. https://www.ncbi.nlm.nih.gov/pubmed/22482940.

Chau, C. H., P. S. Steeg, and W. D. Figg. "Antibody-Drug Conjugates for Cancer." *Lancet* 394, no. 10200 (2019): 793–804. doi:10.1016/S0140-6736(19)31774-X. https://www.ncbi.nlm.nih.gov/pubmed/31478503.

Cheson, B. D., N. Chua, J. Mayer, G. Dueck, M. Trněný, K. Bouabdallah, N. Fowler, V. Delwail, O. Press, G. Salles, J. G. Gribben, A. Lennard, P. J. Lugtenburg, G. Fingerle-Rowson, F. Mattiello, A. Knapp, and L. H. Sehn. "Overall Survival Benefit in Patients with Rituximab-Refractory Indolent Non-Hodgkin Lymphoma Who Received Obinutuzumab plus Bendamustine Induction and Obinutuzumab Maintenance in the GADOLIN Study." *Journal of Clinical Oncology* 36, no. 22 (2018): 2259–66. doi:10.1200/JCO.2017.76.3656. https://www.ncbi.nlm.nih.gov/pubmed/29584548.

Chien, A. J., and H. S. Rugo. "Tyrosine Kinase Inhibitors for Human Epidermal Growth Factor receptor 2-Positive Metastatic Breast Cancer: Is Personalizing Therapy Within Reach?. " *Journal of Clinical Oncology* 35, no. 27 (2017): 3089–91. doi:10.1200/JCO.2017.73.5670. https://www.ncbi.nlm.nih.gov/pubmed/28783451.

Ciruelos Gil, E. M. "Targeting the PI3K/AKT/mTOR Pathway in Estrogen Receptor-Positive Breast Cancer." *Cancer Treatment Reviews* 40, no. 7 (2014): 862–71. doi:10.1016/j.ctrv.2014.03.004. https://www.ncbi.nlm.nih.gov/pubmed/24774538.

Cocco, E., M. Scaltriti, and A. Drilon. "NTRK Fusion-Positive Cancers and TRK Inhibitor Therapy." *Nature Reviews. Clinical Oncology* 15, no. 12 (2018): 731–47. doi:10.1038/s41571-018-0113-0. https://www.ncbi.nlm.nih.gov/pubmed/30333516.

Cortes, J. E., F. H. Heidel, A. Hellmann, W. Fiedler, B. D. Smith, T. Robak, P. Montesinos, D. A. Pollyea, P. DesJardins, O. Ottmann, W. W. Ma, M. N. Shaik, A. D. Laird, M. Zeremski, A. O'Connell, G. Chan, and M. Heuser. "Randomized Comparison of Low Dose Cytarabine with or Without Glasdegib in Patients with Newly Diagnosed Acute Myeloid Leukemia or High-Risk Myelodysplastic Syndrome." *Leukemia* 33, no. 2 (2019a): 379–89. doi:10.1038/s41375-018-0312-9. https://www.ncbi.nlm.nih.gov/pubmed/30555165.

Cortes, J. E., R. Gutzmer, M. W. Kieran, and J. A. Solomon. "Hedgehog Signaling Inhibitors in Solid and Hematological Cancers." *Cancer Treatment Reviews* 76 (2019b): 41–50. doi:10.1016/j.ctrv.2019.04.005. https://www.ncbi.nlm.nih.gov/pubmed/31125907.

Costa, R. B., R. L. B. Costa, S. M. Talamantes, J. B. Kaplan, M. A. Bhave, A. Rademaker, C. Miller, B. A. Carneiro, D. Mahalingam, and Y. K. Chae. "Systematic Review and Meta-Analysis of Selected Toxicities of Approved." *Oncotarget* 9, no. 31 (2018): 22137–46. doi:10.18632/oncotarget.25154. https://www.ncbi.nlm.nih.gov/pubmed/29774128.

Crawford, E. D., A. Heidenreich, N. Lawrentschuk, B. Tombal, A. C. L. Pompeo, A. Mendoza-Valdes, K. Miller, F. M. J. Debruyne, and L. Klotz. "Androgen-Targeted Therapy in Men with Prostate Cancer: Evolving Practice and Future Considerations." *Prostate Cancer & Prostatic Diseases* 22, no. 1 (2019): 24–38. doi:10.1038/s41391-018-0079-0. https://www.ncbi.nlm.nih.gov/pubmed/30131604.

Curtin, J. A., K. Busam, D. Pinkel, and B. C. Bastian. "Somatic Activation of KIT in Distinct Subtypes of Melanoma." *Journal of Clinical Oncology* 24, no. 26 (2006): 4340–6. doi:10.1200/JCO.2006.06.2984. https://www.ncbi.nlm.nih.gov/pubmed/16908931.

Cyramza [Package Insert]. Indianapolis, IN: Eli Lilly and Company, Jun. 2020.

Dagogo-Jack, I., and A. T. Shaw. "Tumour Heterogeneity and Resistance to Cancer Therapies." *Nature Reviews. Clinical Oncology* 15, no. 2 (2018): 81–94. doi:10.1038/nrclinonc.2017.166. https://www.ncbi.nlm.nih.gov/pubmed/29115304.

Daratumumab [Package Insert]. Horsham, PA: Janssen Biotech, Inc., Aug. 2020.

Davey, R. A., and M. Grossmann. "Androgen Receptor Structure, Function and Biology: From Bench to Bedside." *Clinical Biochemist Reviews* 37, no. 1 (2016): 3–15. https://www.ncbi.nlm.nih.gov/pubmed/27057074.

de Weers, M., Y. T. Tai, M. S. van der Veer, J. M. Bakker, T. Vink, D. C. Jacobs, L. A. Oomen, M. Peipp, T. Valerius, J. W. Slootstra, T. Mutis, W. K. Bleeker, K. C. Anderson, H. M. Lokhorst, J. G. van de Winkel, and P. W. Parren. "Daratumumab: A Novel Therapeutic Human CD38 Monoclonal Antibody, Induces Killing of Multiple Myeloma and Other Hematological Tumors." *Journal of Immunology* 186, no. 3 (2011): 1840–8. doi:10.4049/jimmunol.1003032. https://www.ncbi.nlm.nih.gov/pubmed/21187443.

Deeks, E. D. "Polatuzumab Vedotin: First Global Approval." *Drugs* 79, no. 13 (2019): 1467–75. doi:10.1007/s40265-019-01175-0. https://www.ncbi.nlm.nih.gov/pubmed/31352604.

Del Gaizo Moore, V., J. R. Brown, M. Certo, T. M. Love, C. D. Novina, and A. Letai. "Chronic Lymphocytic Leukemia Requires BCL2 to Sequester Prodeath BIM, Explaining Sensitivity to BCL2 Antagonist ABT-737." *Journal of Clinical Investigation* 117, no. 1 (2007): 112–21. doi:10.1172/JCI28281. https://www.ncbi.nlm.nih.gov/pubmed/17200714.

DeVita, V. T., and E. Chu. "A History of Cancer Chemotherapy." *Cancer Research* 68, no. 21 (2008): 8643–53. doi:10.1158/0008-5472.CAN-07-6611. https://www.ncbi.nlm.nih.gov/pubmed/18974103.

Dillon, L. M., and T. W. Miller. "Therapeutic Targeting of Cancers with Loss of PTEN Function." *Current Drug Targets* 15, no. 1 (2014): 65–79. doi:10.2174/1389450114666140106100909. https://www.ncbi.nlm.nih.gov/pubmed/24387334.

Dimopoulos, M. A., D. Dytfeld, S. Grosicki, P. Moreau, N. Takezako, M. Hori, X. Leleu, R. LeBlanc, K. Suzuki, M. S. Raab, P. G. Richardson, M. Popa McKiver, Y. M. Jou, S. G. Shelat, M. Robbins, B. Rafferty, and J. San-Miguel. "Elotuzumab plus Pomalidomide and Dexamethasone for Multiple Myeloma." *New England Journal of Medicine* 379, no. 19 (2018): 1811–22. doi:10.1056/NEJMoa1805762. https://www.ncbi.nlm.nih.gov/pubmed/30403938.

DiNardo, C. D., K. Pratz, V. Pullarkat, B. A. Jonas, M. Arellano, P. S. Becker, O. Frankfurt, M. Konopleva, A. H. Wei, H. M. Kantarjian, T. Xu, W. J. Hong, B. Chyla, J. Potluri, D. A. Pollyea, and A. Letai. "Venetoclax Combined with Decitabine or Azacitidine in Treatment-Naive, Elderly Patients with Acute Myeloid Leukemia." *Blood* 133, no. 1 (2019): 7–17. doi:10.1182/blood-2018-08-868752. https://www.ncbi.nlm.nih.gov/pubmed/30361262.

DiNardo, C. D., B. A. Jonas, V. Pullarkat, M. J. Thirman, J. S. Garcia, A. H. Wei, M. Konopleva, H. Döhner, A. Letai, P. Fenaux, E. Koller, V. Havelange, B. Leber, J. Esteve, J. Wang, V. Pejsa, R. Hájek, K. Porkka, Á. Illés, D. Lavie, R. M. Lemoli, K. Yamamoto, S. S. Yoon, J. H. Jang, S. P. Yeh, M. Turgut, W. J. Hong, Y. Zhou, J. Potluri, and K. W. Pratz. "Azacitidine and Venetoclax in Previously Untreated Acute Myeloid Leukemia." *New England Journal of Medicine* 383, no. 7 (2020): 617–29. doi:10.1056/NEJMoa2012971. https://www.ncbi.nlm.nih.gov/pubmed/32786187.

Doebele, R. C., A. Drilon, L. Paz-Ares, S. Siena, A. T. Shaw, A. F. Farago, C. M. Blakely, T. Seto, B. C. Cho, D. Tosi, B. Besse, S. P. Chawla, L. Bazhenova, J. C. Krauss, Y. K. Chae, M. Barve, I. Garrido-Laguna, S. V. Liu, P. Conkling, T. John, M. Fakih, D. Sigal, H. H. Loong, G. L. Buchschacher, P. Garrido, J. Nieva, C. Steuer, T. R. Overbeck, D. W. Bowles, E. Fox, T. Riehl, E. Chow-Maneval, B. Simmons, N. Cui, A. Johnson, S. Eng, T. R. Wilson, G. D. Demetri, and Trial Investigators. "Entrectinib in Patients with Advanced or Metastatic NTRK Fusion-Positive Solid Tumours: Integrated Analysis of Three Phase 1–2 Trials." *Lancet Oncology* 21, no. 2 (2020): 271–82. doi:10.1016/S1470-2045(19)30691-6. https://www.ncbi.nlm.nih.gov/pubmed/31838007.

Drilon, A., F. Cappuzzo, S. I. Ou, and D. R. Camidge. "Targeting MET in Lung Cancer: Will Expectations Finally Be MET?. " *Journal of Thoracic Oncology* 12, no. 1 (2017): 15–26. doi:10.1016/j.jtho.2016.10.014. https://www.ncbi.nlm.nih.gov/pubmed/27794501.

Drilon, A., G. R. Oxnard, D. S. W. Tan, H. H. F. Loong, M. Johnson, J. Gainor, C. E. McCoach, O. Gautschi, B. Besse, B. C. Cho, N. Peled, J. Weiss, Y. J. Kim, Y. Ohe, M. Nishio, K. Park, J. Patel, T. Seto, T. Sakamoto, E. Rosen, M. H. Shah, F. Barlesi, P. A. Cassier, L. Bazhenova, F. De Braud, E. Garralda, V. Velcheti, M. Satouchi, K. Ohashi, N. A. Pennell, K. L. Reckamp, G. K. Dy, J. Wolf, B. Solomon, G. Falchook, K. Ebata, M. Nguyen, B. Nair, E. Y. Zhu, L. Yang, X. Huang, E. Olek, S. M. Rothenberg, K. Goto, and V. Subbiah. "Efficacy of Selpercatinib In." *New England Journal of Medicine* 383, no. 9 (2020a): 813–24. doi:10.1056/NEJMoa2005653. https://www.ncbi.nlm.nih.gov/pubmed/32846060.

Drilon, A., J. W. Clark, J. Weiss, S. I. Ou, D. R. Camidge, B. J. Solomon, G. A. Otterson, L. C. Villaruz, G. J. Riely, R. S. Heist, M. M. Awad, G. I. Shapiro, M. Satouchi, T. Hida, H. Hayashi, D. A. Murphy, S. C. Wang, S. Li, T. Usari, K. D. Wilner, and P. K. Paik. "Antitumor Activity of Crizotinib in Lung Cancers Harboring a MET exon 14 Alteration." *Nature Medicine* 26, no. 1 (2020b): 47–51. doi:10.1038/s41591-019-0716-8. https://www.ncbi.nlm.nih.gov/pubmed/31932802.

Drilon, A., S. Siena, R. Dziadziuszko, F. Barlesi, M. G. Krebs, A. T. Shaw, C. de Braud, C. Rolfo, M. J. Ahn, J. Wolf, T. Seto, B. C. Cho, M. R. Patel, C. H. Chiu, T. John, K. Goto, C. S. Karapetis, H. T. Arkenau, S. W. Kim, Y. Ohe, Y. C. Li, Y. K. Chae, C. H. Chung, G. A. Otterson, H. Murakami, C. C. Lin, D. S. W. Tan, H. Prenen, T. Riehl, E. Chow-Maneval, B. Simmons, N. Cui, A. Johnson, S. Eng, T. R. Wilson, R. C. Doebele, and

Trial investigators. "Entrectinib in ROS1 Fusion-Positive Non-Small-Cell Lung Cancer: Integrated Analysis of Three Phase 1–2 Trials." *Lancet Oncology* 21, no. 2 (2020c): 261–70. doi:10.1016/S1470-2045(19)30690-4. https://www.ncbi.nlm.nih.gov/pubmed/31838015.

Du, X., Y. Shao, H. F. Qin, Y. H. Tai, and H. J. Gao. "ALK-Rearrangement in Non-Small-Cell Lung Cancer (NSCLC)." *Thoracic Cancer* 9, no. 4 (2018): 423–30. doi:10.1111/1759-7714.12613. https://www.ncbi.nlm.nih.gov/pubmed/29488330.

Du, Z., and C. M. Lovly. "Mechanisms of Receptor Tyrosine Kinase Activation in Cancer." *Molecular Cancer* 17, no. 1 (2018): 58. doi:10.1186/s12943-018-0782-4. https://www.ncbi.nlm.nih.gov/pubmed/29455648.

Duvic, M., M. Evans, and C. Wang. "Mogamulizumab for the Treatment of Cutaneous T-Cell Lymphoma: Recent Advances and Clinical Potential." *Therapeutic Advances in Hematology* 7, no. 3 (2016): 171–4. doi:10.1177/2040620716636541. https://www.ncbi.nlm.nih.gov/pubmed/27247757.

El-Kenawi, A. E., and A. B. El-Remessy. "Angiogenesis Inhibitors in Cancer Therapy: Mechanistic Perspective on Classification and Treatment Rationales." *British Journal of Pharmacology* 170, no. 4 (2013): 712–29. doi:10.1111/bph.12344. https://www.ncbi.nlm.nih.gov/pubmed/23962094.

Epstein, E. H. "Basal Cell Carcinomas: Attack of the Hedgehog." *Nature Reviews. Cancer* 8, no. 10 (2008): 743–54. doi:10.1038/nrc2503. https://www.ncbi.nlm.nih.gov/pubmed/18813320.

Fabbrocini, G., L. Panariello, G. Caro, and S. Cacciapuoti. "Acneiform Rash Induced by EGFR Inhibitors: Review of the Literature and New Insights." *Skin Appendage Disorders* 1, no. 1 (2015): 31–7. doi:10.1159/000371821. https://www.ncbi.nlm.nih.gov/pubmed/27171241.

Fava, C., and G. Saglio. "Can We and Should We Improve on Front-Line Imatinib Therapy for Chronic Myeloid Leukemia?" *Seminars in Hematology* 47, no. 4 (2010): 319–26. doi:10.1053/j.seminhematol.2010.06.001. https://www.ncbi.nlm.nih.gov/pubmed/20875548.

Ferrara, N., K. J. Hillan, H. P. Gerber, and W. Novotny. "Discovery and Development of Bevacizumab, an Anti-VEGF Antibody for Treating Cancer." *Nature Reviews. Drug Discovery* 3, no. 5 (2004): 391–400. doi:10.1038/nrd1381. https://www.ncbi.nlm.nih.gov/pubmed/15136787.

Finn, R. S., J. Dering, D. Conklin, O. Kalous, D. J. Cohen, A. J. Desai, C. Ginther, M. Atefi, I. Chen, C. Fowst, G. Los, and D. J. Slamon. "PD 0332991, a Selective Cyclin D Kinase 4/6 Inhibitor, Preferentially Inhibits Proliferation of Luminal Estrogen Receptor-Positive Human Breast Cancer Cell Lines In Vitro." *Breast Cancer Research* 11, no. 5 (2009): R77. doi:10.1186/bcr2419. https://www.ncbi.nlm.nih.gov/pubmed/19874578.

Fischer, K., O. Al-Sawaf, J. Bahlo, A. M. Fink, M. Tandon, M. Dixon, S. Robrecht, S. Warburton, K. Humphrey, O. Samoylova, A. M. Liberati, J. Pinilla-Ibarz, L. Opat, L. Sivcheva, K. Le Dû, L. M. Fogliatto, C. U. Niemann, R. Weinkove, S. Robinson, T. J. Kipps, S. Boettcher, E. Tausch, R. Humerickhouse, B. Eichhorst, C. M. Wendtner, A. W. Langerak, K. A. Kreuzer, M. Ritgen, V. Goede, S. Stilgenbauer, M. Mobasher, and M. Hallek. "Venetoclax and Obinutuzumab in Patients with CLL and Coexisting Conditions." *New England Journal of Medicine* 380, no. 23 (2019): 2225–36. doi:10.1056/NEJMoa1815281. https://www.ncbi.nlm.nih.gov/pubmed/31166681.

Fischer, T., R. M. Stone, D. J. Deangelo, I. Galinsky, E. Estey, C. Lanza, E. Fox, G. Ehninger, E. J. Feldman, G. J. Schiller, V. M. Klimek, S. D. Nimer, D. G. Gilliland, C. Dutreix, A. Huntsman-Labed, J. Virkus, and F. J. Giles. "Phase IIB Trial of Oral Midostaurin (PKC412), the FMS-Like Tyrosine Kinase 3 Receptor (FLT3) and Multi-Targeted Kinase Inhibitor, in Patients with Acute Myeloid Leukemia and High-Risk Myelodysplastic Syndrome with Either Wild-Type or Mutated FLT3." *Journal of Clinical Oncology* 28, no. 28 (2010): 4339–45. doi:10.1200/JCO.2010.28.9678. https://www.ncbi.nlm.nih.gov/pubmed/20733134.

Francisco, J. A., C. G. Cerveny, D. L. Meyer, B. J. Mixan, K. Klussman, D. F. Chace, S. X. Rejniak, K. A. Gordon, R. DeBlanc, B. E. Toki, C. L. Law, S. O. Doronina, C. B. Siegall, P. D., P. D. Senter, and A. F. Wahl Senter, and A. F. Wahl *Blood* 102, no. 4 (2003). "cAC10-vcMMAE, an anti-CD30-monomethyl auristatin E conjugate with potent and selective antitumor activity.": 1458–65. doi:10.1182/blood-2003-01-0039. https://www.ncbi.nlm.nih.gov/pubmed/12714494.

Freeman, C. L., and L. H. Sehn. "A Tale of Two Antibodies: Obinutuzumab Versus Rituximab." *British Journal of Haematology* 182, no. 1 (2018): 29–45. doi:10.1111/bjh.15232. https://www.ncbi.nlm.nih.gov/pubmed/29741753.

Fuentes, N., and P. Silveyra. "Estrogen Receptor Signaling Mechanisms." *Advances in Protein Chemistry & Structural Biology* 116 (2019): 135–70. doi:10.1016/bs.apcsb.2019.01.001. https://www.ncbi.nlm.nih.gov/pubmed/31036290.

Gainor, J. F., G. Curigliano, and D. W. Kim. "Registrational Dataset from the phase I/II ARROW Trial of Pralsetinib (BLU-667) in Patients (pts) with Advanced RET Fusion+ Non-Small Cell Lung Cancer (NSCLC)." *Journal of Clinical Oncology* (2020).

Gambardella, V., N. Tarazona, J. M. Cejalvo, P. Lombardi, M. Huerta, S. Roselló, T. Fleitas, D. Roda, and A. Cervantes. "Personalized Medicine: Recent Progress in Cancer Therapy." *Cancers* 12, no. 4 (2020). doi:10.3390/cancers12041009. https://www.ncbi.nlm.nih.gov/pubmed/32325878.

Geisler, J. "Differences Between the Non-Steroidal Aromatase Inhibitors Anastrozole and Letrozole–of Clinical Importance?" *British Journal of Cancer* 104, no. 7 (2011): 1059–66. doi:10.1038/bjc.2011.58. https://www.ncbi .nlm.nih.gov/pubmed/21364577.

Ghia, P., A. Pluta, M. Wach, D. Lysak, T. Kozak, M. Simkovic, P. Kaplan, I. Kraychok, A. Illes, J. de la Serna, S. Dolan, P. Campbell, G. Musuraca, A. Jacob, E. Avery, J. H. Lee, W. Liang, P. Patel, C. Quah, and W. Jurczak. "ASCEND: Phase III, Randomized Trial of Acalabrutinib Versus Idelalisib plus Rituximab or Bendamustine plus Rituximab in Relapsed or Refractory Chronic Lymphocytic Leukemia." *Journal of Clinical Oncology* 38, no. 25 (2020): 2849–61. doi:10.1200/JCO.19.03355. https://www.ncbi.nlm.nih.gov/pubmed/32459600.

Ghose, Tarunendu. "The Current Status of Tumor Targeting: A Review." In *Tumor Targeting in Cancer Therapy*, edited by Michael Page. Humana Press Inc., 2002.

Gibney, G. T., L. M. Weiner, and M. B. Atkins. "Predictive Biomarkers for Checkpoint Inhibitor-Based Immunotherapy." *Lancet Oncology* 17, no. 12 (2016): e542–e51. doi:10.1016/S1470-2045(16)30406-5. https:// www.ncbi.nlm.nih.gov/pubmed/27924752.

Goede, V., K. Fischer, R. Busch, A. Engelke, B. Eichhorst, C. M. Wendtner, T. Chagorova, J. de la Serna, M. S. Dilhuydy, T. Illmer, S. Opat, C. J. Owen, O. Samoylova, K. A. Kreuzer, S. Stilgenbauer, H. Döhner, A. W. Langerak, M. Ritgen, M. Kneba, E. Asikanius, K. Humphrey, M. Wenger, and M. Hallek. "Obinutuzumab plus Chlorambucil in Patients with CLL and Coexisting Conditions." *New England Journal of Medicine* 370, no. 12 (2014): 1101–10. doi:10.1056/NEJMoa1313984. https://www.ncbi.nlm.nih.gov/pubmed/24401022.

Goekbuget, Nicola, Hervé Dombret, Massimiliano Bonifacio, Albrecht Reichle, Violaine Havelange, Eike C. Buss, Christoph Faul, Monika Bruggemann, Arnold Ganser, Julia Stieglmaier, Hendrik Wessels, Vincent Haddad, Gerhard Zugmaier, Dirk Nagorsen, Ralf C. Bargou, and R. C. Bargou. "BLAST: A Confirmatory, Single-Arm, phase 2 Study of Blinatumomab, a Bispecific T-Cell Engager (BiTE) Antibody Construct, in Patients with Minimal Residual Disease B-Precursor Acute Lymphoblastic Leukemia (ALL)." *Blood* 124, no. 21 (2014): 379.

Goldenberg, D. M., T. M. Cardillo, S. V. Govindan, E. A. Rossi, and R. M. Sharkey. "Trop-2 Is a Novel Target for Solid Cancer Therapy with Sacituzumab Govitecan (IMMU-132), an Antibody-Drug Conjugate (ADC)." *Oncotarget* 6, no. 26 (2015): 22496–512. doi:10.18632/oncotarget.4318. https://www.ncbi.nlm.nih.gov/pubmed /26101915.

Goldman, J. M., and G. Q. Daley. "Chronic Myeloid Leukemia: A Brief History." In *Myeloproliferative Disorders*, edited by Springer, 1–13. Berlin, Heidelberg: Springer, 2007.

Grossmann, M., A. S. Cheung, and J. D. Zajac. "Androgens and Prostate Cancer; Pathogenesis and Deprivation Therapy." *Best Practice & Research in Clinical Endocrinology & Metabolism* 27, no. 4 (2013): 603–16. doi:10.1016/j.beem.2013.05.001. https://www.ncbi.nlm.nih.gov/pubmed/24054933.

Hallberg, B., and R. H. Palmer. "The Role of the ALK Receptor in Cancer Biology." *Annals of Oncology* 27 Suppl. 3 (2016): iii4–iiiii15. doi:10.1093/annonc/mdw301. https://www.ncbi.nlm.nih.gov/pubmed/27573755.

Hamann, P. R., L. M. Hinman, I. Hollander, C. F. Beyer, D. Lindh, R. Holcomb, W. Hallett, H. R. Tsou, J. Upeslacis, D. Shochat, A. Mountain, D. A. Flowers, and I. Bernstein. "Gemtuzumab Ozogamicin: A Potent and Selective Anti-CD33 Antibody-Calicheamicin Conjugate for Treatment of Acute Myeloid Leukemia." *Bioconjugate Chemistry* 13, no. 1 (2002): 47–58. doi:10.1021/bc010021y. https://www.ncbi .nlm.nih.gov/pubmed/11792178.

Hamblett, K. J., P. D., D. F. Senter, M. M. Sun Chace, J. Lenox, C. G. Cerveny, K. M. Kissler, S. X. Bernhardt, A. K. Kopcha, R. F. Zabinski, D. L. Meyer, J. A. Francisco, and J. A. Francisco. "Effects of Drug Loading on the Antitumor Activity of a Monoclonal Antibody Drug Conjugate." *Clinical Cancer Research* 10, no. 20 (2004): 7063–70. doi:10.1158/1078-0432.CCR-04-0789. https://www.ncbi.nlm.nih.gov/pubmed/15501986.

Hanna, K. S. "Clinical Overview of Enfortumab Vedotin in the Management of Locally Advanced or Metastatic Urothelial Carcinoma." *Drugs* 80, no. 1 (2020): 1–7. doi:10.1007/s40265-019-01241-7. https://www.ncbi.nlm .nih.gov/pubmed/31823332.

Harrison, C., J. J. Kiladjian, H. K. Al-Ali, H. Gisslinger, R. Waltzman, V. Stalbovskaya, M. McQuitty, D. S. Hunter, R. Levy, L. Knoops, F. Cervantes, A. M. Vannucchi, T. Barbui, and G. Barosi. "JAK Inhibition with Ruxolitinib Versus Best Available Therapy for Myelofibrosis." *New England Journal of Medicine* 366, no. 9 (2012): 787–98. doi:10.1056/NEJMoa1110556. https://www.ncbi.nlm.nih.gov/pubmed/22375970.

Harrison, C. N., N. Schaap, A. M. Vannucchi, J. J. Kiladjian, R. V. Tiu, P. Zachee, E. Jourdan, E. Winton, R. T. Silver, H. C. Schouten, F. Passamonti, S. Zweegman, M. Talpaz, J. Lager, Z. Shun, and R. A. Mesa. "Janus kinase-2 Inhibitor Fedratinib in Patients with Myelofibrosis Previously Treated with Ruxolitinib (JAKARTA-2): A Single-Arm, Open-Label, Non-Randomised, phase 2, Multicentre Study." *Lancet Haematology* 4, no. 7 (2017): e317–e24. doi:10.1016/S2352-3026(17)30088-1. https://www.ncbi.nlm.nih.gov/pubmed/28602585.

Herbst, R. S. "Review of Epidermal Growth Factor Receptor Biology." *International Journal of Radiation Oncology Biology Physics* 59, no. 2 Suppl. (2004): 21–6. doi:10.1016/j.ijrobp.2003.11.041. https://www.ncbi.nlm.nih.gov /pubmed/15142631.

Hoelzer, D. "Novel Antibody-Based Therapies for Acute Lymphoblastic Leukemia." *Hematology / the Education Program of the American Society of Hematology. American Society of Hematology. Education Program* 2011 (2011): 243–9. doi:10.1182/asheducation-2011.1.243. https://www.ncbi.nlm.nih.gov/pubmed/22160041.

Hong, D. S., S. G. DuBois, S. Kummar, A. F. Farago, C. M. Albert, K. S. Rohrberg, C. M. van Tilburg, R. Nagasubramanian, J. D. Berlin, N. Federman, L. Mascarenhas, B. Geoerger, A. Dowlati, A. S. Pappo, S. Bielack, F. Doz, R. McDermott, J. D. Patel, R. J. Schilder, M. Tahara, S. M. Pfister, O. Witt, M. Ladanyi, E. R. Rudzinski, S. Nanda, B. H. Childs, T. W. Laetsch, D. M. Hyman, and A. Drilon. "Larotrectinib in Patients with TRK Fusion-Positive Solid Tumours: A Pooled Analysis of Three phase 1/2 Clinical Trials." *Lancet Oncology* 21, no. 4 (2020): 531–40. doi:10.1016/S1470-2045(19)30856-3. https://www.ncbi.nlm.nih.gov/pubmed/32105622.

Horton, H. M., M. J. Bernett, E. Pong, M. Peipp, S. Karki, S. Y. Chu, J. O. Richards, I. Vostiar, P. F. Joyce, R. Repp, J. R. Desjarlais, and E. A. Zhukovsky. "Potent In Vitro and In Vivo Activity of an Fc-Engineered Anti-CD19 Monoclonal Antibody Against Lymphoma and Leukemia." *Cancer Research* 68, no. 19 (2008): 8049–57. doi:10.1158/0008-5472.CAN-08-2268. https://www.ncbi.nlm.nih.gov/pubmed/18829563.

Hsi, E. D., R. Steinle, B. Balasa, S. Szmania, A. Draksharapu, B. P. Shum, M. Huseni, D. Powers, A. Nanisetti, Y. Zhang, A. G. Rice, A. van Abbema, M. Wong, G. Liu, F. Zhan, M. Dillon, S. Chen, S. Rhodes, F. Fuh, N. Tsurushita, S. Kumar, V. Vexler, J. D. Shaughnessy, B. Barlogie, F. van Rhee, M. Hussein, D. E. Afar, and M. B. Williams Afar, and M. B.Williams. "CS1: A Potential New Therapeutic Antibody Target for the Treatment of Multiple Myeloma." *Clinical Cancer Research* 14, no. 9 (2008): 2775–84. doi:10.1158/1078-0432.CCR-07-4246. https://www.ncbi.nlm.nih.gov/pubmed/18451245.

Imai, K., and A. Takaoka. "Comparing Antibody and Small-Molecule Therapies for Cancer." *Nature Reviews. Cancer* 6, no. 9 (2006): 714–27. doi:10.1038/nrc1913. https://www.ncbi.nlm.nih.gov/pubmed/16929325.

Javle, M., and N. J. Curtin. "The Role of PARP in DNA Repair and Its Therapeutic Exploitation." *British Journal of Cancer* 105, no. 8 (2011): 1114–22. doi:10.1038/bjc.2011.382. https://www.ncbi.nlm.nih.gov/pubmed/21989215.

Kantarjian, H., A. Stein, N. Gökbuget, A. K. Fielding, A. C. Schuh, J. M. Ribera, A. Wei, H. Dombret, R. Foà, R. Bassan, Ö. Arslan, M. A. Sanz, J. Bergeron, F. Demirkan, E. Lech-Maranda, A. Rambaldi, X. Thomas, H. A. Horst, M. Brüggemann, W. Klapper, B. L. Wood, A. Fleishman, D. Nagorsen, C. Holland, Z. Zimmerman, and M. S. Topp. "Blinatumomab Versus Chemotherapy for Advanced Acute Lymphoblastic Leukemia." *New England Journal of Medicine* 376, no. 9 (2017a): 836–47. doi:10.1056/NEJMoa1609783. https://www.ncbi.nlm.nih.gov/pubmed/28249141.

Kantarjian, H. M., D. J. DeAngelo, A. S. Advani, M. Stelljes, P. Kebriaei, R. D. Cassaday, A. A. Merchant, N. Fujishima, T. Uchida, M. Calbacho, A. A. Ejduk, S. M. O'Brien, E. J. Jabbour, H. Zhang, B. J. Sleight, E. R. Vandendries, and D. I. Marks. "Hepatic Adverse Event Profile of Inotuzumab Ozogamicin in Adult Patients with Relapsed or Refractory Acute Lymphoblastic Leukaemia: Results from the Open-Label, Randomised, phase 3 INO-VATE Study." *Lancet Haematology* 4, no. 8 (2017b): e387–e98. doi:10.1016/S2352-3026(17)30103-5. https://www.ncbi.nlm.nih.gov/pubmed/28687420.

Kantarjian, H. M., D. J. DeAngelo, M. Stelljes, M. Liedtke, W. Stock, N. Gökbuget, S. M. O'Brien, E. Jabbour, T. Wang, J. Liang White, B. Sleight, E. Vandendries, and A. S. Advani. "Inotuzumab Ozogamicin Versus Standard of Care in Relapsed or Refractory Acute Lymphoblastic Leukemia: Final Report and Long-Term Survival Follow-Up from the Randomized, phase 3 INO-VATE Study." *Cancer* 125, no. 14 (2019): 2474–87. doi:10.1002/cncr.32116. https://www.ncbi.nlm.nih.gov/pubmed/30920645.

Kasamon, Y. L., H. Chen, R. A. de Claro, L. Nie, J. Ye, G. M. Blumenthal, A. T. Farrell, and R. Pazdur. "FDA Approval Summary: Mogamulizumab-kpkc for Mycosis Fungoides and Sézary Syndrome." *Clinical Cancer Research* 25, no. 24 (2019): 7275–80. doi:10.1158/1078-0432.CCR-19-2030. https://www.ncbi.nlm.nih.gov/pubmed/31366601.

Kazazi-Hyseni, F., J. H. Beijnen, and J. H. Schellens. "Bevacizumab." *Oncologist* 15, no. 8 (2010): 819–25. doi:10.1634/theoncologist.2009-0317. https://www.ncbi.nlm.nih.gov/pubmed/20688807.

Kazlauskas, A. "PDGFs and Their Receptors." *Gene* 614 (2017): 1–7. doi:10.1016/j.gene.2017.03.003. https://www.ncbi.nlm.nih.gov/pubmed/28267575.

Kedashiro, S., A. Sugiura, K. Mizutani, and Y. Takai. "Nectin-4 cis-Interacts with ErbB2 and Its Trastuzumab-Resistant Splice Variants, Enhancing Their Activation and DNA Synthesis." *Scientific Reports* 9, no. 1 (2019): 18997. doi:10.1038/s41598-019-55460-9. https://www.ncbi.nlm.nih.gov/pubmed/31831814.

Khongorzul, P., C. J. Ling, F. U. Khan, A. U. Ihsan, and J. Zhang. "Antibody-Drug Conjugates: A Comprehensive Review." *Molecular Cancer Research* 18, no. 1 (2020): 3–19. doi:10.1158/1541-7786.MCR-19-0582. https://www.ncbi.nlm.nih.gov/pubmed/31659006.

Kim, Y. H., M. Bagot, L. Pinter-Brown, A. H. Rook, P. Porcu, S. M. Horwitz, S. Whittaker, Y. Tokura, M. Vermeer, P. L. Zinzani, L. Sokol, S. Morris, E. J. Kim, P. L. Ortiz-Romero, H. Eradat, J. Scarisbrick, A. Tsianakas, C. Elmets, S. Dalle, D. C. Fisher, A. Halwani, B. Poligone, J. Greer, M. T. Fierro, A. Khot, A. J. Moskowitz, A.

Musiek, A. Shustov, B. Pro, L. J. Geskin, K. Dwyer, J. Moriya, M. Leoni, J. S. Humphrey, S. Hudgens, D. O. Grebennik, K. Tobinai, M. Duvic, and MAVORIC Investigators. "Mogamulizumab Versus Vorinostat in Previously Treated Cutaneous T-Cell Lymphoma (MAVORIC): An International, Open-Label, Randomised, Controlled phase 3 Trial." *Lancet Oncology* 19, no. 9 (2018): 1192–204. doi:10.1016/S1470-2045(18)30379-6. https://www.ncbi.nlm.nih.gov/pubmed/30100375.

Kiyoi, H., T. Naoe, Y. Nakano, S. Yokota, S. Minami, S. Miyawaki, N. Asou, K. Kuriyama, I. Jinnai, C. Shimazaki, H. Akiyama, K. Saito, H. Oh, T. Motoji, E. Omoto, H. Saito, R. Ohno, and R. Ueda. "Prognostic Implication of FLT3 and N-RAS Gene Mutations in Acute Myeloid Leukemia." *Blood* 93, no. 9 (1999): 3074–80. https://www.ncbi.nlm.nih.gov/pubmed/10216104.

Koch, S., and L. Claesson-Welsh. "Signal Transduction by Vascular Endothelial Growth Factor Receptors." *Cold Spring Harbor Perspectives in Medicine* 2, no. 7 (2012): a006502. doi:10.1101/cshperspect.a006502. https://www.ncbi.nlm.nih.gov/pubmed/22762016.

Konstantinopoulos, P. A., C. Lacchetti, and C. M. Annunziata. "Germline and Somatic Tumor Testing in Epithelial Ovarian Cancer: ASCO Guideline Summary." *JCO Oncol. Pract* 16, no. 8 (2020): e835–e8. doi:10.1200/JOP.19.00773. https://www.ncbi.nlm.nih.gov/pubmed/32074015.

Kopetz, S., A. Grothey, R. Yaeger, E. Van Cutsem, J. Desai, T. Yoshino, H. Wasan, F. Ciardiello, F. Loupakis, Y. S. Hong, N. Steeghs, T. K. Guren, H. T. Arkenau, P. Garcia-Alfonso, P. Pfeiffer, S. Orlov, S. Lonardi, E. Elez, T. W. Kim, J. H. M. Schellens, C. Guo, A. Krishnan, J. Dekervel, V. Morris, A. Calvo Ferrandiz, L. S. Tarpgaard, M. Braun, A. Gollerkeri, C. Keir, K. Maharry, M. Pickard, J. Christy-Bittel, L. Anderson, V. Sandor, and J. Tabernero. "Encorafenib, Binimetinib, and Cetuximab In." *New England Journal of Medicine* 381, no. 17 (2019): 1632–43. doi:10.1056/NEJMoa1908075. https://www.ncbi.nlm.nih.gov/pubmed/31566309.

Kottaridis, P. D., R. E. Gale, S. E. Langabeer, M. E. Frew, D. T. Bowen, and D. C. Linch. "Studies of FLT3 Mutations in Paired Presentation and Relapse Samples from Patients with Acute Myeloid Leukemia: Implications for the Role of FLT3 Mutations in Leukemogenesis, Minimal Residual Disease Detection, and Possible Therapy with FLT3 Inhibitors." *Blood* 100, no. 7 (2002): 2393–8. doi:10.1182/blood-2002-02-0420. https://www.ncbi.nlm.nih.gov/pubmed/12239147.

Kralovics, R., F. Passamonti, A. S. Buser, S. S. Teo, R. Tiedt, J. R. Passweg, A. Tichelli, M. Cazzola, and R. C. Skoda. "A Gain-of-Function Mutation of JAK2 in Myeloproliferative Disorders." *New England Journal of Medicine* 352, no. 17 (2005): 1779–90. doi:10.1056/NEJMoa051113. https://www.ncbi.nlm.nih.gov/pubmed/15858187.

Kumari, A., O. Silakari, and R. K. Singh. "Recent Advances in Colony Stimulating factor-1 Receptor/c-FMS as an Emerging Target for Various Therapeutic Implications." *Biomedicine & Pharmacotherapy* 103 (2018): 662–79. doi:10.1016/j.biopha.2018.04.046. https://www.ncbi.nlm.nih.gov/pubmed/29679908.

Kutova, O. M., E. L. Guryev, E. A. Sokolova, R. Alzeibak, and I. V. Balalaeva. "Targeted Delivery to Tumors: Multidirectional Strategies to Improve Treatment Efficiency." *Cancers* 11, no. 1 (2019). doi:10.3390/cancers11010068. https://www.ncbi.nlm.nih.gov/pubmed/30634580.

Lachowiez, C., C. D. DiNardo, and M. Konopleva. "Venetoclax in Acute Myeloid Leukemia: Current and Future Directions." *Leukemia & Lymphoma* 61, no. 6 (2020): 1313–22. doi:10.1080/10428194.2020.1719098. https://www.ncbi.nlm.nih.gov/pubmed/32031033.

Lamb, Y. N. "Pexidartinib: First Approval." *Drugs* 79, no. 16 (2019): 1805–12. doi:10.1007/s40265-019-01210-0. https://www.ncbi.nlm.nih.gov/pubmed/31602563.

Lavanya, V., M. Adil, N. Ahmed, A. K. Rishi, and S. Jamal. "Small Molecule Inhibitors as Emerging Cancer Therapeutics." *Integrative Cancer Science and Therapeutics* (2014).

Lheureux, S., C. Denoyelle, P. S. Ohashi, J. S. De Bono, and F. M. Mottaghy. "Molecularly Targeted Therapies in Cancer: A Guide for the Nuclear Medicine Physician." *European Journal of Nuclear Medicine & Molecular Imaging* 44, no. Suppl 1 (2017): 41–54. doi:10.1007/s00259-017-3695-3. https://www.ncbi.nlm.nih.gov/pubmed/28396911.

Li, A. Y., M. G. McCusker, A. Russo, K. A. Scilla, K. Gittens, K. Arensmeyer, R. Mehra, V. Adamo, and C. Rolfo. "RET Fusions in Solid Tumors." *Cancer Treatment Reviews* 81 (2019a): 101911. doi:10.1016/j.ctrv.2019.101911. https://www.ncbi.nlm.nih.gov/pubmed/31715421.

Li, C., J. Wang, Y. Wang, H. Gao, G. Wei, Y. Huang, H. Yu, Y. Gan, L. Mei, H. Chen, H. Hu, Z. Zhang, Y. Jin, and Y. Jin. "Recent Progress in Drug Delivery." *Acta Pharmacologica Sinica B* 9, no. 6 (2019b): 1145–62. doi:10.1016/j.apsb.2019.08.003. https://www.ncbi.nlm.nih.gov/pubmed/31867161.

Li, S., R. L. Ilaria, R. P. Million, G. Q. Daley, and R. A. Van Etten. "The P190, P210, and P230 Forms of the BCR/ABL Oncogene Induce a Similar Chronic Myeloid Leukemia-Like Syndrome in Mice but Have Different Lymphoid Leukemogenic Activity." *Journal of Experimental Medicine* 189, no. 9 (1999): 1399–412. doi:10.1084/jem.189.9.1399. https://www.ncbi.nlm.nih.gov/pubmed/10224280.

Liang, J., Y. L. Wu, B. J. Chen, W. Zhang, Y. Tanaka, and H. Sugiyama. "The C-Kit Receptor-Mediated Signal Transduction and Tumor-Related Diseases." *International Journal of Biological Sciences* 9, no. 5 (2013): 435–43. doi:10.7150/ijbs.6087. https://www.ncbi.nlm.nih.gov/pubmed/23678293.

Lim, S. M., H. R. Kim, J. S. Lee, K. H. Lee, Y. G. Lee, Y. J. Min, E. K. Cho, S. S. Lee, B. S. Kim, M. Y. Choi, H. S. Shim, J. H. Chung, Y. La Choi, M. J. Lee, M. Kim, J. H. Kim, S. M. Ali, M. J. Ahn, and B. C. Cho. "Open-Label, Multicenter, phase II Study of Ceritinib in Patients with Non-Small-Cell Lung Cancer Harboring ROS1 Rearrangement." *Journal of Clinical Oncology* 35, no. 23 (2017): 2613–8. doi:10.1200/JCO.2016.71.3701. https://www.ncbi.nlm.nih.gov/pubmed/28520527.

Lin, J. J., and A. T. Shaw. "Recent Advances in Targeting ROS1 in Lung Cancer." *Journal of Thoracic Oncology* 12, no. 11 (2017): 1611–25. doi:10.1016/j.jtho.2017.08.002. https://www.ncbi.nlm.nih.gov/pubmed/28818606.

Lin, J. J., G. J. Riely, and A. T. Shaw. "Targeting ALK: Precision Medicine Takes on Drug Resistance." *Cancer Discovery* 7, no. 2 (2017): 137–55. doi:10.1158/2159-8290.CD-16-1123. https://www.ncbi.nlm.nih.gov/pubmed/28122866.

Lipinski, M., D. R. Parks, R. V. Rouse, and L. A. Herzenberg. "Human Trophoblast Cell-Surface Antigens Defined by Monoclonal Antibodies." *Proceedings of the National Academy of Sciences of the United States of America* 78, no. 8 (1981): 5147–50. doi:10.1073/pnas.78.8.5147. https://www.ncbi.nlm.nih.gov/pubmed/7029529.

Locke, K. W., D. C. Maneval, and M. J. LaBarre. "ENHANZE." *Drug Delivery* 26, no. 1 (2019): 98–106. doi:10.1080/10717544.2018.1551442. https://www.ncbi.nlm.nih.gov/pubmed/30744432.

Lokhorst, H. M., T. Plesner, J. P. Laubach, H. Nahi, P. Gimsing, M. Hansson, M. C. Minnema, U. Lassen, J. Krejcik, A. Palumbo, N. W. van de Donk, T. Ahmadi, I. Khan, C. M. Uhlar, J. Wang, A. K. Sasser, N. Losic, S. Lisby, L. Basse, N. Brun, and P. G. Richardson. "Targeting CD38 with Daratumumab Monotherapy in Multiple Myeloma." *New England Journal of Medicine* 373, no. 13 (2015): 1207–19. doi:10.1056/NEJMoa1506348. https://www.ncbi.nlm.nih.gov/pubmed/26308596.

Long, G. V., K. T. Flaherty, D. Stroyakovskiy, H. Gogas, E. Levchenko, F. de Braud, J. Larkin, C. Garbe, T. Jouary, A. Hauschild, V. Chiarion-Sileni, C. Lebbe, M. Mandalà, M. Millward, A. Arance, I. Bondarenko, J. B. A. G. Haanen, J. Hansson, J. Utikal, V. Ferraresi, P. Mohr, V. Probachai, D. Schadendorf, P. Nathan, C. Robert, A. Ribas, M. A. Davies, S. R. Lane, J. J. Legos, B. Mookerjee, and J. J. Grob. "Dabrafenib plus Trametinib Versus Dabrafenib Monotherapy in Patients with Metastatic BRAF V600E/K-mutant Melanoma: Long-Term Survival and Safety Analysis of a phase 3 Study." *Annals of Oncology* 28, no. 7 (2017): 1631–9. doi:10.1093/annonc/mdx176. https://www.ncbi.nlm.nih.gov/pubmed/28475671.

Lonial, S., M. Dimopoulos, A. Palumbo, D. White, S. Grosicki, I. Spicka, A. Walter-Croneck, P. Moreau, M. V. Mateos, H. Magen, A. Belch, D. Reece, M. Beksac, A. Spencer, H. Oakervee, R. Z. Orlowski, M. Taniwaki, C. Röllig, H. Einsele, K. L. Wu, A. Singhal, J. San-Miguel, M. Matsumoto, J. Katz, E. Bleickardt, V. Poulart, K. C. Anderson, P. Richardson, and ELOQUENT-2 Investigators. "Elotuzumab Therapy for Relapsed or Refractory Multiple Myeloma." *New England Journal of Medicine* 373, no. 7 (2015): 621–31. doi:10.1056/NEJMoa1505654. https://www.ncbi.nlm.nih.gov/pubmed/26035255.

Lonial, S., H. C. Lee, A. Badros, S. Trudel, A. K. Nooka, A. Chari, A. O. Abdallah, N. Callander, N. Lendvai, D. Sborov, A. Suvannasankha, K. Weisel, L. Karlin, E. Libby, B. Arnulf, T. Facon, C. Hulin, K. M. Kortüm, P. Rodríguez-Otero, S. Z. Usmani, P. Hari, R. Baz, H. Quach, P. Moreau, P. M. Voorhees, I. Gupta, A. Hoos, E. Zhi, J. Baron, T. Piontek, E. Lewis, R. C. Jewell, E. J. Dettman, R. Popat, S. D. Esposti, J. Opalinska, P. Richardson, and A. D. Cohen. "Belantamab Mafodotin for Relapsed or Refractory Multiple Myeloma (DREAMM-2): A Two-Arm, Randomised, Open-Label, phase 2 Study." *Lancet Oncology* 21, no. 2 (2020): 207–21. doi:10.1016/S1470-2045(19)30788-0. https://www.ncbi.nlm.nih.gov/pubmed/31859245.

Loriot, Y., A. Necchi, S. H. Park, J. Garcia-Donas, R. Huddart, E. Burgess, M. Fleming, A. Rezazadeh, B. Mellado, S. Varlamov, M. Joshi, I. Duran, S. T. Tagawa, Y. Zakharia, B. Zhong, K. Stuyckens, A. Santiago-Walker, P. De Porre, A. O'Hagan, A. Avadhani, A. O. Siefker-Radtke, and BLC2001 Study Group. "Erdafitinib in Locally Advanced or Metastatic Urothelial Carcinoma." *New England Journal of Medicine* 381, no. 4 (2019): 338–48. doi:10.1056/NEJMoa1817323. https://www.ncbi.nlm.nih.gov/pubmed/31340094.

Lynparza *[package insert]*. Wilmington, DE: AstraZeneca Pharmaceuticals LP, Nov. 2020.

Ma, C., S. Wei, and Y. Song. "T790M and Acquired Resistance of EGFR TKI: A Literature Review of Clinical Reports." *Journal of Thoracic Disease* 3, no. 1 (2011): 10–8. doi:10.3978/j.issn.2072-1439.2010.12.02. https://www.ncbi.nlm.nih.gov/pubmed/22263058.

Mahipal, A., S. H. Tella, A. Kommalapati, J. Yu, and R. Kim. "Prevention and Treatment of FGFR Inhibitor-Associated Toxicities." *Critical Reviews in Oncology/Hematology* 155 (2020): 103091. doi:10.1016/j.critrevonc.2020.103091. https://www.ncbi.nlm.nih.gov/pubmed/32961472.

Makita, S., and K. Tobinai. "Mogamulizumab for the Treatment of T-Cell Lymphoma." *Expert Opinion on Biological Therapy* 17, no. 9 (2017): 1145–53. doi:10.1080/14712598.2017.1347634. https://www.ncbi.nlm.nih.gov/pubmed/28649848.

Mandai, K., Y. Rikitake, M. Mori, and Y. Takai. "Nectins and Nectin-Like Molecules in Development and Disease." *Current Topics in Developmental Biology* 112 (2015): 197–231. doi:10.1016/bs.ctdb.2014.11.019. https://www.ncbi.nlm.nih.gov/pubmed/25733141.

Marcus, R., A. Davies, K. Ando, W. Klapper, S. Opat, C. Owen, E. Phillips, R. Sangha, R. Schlag, J. F. Seymour, W. Townsend, M. Trněný, M. Wenger, G. Fingerle-Rowson, K. Rufibach, T. Moore, M. Herold, and W. Hiddemann. "Obinutuzumab for the First-Line Treatment of Follicular Lymphoma." *New England Journal of Medicine* 377, no. 14 (2017): 1331–44. doi:10.1056/NEJMoa1614598. https://www.ncbi.nlm.nih.gov/pubmed/28976863.

McArthur, G. A., P. B. Chapman, C. Robert, J. Larkin, J. B. Haanen, R. Dummer, A. Ribas, D. Hogg, O. Hamid, P. A. Ascierto, C. Garbe, A. Testori, M. Maio, P. Lorigan, C. Lebbé, T. Jouary, D. Schadendorf, S. J. O'Day, J. M. Kirkwood, A. M. Eggermont, B. Dréno, J. A. Sosman, K. T. Flaherty, M. Yin, I. Caro, S. Cheng, K. Trunzer, and A. Hauschild. "Safety and Efficacy of Vemurafenib in BRAF(V600E) and BRAF(V600K) Mutation-Positive Melanoma (BRIM-3): Extended Follow-Up of a phase 3, Randomised, Open-Label Study." *Lancet Oncology* 15, no. 3 (2014): 323–32. doi:10.1016/S1470-2045(14)70012-9. https://www.ncbi.nlm.nih.gov/pubmed/24508103.

Melo, J. V., and M. W. Deininger. "Biology of Chronic Myelogenous Leukemia: Signaling Pathways of Initiation and Transformation." *Hematology/Oncology Clinics of North America* 18, no. 3 (2004): 545–68, vii–viii. doi:10.1016/j.hoc.2004.03.008. https://www.ncbi.nlm.nih.gov/pubmed/15271392.

Mensah, F. A., J. P. Blaize, and L. J. Bryan. "Spotlight on Copanlisib and Its Potential in the Treatment of Relapsed/Refractory Follicular Lymphoma: Evidence to Date." *OncoTargets & Therapy* 11 (2018): 4817–27. doi:10.2147/OTT.S142264. https://www.ncbi.nlm.nih.gov/pubmed/30147333.

Milojkovic, D., and J. Apperley. "Mechanisms of Resistance to Imatinib and Second-Generation Tyrosine Inhibitors in Chronic Myeloid Leukemia." *Clinical Cancer Research* 15, no. 24 (2009): 7519–27. doi:10.1158/1078-0432.CCR-09-1068. https://www.ncbi.nlm.nih.gov/pubmed/20008852.

Modi, S., C. Saura, T. Yamashita, Y. H. Park, S. B. Kim, K. Tamura, F. Andre, H. Iwata, Y. Ito, J. Tsurutani, J. Sohn, N. Denduluri, C. Perrin, K. Aogi, E. Tokunaga, S. A. Im, K. S. Lee, S. A. Hurvitz, J. Cortes, C. Lee, S. Chen, L. Zhang, J. Shahidi, A. Yver, I. Krop, and DESTINY-Breast01 Investigators. "Trastuzumab Deruxtecan in Previously Treated HER2-Positive Breast Cancer." *New England Journal of Medicine* 382, no. 7 (2020): 610–21. doi:10.1056/NEJMoa1914510. https://www.ncbi.nlm.nih.gov/pubmed/31825192.

Moore, A. R., S. C. Rosenberg, F. McCormick, and S. Malek. "RAS-Targeted Therapies: Is the Undruggable Drugged?" *Nature Reviews. Drug Discovery* 19, no. 8 (2020): 533–52. doi:10.1038/s41573-020-0068-6. https://www.ncbi.nlm.nih.gov/pubmed/32528145.

Morabito, F., A. G. Recchia, E. Vigna, C. Botta, M. Skafi, M. Abu-Rayyan, M. Atrash, S. Galimberti, L. Morabito, H. Al-Janazreh, M. Martino, G. Cutrona, and M. Gentile. "An In-Depth Evaluation of Acalabrutinib for the Treatment of Mantle-Cell Lymphoma." *Expert Opinion on Pharmacotherapy* 21, no. 1 (2020): 29–38. doi:10.1080/14656566.2019.1689959. https://www.ncbi.nlm.nih.gov/pubmed/31738609.

Morgensztern, D., K. Politi, and R. S. Herbst. "EGFR Mutations in Non-Small-Cell Lung Cancer: Find, Divide, and Conquer." *JAMA Oncology* 1, no. 2 (2015): 146–8. doi:10.1001/jamaoncol.2014.278. https://www.ncbi.nlm.nih.gov/pubmed/26181013.

Moskowitz, C. H., A. Nademanee, T. Masszi, E. Agura, J. Holowiecki, M. H. Abidi, A. I. Chen, P. Stiff, A. M. Gianni, A. Carella, D. Osmanov, V. Bachanova, J. Sweetenham, A. Sureda, D. Huebner, E. L. Sievers, A. Chi, E. K. Larsen, N. N. Hunder, J. Walewski, and AETHERA Study Group. "Brentuximab Vedotin as Consolidation Therapy After Autologous Stem-Cell Transplantation in Patients with Hodgkin's Lymphoma At Risk of Relapse or Progression (AETHERA): A Randomised, Double-Blind, Placebo-Controlled, phase 3 Trial." *Lancet* 385, no. 9980 (2015): 1853–62. doi:10.1016/S0140-6736(15)60165-9. https://www.ncbi.nlm.nih.gov/pubmed/25796459.

Mulligan, L. M. "RET Revisited: Expanding the Oncogenic Portfolio." *Nature Reviews. Cancer* 14, no. 3 (2014): 173–86. doi:10.1038/nrc3680. https://www.ncbi.nlm.nih.gov/pubmed/24561444.

Murthy, R. K., S. Loi, A. Okines, E. Paplomata, E. Hamilton, S. A. Hurvitz, N. U. Lin, V. Borges, V. Abramson, C. Anders, P. L. Bedard, M. Oliveira, E. Jakobsen, T. Bachelot, S. S. Shachar, V. Müller, S. Braga, F. P. Duhoux, R. Greil, D. Cameron, L. A. Carey, G. Curigliano, K. Gelmon, G. Hortobagyi, I. Krop, S. Loibl, M. Pegram, D. Slamon, M. C. Palanca-Wessels, L. Walker, W. Feng, and E. P. Winer. "Tucatinib, Trastuzumab, and Capecitabine for HER2-Positive Metastatic Breast Cancer." *New England Journal of Medicine* 382, no. 7 (2020): 597–609. doi:10.1056/NEJMoa1914609. https://www.ncbi.nlm.nih.gov/pubmed/31825569.

Nami, B., H. Maadi, and Z. Wang. "Mechanisms Underlying the Action and Synergism of Trastuzumab and Pertuzumab in Targeting HER2-Positive Breast Cancer." *Cancers* 10, no. 10 (2018). doi:10.3390/cancers10100342. https://www.ncbi.nlm.nih.gov/pubmed/30241301.

Neel, D. S., and T. G. Bivona. "Resistance Is Futile: Overcoming Resistance to Targeted Therapies in Lung Adenocarcinoma." *NPJ Precision Oncology* 1 (2017). doi:10.1038/s41698-017-0007-0. https://www.ncbi.nlm.nih.gov/pubmed/29152593.

Nerlynx [Package Insert]. Los Angeles, CA: Puma Biotechnology, Inc., 2020.

Niemann, C. U., S. E. Herman, I. Maric, J. Gomez-Rodriguez, A. Biancotto, B. Y. Chang, S. Martyr, M. Stetler-Stevenson, C. M. Yuan, K. R. Calvo, R. C. Braylan, J. Valdez, Y. S. Lee, D. H. Wong, J. Jones, C. Sun, G. E. Marti, M. Z. Farooqui, and A. Wiestner. "Disruption of In Vivo Chronic Lymphocytic Leukemia Tumor-Microenvironment Interactions by Ibrutinib: Findings from an Investigator-Initiated phase II Study." *Clinical Cancer Research* 22, no. 7 (2016): 1572–82. doi:10.1158/1078-0432.CCR-15-1965. https://www.ncbi.nlm.nih.gov/pubmed/26660519.

Niu, G., and X. Chen. "Vascular Endothelial Growth Factor as an Anti-Angiogenic Target for Cancer Therapy." *Current Drug Targets* 11, no. 8 (2010): 1000–17. doi:10.2174/138945010791591395. https://www.ncbi.nlm.nih.gov/pubmed/20426765.

Okeley, N. M., J. B. Miyamoto, X. Zhang, R. J. Sanderson, D. R. Benjamin, E. L. Sievers, P. D., P. D. Senter, and S. C. Alley. "Intracellular Activation of SGN-35: A Potent Anti-CD30 Antibody-drug Conjugate." *Clinical Cancer Research* 16, no. 3 (2010): 888–97. doi:10.1158/1078-0432.CCR-09-2069. https://www.ncbi.nlm.nih.gov/pubmed/20086002.

Papadopoulos, N., and J. Lennartsson. "The PDGF/PDGFR Pathway as a Drug Target." *Molecular Aspects of Medicine* 62 (2018): 75–88. doi:10.1016/j.mam.2017.11.007. https://www.ncbi.nlm.nih.gov/pubmed/29137923.

Patel, H. K., and T. Bihani. "Selective Estrogen Receptor Modulators (SERMs) and Selective Estrogen Receptor Degraders (SERDs) in Cancer Treatment." *Pharmacology & Therapeutics* 186 (2018): 1–24. doi:10.1016/j.pharmthera.2017.12.012. https://www.ncbi.nlm.nih.gov/pubmed/29289555.

Pederzoli, F., M. Bandini, L. Marandino, S. M. Ali, R. Madison, J. Chung, J. S. Ross, and A. Necchi. "Targetable Gene Fusions and Aberrations in Genitourinary Oncology." *Nature Reviews. Urology* 17, no. 11 (2020): 613–25. doi:10.1038/s41585-020-00379-4. https://www.ncbi.nlm.nih.gov/pubmed/33046892.

Perl, A. E., G. Martinelli, J. E. Cortes, A. Neubauer, E. Berman, S. Paolini, P. Montesinos, M. R. Baer, R. A. Larson, C. Ustun, F. Fabbiano, H. P. Erba, A. Di Stasi, R. Stuart, R. Olin, M. Kasner, F. Ciceri, W. C. Chou, N. Podoltsev, C. Recher, H. Yokoyama, N. Hosono, S. S. Yoon, J. H. Lee, T. Pardee, A. T. Fathi, C. Liu, N. Hasabou, X. Liu, E. Bahceci, and M. J. Levis. "Gilteritinib or Chemotherapy for Relapsed or Refractory." *New England Journal of Medicine* 381, no. 18 (2019): 1728–40. doi:10.1056/NEJMoa1902688. https://www.ncbi.nlm.nih.gov/pubmed/31665578.

Pernas, S., S. M. Tolaney, E. P. Winer, and S. Goel. "CDK4/6 Inhibition in Breast Cancer: Current Practice and Future Directions." *Therapeutic Advances in Medical Oncology* 10 (2018): 1758835918786451. doi:10.1177/1758835918786451. https://www.ncbi.nlm.nih.gov/pubmed/30038670.

Petersdorf, S. H., K. J. Kopecky, M. Slovak, C. Willman, T. Nevill, J. Brandwein, R. A. Larson, H. P. Erba, P. J. Stiff, R. K. Stuart, R. B. Walter, M. S. Tallman, L. Stenke, and F. R. Appelbaum. "A phase 3 Study of Gemtuzumab Ozogamicin During Induction and Postconsolidation Therapy in Younger Patients with Acute Myeloid Leukemia." *Blood* 121, no. 24 (2013): 4854–60. doi:10.1182/blood-2013-01-466706. https://www.ncbi.nlm.nih.gov/pubmed/23591789.

Pittoni, P., S. Piconese, C. Tripodo, and M. P. Colombo. "Tumor-Intrinsic and -Extrinsic Roles of c-Kit: Mast Cells as the Primary Off-Target of Tyrosine Kinase Inhibitors." *Oncogene* 30, no. 7 (2011): 757–69. doi:10.1038/onc.2010.494. https://www.ncbi.nlm.nih.gov/pubmed/21057534.

Pollyea, D. A., M. Amaya, P. Strati, and M. Y. Konopleva. "Venetoclax for AML: Changing the Treatment Paradigm." *Blood Advances* 3, no. 24 (2019): 4326–35. doi:10.1182/bloodadvances.2019000937. https://www.ncbi.nlm.nih.gov/pubmed/31869416.

Polson, A. G., S. F. Yu, K. Elkins, B. Zheng, S. Clark, G. S. Ingle, D. S. Slaga, L. Giere, C. Du, C. Tan, J. A. Hongo, A. Gogineni, M. J. Cole, R. Vandlen, J. P. Stephan, J. Young, W. Chang, S. J. Scales, S. Ross, D. Eaton, and A. Ebens. "Antibody-Drug Conjugates Targeted to CD79 for the Treatment of Non-Hodgkin Lymphoma." *Blood* 110, no. 2 (2007): 616–23. doi:10.1182/blood-2007-01-066704. https://www.ncbi.nlm.nih.gov/pubmed/17374736.

Pommier, Y., M. J. O'Connor, and J. de Bono. "Laying a Trap to Kill Cancer Cells: PARP Inhibitors and Their Mechanisms of Action." *Science Translational Medicine* 8, no. 362 (2016): 362ps17. doi:10.1126/scitranslmed.aaf9246. https://www.ncbi.nlm.nih.gov/pubmed/27797957.

Porta, C., C. Paglino, and A. Mosca. "Targeting PI3K/Akt/mTOR Signaling in Cancer." *Frontiers in Oncology* 4 (2014): 64. doi:10.3389/fonc.2014.00064. https://www.ncbi.nlm.nih.gov/pubmed/24782981.

Postow, M. A., M. K. Callahan, and J. D. Wolchok. "Immune Checkpoint Blockade in Cancer Therapy." *Journal of Clinical Oncology* 33, no. 17 (2015): 1974–82. doi:10.1200/JCO.2014.59.4358. https://www.ncbi.nlm.nih.gov/pubmed/25605845.

Pratz, K. W., and M. Levis. "How I Treat FLT3-Mutated AML." *Blood* 129, no. 5 (2017): 565–71. doi:10.1182/blood-2016-09-693648. https://www.ncbi.nlm.nih.gov/pubmed/27872057.

Propper, D. J., A. C. McDonald, A. Man, P. Thavasu, F. Balkwill, J. P. Braybrooke, F. Caponigro, P. Graf, C. Dutreix, R. Blackie, S. B. Kaye, T. S. Ganesan, D. C. Talbot, A. L. Harris, and C. Twelves. "Phase I and Pharmacokinetic Study of PKC412, an Inhibitor of Protein Kinase C." *Journal of Clinical Oncology* 19, no. 5 (2001): 1485–92. doi:10.1200/JCO.2001.19.5.1485. https://www.ncbi.nlm.nih.gov/pubmed/11230495.

Raica, M., and A. M. Cimpean. "Platelet-Derived Growth Factor (PDGF)/PDGF Receptors (PDGFR) Axis as Target for Antitumor and Antiangiogenic Therapy." *Pharmaceuticals* 3, no. 3 (2010): 572–99. doi:10.3390/ph3030572. https://www.ncbi.nlm.nih.gov/pubmed/27713269.

Reungwetwattana, T., Y. Liang, V. Zhu, and S. I. Ou. "The Race to Target MET exon 14 Skipping Alterations in Non-Small Cell Lung Cancer: The Why, the How, the Who, the Unknown, and the Inevitable." *Lung Cancer* 103 (2017): 27–37. doi:10.1016/j.lungcan.2016.11.011. https://www.ncbi.nlm.nih.gov/pubmed/28024693.

Ricart, A. D. "Antibody-Drug Conjugates of Calicheamicin Derivative: Gemtuzumab Ozogamicin and Inotuzumab Ozogamicin." *Clinical Cancer Research* 17, no. 20 (2011): 6417–27. doi:10.1158/1078-0432.CCR-11-0486. https://www.ncbi.nlm.nih.gov/pubmed/22003069.

Ricciuti, B., M. Brambilla, G. Metro, S. Baglivo, R. Matocci, M. Pirro, and R. Chiari. "Targeting NTRK Fusion in Non-Small Cell Lung Cancer: Rationale and Clinical Evidence." *Medical Oncology* 34, no. 6 (2017): 105. doi:10.1007/s12032-017-0967-5. https://www.ncbi.nlm.nih.gov/pubmed/28444624.

Rice, M. A., S. V. Malhotra, and T. Stoyanova. "Second-Generation Antiandrogens: From Discovery to Standard of Care in Castration Resistant Prostate Cancer." *Frontiers in Oncology* 9 (2019): 801. doi:10.3389/fonc.2019.00801. https://www.ncbi.nlm.nih.gov/pubmed/31555580.

Riggs, B. L., and L. C. Hartmann. "Selective Estrogen-Receptor Modulators: Mechanisms of Action and Application to Clinical Practice." *New England Journal of Medicine* 348, no. 7 (2003): 618–29. doi:10.1056/NEJMra022219. https://www.ncbi.nlm.nih.gov/pubmed/12584371.

Roberts, P. J., and C. J.Der . "Targeting the Raf-MEK-ERK Mitogen-Activated Protein Kinase Cascade for the Treatment of Cancer." *Oncogene* 26, no. 22 (2007): 3291–310. doi:10.1038/sj.onc.1210422. https://www.ncbi.nlm.nih.gov/pubmed/17496923.

Röllig, C., H. Serve, A. Hüttmann, R. Noppeney, C. Müller-Tidow, U. Krug, C. D. Baldus, C. H. Brandts, V. Kunzmann, H. Einsele, A. Krämer, K. Schäfer-Eckart, A. Neubauer, A. Burchert, A. Giagounidis, S. W. Krause, A. Mackensen, W. Aulitzky, R. Herbst, M. Hänel, A. Kiani, N. Frickhofen, J. Kullmer, U. Kaiser, H. Link, T. Geer, A. Reichle, C. Junghanß, R. Repp, F. Heits, H. Dürk, J. Hase, I. M. Klut, T. Illmer, M. Bornhäuser, M. Schaich, S. Parmentier, M. Görner, C. Thiede, M. von Bonin, J. Schetelig, M. Kramer, W. E. Berdel, G. Ehninger, and Study Alliance Leukaemia. "Addition of Sorafenib Versus Placebo to Standard Therapy in Patients Aged 60 Years or Younger with Newly Diagnosed Acute Myeloid Leukaemia (SORAML): A Multicentre, phase 2, Randomised Controlled Trial." *Lancet Oncology* 16, no. 16 (2015): 1691–9. doi:10.1016/S1470-2045(15)00362-9. https://www.ncbi.nlm.nih.gov/pubmed/26549589.

Romei, C., R. Ciampi, and R. Elisei. "A Comprehensive Overview of the Role of the RET Proto-Oncogene in Thyroid Carcinoma." *Nature Reviews Endocrinology* 12, no. 4 (2016): 192–202. doi:10.1038/nrendo.2016.11. https://www.ncbi.nlm.nih.gov/pubmed/26868437.

Rosenberg, J. E., P. H. O'Donnell, A. V. Balar, B. A. McGregor, E. I. Heath, E. Y. Yu, M. D. Galsky, N. M. Hahn, E. M. Gartner, J. M. Pinelli, S. Y. Liang, A. Melhem-Bertrandt, and D. P. Petrylak. "Pivotal Trial of Enfortumab Vedotin in Urothelial Carcinoma After Platinum and Anti-Programmed Death 1/Programmed Death Ligand 1 Therapy." *Journal of Clinical Oncology* 37, no. 29 (2019): 2592–600. doi:10.1200/JCO.19.01140. https://www.ncbi.nlm.nih.gov/pubmed/31356140.

Roy, R., J. Chun, and S. N. Powell. "BRCA1 and BRCA2: Different Roles in a Common Pathway of Genome Protection." *Nature Reviews. Cancer* 12, no. 1 (2011): 68–78. doi:10.1038/nrc3181. https://www.ncbi.nlm.nih.gov/pubmed/22193408.

Rubraca *[package insert]*. Boulder, CO: Clovis Oncology, Inc, Oct. 2020.

Salgia, R. "MET in Lung Cancer: Biomarker Selection Based on Scientific Rationale." *Molecular Cancer Therapeutics* 16, no. 4 (2017): 555–65. doi:10.1158/1535-7163.MCT-16-0472. https://www.ncbi.nlm.nih.gov/pubmed/28373408.

Salles, G., J. Duell, E. González Barca, O. Tournilhac, W. Jurczak, A. M. Liberati, Z. Nagy, A. Obr, G. Gaidano, M. André, N. Kalakonda, M. Dreyling, J. Weirather, M. Dirnberger-Hertweck, S. Ambarkhane, G. Fingerle-Rowson, and K. Maddocks. "Tafasitamab plus Lenalidomide in Relapsed or Refractory Diffuse Large B-Cell Lymphoma (L-MIND): A Multicentre, Prospective, Single-Arm, phase 2 Study." *Lancet Oncology* 21, no. 7 (2020): 978–88. doi:10.1016/S1470-2045(20)30225-4. https://www.ncbi.nlm.nih.gov/pubmed/32511983.

Salonen, A. J., J. Viitanen, S. Lundstedt, M. Ala-Opas, K. Taari, T. L. Tammela, and FinnProstate Group. "Finnish Multicenter Study Comparing Intermittent to Continuous Androgen Deprivation for Advanced Prostate Cancer: Interim Analysis of Prognostic Markers Affecting Initial Response to Androgen Deprivation." *Journal of Urology* 180, no. 3 (2008): 915–9; discussion 919–20. doi:10.1016/j.juro.2008.05.009. https://www.ncbi.nlm.nih.gov/pubmed/18635219.

Sanchez, J. N., T. Wang, and M. S. Cohen. "BRAF and MEK Inhibitors: Use and Resistance in BRAF-Mutated Cancers." *Drugs* 78, no. 5 (2018): 549–66. doi:10.1007/s40265-018-0884-8. https://www.ncbi.nlm.nih.gov/pubmed/29488071.

Sanford, M. "Blinatumomab: First Global Approval." *Drugs* 75, no. 3 (2015): 321–7. doi:10.1007/s40265-015-0356-3. https://www.ncbi.nlm.nih.gov/pubmed/25637301.

Sattler, M., and R. Salgia. "Targeting c-Kit Mutations: Basic Science to Novel Therapies." *Leukemia Research* 28 Suppl. 1 (2004): S11–S20. doi:10.1016/j.leukres.2003.10.004. https://www.ncbi.nlm.nih.gov/pubmed/15036937.

Scott, L. J. "Brentuximab Vedotin: A Review in CD30-Positive Hodgkin Lymphoma." *Drugs* 77, no. 4 (2017): 435–45. doi:10.1007/s40265-017-0705-5. https://www.ncbi.nlm.nih.gov/pubmed/28190142.

Scott, L. J. "Larotrectinib: First Global Approval." *Drugs* 79, no. 2 (2019): 201–6. doi:10.1007/s40265-018-1044-x. https://www.ncbi.nlm.nih.gov/pubmed/30635837.

Sehn, L. H., A. F. Herrera, C. R. Flowers, M. K. Kamdar, A. McMillan, M. Hertzberg, S. Assouline, T. M. Kim, W. S. Kim, M. Ozcan, J. Hirata, E. Penuel, J. N. Paulson, J. Cheng, G. Ku, and M. J. Matasar. "Polatuzumab Vedotin in Relapsed or Refractory Diffuse Large B-Cell Lymphoma." *Journal of Clinical Oncology* 38, no. 2 (2020): 155–65. doi:10.1200/JCO.19.00172. https://www.ncbi.nlm.nih.gov/pubmed/31693429.

Sekulic, A., A. R. Mangold, D. W. Northfelt, and P. M. LoRusso. "Advanced Basal Cell Carcinoma of the Skin: Targeting the Hedgehog Pathway." *Current Opinion in Oncology* 25, no. 3 (2013): 218–23. doi:10.1097/CCO.0b013e32835ff438. https://www.ncbi.nlm.nih.gov/pubmed/23493193.

Senapati, S., A. K. Mahanta, S. Kumar, and P. Maiti. "Controlled Drug Delivery Vehicles for Cancer Treatment and Their Performance." *Signal Transduction & Targeted Therapy* 3 (2018): 7. doi:10.1038/s41392-017-0004-3. https://www.ncbi.nlm.nih.gov/pubmed/29560283.

Senter, P. D., and E. L. Sievers. "The Discovery and Development of Brentuximab Vedotin for Use in Relapsed Hodgkin Lymphoma and Systemic Anaplastic Large Cell Lymphoma." *Nature Biotechnology* 30, no. 7 (2012): 631–7. doi:10.1038/nbt.2289. https://www.ncbi.nlm.nih.gov/pubmed/22781692.

Seymour, J. F., T. J. Kipps, B. Eichhorst, P. Hillmen, J. D'Rozario, S. Assouline, C. Owen, J. Gerecitano, T. Robak, J. De la Serna, U. Jaeger, G. Cartron, M. Montillo, R. Humerickhouse, E. A. Punnoose, Y. Li, M. Boyer, K. Humphrey, M. Mobasher, and A. P. Kater. "Venetoclax-rituximab in Relapsed or Refractory Chronic Lymphocytic Leukemia." *New England Journal of Medicine* 378, no. 12 (2018): 1107–20. doi:10.1056/NEJMoa1713976. https://www.ncbi.nlm.nih.gov/pubmed/29562156.

Shah, M., M. R. Nunes, and V. Stearns. "CDK4/6 Inhibitors: Game Changers in the Management of Hormone Receptor–Positive Advanced Breast Cancer?" *Oncology* 32, no. 5 (2018): 216–22. https://www.ncbi.nlm.nih.gov/pubmed/29847850.

Sharman, J. P., M. Egyed, W. Jurczak, A. Skarbnik, J. M. Pagel, I. W. Flinn, M. Kamdar, T. Munir, R. Walewska, G. Corbett, L. M. Fogliatto, Y. Herishanu, V. Banerji, S. Coutre, G. Follows, P. Walker, K. Karlsson, P. Ghia, A. Janssens, F. Cymbalista, J. A. Woyach, G. Salles, W. G. Wierda, R. Izumi, V. Munugalavadla, P. Patel, M. H. Wang, S. Wong, and J. C. Byrd. "Acalabrutinib with or Without Obinutuzumab Versus Chlorambucil and Obinutuzmab for Treatment-Naive Chronic Lymphocytic Leukaemia (ELEVATE TN): A Randomised, Controlled, phase 3 Trial." *Lancet* 395, no. 10232 (2020): 1278–91. doi:10.1016/S0140-6736(20)30262-2. https://www.ncbi.nlm.nih.gov/pubmed/32305093.

Shaw, A. T., and J. A. Engelman. "ALK in Lung Cancer: Past, Present, and Future." *Journal of Clinical Oncology* 31, no. 8 (2013): 1105–11. doi:10.1200/JCO.2012.44.5353. https://www.ncbi.nlm.nih.gov/pubmed/23401436.

Shaw, A. T., S. H. Ou, Y. J. Bang, D. R. Camidge, B. J. Solomon, R. Salgia, G. J. Riely, M. Varella-Garcia, G. I. Shapiro, D. B. Costa, R. C. Doebele, L. P. Le, Z. Zheng, W. Tan, P. Stephenson, S. M. Shreeve, L. M. Tye, J. G. Christensen, K. D. Wilner, J. W. Clark, and A. J. Iafrate. "Crizotinib in ROS1-Rearranged Non-Small-Cell Lung Cancer." *New England Journal of Medicine* 371, no. 21 (2014): 1963–71. doi:10.1056/NEJMoa1406766. https://www.ncbi.nlm.nih.gov/pubmed/25264305.

Shibuya, M. "Vascular Endothelial Growth Factor (VEGF) and Its Receptor (VEGFR) Signaling in Angiogenesis: A Crucial Target for Anti- and Pro-Angiogenic Therapies." *Genes & Cancer* 2, no. 12 (2011): 1097–105. doi:10.1177/1947601911423031. https://www.ncbi.nlm.nih.gov/pubmed/22866201.

Shingleton, J. R., and S. S. Dave. "Polatuzumab Vedotin: Honing in on Relapsed or Refractory Diffuse Large B-Cell Lymphoma." *Journal of Clinical Oncology* 38, no. 2 (2020): 166–8. doi:10.1200/JCO.19.02587. https://www.ncbi.nlm.nih.gov/pubmed/31770050.

Shvartsur, A., and B. Bonavida. "Trop2 and Its Overexpression in Cancers: Regulation and Clinical/Therapeutic Implications." *Genes & Cancer* 6, no. 3–4 (2015): 84–105. doi:10.18632/genesandcancer.40. https://www.ncbi .nlm.nih.gov/pubmed/26000093.

Simons, M., E. Gordon, and L. Claesson-Welsh. "Mechanisms and Regulation of Endothelial VEGF Receptor Signalling." *Nature Reviews. Molecular Cell Biology* 17, no. 10 (2016): 611–25. doi:10.1038/nrm.2016.87. https://www.ncbi.nlm.nih.gov/pubmed/27461391.

Soltamox [Package Insert]. Leeds, UK: Rosemont Pharmaceuticals, Limited Company, 2018.

Song, Yuqin, Keshu Zhou, Dehui Zou, Jianfeng Zhou, Jianda Hu, Haiyan Yang, Huilai Zhang, Jie Ji, Wei Xu, Jie Jin, Fangfang Lv, Ru Feng, Sujun Gao, Daobin Zhou, Haiyi Guo, Aihua Wang, James Hilger, Jane Huang, William Novotny, Muhtar Osman, and Jun Zhu. "And Activity of the Investigational Bruton Tyrosine Kinase Inhibitor Zanubrutinib (BGB-3111) in Patients with Mantle Cell Lymphoma from a Phase 2 Trial." *Blood* 132, no. Supplement 1 (2018): 148.

Stone, R. M., S. J. Mandrekar, B. L. Sanford, K. Laumann, S. Geyer, C. D. Bloomfield, C. Thiede, T. W. Prior, K. Döhner, G. Marcucci, F. Lo-Coco, R. B. Klisovic, A. Wei, J. Sierra, M. A. Sanz, J. M. Brandwein, T. de Witte, D. Niederwieser, F. R. Appelbaum, B. C. Medeiros, M. S. Tallman, J. Krauter, R. F. Schlenk, A. Ganser, H. Serve, G. Ehninger, S. Amadori, R. A. Larson, and H. Döhner. "Midostaurin plus Chemotherapy for Acute Myeloid Leukemia with a FLT3 Mutation." *New England Journal of Medicine* 377, no. 5 (2017): 454–64. doi:10.1056/NEJMoa1614359. https://www.ncbi.nlm.nih.gov/pubmed/28644114.

Subbiah, V., D. Yang, V. Velcheti, A. Drilon, and F. Meric-Bernstam. "State-of-the-Art Strategies for Targeting." *Journal of Clinical Oncology* 38, no. 11 (2020): 1209–21. doi:10.1200/JCO.19.02551. https://www.ncbi.nlm .nih.gov/pubmed/32083997.

Syed, Y. Y. "Sacituzumab Govitecan: First Approval." *Drugs* 80, no. 10 (2020): 1019–25. doi:10.1007/s40265-020-01337-5. https://www.ncbi.nlm.nih.gov/pubmed/32529410.

Tafasitamab [Package Insert]. Boston, MA: MorphoSys US Inc., 2020.

Tai, Y. T., P. A. Mayes, C. Acharya, M. Y. Zhong, M. Cea, A. Cagnetta, J. Craigen, J. Yates, L. Gliddon, W. Fieles, B. Hoang, J. Tunstead, A. L. Christie, A. L. Kung, P. Richardson, N. C. Munshi, and K. C. Anderson. "Novel Anti-B-Cell Maturation Antigen Antibody-Drug Conjugate (GSK2857916) Selectively Induces Killing of Multiple Myeloma." *Blood* 123, no. 20 (2014): 3128–38. doi:10.1182/blood-2013-10-535088. https://www.ncbi .nlm.nih.gov/pubmed/24569262.

Taksin, A. L., O. Legrand, E. Raffoux, T. de Revel, X. Thomas, N. Contentin, R. Bouabdallah, C. Pautas, P. Turlure, O. Reman, C. Gardin, B. Varet, S. de Botton, F. Pousset, H. Farhat, S. Chevret, H. Dombret, and S. Castaigne. "High Efficacy and Safety Profile of Fractionated Doses of Mylotarg as Induction Therapy in Patients with Relapsed Acute Myeloblastic Leukemia: A Prospective Study of the Alfa Group." *Leukemia* 21, no. 1 (2007): 66–71. doi:10.1038/sj.leu.2404434. https://www.ncbi.nlm.nih.gov/pubmed/17051246.

Talzenna [Package Insert]. New York: Pfizer Inc., Oct. 2020.

"Tamoxifen for Early Breast Cancer: An Overview of the Randomised Trials." *Lancet* 351, no. 9114 Early Breast Cancer Trialists' Collaborative Group (1998): 1451–67. https://www.ncbi.nlm.nih.gov/pubmed/9605801.

Tarantelli, C., A. Lupia, A. Stathis, and F. Bertoni. "Is There a Role for Dual PI3K/mTOR Inhibitors for Patients Affected with Lymphoma?. " *International Journal of Molecular Sciences* 21, no. 3 (2020). doi:10.3390/ ijms21031060. https://www.ncbi.nlm.nih.gov/pubmed/32033478.

Tedder, T. F., M. Inaoki, and S. Sato. "The CD19-CD21 Complex Regulates Signal Transduction Thresholds Governing Humoral Immunity and Autoimmunity." *Immunity* 6, no. 2 (1997): 107–18. doi:10.1016/s1074-7613(00)80418-5. https://www.ncbi.nlm.nih.gov/pubmed/9047233.

Touzeau, C., J. Ryan, J. Guerriero, P. Moreau, T. N. Chonghaile, S. Le Gouill, P. Richardson, K. Anderson, M. Amiot, and A. Letai. "BH3 Profiling Identifies Heterogeneous Dependency on Bcl-2 Family Members in Multiple Myeloma and Predicts Sensitivity to BH3 Mimetics." *Leukemia* 30, no. 3 (2016): 761–4. doi:10.1038/ leu.2015.184. https://www.ncbi.nlm.nih.gov/pubmed/26174630.

Trenevska, I., D. Li, and A. H. Banham. "Therapeutic Antibodies Against Intracellular Tumor Antigens." *Frontiers in Immunology* 8 (2017): 1001. doi:10.3389/fimmu.2017.01001. https://www.ncbi.nlm.nih.gov/pubmed/28868054.

Trudel, S., N. Lendvai, R. Popat, P. M. Voorhees, B. Reeves, E. N. Libby, P. G. Richardson, A. Hoos, I. Gupta, V. Bragulat, Z. He, J. B. Opalinska, and A. D. Cohen. "Antibody-Drug Conjugate, GSK2857916, in Relapsed/ Refractory Multiple Myeloma: An Update on Safety and Efficacy from Dose Expansion Phase I Study." *Blood Cancer Journal* 9, no. 4 (2019): 37. doi:10.1038/s41408-019-0196-6. https://www.ncbi.nlm.nih.gov/pubmed /30894515.

Van Cutsem, E., J. Tabernero, R. Lakomy, H. Prenen, J. Prausová, T. Macarulla, P. Ruff, G. A. van Hazel, V. Moiseyenko, D. Ferry, J. McKendrick, J. Polikoff, A. Tellier, R. Castan, and C. Allegra. "Addition of Aflibercept to Fluorouracil, Leucovorin, and Irinotecan Improves Survival in a phase III Randomized Trial in

Patients with Metastatic Colorectal Cancer Previously Treated with an Oxaliplatin-Based Regimen." *Journal of Clinical Oncology* 30, no. 28 (2012): 3499–506. doi:10.1200/JCO.2012.42.8201. https://www.ncbi.nlm.nih.gov/pubmed/22949147.

van de Donk, N. W., M. L. Janmaat, T. Mutis, J. J. Lammerts van Bueren, T. Ahmadi, A. K. Sasser, H. M. Lokhorst, and P. W. Parren. "Monoclonal Antibodies Targeting CD38 in Hematological Malignancies and Beyond." *Immunologic Research* 270, no. 1 (2016): 95–112. doi:10.1111/imr.12389. https://www.ncbi.nlm.nih.gov/pubmed/26864107.

Venetoclax [Package Insert]. North Chicago, IL: Abbvie Inc, Oct. 2020.

Verma, S., D. Miles, L. Gianni, I. E. Krop, M. Welslau, J. Baselga, M. Pegram, D. Y. Oh, V. Diéras, E. Guardino, L. Fang, M. W. Lu, S. Olsen, K. Blackwell, and EMILIA Study Group. "Trastuzumab Emtansine for HER2-Positive Advanced Breast Cancer." *New England Journal of Medicine* 367, no. 19 (2012): 1783–91. doi:10.1056/NEJMoa1209124. https://www.ncbi.nlm.nih.gov/pubmed/23020162.

Verstovsek, S., R. A. Mesa, J. Gotlib, R. S. Levy, V. Gupta, J. F. DiPersio, J. V. Catalano, M. Deininger, C. Miller, R. T. Silver, M. Talpaz, E. F. Winton, J. H. Harvey, M. O. Arcasoy, E. Hexner, R. M. Lyons, R. Paquette, A. Raza, K. Vaddi, S. Erickson-Viitanen, I. L. Koumenis, W. Sun, V. Sandor, and H. M. Kantarjian. "A Double-Blind, Placebo-Controlled Trial of Ruxolitinib for Myelofibrosis." *New England Journal of Medicine* 366, no. 9 (2012): 799–807. doi:10.1056/NEJMoa1110557. https://www.ncbi.nlm.nih.gov/pubmed/22375971.

Vitolo, U., M. Trněný, D. Belada, J. M. Burke, A. M. Carella, N. Chua, P. Abrisqueta, J. Demeter, I. Flinn, X. Hong, W. S. Kim, A. Pinto, Y. K. Shi, Y. Tatsumi, M. Z. Oestergaard, M. Wenger, G. Fingerle-Rowson, O. Catalani, T. Nielsen, M. Martelli, and L. H. Sehn. "Obinutuzumab or Rituximab plus Cyclophosphamide, Doxorubicin, Vincristine, and Prednisone in Previously Untreated Diffuse Large B-Cell Lymphoma." *Journal of Clinical Oncology* 35, no. 31 (2017): 3529–37. doi:10.1200/JCO.2017.73.3402. https://www.ncbi.nlm.nih.gov/pubmed/28796588.

von Mehren, M., J. Kane, M. Bui, E. Choy, M. Connelly, S. Dry, K. N. Ganjoo, S. George, R. J. Gonzalez, M. J. Heslin, J. Homsi, V. Keedy, C. M. Kelly, E. Kim, D. Liebner, M. McCarter, S. V. McGarry, C. Meyer, A. S. Pappo, A. M. Parkes, I. B. Paz, I. A. Petersen, M. Poppe, R. F. Riedel, B. Rubin, S. Schuetze, J. Shabason, J. K. Sicklick, M. B. Spraker, M. Zimel, M. A. Bergman, and G. V. George. "Gastrointestinal Stromal Tumors, Version 1.2021." *Journal of the National Comprehensive Cancer Network* (2020).

von Minckwitz, G., C. S. Huang, M. S. Mano, S. Loibl, E. P. Mamounas, M. Untch, N. Wolmark, P. Rastogi, A. Schneeweiss, A. Redondo, H. H. Fischer, W. Jacot, A. K. Conlin, C. Arce-Salinas, I. L. Wapnir, C. Jackisch, M. P. DiGiovanna, P. A. Fasching, J. P. Crown, P. Wülfing, Z. Shao, E. Rota Caremoli, H. Wu, L. H. Lam, D. Tesarowski, M. Smitt, H. Douthwaite, S. M. Singel, C. E. Geyer, and KATHERINE Investigators. "Trastuzumab Emtansine for Residual Invasive HER2-Positive Breast Cancer." *New England Journal of Medicine* 380, no. 7 (2019): 617–28. doi:10.1056/NEJMoa1814017. https://www.ncbi.nlm.nih.gov/pubmed/30516102.

Wacker, B., T. Nagrani, J. Weinberg, K. Witt, G. Clark, and P. J. Cagnoni. "Correlation Between Development of Rash and Efficacy in Patients Treated with the Epidermal Growth Factor Receptor Tyrosine Kinase Inhibitor Erlotinib in Two Large Phase III Studies." *Clinical Cancer Research* 13, no. 13 (2007): 3913–21. doi:10.1158/1078-0432.CCR-06-2610. https://www.ncbi.nlm.nih.gov/pubmed/17606725.

Wang, M., S. Rule, P. L. Zinzani, A. Goy, O. Casasnovas, S. D. Smith, G. Damaj, J. Doorduijn, T. Lamy, F. Morschhauser, C. Panizo, B. Shah, A. Davies, R. Eek, J. Dupuis, E. Jacobsen, A. P. Kater, S. Le Gouill, L. Oberic, T. Robak, T. Covey, R. Dua, A. Hamdy, X. Huang, R. Izumi, P. Patel, W. Rothbaum, J. G. Slatter, and W. Jurczak. "Acalabrutinib in Relapsed or Refractory Mantle Cell Lymphoma (ACE-LY-004): A Single-Arm, Multicentre, phase 2 Trial." *Lancet* 391, no. 10121 (2018): 659–67. doi:10.1016/S0140-6736(17)33108-2. https://www.ncbi.nlm.nih.gov/pubmed/29241979.

Wang, Q., S. Yang, K. Wang, and S. Y. Sun. "MET Inhibitors for Targeted Therapy of EGFR TKI-Resistant Lung Cancer." *Journal of Hematology & Oncology* 12, no. 1 (2019): 63. doi:10.1186/s13045-019-0759-9. https://www.ncbi.nlm.nih.gov/pubmed/31227004.

Wee, P., and Z. Wang. "Epidermal Growth Factor Receptor Cell Proliferation Signaling Pathways." *Cancers* 9, no. 5 (2017). doi:10.3390/cancers9050052. https://www.ncbi.nlm.nih.gov/pubmed/28513565.

Wei, A. H., S. A. Strickland, J. Z. Hou, W. Fiedler, T. L. Lin, R. B. Walter, A. Enjeti, I. S. Tiong, M. Savona, S. Lee, B. Chyla, R. Popovic, A. H. Salem, S. Agarwal, T. Xu, K. M. Fakouhi, R. Humerickhouse, W. J. Hong, J. Hayslip, and G. J. Roboz. "Venetoclax Combined with Low-Dose Cytarabine for Previously Untreated Patients with Acute Myeloid Leukemia: Results from a Phase Ib/II Study." *Journal of Clinical Oncology* 37, no. 15 (2019): 1277–84. doi:10.1200/JCO.18.01600. https://www.ncbi.nlm.nih.gov/pubmed/30892988.

Wei, A. H., P. Montesinos, V. Ivanov, C. D. DiNardo, J. Novak, K. Laribi, I. Kim, D. A. Stevens, W. Fiedler, M. Pagoni, O. Samoilova, Y. Hu, A. Anagnostopoulos, J. Bergeron, J. Z. Hou, V. Murthy, T. Yamauchi, A. McDonald, B. Chyla, S. Gopalakrishnan, Q. Jiang, W. Mendes, J. Hayslip, and P. Panayiotidis. "Venetoclax plus LDAC for

Newly Diagnosed AML Ineligible for Intensive Chemotherapy: A phase 3 Randomized Placebo-Controlled Trial." *Blood* 135, no. 24 (2020): 2137–45. doi:10.1182/blood.2020004856. https://www.ncbi.nlm.nih.gov/pubmed/32219442.

Wells, S. A., B. G. Robinson, R. F. Gagel, H. Dralle, J. A. Fagin, M. Santoro, E. Baudin, R. Elisei, B. Jarzab, J. R. Vasselli, J. Read, P. Langmuir, A. J. Ryan, and M. J. Schlumberger. "Vandetanib in Patients with Locally Advanced or Metastatic Medullary Thyroid Cancer: A Randomized, Double-Blind phase III Trial." *Journal of Clinical Oncology* 30, no. 2 (2012): 134–41. doi:10.1200/JCO.2011.35.5040. https://www.ncbi.nlm.nih.gov/pubmed/22025146.

White Al-Habeeb, N., V. Kulasingam, E. P. Diamandis, G. M. Yousef, G. J. Tsongalis, L. Vermeulen, Z. Zhu, and S. Kamel-Reid. "The Use of Targeted Therapies for Precision Medicine in Oncology." *Clinical Chemistry* 62, no. 12 (2016): 1556–64. doi:10.1373/clinchem.2015.247882. https://www.ncbi.nlm.nih.gov/pubmed/27679436.

Wilcox, R. A. "Mogamulizumab: 2 Birds, 1 Stone." *Blood* 125, no. 12 (2015): 1847–8. doi:10.1182/blood-2015-02-625251. https://www.ncbi.nlm.nih.gov/pubmed/25792728.

Wolf, J., T. Seto, J. Y. Han, N. Reguart, E. B. Garon, H. J. M. Groen, D. S. W. Tan, T. Hida, M. de Jonge, S. V. Orlov, E. F. Smit, P. J. Souquet, J. Vansteenkiste, M. Hochmair, E. Felip, M. Nishio, M. Thomas, K. Ohashi, R. Toyozawa, T. R. Overbeck, F. de Marinis, T. M. Kim, E. Laack, A. Robeva, S. Le Mouhaer, M. Waldron-Lynch, B. Sankaran, O. A. Balbin, X. Cui, M. Giovannini, M. Akimov, R. S. Heist, and GEOMETRY Mono-1 Investigators. "Capmatinib In." *New England Journal of Medicine* 383, no. 10 (2020): 944–57. doi:10.1056/NEJMoa2002787. https://www.ncbi.nlm.nih.gov/pubmed/32877583.

Wu, J., J. Fu, M. Zhang, and D. Liu. "Blinatumomab: A Bispecific T Cell Engager (BiTE) Antibody Against CD19/CD3 for Refractory Acute Lymphoid Leukemia." *Journal of Hematology & Oncology* 8 (2015): 104. doi:10.1186/s13045-015-0195-4. https://www.ncbi.nlm.nih.gov/pubmed/26337639.

Wu, Y., Y. Wang, Y. Gu, J. Xia, X. Kong, Q. Qian, and Y. Hong. "Safety and Efficacy of Ofatumumab in Chronic Lymphocytic Leukemia: A Systematic Review and Meta-Analysis." *Hematology* 22, no. 10 (2017): 578–84. doi:10.1080/10245332.2017.1333974. https://www.ncbi.nlm.nih.gov/pubmed/28580841.

Yang, J., J. Nie, X. Ma, Y. Wei, Y. Peng, and X. Wei. "Targeting PI3K in Cancer: Mechanisms and Advances in Clinical Trials." *Molecular Cancer* 18, no. 1 (2019): 26. doi:10.1186/s12943-019-0954-x. https://www.ncbi.nlm.nih.gov/pubmed/30782187.

Zaman, S., R. Wang, and V. Gandhi. "Targeting the Apoptosis Pathway in Hematologic Malignancies." *Leukemia & Lymphoma* 55, no. 9 (2014): 1980–92. doi:10.3109/10428194.2013.855307. https://www.ncbi.nlm.nih.gov/pubmed/24295132.

Zein, N., A. M. Sinha, W. J. McGahren, and G. A. Ellestad. "Calicheamicin Gamma 1I: An Antitumor Antibiotic That Cleaves Double-Stranded DNA Site Specifically." *Science* 240, no. 4856 (1988): 1198–201. doi:10.1126/science.3240341. https://www.ncbi.nlm.nih.gov/pubmed/3240341.

Zeiser, R., N. von Bubnoff, J. Butler, M. Mohty, D. Niederwieser, R. Or, J. Szer, E. M. Wagner, T. Zuckerman, B. Mahuzier, J. Xu, C. Wilke, K. K. Gandhi, G. Socié, and REACH2 Trial Group. "Ruxolitinib for Glucocorticoid-Refractory Acute Graft-Versus-Host Disease." *New England Journal of Medicine* 382, no. 19 (2020): 1800–10. doi:10.1056/NEJMoa1917635. https://www.ncbi.nlm.nih.gov/pubmed/32320566.

Zejula [Package Insert]. Research Triangle Park, NC: GlaxoSmithKline, Apr. 2020.

Zhou, X., W. Hu, and X. Qin. "The Role of Complement in the Mechanism of Action of Rituximab for B-Cell Lymphoma: Implications for Therapy." *Oncologist* 13, no. 9 (2008): 954–66. doi:10.1634/theoncologist.2008-0089. https://www.ncbi.nlm.nih.gov/pubmed/18779537.

Zhu, Y., J. Yang, D. Xu, X. M. Gao, Z. Zhang, J. L. Hsu, C. W. Li, S. O. Lim, Y. Y. Sheng, Y. Zhang, J. H. Li, Q. Luo, Y. Zheng, Y. Zhao, L. Lu, H. L. Jia, M. C. Hung, Q. Z. Dong, and L. X. Qin. "Disruption of Tumour-Associated Macrophage Trafficking by the Osteopontin-Induced Colony-Stimulating factor-1 Signalling Sensitises Hepatocellular Carcinoma to Anti-PD-L1 Blockade." *Gut* 68, no. 9 (2019): 1653–66. doi:10.1136/gutjnl-2019-318419. https://www.ncbi.nlm.nih.gov/pubmed/30902885.

Zirlik, K., and J. Duyster. "Anti-Angiogenics: Current Situation and Future Perspectives." *Oncology Research & Treatment* 41, no. 4 (2018): 166–71. doi:10.1159/000488087. https://www.ncbi.nlm.nih.gov/pubmed/29562226.

Zobniw, C. M., V. A. Trinh, K. Posey, and N. Somaiah. "Olaratumab in the Management of Advanced Soft Tissue Sarcoma." *Journal of Oncology Pharmacy Practice* 25, no. 2 (2019): 442–8. doi:10.1177/1078155218788135. https://www.ncbi.nlm.nih.gov/pubmed/30032714.

Localizing Therapeutics to the Brain

6

Sakshi Hans, Karrina McNamara, Eoghan Cunnane, Aisling M. Ross, Lara Scheherazade Milane, John J.E. Mulvihill, and Andreas M. Grabrucker

Contents

6.1 INTRODUCTION: BACKGROUND AND DRIVING FORCES

Numerous neurological diseases have been identified that range from neurodegenerative (Alzheimer's, Parkinson's) and neurological (multiple sclerosis, epilepsy) to psychiatric ailments such as schizophrenia. The diagnosis and treatment of these diseases are faced with a unique challenge in biomedicine: although pharmacologically active, many drugs to treat brain disorders cannot exert their actions at the desired site of action, the central nervous system (CNS). This is because the entry of therapeutic substances into the CNS is blocked by multiple tissue barriers, namely the blood–brain barrier (BBB), blood–cerebrospinal fluid barrier (BCSFB or BCB), and brain–CSF barrier. In the case of tumors in the brain, a fourth kind of barrier, called the blood–tumor barrier (BTB), can exist as well (Grabrucker et al., 2013) (Figure 6.1).

Many drug delivery platforms additionally face a significant challenge from the reticuloendothelial system (RES) or mononuclear phagocyte system (MPS). This system (particularly Kupffer cells) recognizes drug delivery systems such as nanoparticles (NPs) as foreign bodies and removes them from the circulation. This is due to specific serum proteins known as opsonins, which bind to the surface of the

DOI: 10.1201/9781003092773-7

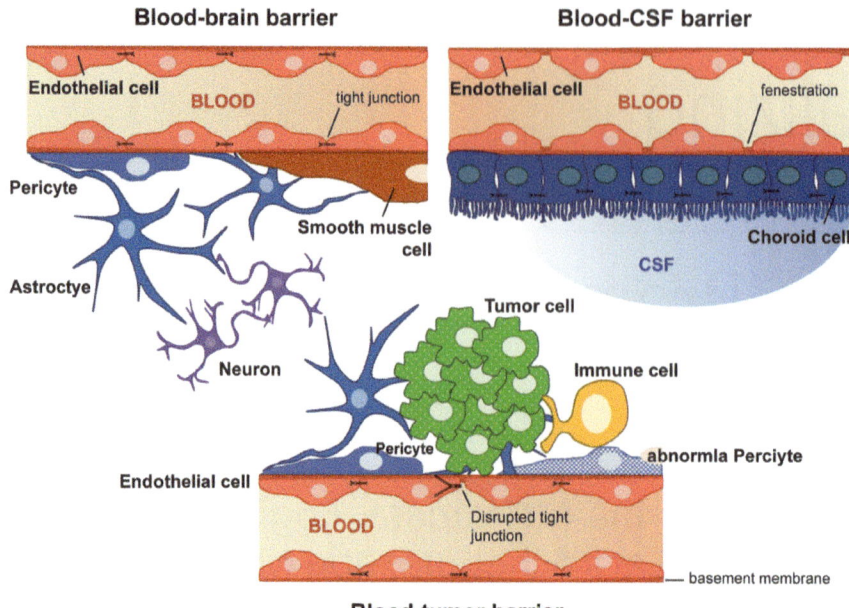

FIGURE 6.1   Top left: diagram of a blood vessel in the brain lined by the blood–brain barrier (BBB). The BBB is a multicellular structure that consists of a monolayer of endothelial cells which are tightly connected through cell adhesion molecules forming tight junctions, smooth muscle cells in case of larger arterioles, pericytes that are connected to the abluminal side of the endothelial cells and are linked to a basement membrane, and astrocytes that have endfeet that ensheath the vessel and have many functions. For example, through cytokine secretion, interaction with neurons occurs, mediating their survival, development, metabolism, and neurotransmission. Top right: diagram of a blood vessel in the brain lined by the cells forming the blood–CSF barrier. These cells are endothelial cells containing fenestrations, and choroid cells that are interconnected through tight junctions (more permeable than those between the endothelial cells of the BBB) and secrete the cerebrospinal fluid (CSF). Microvilli on the CSF-facing side increase surface area. Bottom: diagram of a blood–tumor barrier. The blood–tumor barrier may show decreased expression of tight junction proteins due to cell signaling from the tumor, alterations in pericyte physiology, and disruption of astrocytic interactions with endothelial cells. Additionally, immune cells may invade the structure. Although this may contribute to decreased barrier integrity, the expression of efflux transporters limits drug delivery into the tumor, and permeability varies in different parts of the tumor.

nanocarriers and allow them to be recognized by the RES. It should be noted that positively charged NPs can adsorb opsonins, leading them to be cleared from circulation faster. Coating polymeric NPs with polysorbate-80 can improve targeting to the CNS, for example, by reducing clearance by the RES (Chhabra et al., 2015). Another study by Liu et al. (2013) showed that treatment with intralipid increased the blood half-life of superparamagnetic iron oxide particles.

The method of modifying the NP surface with polyethylene glycol decreases clearance by immune cells but also reduces their uptake by target cells into the brain. In a new study concerning the strategy called RES blockade, engineered enzyme-resistant peptide ligands were bound to D self-peptide labeled liposomes (DSL). Post-administration, the DSLs were adsorbed onto liver phagocytic cells, forming a kind of mask that blocked interactions between NPs and phagocytes (Tang et al., 2019). From these and other studies, it is evident that overcoming clearance of drug delivery systems such as nanocarriers by phagocytic immune cells is a critical additional step besides barrier crossing towards the successful brain-targeted delivery of therapeutic NPs.

Thus, new advances in biomedical science are needed to deliver drugs to this otherwise inaccessible organ (Mulvihill et al., 2020). The delivery systems are based on different strategies, but some exploit physiological transport processes to get past the BBB. These mechanisms are discussed in more detail in the following section. However, more research is needed to assess the *in vivo* efficacy of many of these technologies to create impactful treatments. Factors such as toxicity profiles, possible physiological reactions and interactions with the body, and cost of production need to be considered to achieve safe and highly specific drug targeting for the effective treatment of many brain disorders.

6.2 STRATEGIES FOR BRAIN-TARGETED DRUG DELIVERY

Targeted drug delivery to the brain is faced with several challenges due to the barriers mentioned above that block the penetration of many molecules into the brain parenchyma. Several strategies have been developed to overcome this limitation and facilitate the delivery of therapeutics across the BBB (Figures 6.2 and 6.3). One broad category of methods involves chemical modification of the drug, for example, seen in prodrugs. Prodrugs are inactive molecules of the parent or original drug which are converted to the active form of the drug in a single step after crossing the BBB. Unlike prodrugs, chemical drug delivery systems (CDDS) involve a multi-step process in which the inactive drug is converted to the active form. A step frequently taken to increase the brain uptake of a drug is coupling it to a lipophilizing moiety. After uptake, it is then converted to a lipid-insoluble compound within the brain, effectively "locking in" the drug behind the BBB.

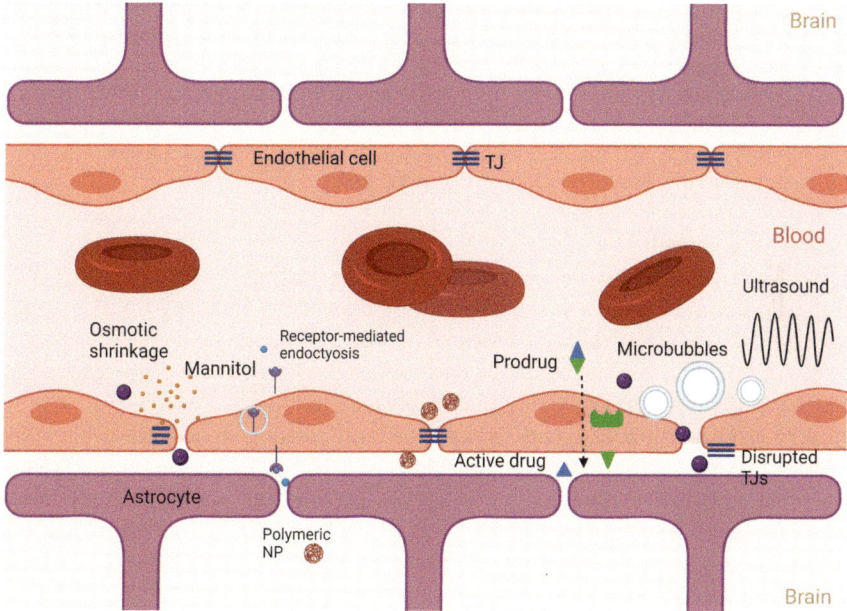

FIGURE 6.2   Various strategies for drug delivery across the BBB. Far-right shows the technique of focused ultrasound paired with microbubbles present at the desired site. The ultrasound wave causes the bubbles to expand and contract, resulting in the temporarily opening of endothelial tight junctions to allow drug entry into the brain. Right: prodrugs can cross the BBB and convert to an active form of the drug inside the brain. The natural endogenous transport systems of the body can be utilized via receptor-mediated endocytosis. A ligand such as transferrin conjugated with the drug molecule binds to its receptor on the cell and is carried across the barrier by transcytosis. Similarly, polymeric NPs (left) can cross the BBB using receptor-mediated endocytosis, among others. Far-left shows osmotic shrinkage: the endothelial cells are induced to shrink upon administration of the hypertonic agent mannitol, allowing molecules to cross the tight junctions (TJs).

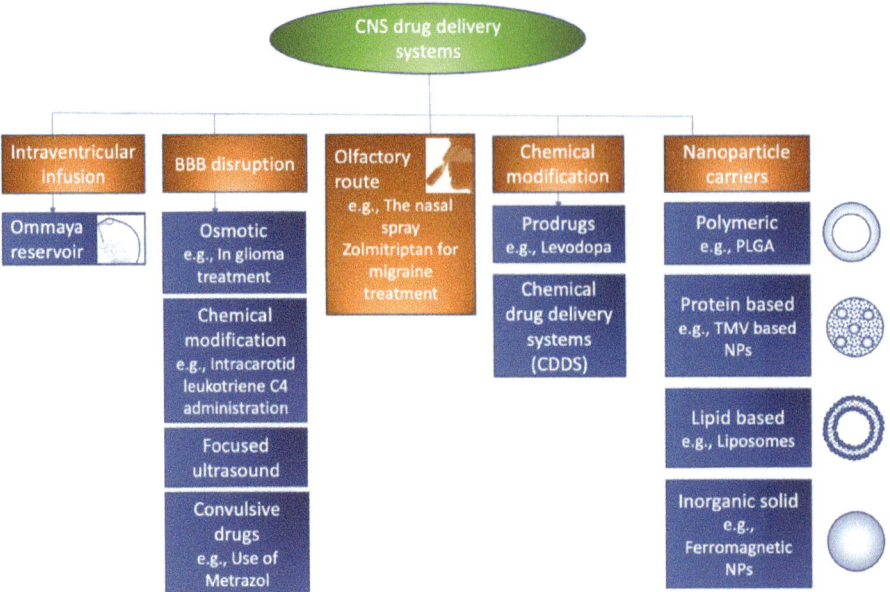

FIGURE 6.3   At a glance: methods of drug delivery to the CNS. The broad categories are depicted. Invasive procedures such as intraventricular infusion have long been used; notably, the Ommaya reservoir catheter system is used to administer drugs directly into the brain. BBB disruption is carried out via chemical means, osmotic shrinkage, and focused ultrasound. BBB disruption is very invasive. Prodrugs and drug delivery systems involving conversion to the active form of the therapeutic drug in the brain are further options for drug delivery across the BBB. Prodrugs involve conversion to the active form in a single step, while CDDs involve multiple steps. Additionally, intranasal delivery may be used for brain-targeted drug delivery. Nanoparticle carriers are a modern advance in nanomedicine and present many advantages. Diverse nanocarrier types are available for use and are proven to be highly suitable for drug delivery in multiple therapeutic areas. NPs may be polymeric in nature, lipid-based, protein-based, or made of inorganic solids.

A more invasive approach is an intraventricular infusion of a drug, for example, via the Ommaya reservoir, an intraventricular pump, or catheter system. This technique is notably used in the treatment of leptomeningeal disease. However, the short diffusion distance of the drug limits its efficacy, making it more suitable for localized drug therapy (Sandberg et al., 2000). Due to the invasiveness, this approach has risks in terms of infection and can be linked to complications such as the occurrence of aseptic chemical meningitis (Chamberlain Kormanik, and Barba, 1997).

Drug delivery using an olfactory route exploits the body's endogenous pathways (via the nose to the brain) and bypasses systemic circulation (Grabrucker et al., 2013). The intranasal (i.n.) route is useful for drugs that are not efficiently absorbed orally and has the added advantage of avoiding degradation in the liver and gastrointestinal tract (first-pass effect). I.n. delivery is used in multiple therapeutic areas, including migraine treatment, cancer therapy, and neurodegenerative disorders, among others (Bahadur and Pathak, 2012; Pawar et al., 2021).

Limitations faced by this method include low pH conditions of the nasal epithelium and inflammation of the nasal mucosal lining. Lipophilic substances are more easily absorbed by this route, as they can cross the lipid bilayer of cell membranes with ease. The molecular weight and charge of a drug are other limiting factors affecting transport, as neutral substances below 300 Da are absorbed easily across the nasal membrane compared to charged, heavier molecules. Molecules weighing over 1000 Da show a much lower uptake rate (Ozsoy, Gungor, and Cevher, 2009). Finally, olfactory delivery is restricted by the volume of formulation that can be administered (about 25–200 μl) (Romeo et al., 1998).

The disruption of the BBB is another method that allows targeted drug delivery to the brain. It is usually achieved by temporarily opening the tight junctions of the BBB. Osmotic disruption of the BBB can be done by inducing the endothelial cells of the blood capillaries to shrink. This leads to the opening of the tight junctions of the CNS, which would usually block the passage of substances between the blood and the brain. Administration of mannitol, a hyperosmotic agent, forces the tight junctions of the CNS to widen by shrinking the endothelial cells (demonstrated *in vivo* in rat models). This technique, for example, was used in the treatment of gliomas (Karmur et al., 2020).

In another approach, the blood–tumor barrier is induced to open by the intracarotid administration of leukotriene C4 as demonstrated in an investigation by Chio, Baba, and Black (1992). It was found that administration of the leukotriene led to selective permeabilization of the BBB within RG-2 rat tumors. Alternatively, microbubbles can be injected into the bloodstream along with a focused ultrasound application. The physical movement of the microbubbles as they expand and contract due to the ultrasound waves causes the tight junctions to temporarily open, allowing the entry of therapeutic drugs into the brain (Konofagou et al., 2012). Magnetic resonance imaging (MRI) can be used to visualize and assess BBB opening, improving precise targeting of the brain via this method. Ultrasound sonication is useful to target relatively confined areas of the brain and is a non-invasive method that does not rely on riskier surgery and/or catheter insertion (Burgess et al., 2015).

Generating conditions such as hypertension and ischemia and the use of convulsive drugs such as Metrazol plus anti-convulsive agents are some more methods to disrupt the BBB temporarily. However, there are serious disadvantages to all methods disrupting the BBB, as disturbing the brain's protective mechanisms significantly increases its vulnerability to infection and disease (Chhabra et al., 2015).

Thus, it is clear there are significant challenges to safe and efficient targeted drug delivery to the brain. However, nanocarriers are a promising emerging technology that can facilitate brain-targeted drug delivery without harmful disruption to the BBB. To be safe, nanocarriers must be non-thrombogenic and non-immunogenic and remain stable in the blood circulation. Several nano-delivery platforms have been developed that fulfill these criteria – for example, polymeric NPs, protein-based NPs, liposomes, and solid NPs (Figure 6.3). The nanosystems present several advantages. Many nanocarriers exploit the physiological mechanisms of blood-to-brain transport mediated by the BBB cells, such as transcytosis. The use of NPs makes drug delivery highly accessible to otherwise confined organs such as the brain. NPs are also capable of specific targeting of the therapeutic to the desired site of action, up to the subcellular level in case of organelle-specific disease. A diversity of molecules of different molecular weights and chemical properties can be encapsulated within the NP layer. Both hydrophilic and hydrophobic substances can be encapsulated within the nanocarrier coating. For example, as hydrophilic molecules cannot cross the BBB, a hydrophilic drug may be encapsulated by a lipophilic sphere, known as a liposome. However, the increased lipophilicity of the nanocarrier also increases its efflux from the brain parenchyma. It is also essential to engineer some nanocarriers with specific ligands to avoid them being phagocytosed by the RES, which is the basis of the blockade strategy to evade phagocytosis (see Section 6.1).

The nanocarrier outer coating offers protection to the therapeutic drug from enzymatic degradation as well. Polymeric nanocarriers such as polylactide-co-glycolide or PLGA are also sustainable and biodegradable. Finally, nanomedicine can be used to treat a wide range of diseases, from neurological disorders to tumors, and is crucial in research ventures such as gene therapy (Chhabra et al., 2015).

NPs used in drug delivery are often lipid- or polymer-based. Polymeric NPs can be natural or synthetic and are advantageous in that they can carry a high amount of a drug. The synthetic, biodegradable nanocarrier poly(n-butylcyanoacrylate) (PBCA) is an effective vehicle for drug delivery. It is taken up via an endocytotic mechanism involving apolipoprotein E, which adsorbs onto NPs coated with polysorbate (Wagner et al., 2012). Combining this NP with the surfactant polysorbate-80 reduces clearance by the RES, thereby increasing the drug's systemic circulation. A downside of these NPs is that higher doses of PBCA NPs with polysorbate surfactant are damaging to the BBB, and the pharmacological effects of the drug delivered by this method are brief, making this carrier more suitable for drugs with frequent administration. Therefore, there are certain benefits and risks of using PBCA nanocarriers, and these should be appropriately evaluated while using this approach (Olivier, 2005).

The natural polymer PLGA is ideal for penetration into the CNS and can carry a high volume of therapeutic drug. Here, the drug of interest is released in the brain by degrading the PLGA layer by autocatalytic cleavage of ester bonds. Like that of other polymeric or solid NPs, the PLGA NP surface can be modified, and ligands attached. Thus, they can enter the brain through ligand-mediated transcytosis, carrier-mediated transport, or endocytosis (Grabrucker et al., 2013). For example, NPs can be modified with a surface-bound ligand, such as transferrin receptor binding antibodies and peptides. This engineering facilitates the transport of the NPs across the BBB to the brain. In receptor-mediated endocytosis, the NP-bound ligand interacts with a specific cell membrane receptor, causing the formation of endocytic vesicles and their passage via transcytosis across the BBB. Other frequently used ligands are transferrin, lactoferrin, folic acid, and a-mannose. The conjugation of multiple ligands to the NP may provide further specificity that allows cell-type-specific targeting or the targeting of cellular organelles. For example, in a recent study, angiopep-conjugated polymersomes loaded with doxorubicin were developed to target the LRP-1 receptor. This receptor is overexpressed in glioma and BBB cells and is an example of cell-type-specific targeting that resulted in a high accumulation of nanomedicine in the target tissue (Mulvihill et al., 2020). However, an aspect of nanocarriers that is often overlooked due to few *in vivo* studies is the presence of protein coronas. A protein corona (PC) is a layer of absorbed plasma proteins that forms around the surface of the NP and is unique for each nanocarrier type. This particular subset of serum proteins on the nanocarrier surface is known as the NP's adsorbome (Walkey et al., 2012). The PC confers unique properties to the NP regarding its cellular uptake, toxicity, shape circulation, and distribution in the body. Factors that influence the type of PC formed include the composition of the NP and its surface charge and significantly the hydrophilicity or hydrophobicity of the NP. Hydrophobic carrier particles are opsonized with proteins faster than hydrophilic NPs since proteins can better adsorb onto their surface (Aggarwal et al., 2009).

Other limitations of NPs exist, such as competitive binding of endogenous ligands with the specific receptor versus the ligand associated with the NP. Overly tight receptor-ligand bonding leads to a low exocytosis rate and fewer NPs entering the CNS. It is, therefore, vital that a suitable ligand is selected to be coupled to the nanocarrier.

Solid, metal-based NPs have also been investigated in the context of drug delivery to the brain and present several interesting advantages that could be exploited for targeted drug delivery. Namely, these NPs are generally considered to experience minimal clearance by the RES (Adabi et al., 2017; Iravani, 2017), thereby maximizing time in circulation and improving the probability of BBB penetration (Cupaioli et al., 2014; Ross et al., 2019). Further, the systems for the synthesis of metallic NPs are highly sophisticated and controllable, presenting the opportunity to create NPs sub 10 nm in size, which will potentially pass more easily across the BBB (Ross et al., 2019). Additionally, the multivalent properties of metallic NPs could facilitate functionalization with a variety of ligands for site-specific targeting, further enhancing transport across the BBB, as well as direct drug conjugation (Yim et al., 2012). Finally, and perhaps most interestingly, many metallic NPs are suitable for use as contrast imaging agents, presenting an avenue for diagnostic as well as therapeutic capabilities – also known as theranostic NPs (Chen et al., 2014; Cupaioli et al., 2014; McNamara and Tofail, 2015; Das et al., 2016; Guo et al., 2017; Ma et al., 2017, Nair et al., 2021).

6.3 RECENT ADVANCES TOWARDS BRAIN-TARGETED NANOMEDICINES

Nanocarriers are a newly emerging technology in biomedicine and hold much potential for highly specific, targeted delivery of a wide variety of therapeutics. Different pathways and mechanisms of action can be used that all have their advantages and drawbacks of use. Disadvantages often relate to the efficiency of the formulation, its toxicity profile, translation from *in vitro* to *in vivo* experiments, and challenges in scaling up from initial research setting to industrial production. Additionally, nanocarriers' high cost of design and production is another potential limitation (Chhabra et al., 2015). Nevertheless, several promising developments in preclinical and sometimes clinical research using nanocarriers have been made, especially in the area of brain cancers and neurodegenerative disorders.

6.3.1 Crossing the Blood–Brain Barrier

The BBB is a dynamic, biological barrier between the circulation and the CNS and comprises endothelial cells, pericytes, astrocytes, and the basement membrane. It functions as a layer of protection against potentially neurotoxic substances due to the presence of tight junctions between cells called *zonulae occludentes*. While being protective, at the same time, the BBB presents a significant obstacle to treating disorders of the CNS. The tight junctions of the BBB block the passage of molecules via passive diffusion between the epithelial cells of the capillaries of the CNS. The BBB is further bolstered by the presence of pericytes and glial cells, which overall gives the barrier cells a very high degree of electrical resistance (1,500–2,000 ohm) compared to systemic endothelial cells. Notably, the BBB cells mediating capillary exchange also lack an intercellular cleft, fenestrae, and a mechanism of pinocytosis. Therefore, the passive diffusion of lipid-insoluble (such as small ions) and large hydrophilic molecules into the brain is complex, and an active mechanism of transport is required. Under physiological conditions, several substances are continuously transported across the BBB. For example, the glucose transporter protein (GLUT-1) regulates the transport of glucose through the BBB.

Another feature of the BBB that blocks the passage of substances is the presence of degrading enzymes that metabolize drugs. Several phase I and phase II metabolic enzymes have been identified in the endothelial cells of the BBB. Although certain lipophilic molecules such as benzodiazepines can cross the barrier, factors such as molecular weight and affinity for a specific transport system govern which molecules can cross the BBB. For example, molecules under 400 Da cannot cross the BBB. Transport proteins associated with the BBB include P-glycoprotein (Pgp) and multidrug resistance-associated proteins (MRPs), and these also limit the entry and retention of substances in the brain.

Additionally, some chemicals, including neurotransmitters (among them serotonin and adrenaline), can act on endothelial cells and their receptors in the brain, as well as astrocytes. This mechanism modulates aspects of the BBB, such as tightness of the tight junctions and the expression of transporter proteins (Grabrucker et al., 2016). However, it is important to note that the integrity of the BBB may be altered in conditions such as Alzheimer's disease and after a stroke or brain trauma.

In vitro models are helpful to study the characteristics of the BBB in an artificial, highly controllable environment at a relatively low cost. For example, one of the most widely used models of the BBB is the Transwell apparatus. This simplified model is comprised of a monolayer of brain microvascular endothelial cells (ECs) on either side of a semipermeable, microporous membrane. These ECs simulate the luminal/vascular and abluminal/parenchymal sides of the BBB, and they are immersed in growth media while the membrane facilitates the passage of cellular substances and nutrients across the two compartments. The Transwell model is used to study drug permeability and receptor-ligand binding affinity (Naik and Cucullo, 2012).

The dynamic cone and plate model was designed to simulate the endothelial shear stress that occurs *in vitro*. The EC monolayer is seeded onto a plate and exposed to shear stress (SS) generated by a rotating cone. This model explores laminar or turbulent flow in the context of the BBB, as flow is a key modulator of its characteristics. Still, this model is limited as the shear stress experienced by the ECs is not evenly distributed, and it also lacks other components of the *in vivo* BBB such as astrocytes and pericytes (He et al., 2014).

Three-dimensional, dynamic models of the BBB are a more realistic simulation of the *in situ* organ. This system, also known as the DIV-BBB, involves the culture of brain ECs with abluminal astrocytes along with exposure to laminar shear stress. Thus, this model incorporates the functional and physiological components of the BBB environment (Santaguida et al., 2006).

Another model designed to simulate the BBB is the 3D ECM-based cell culture model. The advantage of these models is that they allow for close cell-to-cell signaling and the release of physiological factors and biochemical substances. This technology can be paired with high-resolution imaging techniques to investigate changes occurring over time in the 3D culture microenvironment (Naik and Cucullo, 2012).

However, there are certain flaws associated with the current models, for example, with regards to altered cell physiology due to an *in vitro* environment. Cells cultured in an artificial environment lack exposure to physiological factors and stimuli that they would typically receive and therefore tend to undergo dedifferentiation. Such cells may not express the biological features exhibited in the BBB. Considering these issues, it is important to validate *in vitro* studies by conducting *in vivo* investigations.

Recent investigations of inorganic nanoparticle delivery systems capable of crossing the BBB have shown that, in particular, iron oxide and gold NPs could be helpful in both drug delivery and diagnostics. The use of nanosystems for *in vivo* diagnosis gained traction after the 2002 paper by Poduslo et al. showed that gadolinium-loaded NPs could potentially be used to cross the BBB, bind to amyloid-beta plaques, and enhance MRI signal (Poduslo et al., 2002; Luo et al., 2020). Subsequently, functionalized ultra-small superparamagnetic iron oxide NPs were identified as similarly capable of reaching and targeting amyloid-beta plaques for enhanced imaging and diagnosis of Alzheimer's disease (Yang et al., 2011; Chen et al., 2014). From here, advancements have been made to further conjugate therapeutic moieties to the NP surface for simultaneous treatment and imaging. This technique is being explored for CNS diseases, including glioblastoma (Israel et al., 2020; Norouzi et al., 2020; Shen et al., 2020; Sheervalilou et al., 2021; Tu et al., 2021), Alzheimer's disease (Poduslo et al., 2002; Lai et., 2016; Luo et al., 2020), and Parkinson's disease (Niu et al., 2017; Hu et al., 2018; Liu et al., 2020).

Polymer or polymeric-based NPs are particles that range in size from 1 to 1,000 nm. Polymer-based NPs are popular for use in many applications, particularly drug delivery, as active compounds can be either captured in the particle or absorbed onto the particle's surface (Zielińska et al., 2020). These NPs are popular for use as biomaterials as they are biocompatible, non-toxic, and biodegradable (Mahmoud et al., 2020). Polymer-based NPs can be divided into natural (chitosan, collagen, alginate, gelatin, hyaluronan, and albumin) or synthetic (polyethylene glycol (PEG), polylactic acid (PLA), PLGA, poly(butylcyanoacrylate) (PBCA)) polymers (Calzoni et al., 2019). The most utilized NPs for delivering therapeutics to the brain are PLGA, PLA, and PEG-PLGA. Coating NPs with an inert polymer such as PEG or poloxamers is used to increase the circulation lifetime and delivery of the drug across the BBB (Spandana et al., 2020). Polymer or polymeric-based NPs are functionalized with ligands such as transferrin, insulin, and lipoprotein receptors to enable targeting and crossing the BBB (Anthony et al., 2021). The physicochemical properties such as size, shape, surface charge, and coating material of the NPs play an important role in crossing the BBB (Mahmoud et al., 2020).

For example, PLGA NPs have been used to deliver various therapeutics such as doxorubicin (DOX) (Malinovskaya et al., 2017; Wohlfart et al., 2011; Gelperina et al., 2010), methotrexate (Jain et al., 2015), temozolomide (TMZ) (Ananta et al., 2016; Fourniols et al., 2015), paclitaxel (PTX) (Ganipineni et al., 2019; Li et al., 2018; Cui et al., 2016), curcumin (Cur) (Cui et al., 2016; Orunoğlu et al., 2017; Mathew et al., 2012), rapamycin (Escalona-Rayo et al., 2019), Co-Q10 (Wang et al., 2010), and 6-coumarin (Tahara et al., 2011; Jin et al., 2012) across the BBB to treat diseases such as brain tumors and neurodegenerative diseases such as Alzheimer's disease (Del Amo et al., 2021; Mahmoud et al., 2020). Other popular polymer-based NPs used to deliver drugs across the BBB to treat brain tumors and neurodegenerative diseases are PEG-PLGA NPs. Drugs such as 6-coumarin (Hu et al., 2011; Li et al., 2011), TMZ (Ramalho et al., 2018), DOX (Geldenhuys et al., 2015), Cur (Fan et al., 2018; Paka and Ramassamy, 2017), PTX (Guo et al., 2011), and memantine (Sánchez-López et al., 2018) have successfully crossed the BBB to treat these diseases.

Extracellular vesicles (EVs) have also been investigated as NP delivery systems intended to cross the BBB. EVs are lipid-bilayered NPs released by most cell types in the body. They can deliver cargo to target cells by transferring protein/nucleic acid species and the presentation of cell-targeting surface markers. EVs are further stratified into three categories based on size and biogenesis: apoptotic bodies (1 to 5 μm), shedding microvesicles (200 to 1,000 nm), and exosomes (30 to 200 nm) (Cunnane et al., 2018). Recent literature has highlighted the ability of EVs to cross the BBB via transcytosis (Morad et al., 2019; Matsumoto et al., 2017). A comprehensive study by Morad et al. employed a combination of *in vitro* and *in vivo* models to demonstrate that tumor-derived EVs can breach the intact BBB via transcytosis (Morad et al., 2019).

The endothelial recycling endocytic pathway is identified as the transcellular transport mechanism with EVs circumventing the low transcytosis by decreasing brain endothelial expression of rab7 and therefore increasing transport efficiency (Morad et al., 2019). In addition to being able to cross the BBB, EV-based delivery is advantageous compared to traditional drug delivery due to inherent cell targeting, protection of cargo, immune evasion, non-cytotoxicity, and ease of loading, whereby the cargo of EVs can be manipulated to contain specific therapeutics (macromolecules or pharmacological agents) (Nagelkerke et al., 2021; Cunnane et al., 2018). As a result, EVs have been extensively studied as vehicles to target neurodegenerative disease by delivering therapeutics across the BBB. EVs can be engineered to express nervous system-specific proteins (such as rabies viral glycoprotein) (Yang et al., 2020; Alvarez-Erviti et al., 2011) or peptides that exhibit high affinity to reactive cerebral vascular endothelial cells after ischemia (cyclo(Arg-Gly-Asp-D-Tyr-Lys)) (Tian et al., 2018). Such engineered EVs have shown an increased ability to target brain cells and tissue following intravenous administration in animal models. The cargo of EVs has also been manipulated via transfection of the parent cell to contain circSCMH1 (Yang et al., 2020), WW-Cre, and Ndfip1 (Sterzenbach et al., 2017) or via direct loading of EVs with agents such as Cur (Tian et al., 2018; Zhuang et al., 2011), PTX, or DOX (Yang et al., 2015). All of the studies mentioned above demonstrate that EV-loaded cargo crosses the BBB and has a therapeutic effect on the chosen model.

6.3.2 Crossing the Blood–CSF Barrier (Arachnoid Cells)

Unlike the rest of the CNS, areas of the CNS adjacent to the ventricles of the brain lack a blood–brain barrier. The parts are known as the circumventricular organs (CVOs) and include the choroid plexus, pineal gland, neurohypophysis, and medial eminence, among others. The blood capillaries of the choroid plexus lack tight junctions, while the epithelial cells possess tight junctions, forming the blood–cerebrospinal fluid barrier (BCB). The arachnoid mater is one of the three layers within the meninges which surrounds the brain, the other two being the dura mater and the pia mater. The arachnoid barrier (AB) is a part of the BCB. The cells of the AB are located adjacent to the subarachnoid space surrounding the CNS, and they are bathed in CSF. The AB, therefore, restricts the passage of drug molecules from the CSF into the brain (Chhabra et al., 2015). The AB cells have been shown to possess drug transporters proteins that restrict the entry of therapeutics into the brain. A major study by Yasuda et al. in 2013 found that the drug transporters p-glycoprotein (P-gp) and breast cancer resistance protein (BCRP) were highly expressed in cultured AB mouse cells. This is significant considering that many drugs are injected into the CSF of the subarachnoid space (SAS), for example, intrathecal chemotherapy to treat childhood acute lymphoblastic leukemia (Pui et al., 2009).

Therapeutics have limited movement from the CSF compartment to the brain parenchyma, as transport occurs via passive diffusion, which is only possible over short distances. Thus, the BCSFB is defined mainly by long diffusion distances. The bulk flow of the CSF is another factor that prevents drug molecules from reaching the brain. The CSF volume in an adult human is around 140 mL, and this is wholly replaced four to five times a day. In this process, a large number of drugs are lost (Grabrucker et al., 2013).

In vitro models of the BCSFB have been developed for use in leukemia research, as leukemia cells or blasts have been demonstrated to cross the BCB within the choroid plexus. These are usually cell-culture-based and can be prepared using primary cultures of epithelial cells, which have several morphological and biological similarities to the actual blood–cerebrospinal fluid barrier. Immortalized tumorous cell lines may be used as an alternative to primary cultures since they are easier to handle and manipulate. On the other hand, these cells may have differing properties and a higher likelihood of genetic mutations (Erb et al., 2020). Standard and inverted culture models have been designed to simulate the BCB, with an apical side and basolateral side to mimic the CSF and blood compartments, respectively.

A newly emerging, complex technique is the brain organoid, a 3D culture of cells from embryonic stem cells or induced pluripotent cells (Pellegrini et al., 2020). This advanced model more closely simulates the *in vivo* environment of the BBB.

Compared to the BBB, the use of NPs for delivery across the BCB has been largely overlooked as a treatment strategy (Strazielle and Ghersi-Egea, 2016). This is predominantly because it is expected that if NPs cross the BCB, they may still have poor penetration across the brain–CSF barrier into the brain parenchyma (Yokel, 2020). Despite this, targeting this barrier could be promising for treating metastatic tumors (Engelhard et al., 2020). Employing magnetic NPs could be useful in combating the rapid flow of CSF by applying an external magnet to target the nanoparticle drug carriers to the site of action (Engelhard et al., 2020). However, further work is still required to address this *in vivo* and evaluate if these systems can cross the BCB.

6.3.3 Crossing the Brain–CSF Barrier (Leptomeningeal Cells)

The leptomeninges is a composite layer of tissues surrounding the brain, of which the arachnoid mater layer contains the CSF within the subarachnoid space (SAS). The SAS has barriers at either side of it, the arachnoid barrier cell layer (or the blood-arachnoid barrier or the outer CSF–arachnoid barrier layer), on the dura side, and the brain-CSF barrier on the brain side (Brøchner et al., 2015). On the dura side, this SAS contains the leptomeningeal cells and tightly packed epithelial cells that form an impermeable barrier that separates CSF from blood vessels in the dura (Chamberlin, 2010). On the brain side, the brain-CSF barrier contains a multitude of non-tight-junctioned cells such as the arachnoid barrier cells and glial endfeet barriers. There are many names for these barriers, and some have been confused with each other (Brøchner et al., 2015). Regardless of their names, little is known of these barriers mentioned above even though they account for a large area of the brain surface during human development and should not be ignored in studying and investigating potential methods of drug delivery of pharmaceuticals to the brain (Weller et al., 2018).

The CSF spaces are lined with leptomeningeal cells, which act as protective barriers and facilitators for substances such as solutes, fluids, and cells to enter the brain parenchyma from the CSF. The brain–CSF barrier has been subjected to considerably less investigation than the BBB and blood–CSF barrier. However, leptomeningeal cells have been successfully cultured in a serum-free medium (Motohashi et al., 1994). Similarly, a 1991 study by Murphy, Chen, and George established an immortalized cell line derived from primary leptomeningeal cultures almost identical to the original cell line. Designated as LTAg2B, this cell line holds potential for developing *in vitro* models to study the functions and characteristics of leptomeningeal cells. This immortalized cell line is significant considering the rapid rate of senescence of leptomeningeal cells in culture, making them relatively difficult to study. The LTAg2B line also expressed all the genes usually expressed in primary leptomeningeal cells, making it an ideal model for *in vitro* studies.

To conclude, further investigations are required to define the properties of the brain–CSF barrier, and suitable cell culture models are crucial to fulfilling this.

As mentioned in Section 6.3.2, the delivery of NPs across the brain–CSF barrier has largely been ignored due to concerns regarding the penetration of drugs into the brain parenchyma once the BCB and brain–CSF barrier have been overcome. Even though this barrier is considered relatively leaky compared to the BBB and BCB, it requires movement of the nanosystems across the leptomeningeal cells by passive diffusion against the flow of fluid out of the brain and into the CSF (Yokel, 2020). Therefore, it is thought that any NPs that do cross this barrier will penetrate short distances into the parenchyma before being removed from the brain via the arachnoid granulations back into the CSF (Yokel, 2020). For this reason, this barrier has been ignored as a route for the delivery of solid, inorganic NPs to the brain.

Few studies have examined the ability of polymeric NPs to traverse these barriers (Strazielle and Ghersi-Egea, 2016; Yasuda et al., 2013) compared to the BBB. Even though there is a push toward intrathecally administered drugs, few studies on the arachnoid barrier cells and the leptomeningeal cells on the effect of these drugs on the cells and their ability to permeate through exist (Pui et al., 2009). As arachnoid barrier cells express drug transport proteins, similar to the BBB cells and choroid plexus cells, they likely contribute to the blood–CSF drug permeation barrier. There are few *in vitro* models of these to study the interaction of NPs with these barriers (Gomez-Zepeda et al., 2020), and future work should attempt to implement arachnoid barrier cells and test these NPs (Holman et al., 2005; Janson et al., 2011).

6.3.4 Crossing the Blood–Tumor Barrier

The global incidence of malignant brain tumors is 4.25 people per 100,000 (Bell et al., 2019). Although the global incidence is low, brain tumors are the main cancer-related death in children under 14 years old (Bell et al., 2019). Crossing the blood–brain barrier, crossing the tumor barrier, and off-target toxicity are significant challenges to treating brain tumors. The standard of care for brain tumors is usually surgery followed by radiation or chemotherapy. Some of the most recent advancements in treating brain tumors include advanced imaged guided surgeries and immunotherapies (Haumann et al., 2020). The strategies for localizing therapies to the brain to treat brain tumors are depicted in Figure 6.4 (Haumann et al., 2020). These include intranasal delivery, nanomedicine, focused ultrasound, convection-enhanced delivery, and intra-arterial delivery. Although there are advantages and disadvantages to each strategy, an essential consideration for most brain tumor drug delivery strategies is that two difficult barriers must be crossed or diverted: the blood–brain barrier and the tumor barrier.

In the context of brain cancer, the tumor barrier is often referred to simply as the blood–tumor barrier (Arvanitis et al., 2020; Belykh et al., 2020), but it is essential to recognize that the tumor barrier has three interfaces: the vasculature, the lymphatics, and the brain. In the simplest terms, a cancer cell (regardless of tissue origin) is a cell that will adapt and change however necessary to confer survival. In this sense, cancer is a disease of molecular evolution and survival of the fittest at its finest (Milane, 2017). Considering this, an important characteristic of the three brain tumor interfaces is that they are all constantly changing. The perpetual

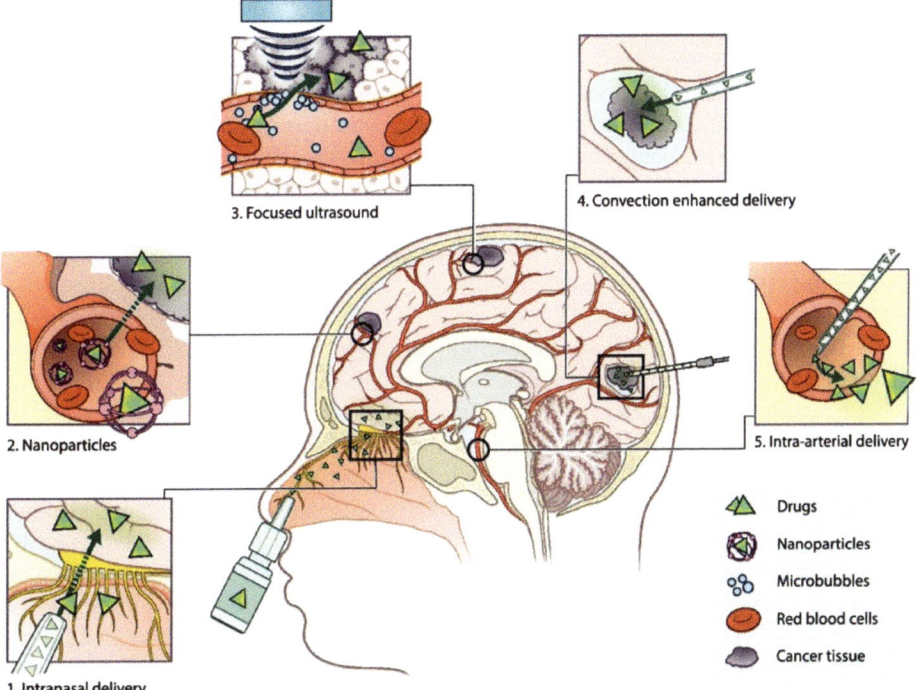

FIGURE 6.4 The various approaches to effectively cross the blood–brain barrier include intranasal delivery, NPs, focused ultrasound, convection-enhanced delivery, and intra-arterial delivery. Standard systemic delivery is also an approach, as are combination approaches such as intranasally administered NPs (from Haumann et al. (2020) and reprinted under permission of the Creative Commons license 4.0).

adaptations and changes that brain tumor cells and the three interfaces undergo further complicate effective treatment.

The brain tumor–blood interface is most notably characterized by constant remodeling (angiogenesis and vessel damage and destruction), increased vascular permeability, altered pericyte morphology and distribution, and loss of astrocyte endfeet connections (Arvanitis et al., 2020; Belykh et al., 2020). Metastatic brain cancer also permanently disrupts the BBB (Achrol et al., 2019). Likewise, although the meningeal lymphatic network is not well characterized, the tumor–lymphatic interface is characterized by constant remodeling and poor lymphatic drainage (Hu et al., 2020b). The poor lymphatic drainage increases the intra-tumoral pH, which creates an impenetrable and toxic barrier at the tumor–normal brain cell interface. These vascular and lymphatic characteristics of solid tumors contribute to the enhanced permeability and retention (EPR) effect (Milane, 2017). The enhanced permeability is due to the loss of vascular tight junctions and the haphazard growth and destruction of tumor neo-vasculature, and the improved retention is due to the lack of lymphatic drainage. Nanomedicine is ideal for exploiting the EPR effect as systemically administered nanomedicine preferentially accumulates at the tumor site due to increased vascular permeability, and the nanomedicine is retained for a prolonged duration due to lack of lymphatic clearance (Milane, 2017).

Exploiting the EPR effect is a critical strategy for localizing therapeutics to brain tumors. A current phase I/II clinical trial (NCT04881032) for newly diagnosed glioblastoma patients is examining the combination of polysiloxane gadolinium-chelates based NPs (AGuIX®) with radiation and temozolomide (Lux et al., 2019). AGuIX® is designed to target, image, and treat brain tumors (Lux et al., 2019). Gadolinium is a common MRI contrast agent; AGuIX® has surface absorbed cyclic gadolinium chelates that increase the MRI signal more effectively than current commercial gadoliniums (Lux et al., 2019). The principle of AGuIX® treatment is radiosensitization (Lux et al., 2019). The cyclic gadolinium chelates increase the efficacy of radiation by producing toxic radical species, electrons, photons, and photoelectrons (Lux et al., 2019). AGuIX® NPs have demonstrated success in multiple rodent models, monkeys, and first in human studies for various types of cancer (Lux et al., 2019).

AGuIX® is a remarkable approach to brain tumor treatment, combining nanomedicine with standard radiation. Although the current phase I/II AGuIX® is promising, there is no perfect therapy, and the risk of off-target effects and residual toxicity from AGuIX® is high. When tumor cells are radically ablated through radiation and enhanced radiation, efferocytosis cannot occur. Indeed, glioblastomas have been shown to upregulate CD47 to avoid efferocytosis (Hu et al., 2020a). Without efferocytosis during large-scale cell ablation, cellular debris accumulates and can damage and kill surrounding cells, leading to further neuronal cell death (Hu et al., 2020a). This is a benefit of immune-activating therapies compared to other approaches to treating cancer. When a patient's immune system is activated to recognize, fight, and clear cancer, the tumor cells are not left as a mass of cellular debris. Still, they are effectively digested and cleared by the immune system. Cell death is one aspect of cancer treatment; clearance of apoptotic bodies, ruptured cells, and cellular debris is another important and often neglected aspect of cancer treatment. As mentioned, no therapy is perfect, and although efficacy has been demonstrated for AGuIX®, there has yet to be a cancer treatment that is 100% effective in eliminating all cancer cells.

Another current clinical trial (NCT02022644) examines the application of irinotecan liposomes with convection-enhanced delivery for treating high-grade, recurrent glioma (Butowski et al., 2014). The approach of this treatment is to administer the liposomes with irinotecan (a topoisomerase I inhibitor) via multiple intra-tumoral catheters that establish a pressure gradient, increasing the distribution of the liposomes in the tumor (Butowski et al., 2014). The current trial uses liposomes loaded with irinotecan and the contrast agent gadoteridol; MRI is used to perform real-time convection-enhanced delivery to localize the liposomes to the tumor effectively (Butowski et al., 2014). This dose-escalation study is a promising combination of nanomedicine, imaging, and convection-enhanced delivery. The drawbacks of this therapy are the invasive procedure and the risk of cancer cell spread from the intra-tumoral injection. Whenever a tumor is directly and physically penetrated, the device must be removed from the patient. Upon removal, cancer cells can be carried through the exit process and relocated to new regions of the brain. These two current clinical trials of nanomedicine for treating brain tumors highlight the advancements in the field. There are numerous exploratory/investigational nanomedicines for treating brain tumors that have been evaluated in pre-clinical models.

In addition to nanomedicine approaches, immunotherapy approaches are also explored in clinical trials (Feldmann et al., 2021). A common immunotherapy approach is chimeric antigen receptor (CAR) T-cell therapy. The principle of CAR-T therapy is to extract a patient's peripheral blood monocytes, select for and stimulate T-cells, engineer the T-cells to express the CAR (with a tumor-specific domain), expand the T-cells, and infuse the cells back into the patient. There are currently numerous CAR-T clinical trials for treating brain tumors. The route of administration varies from intravenous, intracranial tumor injection and intracranial ventricle administration (Feldmann et al., 2021). Current clinical trials include CARs for Her2, EGFRvIII, and IL-13Rα2 (Feldmann et al., 2021). The expression of these receptors is high in glioblastoma multiforme. Her2 is a tyrosine kinase upregulated in many cancers and is important for proliferation. EGFRvIII is a mutant of the wild-type Epidermal Growth Factor Receptor expressed in a high percentage of glioblastoma multiforme patients and is important for proliferation (Feldmann et al., 2021). IL-13Rα2 is neoantigen expressed in some cancers. IL-13Rα2 signaling activates the mTOR pathway and invasion (Feldmann et al., 2021). As demonstrated with these different CARs, many other targets can be selected for treating brain tumors. A clear benefit of CAR-T cell therapy and immune-activating approaches is the complete resolution and clearance of dead cells. However, an apparent downfall of these approaches is over-stimulation of the immune system and the possibility of severe immune reactions such as cytokine storms that lead to systemic inflammation and can result in organ dysfunction and death.

Although there are multiple strategies for localizing therapeutics to brain tumors, two of the most promising approaches currently advancing in the clinic are nanomedicine approaches and immunotherapies. The future will likely include promising nanomedicine-based immunotherapies for activating a patient's immune system to recognize, destroy, and clear brain cancer cells.

6.4 CONCLUSION

Currently, few strategies exist that allow efficient drug delivery into the brain of molecules that cannot cross the BBB or are poorly soluble. However, nanocarriers such as inorganic solid NPs, lipid-based liposomes, polymer-based NPs, protein-based NPs, dendrimers, nanoemulsions, nanosuspensions, nanogels, and the more recently developed nanomicelles, exosomes, and metal-organic frameworks are offering new designs that exploit specific cellular pathways for BBB crossing. Hopefully, this will allow the generation of novel nanomedicines that ideally will enable precise targeting, visualization, and drug delivery, thus treating brain disorders while at the same time allowing monitoring of disease progression and therapeutic efficacy.

To reach this goal, new and improved biomimetics for the BBB that incorporate multiple cell types and basement membranes, integrate dynamic flow, and consider electrical resistance, better standardization of NP characterization enabling traversal of the BBB, and better knowledge about the protein corona acquired by nanocarriers in the circulation are needed.

REFERENCES

Achrol, A. S., R. C. Rennert, C. Anders, R. Soffietti, M. S. Ahluwalia, L. Nayak, S. Peters, N. D. Arvold, G. R. Harsh, P. S. Steeg, and S. D. Chang. "Brain Metastases." *Nature Reviews Disease Primers* 5, no. 1 (2019): 5. doi:10.1038/s41572-018-0055-y.

Adabi, M., M. Naghibzadeh, M. Adabi, M. A. Zarrinfard, S. S. Esnaashari, A. M. Seifalian, R. Faridi-Majidi, H. Tanimowo Aiyelabegan, and H. Ghanbari. "Biocompatibility and Nanostructured Materials: Applications in Nanomedicine." *Artificial Cells, Nanomedicine, and Biotechnology* 45, no. 4 (2017): 833–842. doi:10.1080/2 1691401.2016.1178134.

Aggarwal, P., J. B. Hall, C. B. McLeland, M. A. Dobrovolskaia, and S. E. McNeil. "Nanoparticle Interaction with Plasma Proteins as It Relates to Particle Biodistribution, Biocompatibility and Therapeutic Efficacy." *Advanced Drug Delivery Reviews* 61, no. 6 (2009): 428–37. doi:10.1016/j.addr.2009.03.009.

Alvarez-Erviti, L., Y. Seow, H. Yin, C. Betts, S. Lakhal, and M. J. Wood. "Delivery of siRNA to the Mouse Brain by Systemic Injection of Targeted Exosomes." *Nature Biotechnology* 29, no. 4 (2011): 341–5. doi:10.1038/nbt.1807.

Ananta, J. S., R. Paulmurugan, and T. F. Massoud. "Temozolomide-Loaded PLGA Nanoparticles to Treat Glioblastoma Cells: A Biophysical and Cell Culture Evaluation." *Neurological Research* 38, no. 1 (2016): 51–9. doi:10.1080/01616412.2015.1133025.

Anthony, D. P., M. M. Hegde, S. S. Shetty, T. Rafic, S. Mutalik, and B. S. Rao. "Targeting Receptor-Ligand Chemistry for Drug Delivery Across Blood-Brain Barrier in Brain Diseases." *Life Sciences* 274 (2021): 119326. doi:10.1016/j.lfs.2021.119326.

Arvanitis, C. D., G. B. Ferraro, and R. K. Jain. "The Blood-Brain Barrier and Blood-Tumour Barrier in Brain Tumours and Metastases." *Nature Reviews. Cancer* 20, no. 1 (2020): 26–41. doi:10.1038/s41568-019-0205-x.

Bahadur, S., and K. Pathak. "Physicochemical and Physiological Considerations for Efficient Nose-to-Brain Targeting." *Expert Opinion on Drug Delivery* 9, no. 1 (2012): 19–31. doi:10.1517/17425247.2012.636801.

Bell, J. S., R. M. Koffie, A. Rattani, M. C. Dewan, R. E. Baticulon, M. M. Qureshi, E. J. Wahjoepramono, G. Rosseau, K. Park, and B. V. Nahed. "Global Incidence of Brain and Spinal Tumors by Geographic Region and Income Level Based on Cancer Registry Data." *Journal of Clinical Neuroscience* 66 (2019): 121–7. doi:10.1016/j.jocn.2019.05.003.

Belykh, E., K. V. Shaffer, C. Lin, V. A. Byvaltsev, M. C. Preul, and L. Chen. "Blood-Brain Barrier, Blood-Brain Tumor Barrier, and Fluorescence-Guided Neurosurgical Oncology: Delivering Optical Labels to Brain Tumors." *Frontiers in Oncology* 10 (2020): 739. doi:10.3389/fonc.2020.00739.

Brøchner, C. B., C. B. Holst, and K. Møllgård. "Outer Brain Barriers in Rat and Human Development." *Frontiers in Neuroscience* 9 (2015): 75. doi:10.3389/fnins.2015.00075.

Burgess, A., K. Shah, O. Hough, and K. Hynynen. "Focused Ultrasound-Mediated Drug Delivery Through the Blood-Brain Barrier." *Expert Review of Neurotherapeutics* 15, no. 5 (2015): 477–91. doi:10.1586/14737175.2015.1028369.

Butowski, N., K. Bankiewicz, A. Kells, A. Martin, M. Berger, M. Aghi, M. Prados, S. Chang, and J. Clarke. "A Phase i Study of Convection-Enhanced Delivery of Liposomal-Irinotecan Using Real-Time Imaging with Gadolinium in Patients with Recurrent High Grade Glioma." *Neuro-Oncology* 16, no. 3 (2014): iii13. doi:10.1093/neuonc/nou206.46.

Calzoni, E., A. Cesaretti, A. Polchi, A. Di Michele, B. Tancini, and C. Emiliani. "Biocompatible Polymer Nanoparticles for Drug Delivery Applications in Cancer and Neurodegenerative Disorder Therapies." *Journal of Functional Biomaterials* 10, no. 1 (2019): 4. doi:10.3390/jfb10010004.

Chamberlain, M. C. "Anticancer Therapies and CNS Relapse: Overcoming Blood–Brain and Blood–Cerebrospinal Fluid Barrier Impermeability." *Expert Review of Neurotherapeutics* 10, no. 4 (2010): 547–61. doi:10.1586/ern.10.14.

Chamberlain, M. C., P. A. Kormanik, and D. Barba. "Complications Associated with Intraventricular Chemotherapy in Patients with Leptomeningeal Metastases." *Journal of Neurological Surgery* 87, no. 5 (1997): 694–9. doi:10.3171/jns.1997.87.5.0694.

Chen, F., E. B. Ehlerding, and W. Cai. "Theranostic Nanoparticles." *Journal of Nuclear Medicine* 55, no. 12 (2014): 1919–22. doi:10.2967/jnumed.114.146019.

Chen, G. J., Y. Z. Su, C. Hsu, Y. L. Lo, S. J. Huang, J. H. Ke, Y. C. Kuo, and L. F. Wang. "Angiopep-pluronic F127-Conjugated Superparamagnetic Iron Oxide Nanoparticles as Nanotheranostic Agents for BBB Targeting." *Journal of Materials Chemistry B* 2, no. 34 (2014): 5666–75. doi:10.1039/c4tb00543k.

Chhabra, R., G. Tosi, and A. M. Grabrucker. "Emerging Use of Nanotechnology in the Treatment of Neurological Disorders." *Current Pharmaceutical Design* 21, no. 22 (2015): 3111–30. doi:10.2174/1381612821666150531164124.

Chio, C. C., T. Baba, and K. L. Black. "Selective Blood-Tumor Barrier Disruption by Leukotrienes." *Journal of Neurological Surgery* 77, no. 3 (1992): 407–10. doi:10.3171/jns.1992.77.3.0407.

Cui, Y., M. Zhang, F. Zeng, H. Jin, Q. Xu, and Y. Huang. "Dual-Targeting Magnetic PLGA Nanoparticles for Codelivery of Paclitaxel and Curcumin for Brain Tumor Therapy." *ACS Applied Materials & Interfaces* 8, no. 47 (2016): 32159–69. doi:10.1021/acsami.6b10175.

Cunnane, E. M., J. S. Weinbaum, F. J. O'Brien, and D. A. Vorp. "Future Perspectives on the Role of Stem Cells and Extracellular Vesicles in Vascular Tissue Regeneration." *Frontiers in Cardiovascular Medicine* 5 (2018): 86. doi:10.3389/fcvm.2018.00086.

Cupaioli, F. A., F. A. Zucca, D. Boraschi, and L. Zecca. "Engineered Nanoparticles. How Brain Friendly Is This New Guest?." *Progress in Neurobiology* 119–120 (2014 Aug.–Sep.): 20–38. doi:10.1016/j.pneurobio.2014.05.002.

Das, S., A. Carnicer-Lombarte, J. W. Fawcett, and U. Bora. "Bio-Inspired Nano Tools for Neuroscience." *Progress in Neurobiology* 142 (2016): 1–22. doi:10.1016/j.pneurobio.2016.04.008.

Del Amo, L., A. Cano, M. Ettcheto, E. B. Souto, M. Espina, A. Camins, M. L. García, and E. Sánchez-López. "Surface Functionalization of PLGA Nanoparticles to Increase Transport Across the BBB for Alzheimer's Disease." *Applied Sciences* 11, no. 9 (2021): 4305. doi:10.3390/app11094305.

Engelhard, H. H., A. J. Willis, S. I. Hussain, G. Papavasiliou, D. J. Banner, A. Kwasnicki, S. S. Lakka, S. Hwang, T. Shokuhfar, S. C. Morris, and B. Liu. "Etoposide-Bound Magnetic Nanoparticles Designed for Remote Targeting of Cancer Cells Disseminated Within Cerebrospinal Fluid Pathways." *Frontiers in Neurology* 11 (2020): 596632. doi:10.3389/fneur.2020.596632.

Erb, U., C. Schwerk, H. Schroten, and M. Karremann. "Review of Functional In Vitro Models of the Blood-Cerebrospinal Fluid Barrier in Leukaemia Research." *Journal of Neuroscience Methods* 329 (2020): 108478. doi:10.1016/j.jneumeth.2019.108478.

Escalona-Rayo, O., P. Fuentes-Vázquez, S. Jardon-Xicotencatl, C. G. García-Tovar, S. Mendoza-Elvira, and D. Quintanar-Guerrero. "Rapamycin-Loaded Polysorbate 80-Coated PLGA Nanoparticles: Optimization of Formulation Variables and In Vitro Anti-Glioma Assessment." *Journal of Drug Delivery Science & Technology* 52 (2019): 488–99. doi:10.1016/j.jddst.2019.05.026.

Fan, S., Y. Zheng, X. Liu, W. Fang, X. Chen, W. Liao, X. Jing, M. Lei, E. Tao, Q. Ma, X. Zhang, R. Guo, and J. Liu. "Curcumin-Loaded PLGA-PEG Nanoparticles Conjugated with B6 Peptide for Potential Use in Alzheimer's Disease." *Drug Delivery* 25, no. 1 (2018): 1044–55. doi:10.1080/10717544.2018.1461955.

Feldman, L., C. Brown, and B. Badie. "Chimeric Antigen Receptor T-Cell Therapy: Updates in Glioblastoma Treatment." *Neurosurgery* 88, no. 6 (2021): 1056–64. doi:10.1093/neuros/nyaa584.

Fourniols, T., L. D. Randolph, A. Staub, K. Vanvarenberg, J. G. Leprince, V. Préat, A. des Rieux, and F. Danhier. "Temozolomide-Loaded Photopolymerizable PEG-DMA-Based Hydrogel for the Treatment of Glioblastoma." *Journal of Controlled Release* 210 (2015): 95–104. doi:10.1016/j.jconrel.2015.05.272.

Ganipineni, L. P., B. Ucakar, N. Joudiou, R. Riva, C. Jérôme, B. Gallez, F. Danhier, and V. Préat. "Paclitaxel-Loaded Multifunctional Nanoparticles for the Targeted Treatment of Glioblastoma." *Journal of Drug Targeting* 27, no. 5–6 (2019): 614–23. doi:10.1080/1061186X.2019.1567738.

Geldenhuys, W., D. Wehrung, A. Groshev, A. Hirani, and V. Sutariya. "Brain-Targeted Delivery of Doxorubicin Using Glutathione-Coated Nanoparticles for Brain Cancers." *Pharmaceutical Development & Technology* 20, no. 4 (2015): 497–506. doi:10.3109/10837450.2014.892130.

Gelperina, S., O. Maksimenko, A. Khalansky, L. Vanchugova, E. Shipulo, K. Abbasova, R. Berdiev, S. Wohlfart, N. Chepurnova, and J. Kreuter. "Drug Delivery to the Brain Using Surfactant-Coated Poly (Lactide-Co-Glycolide) Nanoparticles: Influence of the Formulation Parameters." *European Journal of Pharmaceutics & Biopharmaceutics* 74, no. 2 (2010): 157–63. doi:10.1016/j.ejpb.2009.09.003Get.

Gomez-Zepeda, D., M. Taghi, J. M. Scherrmann, X. Decleves, and M. C. Menet. "ABC Transporters at the Blood–Brain Interfaces, Their Study Models, and Drug Delivery Implications in Gliomas." *Pharmaceutics* 12, no. 1 (2020): 20. doi:10.3390/pharmaceutics12010020.

Grabrucker, A. M., R. Chhabra, D. Belletti, F. Forni, M. Vandelli, B. Ruozi, and G. Tosi. "Nanoparticles as Blood–Brain Barrier Permeable CNS Targeted Drug Delivery Systems." In *Topics in Medicinal Chemistry* vol. 10, edited by G. Fricker, M. Ott, A. Mahringer *The Blood Brain Barrier (BBB)*. Berlin, Heidelberg: Springer, 2013. doi:10.1007/7355_2013_22.

Grabrucker, A. M., B. Ruozi, D. Belletti, F. Pederzoli, F. Forni, M. A. Vandelli, and G. Tosi. "Nanoparticle Transport Across the Blood Brain Barrier." *Tissue Barriers* 4, no. 1 (2016 Jan.–Mar.): e1153568. doi:10.1080/21688370.2016.1153568.

Guo, J., X. Gao, L. Su, H. Xia, G. Gu, Z. Pang, X. Jiang, L. Yao, J. Chen, and H. Chen. "Aptamer-Functionalized PEG–PLGA Nanoparticles for Enhanced Anti-Glioma Drug Delivery." *Biomaterials* 32, no. 31 (2011): 8010–20. doi:10.1016/j.biomaterials.2011.07.004.

Guo, J., K. Rahme, Y. He, L. L. Li, J. D. Holmes, and C. M. O'Driscoll. "Gold Nanoparticles Enlighten the Future of Cancer Theranostics." *International Journal of Nanomedicine* 12 (2017): 6131–52. doi:10.2147/IJN.S140772.

Haumann, R., J. C. Videira, G. J. L. Kaspers, D. G. van Vuurden, and E. Hulleman. "Overview of Current Drug Delivery Methods Across the Blood-Brain Barrier for the Treatment of Primary Brain Tumors." *CNS Drugs* 34, no. 11 (2020): 1121–31. doi:10.1007/s40263-020-00766-w.

He, Y., Y. Yao, S. E. Tsirka, and Y. Cao. "Cell-Culture Models of the Blood-Brain Barrier." *Stroke* 45, no. 8 (2014): 2514–26. doi:10.1161/STROKEAHA.114.005427.

Holman, D. W., D. M. Grzybowski, B. C. Mehta, S. E. Katz, and M. Lubow. "Characterization of Cytoskeletal and Junctional Proteins Expressed by Cells Cultured from Human Arachnoid Granulation Tissue." *Cerebrospinal Fluid Research* 2 (2005): 1–12. doi:10.1186/1743-8454-2-9.

Hu, J., Q. Xiao, M. Dong, D. Guo, X. Wu, and B. Wang. "Glioblastoma Immunotherapy Targeting the Innate Immune Checkpoint CD47-SIRPα Axis." *Frontiers in Immunology* 11 (2020a): 593219. doi:10.3389/fimmu.2020.593219.

Hu, K., Y. Shi, W. Jiang, J. Han, S. Huang, and X. Jiang. "Lactoferrin Conjugated PEG-PLGA Nanoparticles for Brain Delivery: Preparation, Characterization and Efficacy in Parkinson's Disease." *International Journal of Pharmacy* 415, no. 1–2 (2011): 273–83. doi:10.1016/j.ijpharm.2011.05.062.

Hu, K., X. Chen, W. Chen, L. Zhang, J. Li, J. Ye, Y. Zhang, L. Zhang, C. H. Li, L. Yin, and Y. Q. Guan. "Neuroprotective Effect of Gold Nanoparticles Composites in Parkinson's Disease Model." *Nanomedicine* 14, no. 4 (2018): 1123–36. doi:10.1016/j.nano.2018.01.020.

Hu, X., Q. Deng, L. Ma, Q. Li, Y. Chen, Y. Liao, F. Zhou, C. Zhang, L. Shao, J. Feng, T. He, W. Ning, Y. Kong, Y. Huo, A. He, B. Liu, J. Zhang, R. Adams, Y. He, F. Tang, X. Bian, and J. Luo. "Meningeal Lymphatic Vessels Regulate Brain Tumor Drainage and Immunity." *Cell Research* 30, no. 3 (2020b): 229–43. doi:10.1038/s41422-020-0287-8.

Iravani, S. "EMR of Metallic Nanoparticles." In *EMR/ESR/EPR Spectroscopy for Characterization of Nanomaterials*, edited by A. K. Shukla, 79–90. Berlin, Heidelberg: Springer, 2017.

Israel, L. L., A. Galstyan, E. Holler, and J. Y. Ljubimova. "Magnetic Iron Oxide Nanoparticles for Imaging, Targeting and Treatment of Primary and Metastatic Tumors of the Brain." *Journal of Controlled Release* 320 (2020): 45–62. doi:10.1016/j.jconrel.2020.01.009.

Jain, A., A. Jain, N. K. Garg, R. K. Tyagi, B. Singh, O. P. Katare, T. J. Webster, and V. Soni. "Surface Engineered Polymeric Nanocarriers Mediate the Delivery of Transferrin–Methotrexate Conjugates for an Improved Understanding of Brain Cancer." *Acta Biomaterialia* 24 (2015): 140–51. doi:10.1016/j.actbio.2015.06.027.

Janson, C., L. Romanova, E. Hansen, A. Hubel, and C. Lam. "Immortalization and Functional Characterization of Rat Arachnoid Cell Lines." *Neuroscience* 177 (2011): 23–34. doi:10.1016/j.neuroscience.2010.12.035.

Jin, Y., A. Xu, M. Yao, B. Li, J. Ying, G. Xu, and W. Ma. "A Physical Model for the Size-Dependent Cellular Uptake of Nanoparticles Modified with Cationic Surfactants." *International Journal of Nanomedicine* 7 (2012): 3547–54. doi:10.2147/IJN.S32188.

Karmur, B. S., J. Philteos, A. Abbasian, B. E. Zacharia, N. Lipsman, V. Levin, S. Grossman, and A. Mansouri. "Blood-Brain Barrier Disruption in Neuro-Oncology: Strategies, Failures, and Challenges to Overcome." *Frontiers in Oncology* 10 (2020): 563840. doi:10.3389/fonc.2020.563840.

Konofagou, E. E., Y. S. Tung, J. Choi, T. Deffieux, B. Baseri, and F. Vlachos. "Ultrasound-Induced Blood-Brain Barrier Opening." *Current Pharmaceutical Biotechnology* 13, no. 7 (2012): 1332–45. doi:10.2174/138920112800624364.

Lai, L., C. Zhao, X. Li, X. Liu, H. Jiang, M. Selke, and X. Wang. "Fluorescent Gold Nanoclusters for In Vivo Target Imaging of Alzheimer's Disease." *RSC Advances* 6, no. 36 (2016): 30081–8.

Li, J., L. Feng, L. Fan, Y. Zha, L. Guo, Q. Zhang, J. Chen, Z. Pang, Y. Wang, X. Jiang, V. C. Yang, and L. Wen. "Targeting the Brain with PEG–PLGA Nanoparticles Modified with Phage-Displayed Peptides." *Biomaterials* 32, no. 21 (2011): 4943–50. doi:10.1016/j.biomaterials.2011.03.031.

Li, J., J. Zhao, T. Tan, M. Liu, Z. Zeng, Y. Zeng, L. Zhang, C. Fu, D. Chen, and T. Xie. "Nanoparticle Drug Delivery System for Glioma and Its Efficacy Improvement Strategies: A Comprehensive Review." *International Journal of Nanomedicine* 15 (2020): 2563–82. doi:10.2147/IJN.S243223.

Li, Y., M. Wu, N. Zhang, C. Tang, P. Jiang, X. Liu, F. Yan, and H. Zheng. "Mechanisms of Enhanced Antiglioma Efficacy of Polysorbate 80-Modified Paclitaxel-Loaded PLGA Nanoparticles by Focused Ultrasound." *Journal of Cellular & Molecular Medicine* 22, no. 9 (2018): 4171–82. doi:10.1111/jcmm.13695.

Liu, L., T. K. Hitchens, Q. Ye, Y. Wu, B. Barbe, D. E. Prior, W. F. Li, F. C. Yeh, L. M. Foley, D. J. Bain, and C. Ho. "Decreased Reticuloendothelial System Clearance and Increased Blood Half-Life and Immune Cell Labeling for Nano- and Micron-Sized Superparamagnetic Iron-Oxide Particles upon Pre-Treatment with Intralipid." *Biochimica & Biophysica Acta* 6, no. 6 (2013); 1830: 3447–53. doi:10.1016/j.bbagen.2013.01.021.

Liu, L., M. Li, M. Xu, Z. Wang, Z. Zeng, Y. Li, Y. Zhang, R. You, C. H. Li, and Y. Q. Guan. "Actively Targeted Gold Nanoparticle Composites Improve Behavior and Cognitive Impairment in Parkinson's Disease Mice." *Materials Science & Engineering C – Materials for Biological Applications* 114 (2020): 111028. doi:10.1016/j.msec.2020.111028.

Luo, S., C. Ma, M. Q. Zhu, W. N. Ju, Y. Yang, and X. Wang. "Application of Iron Oxide Nanoparticles in the Diagnosis and Treatment of Neurodegenerative Diseases with Emphasis on Alzheimer's Disease." *Frontiers in Cellular Neuroscience* 14 (2020): 21. doi:10.3389/fncel.2020.00021.

Lux, F., V. L. Tran, E. Thomas, S. Dufort, F. Rossetti, M. Martini, C. Truillet, T. Doussineau, G. Bort, F. Denat, F. Boschetti, G. Angelovski, A. Detappe, Y. Crémillieux, N. Mignet, B. T. Doan, B. Larrat, S. Meriaux, E. Barbier, S. Roux, P. Fries, A. Müller, M. C. Abadjian, C. Anderson, E. Canet-Soulas, P. Bouziotis, M. Barberi-Heyob, C. Frochot, C. Verry, J. Balosso, M. Evans, J. Sidi-Boumedine, M. Janier, K. Butterworth, S. McMahon, K. Prise, M. T. Aloy, D. Ardail, C. Rodriguez-Lafrasse, E. Porcel, S. Lacombe, R. Berbeco,

A. Allouch, J. L. Perfettini, C. Chargari, E. Deutsch, G. Le Duc, and O. Tillement. "AGuIX® from Bench to Bedside-Transfer of an Ultrasmall Theranostic Gadolinium-Based Nanoparticle to Clinical Medicine." *British Journal of Radiology* 92, no. 1093 (2019): 20180365. doi:10.1259/bjr.20180365.

Ma, Y. Y., K. T. Jin, S. B. Wang, H. J. Wang, X. M. Tong, D. S. Huang, and X. Z. Mou. "Molecular Imaging of Cancer with Nanoparticle-Based Theranostic Probes." *Contrast Media & Molecular Imaging* 2017 (2017): 1026270. doi:10.1155/2017/1026270.

Mahmoud, B. S., A. H. AlAmri, and C. McConville. "Polymeric Nanoparticles for the Treatment of Malignant Gliomas." *Cancers* 12, no. 1 (2020): 175. doi:10.3390/cancers12010175.

Malinovskaya, Y., P. Melnikov, V. Baklaushev, A. Gabashvili, N. Osipova, S. Mantrov, Y. Ermolenko, O. Maksimenko, M. Gorshkova, V. Balabanyan, J. Kreuter, and S. Gelperina. "Delivery of Doxorubicin-Loaded PLGA Nanoparticles into U87 Human Glioblastoma Cells." *International Journal of Pharmacy* 524, no. 1–2 (2017): 77–90. doi:10.1016/j.ijpharm.2017.03.049.

Mathew, A., T. Fukuda, Y. Nagaoka, T. Hasumura, H. Morimoto, Y. Yoshida, T. Maekawa, K. Venugopal, and D. S. Kumar. "Curcumin Loaded-PLGA Nanoparticles Conjugated with Tet-1 Peptide for Potential Use in Alzheimer's Disease." *PLOS ONE* 7, no. 3 (2012): e32616. doi:10.1371/journal.pone.0032616.

Matsumoto, J., T. Stewart, L. Sheng, N. Li, K. Bullock, N. Song, M. Shi, W. A. Banks, and J. Zhang. "Transmission of α-Synuclein-Containing Erythrocyte-Derived Extracellular Vesicles Across the Blood-Brain Barrier via Adsorptive Mediated Transcytosis: Another Mechanism for Initiation and Progression of Parkinson's Disease?." *Acta Neuropathologica Communications* 5, no. 1 (2017): 71. doi:10.1186/s40478-017-0470-4.

McNamara, K., and S. A. Tofail. "Nanosystems: The Use of Nanoalloys, Metallic, Bimetallic, and Magnetic Nanoparticles in Biomedical Applications." *Physical Chemistry Chemical Physics* 17, no. 42 (2015): 27981–95. doi:10.1039/c5cp00831j.

Milane, L. Chapter 9. "Cancer." In *Nanomedicine for Inflammatory Diseases*, edited by L. Milane, and M. Amiji, 319–31. Boca Raton, FL: CRC Press, 2017.

Morad, G., C. V. Carman, E. J. Hagedorn, J. R. Perlin, L. I. Zon, N. Mustafaoglu, T. E. Park, D. E. Ingber, C. C. Daisy, and M. A. Moses. "Tumor-Derived Extracellular Vesicles Breach the Intact Blood-Brain Barrier Viatranscytosis." *ACS Nano* 13, no. 12 (2019): 13853–65. doi:10.1021/acsnano.9b04397.

Motohashi, O., M. Suzuki, N. Yanai, K. Umezawa, N. Shida, R. Shirane, and T. Yoshimoto. "Primary Culture of Human Leptomeningeal Cells in Serum-Free Medium." *Neuroscience Letters* 165, no. 1–2 (1994): 122–4. doi:10.1016/0304-3940(94)90724-2.

Mulvihill, J. J., E. M. Cunnane, A. M. Ross, J. T. Duskey, G. Tosi, and A. M. Grabrucker. "Drug Delivery Across the Blood-Brain Barrier: Recent Advances in the Use of Nanocarriers." *Nanomedicine* 15, no. 2 (2020): 205–14. doi:10.2217/nnm-2019-0367.

Murphy, M., J. N. Chen, and D. L. George. "Establishment and Characterization of a Human Leptomeningeal Cell Line." *Journal of Neuroscience Research* 30, no. 3 (1991): 475–83. doi:10.1002/jnr.490300304.

Nagelkerke, A., M. Ojansivu, L. van der Koog, T. E. Whittaker, E. M. Cunnane, A. M. Silva, N. Dekker, and M. M. Stevens. "Extracellular Vesicles for Tissue Repair and Regeneration: Evidence, Challenges and Opportunities." *Advanced Drug Delivery Reviews* 175 (2021): 113775. doi:10.1016/j.addr.2021.04.013.

Naik, P., and L. Cucullo. "In Vitro Blood-Brain Barrier Models: Current and Perspective Technologies." *Journal of Pharmaceutical Sciences* 101, no. 4 (2012): 1337–54. doi:10.1002/jps.23022.

Nair, A. B., M. A. Morsy, P. Shinu, S. Kotta, M. Chandrasekaran, and A. Tahir. "Advances of Non-Iron Metal Nanoparticles in Biomedicine." *Journal of Pharmacy & Pharmaceutical Sciences* 24 (2021): 41–61. doi:10.18433/jpps31434.

Niu, S., L. K. Zhang, L. Zhang, S. Zhuang, X. Zhan, W. Y. Chen, S. Du, L. Yin, R. You, C. H. Li, and Y. Q. Guan. "Inhibition by Multifunctional Magnetic Nanoparticles Loaded with Alpha-Synuclein RNAi Plasmid in a Parkinson's Disease Model." *Theranostics* 7, no. 2 (2017): 344–56. doi:10.7150/thno.16562.

Norouzi, M., V. Yathindranath, J. A. Thliveris, B. M. Kopec, T. J. Siahaan, and D. W. Miller. "Doxorubicin-Loaded Iron Oxide Nanoparticles for Glioblastoma Therapy: A Combinational Approach for Enhanced Delivery of Nanoparticles" *Scientific Report* 10, no. 1 (2020): 11292. doi:10.1038/s41598-020-68017-y.

Olivier, J. C. "Drug Transport to Brain with Targeted Nanoparticles." *Neurorx* 2, no. 1 (2005): 108–19. doi:10.1602/neurorx.2.1.108.

Orunoğlu, M., A. Kaffashi, S. B. Pehlivan, S. Şahin, F. Söylemezoğlu, K. K. Oğuz, and M. Mut. "Effects of Curcumin-Loaded PLGA Nanoparticles on the RG2 Rat Glioma Model." *Materials Science & Engineering. Part C* 78 (2017): 32–8. doi:10.1016/j.msec.2017.03.292.

Ozsoy, Y., S. Gungor, and E. Cevher. "Nasal Delivery of High Molecular Weight Drugs." *Molecules* 14, no. 9 (2009): 3754–79. doi:10.3390/molecules14093754.

Paka, G. D., and C. Ramassamy. "Optimization of Curcumin-Loaded PEG-PLGA Nanoparticles by GSH Functionalization: Investigation of the Internalization Pathway in Neuronal Cells." *Molecular Pharmaceutics* 14, no. 1 (2017): 93–106. doi:10.1021/acs.molpharmaceut.6b00738.

Pawar, G., N. N. Parayath, A. A. Sharma, C. Coito, O. Khorkova, J. Hsiao, W. T. Curry, M. M. Amiji, and B. S. Bleier. "Endonasal CNS Delivery System for Blood-Brain Barrier Impermeant Therapeutic Oligonucleotides Using Heterotopic Mucosal Engrafting." *Frontiers in Pharmacology* 12 (2021): 660841. doi:10.3389/fphar.2021.660841.

Pellegrini, L., A. Albecka, D. L. Mallery, M. J. Kellner, D. Paul, A. P. Carter, L. C. James, and M. A. Lancaster. "SARS-CoV-2 Infects the Brain Choroid Plexus and Disrupts the Blood-CSF Barrier in Human Brain Organoids." *Cell Stem Cell* 27, no. 6 (2020): 951–961.e5. doi:10.1016/j.stem.2020.10.001.

Poduslo, J. F., T. M. Wengenack, G. L. Curran, T. Wisniewski, E. M. Sigurdsson, S. I. Macura, B. J. Borowski, and C. R. Jack Jr. "Molecular Targeting of Alzheimer's Amyloid Plaques for Contrast-enhanced Magnetic Resonance Imaging." *Neurobiology of Disease* 11, no. 2 (2002): 315–329. doi:10.1006/nbdi.2002.0550.

Pui, C. H., D. Campana, D. Pei, W. P. Bowman, J. T. Sandlund, S. C. Kaste, R. C. Ribeiro, J. E. Rubnitz, S. C. Raimondi, M. Onciu, E. Coustan-Smith, L. E. Kun, S. Jeha, C. Cheng, S. C. Howard, V. Simmons, A. Bayles, M. L. Metzger, J. M. Boyett, J. M. Boyett, W. Leung, R. Handgretinger, J. R. Downing, W. E. Evans, and M. V. Relling. "Treating Childhood Acute Lymphoblastic Leukemia Without Cranial Irradiation." *New England Journal of Medicine* 360, no. 26 (2009): 2730–41. doi:10.1056/NEJMoa0900386.

Ramalho, M., E. Sevin, F. Gosselet, J. Lima, M. Coelho, J. Loureiro, and M. Pereira. "Receptor-Mediated PLGA Nanoparticles for Glioblastoma multiforme Treatment." *International Journal of Pharmacy* 545, no. 1–2 (2018): 84–92. doi:10.1016/j.ijpharm.2018.04.062.

Romeo, V. D., J. deMeireles, A. P. Sileno, H. K. Pimplaskar, and C. R. Behl. "Effects of Physicochemical Properties and Other Factors on Systemic Nasal Drug Delivery." *Advanced Drug Delivery Reviews* 29, no. 1–2 (1998): 89–116. doi:10.1016/s0169-409x(97)00063-x.

Ross, A. M., D. Mc Nulty, C. O'Dwyer, A. M. Grabrucker, P. Cronin, and J. J. E. Mulvihill. "Mulvihill JJE. Standardization of Research Methods Employed in Assessing the Interaction Between Metallic-Based Nanoparticles and the Blood-Brain Barrier: Present and Future Perspectives." *Journal of Controlled Release* 296 (2019): 202–24. doi:10.1016/j.jconrel.2019.01.022.

Sánchez-López, E., M. Ettcheto, M. A. Egea, M. Espina, A. Cano, A. C. Calpena, A. Camins, N. Carmona, A. M. Silva, E. B. Souto, and M. L. García. "Memantine Loaded PLGA Pegylated Nanoparticles for Alzheimer's Disease: In Vitro and In Vivo Characterization." *Journal of Nanobiotechnology* 16, no. 1 (2018): 1–16. doi:10.1186/s129510180356z.

Sandberg, D. I., M. H. Bilsky, M. M. Souweidane, J. Bzdil, and P. H. Gutin. "Ommaya Reservoirs for the Treatment of Leptomeningeal Metastases." *Neurosurgery* 47, no. 1 (2000): 49–54; discussion 54–5. doi:10.1097/00006123-200007000-00011.

Santaguida, S., D. Janigro, M. Hossain, E. Oby, E. Rapp, and L. Cucullo. "Side by Side Comparison Between Dynamic Versus Static Models of Blood-Brain Barrier In Vitro: A Permeability Study." *Brain Research* 1109, no. 1 (2006): 1–13. doi:10.1016/j.brainres.2006.06.027.

Sheervalilou, R., M. Shirvaliloo, S. Sargazi, and H. Ghaznavi. "Recent Advances in Iron Oxide Nanoparticles for Brain Cancer Theranostics: From in Vitroto Clinical Applications." *Expert Opinion on Drug Delivery* (2021): 1–29. doi:10.1080/17425247.2021.1888926.

Shen, Z., T. Liu, Z. Yang, Z. Zhou, W. Tang, W. Fan, Y. Liu, J. Mu, L. Li, V. I. Bregadze, S. K. Mandal, A. A. Druzina, Z. Wei, X. Qiu, A. Wu, and X. Chen. "Small-Sized Gadolinium Oxide Based Nanoparticles for High-Efficiency Theranostics of Orthotopic Glioblastoma." *Biomaterials* 235 (2020): 119783. doi:10.1016/j.biomaterials.2020.119783.

Spandana, K. A., M. Bhaskaran, V. R. Karri, and J. Natarajan. "A Comprehensive Review of Nano Drug Delivery System in the Treatment of CNS Disorders." *Journal of Drug Delivery Science & Technology* 57 (2020). PubMed: 101628.

Sterzenbach, U., U. Putz, L. H. Low, J. Silke, S. S. Tan, and J. Howitt. "Engineered Exosomes as Vehicles for Biologically Active Proteins." *Molecular Therapy* 25, no. 6 (2017): 1269–78. doi:10.1016/j.ymthe.2017.03.030.

Strazielle, N., and J. F. Ghersi-Egea. "Potential Pathways for CNS Drug Delivery Across the Blood-Cerebrospinal Fluid Barrier." *Current Pharmaceutical Design* 22, no. 35 (2016): 5463–76. doi:10.2174/138161282266616072611215.

Tahara, K., Y. Miyazaki, Y. Kawashima, J. Kreuter, and H. Yamamoto. "Brain Targeting with Surface-Modified Poly(D,L-Lactic-Coglycolic Acid) Nanoparticles Delivered via Carotid Artery Administration." *European Journal of Pharmaceutics & Biopharmaceutics* 77, no. 1 (2011): 84–8. doi:10.1016/j.ejpb.2010.11.002.

Tang, Y., X. Wang, J. Li, Y. Nie, G. Liao, Y. Yu, and C. Li. "Overcoming the Reticuloendothelial System Barrier to Drug Delivery with a "Don't-Eat-Us" Strategy." *ACS Nano* 13, no. 11 (2019): 13015–26. doi:10.1021/acsnano.9b05679.

Tian, T., H. X. Zhang, C. P. He, S. Fan, Y. L. Zhu, C. Qi, N. P. Huang, Z. D. Xiao, Z. H. Lu, B. A. Tannous, and J. Gao. "Surface Functionalized Exosomes as Targeted Drug Delivery Vehicles for Cerebral Ischemia Therapy." *Biomaterials* 150 (2018): 137–49. doi:10.1016/j.biomaterials.2017.10.012.

Tu, L., Z. Luo, Y. L. Wu, S. Huo, and X. J. Liang. "Gold-Based Nanomaterials for the Treatment of Brain Cancer." *Cancer Biology & Medicine* (2021) [forthcoming]. doi:10.20892/j.issn.2095-3941.2020.0524.

Wagner, S., A. Zensi, S. L. Wien, S. E. Tschickardt, W. Maier, T. Vogel, F. Worek, C. U. Pietrzik, J. Kreuter, and H. von Briesen. "Uptake Mechanism of ApoE-Modified Nanoparticles on Brain Capillary Endothelial Cells as a Blood-Brain Barrier Model." *PLOS ONE* 7, no. 3 (2012): e32568. doi:10.1371/journal.pone.0032568.

Walkey, C. D., J. B. Olsen, H. Guo, A. Emili, and W. C. Chan. "Nanoparticle Size and Surface Chemistry Determine Serum Protein Adsorption and Macrophage Uptake." *Journal of the American Chemical Society* 134, no. 4 (2012): 2139–47. doi:10.1021/ja2084338.

Wang, Z. H., Z. Y. Wang, C. S. Sun, C. Y. Wang, T. Y. Jiang, and S. L. Wang. "Trimethylated Chitosan-Conjugated PLGA Nanoparticles for the Delivery of Drugs to the Brain." *Biomaterials* 31, no. 5 (2010): 908–15. doi:10.1016/j.biomaterials.2009.09.104.

Weller, R. O., M. M. Sharp, M. Christodoulides, R. O. Carare, and K. Møllgård. "The Meninges as Barriers and Facilitators for the Movement of Fluid, Cells and Pathogens Related to the Rodent and Human CNS." *Acta Neuropathology* 135, no. 3 (2018): 363–85. doi:10.1007/s00401-018-1809-z.

Wohlfart, S., A. S. Khalansky, S. Gelperina, O. Maksimenko, C. Bernreuther, M. Glatzel, and J. Kreuter. "Efficient Chemotherapy of Rat Glioblastoma Using Doxorubicin-Loaded PLGA Nanoparticles with Dierent Stabilizers." *PLOS ONE* 6, no. 5 (2011): e19121. doi:10.1371/journal.pone.0019121.

Yang, J., Y. Z. Wadghiri, D. M. Hoang, W. Tsui, Y. Sun, E. Chung, Y. Li, A. Wang, M. de Leon, and T. Wisniewski. "Detection of Amyloid Plaques Targeted by USPIO-Aβ1-42 in Alzheimer's Disease Transgenic Mice Using Magnetic Resonance Microimaging." *Neuroimage* 55, no. 4 (2011): 1600–9. doi:10.1016/j.neuroimage.2011.01.023.

Yang, L., B. Han, Z. Zhang, S. Wang, Y. Bai, Y. Zhang, Y. Tang, L. Du, L. Xu, F. Wu, L. Zuo, X. Chen, Y. Lin, K. Liu, Q. Ye, B. Chen, B. Li, T. Tang, Y. Wang, L. Shen, G. Wang, M. Ju, M. Yuan, W. Jiang, J. H. Zhang, G. Hu, J. Wang, and H. Yao. "Extracellular Vesicle-Mediated Delivery of Circular RNA SCMH1 Promotes Functional Recovery in Rodent and Nonhuman Primate Ischemic Stroke Models." *Circulation* 142, no. 6 (2020): 556–74. doi:10.1161/CIRCULATIONAHA.120.045765.

Yang, T., P. Martin, B. Fogarty, A. Brown, K. Schurman, R. Phipps, V. P. Yin, P. Lockman, and S. Bai. "Exosome Delivered Anticancer Drugs Across the Blood-Brain Barrier for Brain Cancer Therapy in Danio rerio." *Pharmaceutical Research* 32, no. 6 (2015): 2003–14. doi:10.1007/s11095-014-1593-y.

Yasuda, K., C. Cline, P. Vogel, M. Onciu, S. Fatima, B. P. Sorrentino, R. K. Thirumaran, S. Ekins, K. Urade, K. Fujimori, and E. G. Schuetz. "Drug Transporters on Arachnoid Barrier Cells Contribute to the Blood-Cerebrospinal Fluid Barrier." *Drug Metabolism & Disposition* 41, no. 4 (2013): 923–31. doi:10.1124/dmd.112.050344.

Yim, Y. S., J. S. Choi, G. T. Kim, C. H. Kim, T. H. Shin, D. G. Kim, and J. Cheon. "A Facile Approach for the Delivery of Inorganic Nanoparticles into the Brain by Passing Through the Blood-Brain Barrier (BBB)." *Chemical Communications* 48, no. 1 (2012): 61–3. doi:10.1039/c1cc15113d.

Yokel, R. A. "Nanoparticle Brain Delivery: A Guide to Verification Methods." *Nanomedicine* 15, no. 4 (2020): 409–32. doi:10.2217/nnm-2019-0169.

Zhuang, X., X. Xiang, W. Grizzle, D. Sun, S. Zhang, R. C. Axtell, S. Ju, J. Mu, L. Zhang, L. Steinman, D. Miller, and H. G. Zhang. "Treatment of Brain Inflammatory Diseases by Delivering Exosome Encapsulated Anti-Inflammatory Drugs from the Nasal Region to the Brain." *Molecular Therapy* 19, no. 10 (2011): 1769–79. doi:10.1038/mt.2011.164.

Zielińska, A., F. Carreiró, A. M. Oliveira, A. Neves, B. Pires, D. N. Venkatesh, A. Durazzo, M. Lucarini, P. Eder, A. M. Silva, A. Santini, and E. B. Souto. "Polymeric Nanoparticles: Production, Characterization, Toxicology and Ecotoxicology." *Molecules* 25, no. 16 (2020): 3731. doi:10.3390/molecules25163731.

Pulmonary Drug Delivery

7

Basanth Babu Eedara, Wafaa Alabsi,
David Encinas-Basurto, Robin Polt, Don Hayes Jr,
Stephen M. Black, and Heidi M. Mansour

Contents

DOI: 10.1201/9781003092773-8

7.1 INTRODUCTION

Pulmonary delivery of drugs has been one of the important routes of drug administration for the treatment of respiratory disorders (1, 2). Inhalation therapy for asthma and other diseases had a traditional place in Ayurvedic medicine, whose origins date back 4000 years (3). In addition, Benette used the inhalation route for treating tuberculosis nearly four centuries ago (4). The key advantages of pulmonary delivery of drugs for treatment of localized lung diseases are pain-free administration, reduced systemic side effects, higher concentrations of drug in the lungs, reduced frequency of administration and lower dose required for effective treatment, and improved patient compliance (1, 5, 6). The development of modern-day inhalers, such as pressurized metered-dose inhalers (pMDIs), dry powder inhalers (DPIs), jet and vibrating mesh nebulizers, and soft mist inhalers (SMIs), has given pulmonary drug delivery a momentum boost that transformed a therapeutic niche into a market predicted to approach US$41.5 billion by 2026 (7).

Pulmonary drug delivery has been used not only for delivery of drugs for the treatment of localized lung diseases but also for the systemic delivery of drugs, taking advantage of large surface area in the alveolar region, high blood perfusion, thin epithelial membrane, minimal degradative enzymes, and avoidance of first pass metabolism (8, 9). In recent years, inhalation delivery into the lung has been studied as a possible route of administration for systemic diseases, such as diabetes mellitus (10). Two inhaled insulins, Exubera® (Nektar Therapeutics/Aventis/Pfizer, approved in 2006) and Afrezza® (MannKind, USA, approved in 2014), have been approved by the Food and Drug Administration (FDA) for treatment of type 1 and type 2 diabetes in adults (11).

This chapter will describe pulmonary drug delivery for treating local and systemic diseases. It covers a summary of the anatomy and physiology of lungs, lung diseases, mechanisms of aerosol deposition, factors affecting the therapeutic effectiveness of drugs delivered by the pulmonary route, and pulmonary inhalation aerosol delivery devices. Then, various particle engineering techniques used to prepare dry powder particles and characterization of aerosol formulations will be discussed. In addition, the innovations in mitochondrial targeted therapeutics in lung diseases and their current status will be briefly discussed.

7.2 ANATOMY AND PHYSIOLOGY OF LUNGS

The anatomy and physiology of the respiratory tract are complex. The respiratory system is comprised of many components, including the neural contribution, the interstitium, the chest wall, the pulmonary circulation, and the respiratory tract (12). The respiratory tract is divided into two main parts: the upper respiratory tract, including the nose, nasal cavity, and pharynx; and the lower respiratory tract, consisting of the larynx, trachea, right and left bronchi, and lungs (Figure 7.1) (12–14). The bronchial tree is divided into the primary (main) bronchus, secondary bronchus (lobar) for each lobe, tertiary bronchus for each segment (segmental), conducting bronchiole (lobular), terminal bronchiole, respiratory bronchiole, and alveolar duct as well as the alveoli deep in the lung (13, 14).

7.2.1 Airways and Alveoli Structure

The lung's primary component is a system of branching air tubes ending in compound sacs (15). The airways are divided into two specific functional regions: the conducting airways and the respiratory airways (14). Weibel-A is a mathematical model developed to simulate the function of the lungs (14). It is a symmetrical lung model that divides the lungs into 24 compartments. Each compartment corresponds to a generation of the model, and each generation branches symmetrically into two similar smaller branches. The airway conducting region contains trachea (generations 0) to terminal bronchioles (generations 16). The respiratory region comprises generations 17 to 23, including respiratory bronchioles, alveolar ducts, and alveolar sacs. Each compartment will respond differently to aerosol flow and deposition because of the different biological properties and the various dimensions of divisions along the respiratory tract (14).

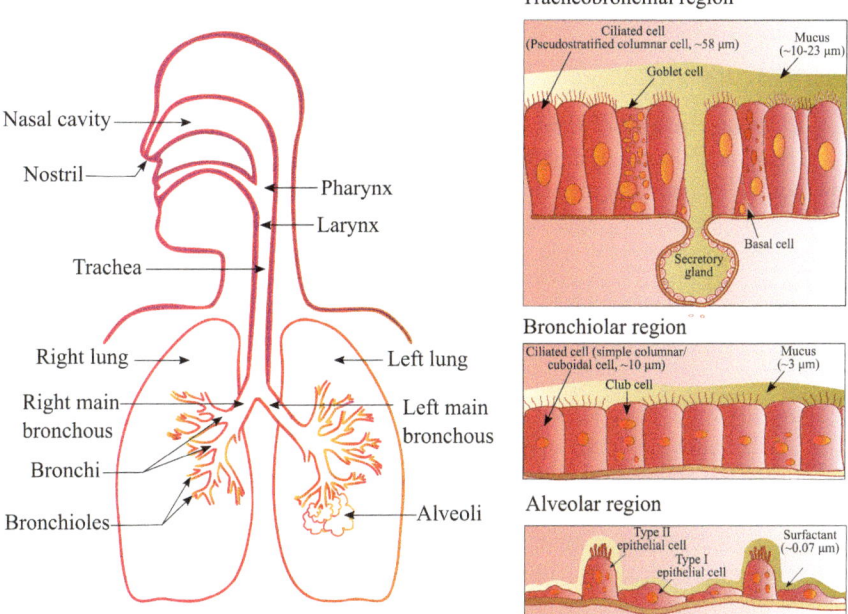

FIGURE 7.1   Anatomy of the lungs and comparison of tracheobronchial, bronchiolar, and alveolar regions of the lungs.

7.2.1.1 Conducting Airways

The conducting airways contain the nasal cavity, pharynx, larynx, trachea, bronchi, and terminal bronchioles; these airways condition and filter the air (14). The airway dimensions are reduced with each bifurcation by moving from the trachea to the terminal bronchioles while the number of airways multiplies in a dichotomous branching pattern (14). The trachea is a fibrocartilaginous tube extending from the inferior end of the larynx (15). It repeatedly branches to form approximately 14 generations of conduits for air to many distinct pulmonary segments (12).

The trachea facilitates the air passage from the nasopharyngeal region to the bronchi and the lungs. It starts at the larynx's edge and divides into right and left bronchi, going to each lung (14, 15). The tracheal epithelium is composed of ciliated cells, mucus-secreting goblet cells, and mucus-secreting glands (Figure 7.1) (14–16). A high proportion of the epithelial cells in the tracheobronchial region are ciliated. Cilia are hair-like projections of about 0.25 µm in diameter and 5 µm in length (14). They are submerged in an epithelial lining fluid, secreted mainly from the serous cells in the submucosal glands. Mucin is a glycoprotein that gives mucus a sticky nature. The mucus with the entrapped particles is moved up out of the respiratory tract during mucociliary clearance by the cilia's synchronized movements toward the pharynx; thus, the layer of mucus and the perciliary fluid through which the cilia beat must be consistent to allow efficient movement of the cilia (14, 16). The movement of cilia in the upward direction pushes the mucus together with foreign particles to the larynx, where they are taken away either by swallowing or by coughing (14, 16). Thus, the trachea performs simple conduction of air between the larynx and the lungs and plays an essential role in protecting the sensitive lung tissue from injuries and invasion by microorganisms or inspired particles (16).

The bronchi undergo further division into smaller airways and have the same tissue structure as the trachea; the bronchi epithelia contain serous cells, brush cells, and club cells (14, 15). The bronchioles are mainly lined with ciliated cuboidal cells without cartilage or glands (Figure 7.1). Moving down more distally, the cartilage becomes irregular in shape and disappears at the bronchiolar level. Furthermore, the number of goblet and serous cells decreases with an increase in club cells. The terminal bronchioles are at the end of the conducting zone; their principal function is to allow airflow into and out of the lungs during breathing (14).

7.2.1.2 Respiratory Airways

The respiratory division consists of respiratory bronchioles, alveolar ducts, alveolar sacs, and alveoli. Also, interstitial lymphatic tissues, lymph vessels, bronchial lymph nodes, fibrous tissue, smooth muscles, vessels, and nerves accompany the air passages (14, 15). Respiratory bronchioles have a diameter of 0.5 mm or less, and their epithelium ranges from simple columnar to simple cuboidal cells with no goblet cells, no cartilage, and no glands (15). The alveolar sacs represent the gas exchange region, which finishes with the alveoli in the periphery.

7.2.1.3 Alveoli

Alveoli have a tiny structure and a large surface area; there are almost 300 million alveoli, providing at least 160 m^2 of surface area, which results in efficient gas exchange in adult lungs (13). Moreover, the blood barrier between the alveoli and the pulmonary capillaries is very thin, allowing rapid gas exchange (14, 15). The alveoli have flatter epithelium and no mucus. The alveolar surface is lined with lung surfactant, which is a surface-active component that contains phospholipids. The surface of the alveoli is lined with two types of pneumocytes (Figure 7.1): type I pneumocytes, which are thin squamous cells composing part of the barrier to gas exchange, and type II pneumocytes, which are larger cuboidal cells; they occur more diffusely than type I cells and are responsible for secreting lung surfactant (14, 15). As is clear from the above, the epithelial thickness and cell population in the airways and alveolar region are different. The airway epithelium is covered by a mucus gel, while the alveolar surface is coated with a surfactant layer. The presence of mucus and surfactant influences deposition, dissolution, solubility, absorption, and clearance of aerosolized particles. Together with the mucus, the ciliated cells provide a major drug clearance mechanism from the trachea and bronchi. In contrast, macrophages play an essential role in clearance from the deep lung (12, 14). All these clearance processes are considered a physical barrier to aerosolized drug delivery to the airways. As a result, knowing the lung's physiology and anatomy is crucial for understanding each physiological region and its role concerning the final drug absorption (14).

7.2.2 Lung Surfactant

Lung surfactant (17) is a lipoprotein complex that contains 10% protein and 90% lipid. Lung surfactant is synthesized, secreted, and recycled by type II epithelial cells in the alveoli. The pulmonary airways are lined with a pulmonary surfactant, which plays a dual role in reducing surface tension and as a host defense mechanism against inhaled pathogens. The alveoli are stabilized against collapse, maintaining a large surface area for gas exchange, by reducing the alveolar surface tension of the air-liquid interface (14). Additionally, surfactant assists oxygen penetration through the lung surface lining and into the blood, thus facilitating the breathing process. Moreover, lung surfactant has anti-inflammatory and antioxidant effects. When aerosol particles settle in the lung, they become enveloped by a monolayer of lung surfactant, which is rapidly digested by macrophages and cleared from the alveolar region (14).

7.2.3 Pulmonary Blood Circulation

The lung is the most perfused organ of the body since it receives the entire cardiac output. The alveolar and respiratory bronchioles receive most of the pulmonary circulation. In contrast, the blood flow in the trachea to terminal bronchioles (i.e., larger airways) is through the systemic circulation, which receives only 1% of the cardiac output (14). The blood that pumps to the lung bronchi and smaller air passages is supplied by branches of the right and left bronchial arteries, whereas the venous return is mostly through the bronchial veins (14, 15). It is likely that aerosolized drugs absorbed into the pulmonary circulation from the upper airway region can be redistributed into remote areas of the lung, which might enhance aerosolized drug efficacy (14).

7.3 RESPIRATORY DISEASES

Respiratory diseases are among the major causes of severe illness and death worldwide. Lung diseases such as chronic obstructive pulmonary disease (COPD), acute lower respiratory infections, asthma, lung cancer, and tuberculosis (TB) are among the leading causes of morbidity and mortality globally (18). According to the World Health Organization (WHO), COPD affects more than 200 million people and is responsible for about 3 million deaths each year; asthma afflicts about 334 million people and is responsible for about 0.49 million deaths per year; lower respiratory infections account for more than 4 million deaths annually; 10 million fall ill and 1.2 million people die from TB annually; and lung cancer accounts for an estimated 2.09 million new cases and 1.76 million deaths per year (19–21). In addition to the above-mentioned lung diseases, there are several other lung diseases, such as sleep-disordered breathing, pulmonary hypertension, and occupational lung diseases. The most common respiratory diseases and treatment are briefly discussed in the following subsections.

7.3.1 Asthma

Asthma is a chronic airway inflammatory airway disease that is characterized by airway obstruction with respiratory symptoms such as cough, chest tightness, dyspnea, and wheezing. Asthma is characterized by infiltration of the lung by eosinophil, T-helper type-2 (Th2) cells, type-2 innate lymphoid (ILC2) cells, mast cells, CD8+ T-lymphocytes, B cells, and dendritic cells (22). Current treatment for asthma includes the use of inhaled corticosteroids (ICS) (beclomethasone dipropionate, fluticasone propionate, budesonide, ciclesonide, mometasone furoate, and fluticasone furoate) in combination with long-acting β-agonists (e.g., salmeterol xinafoate and formoterol fumarate hydrochloride), short-acting β-agonists (albuterol, metaproterenol, levalbuterol, and pirbuterol), mast cell inhibitors (e.g., cromolyn sodium), and anticholinergic agents (ipratropium and tiotropium) (23). Along with these agents, treatment options for treating certain types of asthma include the use of protein- and peptide-based biologicals such as omalizumab, mepolizumab, reslizumab, benralizumab, and dupilumab.

7.3.2 Chronic Obstructive Pulmonary Disease (COPD)

COPD is a complex and multifactorial respiratory disease, characterized by persistent airflow limitation and chronic airway inflammation (24). It is caused by environmental factors (such as tobacco smoking, air pollution, occupational dusts and chemicals, biomass fuel, and allergens) and genetic factors (25, 26). The treatment for COPD includes almost the same drugs used for asthma. Bronchodilation with muscarinic antagonists (tiotropium, glycopyrrolate, umeclidinium), β-agonists (salmeterol, formoterol, indacaterol), and ICS are the foundation of pharmacological treatment in patients with COPD (26).

7.3.3 Lung Infections: Bacterial and Viral

As a major port of entry, the lung is the most common organ of serious infections caused by bacteria (e.g., *Mycobacterium tuberculosis (Mtb)*, *Streptococcus pneumoniae*, *Pseudomonas aeruginosa*) and viruses (e.g., respiratory syncytial virus (RSV), coronaviruses, and influenza viruses). Some of the serious infectious lung diseases will be briefly discussed here.

TB, caused by Mtb, is an airborne infectious disease (27). Mtb is an intracellular, aerobic bacterium that most commonly affects the lungs but can damage any tissue. TB is transmitted from an infected person to another via inhalation of bacteria-containing aerosol droplets emitted to the immediate surroundings during coughing or sneezing. Standard therapy of at least 6 months with an initial intensive phase of treatment (isoniazid, rifampicin, pyrazinamide, and ethambutol) followed by a continuation phase (isoniazid and rifampicin) is recommended for treating drug-susceptible TB in a new patient (28). The resistance of Mtb to available antibiotics with the subsequent development of multi-drug resistance, together with an increasing economic burden, has promptedthe development of new anti-TB drugs and alternative routes of administration (26, 29–32).

Pneumonia is a common acute respiratory infection, causing lung infiltrates visible on chest radiography. Bacteria are among the leading causes of severe pneumonia. *Pseudomonas aeruginosa*, *Acinetobacter*, *Enterobacter* spp., *Klebsiella* sp., *Haemophilus influenzae*, *Staphylococcus aureus*, and *Streptococcus pneumoniae* are the most common bacteria that cause pneumonia. The treatment depends on the type and severity of pneumonia. Somecommonly used antibiotics include vancomycin, linezolid, ceftazidime, ciprofloxacin, amikacin, and tobramycin. Aerosolized tobramycin (TOBI®, an inhalation solution; TOBI® Podhaler®, a PulmoSphere-based DPI formulation) and aerosolized amikacin are effective against common ventilator-associated pneumonia caused by *Pseudomonas aeruginosa* (33, 34).

Human RSV, a member of the *Pneumoviridae* family, is the predominant pathogen identified in hospitalized infants and young children with acute respiratory tract infections. Currently, there are two FDA-approved drugs (palivizumab and ribavirin) available in the market for the management of disease due to severe RSV infection (35, 36). In the united states, ribavirin (Virazole1®, ICN Pharmaceuticals) is marketed as an inhalation solution and is used with a small particle aerosol generator model-2 (SPAG-2) device (36).

Coronaviruses (CoVs) are single-stranded positive-sense RNA viruses that can infect the respiratory, gastrointestinal, hepatic, and central nervous systems of humans and animals (37). At present, there are three coronaviruses, comprising severe acute respiratory syndrome CoV (SARS-CoV; 2002/2003), middle east respiratory syndrome CoV (MERS-CoV; 2012), and SARS-CoV 2 (COVID-19, 2019), that infect the lower respiratory tract and cause severe respiratory disease and pneumonia in humans (38). Currently, there is no specific antiviral therapy for CoV infections, and the main treatments are supportive. However, several vaccine strategies, such as using inactivated viruses, live-attenuated viruses, viral vector-based vaccines, subunit vaccines, recombinant proteins, and DNA vaccines, have been developed. Currently, Pfizer-BioNTech COVID-19 vaccine, Moderna's COVID-19 vaccine, AstraZeneca's Covishield vaccine, and Bharat Biotech's Covaxin™ vaccine are authorized and recommended to prevent COVID-19.

As the lung is the primary site for these infections, inhalation delivery of drugs has a greater potential for effective therapy ofthese diseases. Recently, the members of the International Society for Aerosols in Medicine (ISAM) have reported an urgent need to accelerate the development of inhaled therapies for treating COVID-19 (39). Currently, there are many approved inhaled antibiotics and antiviral therapies for treating lung infections; examples include inhaled ribavarin (Virazole1®, ICN Pharmaceuticals) for RSV infection, inhaled zanamivir (Relenza®, Glaxo Wellcome, Middlesex, UK) for influenza infection, and inhaled amikacin (Arikayce®, Insmed, USA) for *Mycobacterium avium complex* (MAC) lung disease (39–41). Further, several antibiotic drugs have been investigated for targeted pulmonary inhalation aerosol drug delivery for the treatment of pulmonary infections (42–45).

7.3.4 Lung Cancer

Lung cancer remains the most frequently diagnosed cancer, accounting for an estimated 1.76 million deaths in 2018. Non-small cell lung cancer (NSCLC) accounts for ~85% of lung cancer cases (46). Tobacco smoking is the main risk factor for the development of lung cancer. Conventional treatment for lung cancer includes surgical treatment, radiotherapy, and chemotherapy. In recent years, several immunotherapeutic approaches have been tested for treating NSCLC. Aerosolized anticancer therapeutics as DPI have been reported (47, 48).

7.3.5 Lung transplant

Lung transplantation is a surgical option for the treatment of certain advanced lung diseases when patients are determined to be appropriate candidates. Although lung transplant is not curative, it provides the opportunity for patients to have a better quality of life and possibly provides a survival advantage for certain patient populations, including people with cystic fibrosis, pulmonary fibrotic diseases, or pulmonary vascular disorders. Current therapies in lung transplant involve induction (non-specific T cell depletion or cell-cycle arrest) followed by lifelong maintenance immunosuppression with a calcineurin inhibitor, an anti-metabolite, and corticosteroid therapy (49, 50). The rate of acute cellular rejection is highest in lung transplant recipients compared with other solid organ transplant recipients (51), in large part due to direct exposure of the allograft to the external environment. Despite significant immunosuppression used in lung transplant recipients, long-term survival remains limited by chronic lung allograft dysfunction (CLAD), including bronchiolitis obliterans syndrome and restrictive allograft syndrome (52). With direct delivery to the allograft, aerosols including immunosuppressants and antimicrobials offer an opportunity to improve the life of the transplanted organ while reducing systemic side effects. Calcineurin inhibitors are immunosuppressants under development for targeted lung allograft delivery, with cyclosporine being the most studied (53–64). Beyond immunosuppression, aerosolized antimicrobials are used clinically to reduce the risk of airway infection of the lung allografts (65–75). Aerosol development has the potential to greatly affect the future of lung transplantation.

7.3.6 Chronic Bronchitis

Chronic bronchitis is a long-term inflammation of the airways that results in a productive cough lasting more than 3 months in a year for 2 consecutive years (76). It is caused by long-term exposure to inhaled irritants such as cigarette smoke, smog, industrial pollutants, and toxic chemicals. Chronic bronchitis and emphysema are the hallmarks of COPD and often coexist in a patient. Mucous metaplasia, a process in which mucus is overproduced in response to inflammatory signals, is the pathological hallmark of chronic bronchitis (77). The disease starts when damage to the airways initiates inflammation and remodeling of the airway epithelium, leading to mucus hypersecretion, obstruction of the airways, and increased susceptibility to bacterial colonization. The treatment for chronic bronchitis aims to reduce the overproduction of mucus, control inflammation, and easecoughing. Current therapeutic options for treating chronic bronchitis include smoking cessation and administration of expectorants, mucolytics, anticholinergics, glucocorticoids, phosphodiesterase-4 inhibitors, and antioxidants (76).

7.3.7 Cystic Fibrosis (CF)

CF is an inherited multisystem disease characterized by the accumulation of viscous and sticky mucus in organs with epithelial surfaces including lungs, gut, pancreas, and testes (78). It is caused by a mutation in the CF transmembrane conductance regulator (CFTR) gene, which codes for a chloride channel located on the epithelial cell surface. When the CFTR is not functional, the secretions become thick and viscous. There is no cure for CF, but the treatment includes anti-inflammatory therapy, antimicrobial therapy, and airway clearance following respiratory physiotherapy and inhaled mucolytics (79). CFTR modulators are new class of drugs which directly target the defective CFTR protein in CF (80). They can either potentiate the activity of the CFTR channel that is at the epithelial cell surface or correct the defect by allowing CFTR to reach the cell surface (81). Currently, only four CFTR modulators such as ivacaftor, lumacaftor, tezacaftor, elexacaftor, are approved for clinical use in CF patients with certain CFTR mutations (82).

7.3.8 Emphysema

Emphysema is a progressive lung disease that causes permanent enlargement of distal airspaces, leading to obstruction of small airways. The principal cellular mechanism by which lung damage occurs in emphysema is an imbalance between the protease and anti-protease systems in the lung, either as a result of smoking (increasing lung protease activity) or from inherited conditions such as alpha-1 antitrypsin (an anti-protease enzyme) deficiency (83). Medical management of emphysema includes administration of bronchodilators, anti-inflammatory drugs including corticosteroids, and mucolytic agents; oxygen therapy; protein (α-1 antitrypsin) therapy; and surgery or lung transplant (84).

7.3.9 Bronchospastic Pulmonary Disease

Bronchospastic pulmonary disease, called bronchospasm, is a reversible narrowing of the airways in response to a stimulus. Patients who have asthma and chronic bronchitis may exhibit severe bronchoconstriction upon exposure to allergens, toxic chemicals, and cold air (85). The characteristic symptoms and signs of bronchospasm are wheezing, prolonged expiration, reduced breath sounds, and increased pressure during positive pressure ventilation. Treatment for bronchospasm includes administration of β-agonist bronchodilators, epinephrine, isoproterenol, and corticosteroids (86).

7.3.10 Idiopathic Pulmonary Fibrosis

Idiopathic pulmonary fibrosis (IPF) is the most common, fatal, chronic progressive fibrotic interstitial pneumonia, which mainly occurs in older, smoking adults (87). IPF is characterized by shortness of breath, dry cough, and less common symptoms such as discomfort in the chest, fatigue, low-grade fever, and weight loss. The major mechanism involved in the progression of this disease appears to be driven by abnormal and/or dysfunctional alveolar epithelial cells that promote fibroblast recruitment, proliferation, and differentiation, resulting in scarring of the lung, architectural distortion, and irreversible loss of pulmonary function (88). Unfortunately, no effective treatment is available for patients with IPF. However, the mainstay of therapy for IPF includes corticosteroids and immunosuppressive agents. Pulmonary fibrosis (PF) has been described in detail recently (89).

7.3.11 Airway Oxidative Stress

Oxidative stress is a state of imbalance in oxidants (reactive oxygen species, ROS) and antioxidants in a biological system in favor of oxidants, leading to cell damage. ROS such as superoxide anions (O_2^-) and the hydroxyl radical ($\bullet OH$) with unpaired electrons are unstable molecules and participate in oxidation reactions. Biological systems are exposed to oxidants that are generated endogenously (mitochondria, peroxisomes, enzymes of cytochrome P_{450}, NADPH oxidases, nitrogen oxide synthases, and xanthine oxidases) and exogenous sources (compounds present in the air such as ozone, asbestos, and cigarette smoke) (90). Increased lung oxidative stress with higher levels of ROS leads to oxidation of lipids, proteins, and DNA, which may cause direct lung injury. The elimination of ROS using exogenous antioxidants could be an effective preventive measure against various diseases. The most important enzymatic antioxidants that protect against ROS include superoxide dismutase, catalase, and glutathione peroxidase.

7.3.12 Respiratory Distress Syndrome (RDS)/Acute Respiratory Distress Syndrome (ARDS)

RDS is a breathing disorder that affects preterm infants born before 32 weeks of pregnancy (17, 91). RDS is characterized by radiographic diffuse bilateral infiltrates, decreased respiratory compliance, small lung volumes, and severe hypoxemia. Physiological and anatomical immaturity of the lung and surfactant deficiency are the main causes of RDS. Lung surfactant, a lipid-rich fluid, is produced by the alveolar epithelial type II cells that cover the inner surface of alveoli. Lung surfactant reduces the surface tension at the alveolar air-liquid interface and maintains the lung function of gaseous exchange. Treatment for RDS includes exogenous surfactant therapy and positive pressure ventilation. Both natural (Infacsurf®, USA; Alveofact®, Germany; Surfacten®, Japan; Survanta®, USA; Curosurf® Italy) and synthetic (Exosurf®, USA; ALEC®, UK; Surfaxin®, USA) surfactants are effective in the treatment of RDS in preterm infants (91).

ARDS is a lung condition characterized by impaired oxygenation due to fluid accumulation in the alveoli. Etiologies of ARDS include but are limited to pneumonia, trauma, sepsis, pancreatitis, aspiration, inhalation injury, and burns (92). The treatment for ARDS includes treating the underlying risk condition, treating lung injury, and supportive treatment of critically ill patients. Pneumonia is an important cause of ARDS; therefore, treatment with broad spectrum antibiotics and antiviral drugs is critical (92).

7.3.13 Pulmonary Hypertension (PH)

PH, characterized by progressive increase in pulmonary vascular resistance and pulmonary arterial pressure, is associated with significant morbidity and mortality. PH is defined as an abnormal elevation of mean pulmonary artery pressure (mPAP) >20 mmHg at rest, a pulmonary artery wedge pressure ≤15 mmHg, and a pulmonary vascular resistance (PVR) of ≥3 Wood units (93). The WHO categorizes PH into five groups based on causes resulting in similar histopathologic changes: 1. Pulmonary arterial hypertension (PAH); 2. Pulmonary venous hypertension (PVH) due to left heart disease; 3. PH due to lung disease/

hypoxia; 4. Chronic thromboembolic pulmonary hypertension (CTEPH); and 5. PH due to unclear multifactorial mechanisms (94, 95). PAH features precapillary PH, which results in vasoconstriction and stiffening of the small arteries in the lungs secondary to cell proliferation and fibrosis, as well as the development of in situ thrombi or plexiform lesions (96). The current approved drugs target endothelial function and vasodilation via three major mechanisms: the prostacyclin pathway (epoprostenol, iloprost, treprostinil, beraprost), the nitric oxide pathway (sildenafil, tadalafil, vardenafil, riociguat), and the endothelin pathway (bosentan ambrisentan macitentan selexipag) (97). PH and PH therapeutics have been described in detail previously (98, 99).

7.4 THE THREE MAJOR MECHANISMS OF AEROSOL DEPOSITION

The effectiveness of inhalation therapy depends not only on the pharmacology of the drug being inhaled but also on the location and degree of respiratory tract deposition. The phenomenon of aerosol deposition of inhaled particles in distinct regions of the respiratory system is influenced by many elements, such as particle size, particle shape, respiratory rate, lung respiratory volume, and the health situation of the individual (100). Similarly, not only the composition of the aerosol but also the volume and spatial distribution of accumulated particles in the lung influence the pharmacological effect of the inhaled therapy (101, 102). Deposition within the human lung can therefore indicate strategies for the prevention or alleviation of health effects from inhaled toxic particles or new drug aerosol delivery approaches that will overcome the constraints of inhalers (103).

Depending on the particle size, airflow, and location in the respiratory system, particle deposition can occur via the mechanisms of inertial impaction, sedimentation, and Brownian diffusion (Figure 7.2), and to a lesser degree, turbulence, electrostatic precipitation, and interception primarily regulate aerosol deposition (104).

The relative contribution of these various mechanisms is a function of the particle's physical characteristics, the composition of the lungs, and the pattern of the flow. There are three major mechanisms of aerosol particle deposition in the lungs: inertial impaction, sedimentation due to gravitational settling, and diffusion due to Brownian motion (9) Large particles >10 μm) will not enter the lungs but will be deposited in the oropharyngeal region by inertial impaction. Inhaled particles smaller than 10 μm can enter the lungs. Smaller particles <2 μm are primarily deposited in the alveolar region, while particles in the 2-5 μm size range are mainly deposited in the central and small airways.

7.4.1 Inertial Impaction

In the respiratory tract, the predominant mechanism of deposition of particles >10 μm is in the oropharyngeal region. If there is a rapid change in the direction of the flow, inertial forces dominate over gravitational forces, causing particles to maintain their original directional path and not deviate with the change in directional flow (105, 106). In the complex structure of the upper respiratory tract (which stretches from the nasal and mouth cavities to the entry of the trachea) and oropharyngeal region are the most possible locations of deposition by inertial impaction (107, 108).

7.4.2 Sedimentation by Gravitational Settling

Sedimentation, under the action of gravity, refers to the deposition of particles. Deposition by sedimentation due to gravity is the predominant mechanism of aerosol particle deposition in the lungs for current

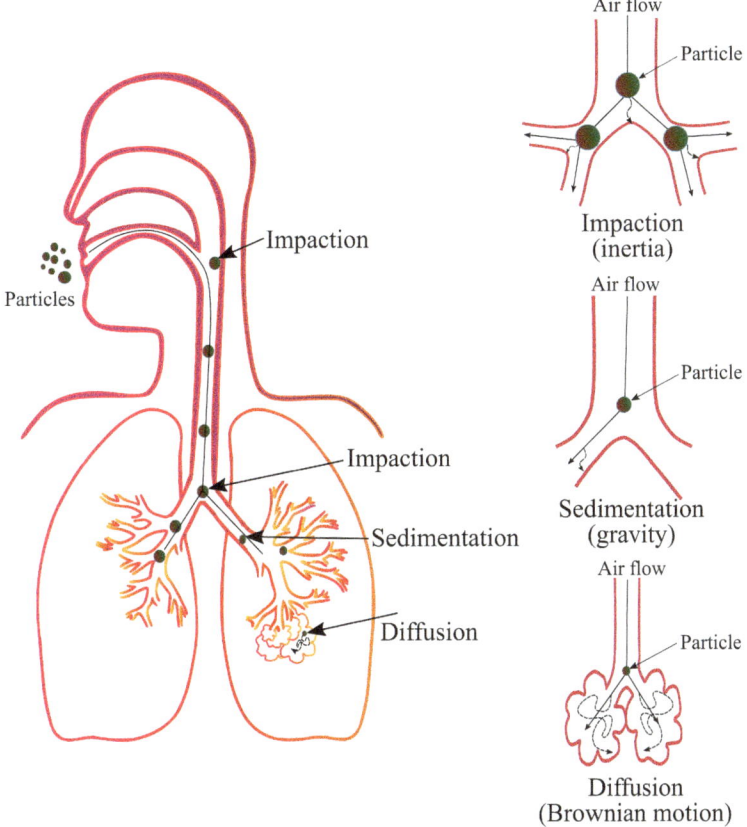

FIGURE 7.2   Deposition mechanisms in the respiratory tract (RT).

therapeutic marketed aerosol products. Airflow is slower, and directional change is less sharp; particle deposition via sedimentation occurs as gravitational forces dominate.

7.4.3 Diffusion

Brownian diffusion, which arises from spontaneous movements of particles caused by encounters with gas molecules, is the third major deposition process in the lung. In comparison with impaction and sedimentation, Brownian diffusion deposition increases with decreasing particle size and becomes the dominant particle deposition process at a size smaller than < 0.01μm; diffusion deposition in the nose, mouth, and pharyngeal airways is also important (101). This mechanism is governed by the geometric rather than the aerodynamic size of the particles (109).

7.4.4 Minor Mechanisms of Aerosol Deposition

Electrostatic attraction and turbulent flow are two minor mechanisms in the lungs and are regarded as having a low probability of occurring with medical aerosols. The airstream flow is transported through the upper airway before reaching the trachea, which is accompanied by drastic changes in cross-sectional areas with major contraction at glottis level. A laryngeal jet is generated by this contraction and can be propagated deep into the bronchial tree, creating local turbulence of the flow. Changes in both magnitude and direction of the trajectories of particles, caused by flow fluctuations and turbulence, will eventually deposit them on the airway walls (101). Turbulent fluctuation has been found to pass the throat and continue downstream to the first three generations of the upper airways (110).

Furthermore, although human airways are electrically neutral, electrostatic charges are introduced via induction or conduction in most aerosol generation and transport processes. Pharmaceutical powders are composed of fine particles in contact with each other or with device walls, which can acquire charges via electron exchange due to different surface potentials. Such electrostatic effects are expected to be significant in the upper airways before these electric charges dissipate due to high humidity. Surface charges in solid particles arise from physical contact between each other and between particles and inhaler device walls during inhalation. Xi, Si (111) measured the electrostatic effects of inhaled aerosol using image-based computational approach, finding for micron-size particles that total and local deposition could be altered by aerosol charge.

7.5 FACTORS AFFECTING THE THERAPEUTIC EFFECTIVENESS OF DRUGS DELIVERED BY THE PULMONARY ROUTE

There are many anatomical, physiological, and immunological obstacles, including the strongly branched composition of the airways, mucosal clearance, macrophage uptake, lung surfactant, alveolar epithelium, and enzymatic metabolism, influencing the absorption and permeation effectiveness of inhaled drugs (112). The greatest challenge for inhaled drugs is being able to deliver enough active pharmaceutical ingredient (API) to the lung. Also, physicochemical properties of the aerosol-containing particles (shape, density, charge, and aerodynamic diameter) will significantly affect the site of deposition and its efficiency (113).

The main parameter that will predict efficient lung deposition is the aerodynamic diameter (114, 115), which is the diameter below which 50% of the total mass of aerosol particles lies. In general, particles with a diameter between 1 and 5 µm will preferentially deposit in the lungs, whereas particles with a larger diameter will deposit in the upper airways or oropharyngeal region. For targeting the alveolar region, particles with a diameter lower than 3 µm are required. However, patient inhalation also has a critical effect on lung deposition, as a poor inhaled flow rate, inhaled volume, and breath hold pause will affect drug quantity in the lungs (116, 117).

The lungs consist of a dynamic branching airway network, also referred to as the bronchial tree. If a particle is to enter the alveolar area and obtain entry to the large epithelial target site, several airway bifurcations must be crossed, where it is likely to be deposited (116). Once a drug is deposited, the aerosol particle must dissolve to release the API for pharmacological effect or for systematic absorption. Fluid in the lung is very limited; only 10-30 mL is available for particle dissolution (118).

The variety of clearance mechanisms that are used in the different stages of the respiratory tract to eliminate foreign particles are mucociliary, mechanical, and alveolar macrophage (AM) clearance and enzymatic degradation. In a healthy lung, one of the defense mechanisms is mucociliary clearance, which is used to remove deposited materials from the conducting airways and deliver them to the oropharynx, where they are swallowed or exhaled. Mucus replacement and clearance should be completed within 24 h. This phenomenon is more prevalent in the upper airway than in the lower airway region (116, 119). On the other hand, in a disease state, where airways can be narrowed by bronchoconstriction, mucus hypersecretion, and inflammation, or even blocked by the mucus layer, the mucociliary clearance becomes impaired and the mechanical clearance (i.e. coughing, sneezing or swallowing) becomes a more prominent clearance mechanism. After lung inhalation, the fate of aerosol-particles is cleared from the lungs, absorbed into blood/lymphatic circulation, or degraded via drug metabolism (120).

AMs recognize and internalize inhaled pathogens and foreign particles by a phagocytic process, which is an important element of the innate immune response. It has been reported that AMs are crucial for the fast clearance of many pulmonary pathogens, such as *P. aeruginosa* and *Klebsiella pneumoniae* (121–123). Macrophages can easily phagocyte particles with a geometric diameter in the range of 1-2 μm, while those with a smaller size are taken up less effectively (102). Clearance by AMs is still the main obstacle to achieving controlled drug release in the alveoli. Rapid alveolar clearance has been shown to occur within 30 min of microparticle administration to the lung in animal models and hinders drug delivery.

Another challenge to efficient inhaled therapy is the susceptibility of drugs to degradation by an enzymatic system:the cytochrome P450 (CYP) family, which can degrade a broad spectrum of inhalable xenobiotics, different inhalable drugs, pollutants, and toxicants. In addition, biopharmaceutics such as inhaled peptides and proteins are highly vulnerable to peptidase and protease activity (118). Although the lung has a low metabolic activity, in contrast to different organs such as the liver, enzymatic degradation notably influences drug local bioavailability and therefore, needs to be carefully assessed at some point in the development of formulations intended for inhalation (124). In lung disease states such as COPD, CF, and asthma, a heavy enzymatic burden due to proteases such as matrix metalloproteinases and elastases is imposed by the high influx of innate immune cells, including macrophages, neutrophils, and eosinophils (125).

7.6 PULMONARY INHALATION AEROSOL DELIVERY DEVICES

Inhalation therapy is the preferred route for delivering drugs for the management of lung diseases such as asthma, COPD, and lower respiratory infections (126, 127). Local therapies offer several advantages for the treatment of lung diseases, including rapid onset of action, lower systemic exposure, and reduced side effects. Historically, inhalation therapy has been used for thousands of years in various cultures and may have originated in the smoking of datura leaves for treating cough in India 4000 years ago (128).

The deposition pattern of the aerosol dose is determined mainly by the physicochemical properties of the formulation and the device used for inhalation. The main devices used for drug delivery via the lung route are the following platforms: nebulizers, metered-dose inhalers (MDIs), and soft mist inhalers for liquid formulations, and DPIs for solid formulations. Table 7.1 highlights the advantages and disadvantages of the aerosol systems used for inhalation delivery. The most important criteria for a medical inhalation device are to produce a reproducible and accurate dose, to generate suitable particles for lung deposition (1-5 μm), to be available in multiple forms for continuous dose, to stabilize the API, and to be cost-effective (129, 130).

7.6.1 Nebulizers

A nebulizer is a commonly used aerosol generator device that does not depend on a patient's inspiratory force to generate the power needed to create the aerosol. Hence, these aerosol devices are active devices, which actively generate the aerosol independently of the patient. This device platform is used in many important pulmonary diseases, including asthma, COPD (24), CF, pulmonary infections (131, 132), and pulmonary hypertension (99). These devices are commonly used to deliver pharmaceutical aerosols in patient populations such as infants, small children, and the elderly who are unable to operate, coordinate, or cooperate with the use of a pMDI or a DPI (133). A primary characteristic of a pharmaceutical nebulizer is the conversion of a liquid drug formulation by mechanical (including ultrasonic) or thermal energy into droplets that can be inhaled and deposited into the lungs. A nebulizer system consists of a nebulizer handset, compressor, tubing, and accessories. The formulations used with nebulizers are either solutions

TABLE 7.1   Advantages and Disadvantages of the Aerosol Systems Used for Inhalation Delivery

AEROSOL SYSTEM	ADVANTAGES	DISADVANTAGES/LIMITATIONS/CHALLENGES
Nebulizer	• Relatively simple liquid formulations and less expensive to manufacture • Versatility in the types of liquid dosage forms (e.g., aqueous solution, aqueous/alcohol cosolvent, suspension, colloidal dispersion, or an emulsion) • No propellant needed • No patient coordination required • Avoids drying process during manufacture • Suitable for patients of all ages • Active device that generates the aerosol independently of the patient's inspiratory force • Does not depend on the patient's inspiratory force to generate the aerosol • Uniquely serves niche populations including infants, the elderly, and those with compromised lung function • Hand-held devices are currently available • Can be used in patients in the intensive care unit in hospitals (e.g., mechanically ventilated patients) • Multiple drugs can exist in the same formulation	• Limited to drugs with high to moderate water solubility • Drug solubility challenges • Formulation must be a liquid dosage form • Physicochemical stability challenges due to the liquid state • Microbial growth potential in the liquid formulation • Must be unit-dose ampules to prevent microbial growth or powder reconstituted just prior to administration • Relatively long administration time compared with other devices • Exact dose delivered to the lungs is a challenge to quantify • Drug loss and higher amounts of formulation wastage • Some types, such as air jet nebulizer systems, are bulky, heavy, and not hand-held • Larger than other aerosol devices • Must be powered by an electrical power supply (e.g., portable battery or plugged electrical outlet) to generate the aerosol • Assembly required • Contamination potential • Time for assembly/disassembly required • Cleaning and drying required after each dose administration
pMDI	• Compact, hand-held, lightweight, and portable • Multidose • Metered dose • Does not require an electrical power source to generate the aerosol • Active device that generates the aerosol independent of the patient's inspiratory force • Does not depend on the patient's inspiratory force to generate the aerosol • Formulation is protected in a metal canister and sealed container environment (when not being actuated by the patient) • Multiple drugs can exist in the same formulation • Minimal preparation time needed prior to dose administration • Device is relatively easy and low-cost to manufacture	• Requires an organic propellant in the formulation to provide the power to generate the aerosol • A dispersed liquid dosage form that readily phase separates • Requires shaking by the patient prior to each administered dose • Drug–propellant incompatibility issues • Drug solubility challenges • Physicochemical stability challenges due to the liquid state • Development of the formulation is costly and time-consuming due to compatibility, solubility, and physicochemical challenges • Microbial growth potential in the liquid formulation • Highly variable aerodynamic droplet particle size produced depending on evaporation rate of the propellant and solvent relative to the aerosol path length • A spacer device is required to improve aerodynamic particle size needed for lung deposition

(Continued)

TABLE 7.1 (Continued)   Advantages and Disadvantages of the Aerosol Systems Used for Inhalation Delivery

AEROSOL SYSTEM	ADVANTAGES	DISADVANTAGES/LIMITATIONS/CHALLENGES
	• Device can be electronic/digital and supports Wi-Fi for patient monitoring and patient compliance with drug therapy • Device has a dose counter that is readily visible to monitor doses remaining	• Hand–lung coordination required • Inhaled aerosol dose is highly dependent on patient hand–lung coordination • High oropharyngeal deposition • Propellant taste detected by patients due to high mouth deposition • Flammability potential of propellants • Inhaled propellant abuse potential • Priming needed before first use of a pMDI product • High variability in aerosol output/drug content
SMI	• Compact, hand-held, lightweight, and portable • Multidose • Metered dose • Propellant free • Generates a slow-moving aerosol mist • Long spray duration (1.5 s) • High proportion of fine liquid droplets • High lung deposition • No shaking required prior to dose administration by the patient • Active device that generates the aerosol independently of the patient's inspiratory force • Does not depend on the patient's inspiratory force to generate the aerosol • Multiple drugs can exist in the same formulation • Relatively easy for patients to administer (i.e., patient-friendly) • Device has a dose counter that is readily visible to monitor doses remaining	• Priming needed before first use of an SMI product • Costs more than pMDIs • Limited to drugs with high to moderate water solubility • Drug solubility challenges • Formulation must be a liquid dosage form • Physicochemical stability challenges due to the liquid state • Formulation must be in solution as an aqueous or aqueous/alcohol cosolvent system • Microbial growth potential in the liquid formulation • The metered volume of 15 μL limits the dose delivery capacity in relation to dose needed for efficacy.
DPI	• Compact, hand-held, lightweight, and portable • Multidose • Metered dose • Propellant free • Easy operation • FDA approved for use by children as young as 4 years old • Device design versatility with different shear stress properties • Propellant free (green, environmentally friendly)	• Relatively expensive to prepare • Surface properties of solid-state particles can significantly impact aerosol dispersion properties • Interparticulate forces in the solid state affect aerosol dispersion • Moisture may cause powders to aggregate due to capillary condensation between the particles affecting aerosol properties • Oropharyngeal drug deposition can occur based on patient's inspiratory force for passive DPI devices

(Continued)

TABLE 7.1 (Continued)   Advantages and Disadvantages of the Aerosol Systems Used for Inhalation Delivery

AEROSOL SYSTEM	ADVANTAGES	DISADVANTAGES/LIMITATIONS/CHALLENGES
	• No hand–mouth coordination required • No microbial growth potential, so no preservatives are needed • Most physically and chemically stable dosage form in the solid state relative to liquid aerosol formulations • Spacers are not needed and are contraindicated • Multiple drugs can exist in the same formulation • Hydrophobic drugs, peptides, and proteins can be delivered • Device has a dose counter that is readily visible to monitor doses remaining • Can be physical mixtures of individual drug and excipient particles • Can be molecular mixtures of molecularly mixed drug with excipient in the same particle • Solid-state particles can be designed with particle properties by particle engineering • Can be active where aerosol generation is independent of the patient's inspiratory force • Can be passive where aerosol generation is dependent on the patient's inspiratory force	

Abbreviations: DPIs, dry powder inhalers; HFA, hydrofluoroalkane; pMDIs, pressurized metered-dose inhalers; SMIs, soft mist inhalers.

or suspensions composed of sterile water for injection as a solvent, glycerin, ethanol, and propylene glycol as a cosolvent, sodium chloride to adjust the isotonicity, and an acid (hydrochloric acid) or base (sodium hydroxide) to adjust the pH. Table 7.2 lists the currently available nebulizer products, their formulation compositions, and their therapeutic applications.

Commercially available nebulizers are classified as air jet nebulizers, ultrasonic nebulizers, and vibrating mesh nebulizers. Air jet nebulizers are powered by compressed air or oxygen to aerosolize liquid medications. The mechanism of aerosol dispersion from an air jet nebulizer is based on the Venturi's rule, according to which the pressure of a fluid decreases as it flows through a narrow sectional region. In an air jet nebulizer, the solution to be aerosolized is entrained into the gas stream and is sheared into a liquid film. This film is unstable and breaks into droplets due to surface tension forces. A baffle located in the aerosol stream impacts these droplets, producing smaller particles. Figure 7.3 shows an air jet nebulizer device, the Pari LC Plus nebulizer and its components. Air jet nebulizers can be classified into jet nebulizers with a reservoir tube (e.g., Sidestream Nebulizers™ (Philips, Murrysville, PA) and the Micro Mist® (Teleflex Medical, Research Triangle Park, NC)), jet nebulizers with a collection bag (Circulaire® II (Westmed, Tucson, AZ)), breath-enhanced jet nebulizers (Pari LC® Sprint (Pari, Midlothian, VA), NebuTech HDN® (Salter Labs, Arvin, CA), and SideStream Plus® (Philips, Murrysville, PA)), and breath-actuated jet

TABLE 7.2   List of Currently Marketed (FDA Approved) Nebulizer Products

PRODUCT NAME (MANUFACTURER)	DRUG NAME (S) (DOSE STRENGTH)	INACTIVE INGREDIENTS/ EXCIPIENTS	DOSAGE FORM	DISEASE APPLICATION
Intal® (Aventis Pharmaceuticals Inc., USA)	Cromolyn sodium (20 mg in 2 mL)	-	Solution	Asthma
Pulmicort Respules® (AstraZeneca Pharmaceuticals LP, USA)	Budesonide (0.25 mg and 0.5 mg in 2 mL)	Disodium edetate, sodium chloride, sodium citrate, citric acid, and polysorbate 80	Suspension	Asthma
Xopenex® (Sepracor Inc., USA)	Levalbuterol HCl (0.31 mg or 0.63 mg or 1.25 mg in 3 mL)	Sodium chloride and sulfuric acid	Solution	Bronchospasm
Ventolin solution (GlaxoSmithKline, USA)	Albuterol sulfate (5 mg/mL)	Benzalkonium chloride, sulfuric acid	Solution	Bronchospasm
AccuNeb® (Dey. L.P., USA)	Albuterol sulfate (0.75 mg or 1.50 mg in 3 mL)	Sodium chloride and sulfuric acid	Solution	Bronchospasm caused by asthma
DuoNeb® (Dey. L.P., USA)	Ipratropium bromide/albuterol sulfate (0.5 mg/3.0 mg in 3 mL)	Sodium chloride, hydrochloric acid, and edetate disodium	Solution	Bronchospasm associated with COPD
Brovana® (Sunovion Pharmaceuticals Inc., USA)	Arformoterol tartrate (22 µg in 2 mL)	Citric acid and sodium citrate	Solution	COPD, chronic bronchitis, and emphysema
Perforomist® (Dey. L.P., USA, 2001)	Formoterol fumarate dihydrate (20 µg in 2 mL)	Sodium chloride, citric acid, and sodium citrate	Solution	COPD, chronic bronchitis, and emphysema
Pulmozyme® (Genentech, Inc., USA, 1993)	Dornase alfa (2.5 mg/2.5 mL)	Calcium chloride dihydrate and sodium chloride	Solution	Cystic fibrosis
Tobi® (Novartis Pharmaceuticals Corporation, USA, 1975)	Tobramycin (300 mg in 5 mL)	Sodium chloride, sulfuric acid, and sodium hydroxide	Solution	Cystic fibrosis
Bethkis® (Cornerstone Therapeutics Inc., USA, 1980)	Tobramycin (300 mg in 4 mL)	Sodium chloride and sulfuric acid	Solution	Cystic fibrosis
Kitabis™ Pak (Pari Innovative Manufacturers, Inc., USA)	Tobramycin (300 mg in 5 mL)	Sodium chloride, sulfuric acid, and sodium hydroxide	Solution	Cystic fibrosis
Cayston® (Gilead Sciences, Inc., USA, 1986)	Lyophilized aztreonam (75 mg) (reconstituted with sterile diluent)	Lysine and sodium chloride	Solution	Cystic fibrosis

(Continued)

TABLE 7.2 (Continued)   List of Currently Marketed (FDA Approved) Nebulizer Products

PRODUCT NAME (MANUFACTURER)	DRUG NAME (S) (DOSE STRENGTH)	INACTIVE INGREDIENTS/ EXCIPIENTS	DOSAGE FORM	DISEASE APPLICATION
HyperSal® (Pari Innovative Manufacturers, Inc., USA)	–	Sodium chloride (3.5%, 6%, and 7%)	Solution	Osmotic, mucolytic in cystic fibrosis
Virazole® (Valeant Pharmaceuticals International Inc., USA)	Lyophilized ribavirin (6 g) (reconstituted with sterile water)	–	Solution	Lower respiratory tract infection
Arikayce® (Insmed Incorporated, USA)	Amikacin liposome inhalation suspension (590 mg/8.4 mL)	Cholesterol, DPPC, sodium chloride, sodium hydroxide, and water for injection	Suspension	MAC lung disease
Ventavis® (Actelion Pharmaceuticals US, Inc., USA)	Iloprost (10 μg/mL)	Ethanol, tromethamine, sodium chloride, and hydrochloric acid	Solution	PAH
Tyvaso® (United Therapeutics Corp., USA)	Treprostinil (1.74 mg/2.9 mL)	Sodium chloride, sodium citrate, sodium hydroxide, hydrochloric acid, and water for injection	Solution	PAH

Abbreviations: COPD, chronic obstructive pulmonary disease; DPPC, dipalmitoyl phosphatidylcholine; HCl, hydrochloric acid; MAC, mycobacterium avium complex; PAH, pulmonary arterial hypertension.

nebulizers (AeroEclipse® II BAN (Monaghan Medical Corporation, Plattsburgh, NY)). Ultrasonic nebulizers generate small liquid droplets by electronically induced vibration of a ceramic piezoelectric crystal and nebulize them as an inhalable aerosol. An ultrasonic nebulizer is compact and silent, and the dosing time is shorter than that of the jet nebulizers. However, they tend to generate heat and are not suitable for heat-sensitive drugs and biopharmaceuticals.

Recent adaptations of ultrasonic devices led to the development of a new class of nebulizers called vibrating mesh nebulizers or vibrating membrane nebulizers, which use micropump technology for

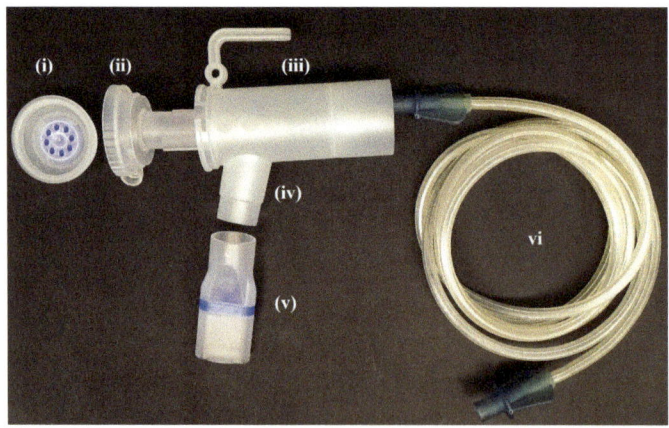

FIGURE 7.3   Pari LC Plus nebulizer and its components. (i) Inspiratory valve cup, (ii) nebulizer insert, (iii) nebulizer cup, (iv) nebulizer outlet, (v) mouthpiece, (vi) Wing-tip™ tubing.

aerosol production (134). The liquid in the reservoir is forced through micron-sized, multiple apertures in the vibrating mesh, which has been described as a "micropump action," to generate an aerosol (135). Vibrating mesh nebulizers are small, more efficient, battery or electricity powered, and portable. Further, they have silent operation and short treatment times compared with other types of nebulizers (130). Vibrating mesh nebulizers can be classified into active mesh nebulizers and passive mesh nebulizers. In active devices, the mesh is directly attached to the piezoelectric element, which contracts and expands on application of an electric current and vibrates a precisely drilled mesh in contact with the medication to generate an aerosol (136). Examples of active mesh nebulizers include the Aeroneb® (Aerogen, Galway, Ireland) and Pari eFlow® (Pari, Starnberg, Germany). In passive devices, a transducer horn induces passive vibrations in the mesh and generates the aerosol (135). Examples of passive mesh nebulizers include the Microair NE-U22® (Omron, Bannockburn, IL) and I-neb (Philips Respironics, Newark, USA).

7.6.2 Pressurized Metered Dose Inhalers (pMDIs)

Newer atomizing aerosol technologies, such as surface acoustic wave microfluidic atomization or capillary aerosol disperser devices, have been developed over the years to overcome the issues with standard nebulizers and to satisfy the criteria for an ideal inhalation device mentioned previously (137). On the other hand, the pMDI was a revolutionary invention that overcame the problems of the first nebulizer, making it the first portable inhalation device and currently the most frequently used for lung delivery. The mechanism of the pMDI is the emission of an aerosol containing the drug by the activation of a propellant, such as chlorofluorocarbons (CFC) and more recently, hydrofluoroalkanes (HFAs) through a nozzle at high velocity (> 30 m/s). After aerosolization, a particle diameter size of 0.5–10 μm is created, and the HFA propellant will evaporate, resulting in lung deposition with a mass median aerodynamic diameter (MMAD) from 1 to 2 μm (138).

The key components of a pMDI device(139, 140) include the formulation filled in a canister (container), the metering valve, and the actuator. The pMDI formulation is either a solution or a suspension-based formulation composed of drug, propellant, and excipients. The traditional CFC propellants have been banned in pMDI preparations due to their ozone depletion effect and replaced with environmentally friendly, HFA propellants. The use of HFA propellant in the pMDI creates an anhydrous and aseptic environment that is capable of slowing down the degradation of peptides and proteins via hydrolysis and microbial decomposition of the API while also securing chemical stability inside the device (141, 142). However, this non-aqueous environment has a major limitation at the time of use due to the low solubility of hydrophilic small molecules like peptides or proteins in the propellant, leading to sedimentation. Further, peptides can suffer from Ostwald ripening if the particle size is not homogeneous, leading to faster sedimentation (143). Among other drawbacks in the use of pMDIs is the inconsistency in the dose of drug emitted between the shaking and firing steps. Hatley, Parker (144) compared the effects of different shake–fire times with commercial pMDIs used for asthma and COPD to test the dose variability. They found that after device shaking, sedimentation and cream formation took place, affecting all devices tested but only having a minor effect on pMDIs containing excipients (145).

pMDI canisters are containers, commonly made of aluminum, stainless steel, glass, and plastic, that are capable of resisting a pressure of up to 150 psig. Surface treatment of the container's inner walls using chemically inert polymers (e.g., epoxy-phenolic polymer, polytetrafluoroethylene (PTFE), perfluorinated ethylene propylene copolymer (FEP), perfluoroalkoxyalkane polymer (PFA), and polyethersulfone (PES)) avoids drug loss by preventing drug adsorption to the inner walls of the container (146). The metering valve, another key component of a pMDI, is designed to deliver a consistent amount (25 to 100 μL/ actuation) of aerosolized formulation through the mouthpiece. Moreover, it functions as a seal over the container. The mouthpiece or actuator consists of a spray nozzle and an expansion chamber. Depressing the canister into the actuator releases the drug–propellant mixture, which then expands and vaporizes to convert the liquid medication into an aerosol. Figure 7.4 shows some of the commonly used pMDI devices and their components. Table 7.3 lists the currently available pMDI products, their formulation composition, and their therapeutic application.

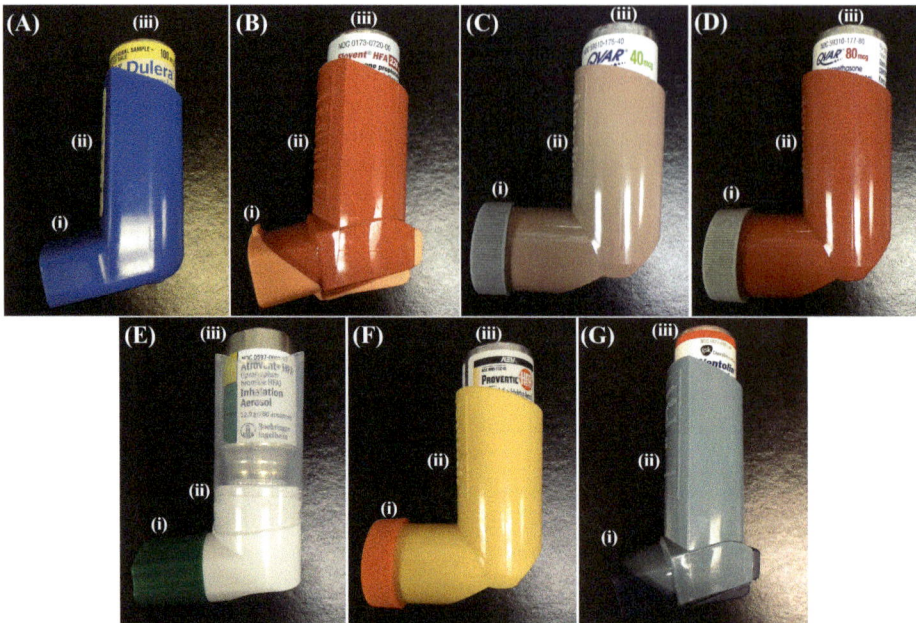

FIGURE 7.4   Examples of pressurized metered-dose inhalers (mDPIs). (A) Dulera® Inhalation Aerosol, (B) Flovent® HFA Inhalation Aerosol, (C) QVAR® 40 µg Inhalation Aerosol, (D) QVAR® 80 µg Inhalation Aerosol, (E) Atrovent® HFA Inhalation Aerosol, (F) Proventil® Inhalation Aerosol, and (G) Ventolin® HFA Inhalation Aerosol. Components of pMDI device: (i) cap, (ii) mouthpiece, and (iii) canister (container containing liquid formulation).

7.6.3 Soft Mist Inhalers (SMIs)

SMIs are a new generation of propellant–free, multi–dose liquid inhalers. They utilize mechanical energy in the form of a tensioned spring to generate a slow-moving aerosol mist through a fine nozzle called a uni-block. The soft mist contains a high proportion of fine liquid droplets with better aerosolization compared with the conventional pMDIs and DPIs. The combination of a high proportion of fine particles (65–80% of <5 µm) with low velocity (0.8 m/s) and long generation time (1.5 s) facilitates improved coordination of inhalation with actuation, high lung deposition (high fine particle fraction (FPF)), and lower oropharyngeal deposition compared with conventional pMDIs (2.0–8.4 m/s, 0.15–0.36 s) (147). The Combivent® Respimat®, Stiolto® Respimat®, Stiverdi® Respimat®, and Spiriva® Respimat® (Boehringer Ingelheim Pharmaceuticals, Inc., USA) are currently available FDA approved SMIs (Table 7.4) (148).

7.6.4 Dry Powder Inhalers (DPIs)

The DPI Market Report examines the increasing potential of formulations for DPIs (149). The design of new inhalers and enhanced particle properties are allowing the delivery of a large range of APIs to the lungs in a more efficient and safe way as DPIs (150). DPIs (151) consist of a powder formulation and a device. Most traditional DPI products on the market are a mixture of micronized drug particles (<5 µm) in combination with large (80–100 µm) carrier particles. However, it is important to note that not all DPI products currently on the market have this formulation approach; several do not use lactose carrier particles as an excipient and are "lactose–carrier free."

Some of the currently marketed DPI products have formulations that contain an additional excipient, magnesium stearate. For example, the commercial products Seebri™ Neohaler®, Incruse® Ellipta®, Anoro® Ellipta®, Utibron Neohaler®, Foster® NEXThaler®, and Breo™ Ellipta™ contain a small amount

TABLE 7.3   List of Currently Marketed (FDA-Approved) Pressurized Metered-Dose Inhaler (pMDI) Products

PRODUCT NAME (MANUFACTURER)	DRUG NAME (S) (DOSE STRENGTH)	INACTIVE INGREDIENTS/ EXCIPIENTS	DOSAGE FORM	DISEASE APPLICATION
Advair HFA® (GlaxoSmithKline, USA)	Fluticasone propionate/salmeterol (45 µg/21 µg, 115 µg/21 µg, or 230 µg/21 µg per actuation)	HFA134a	Suspension	Asthma
Aerospan® (Meda Pharmaceuticals Inc., USA)	Flunisolide (80 µg per actuation)	HFA-134a and ethanol	Solution	Asthma
Alvesco® (Sunovion Pharmaceuticals Inc., USA)	Ciclesonide (80 µg or 160 µg per actuation)	HFA-134a and ethanol	Solution	Asthma
Asmanex® HFA (Merck & Co., Inc., USA)	Mometasone furoate (100 µg or 200 µg per actuation)	HFA134a, ethanol, and oleic acid	Suspension	Asthma
Dulera® (Merck & Co., Inc., USA)	Mometasone furoate/formoterol fumarate dihydrate (100 µg/5 µg or 200 µg/5 µg per actuation)	HFA-227, anhydrous alcohol, and oleic acid	Suspension	Asthma
Flovent HFA® (GlaxoSmithKline, USA)	Fluticasone propionate (44 µg, 110 µg, or 220 µg per actuation)	HFA134a	Suspension	Asthma
Intal® Inhaler (Aventis Pharmaceuticals Inc., USA)	Cromolyn sodium (1 mg per actuation)	Sorbitan trioleate, dichlorotetrafluoroethane, and dichlorodifluoromethane	Solution	Asthma
QVAR® RedihaleR™ (Teva Pharmaceutical Industries Ltd., Israel)	Beclomethasone dipropionate (40 µg or 80 µg per actuation)	HFA-134a and ethanol	Solution	Asthma
Symbicort® (AstraZeneca Pharmaceuticals LP, USA)	Budesonide/formoterol fumarate dihydrate (80 µg/4.5 µg or 160 µg/4.5 µg per actuation)	HFA134a, povidone K25 USP, and polyethylene glycol (PEG) 1000 NF	Suspension	Asthma, COPD, chronic bronchitis, and emphysema
Atrovent HFA® (Boehringer Ingelheim Pharmaceuticals, Inc., USA)	Ipratropium bromide (21 µg per actuation)	HFA-134a, sterile water, dehydrated alcohol, and anhydrous citric acid	Solution	Bronchospasm associated with COPD, chronic bronchitis, and emphysema
ProAir® HFA (Teva Pharmaceutical Industries Ltd., Israel)	Albuterol sulfate (108 µg per actuation)	HFA-134a and ethanol	Suspension	Bronchospasm

(Continued)

TABLE 7.3 (Continued) List of Currently Marketed (FDA-Approved) Pressurized Metered-Dose Inhaler (pMDI) Products

PRODUCT NAME (MANUFACTURER)	DRUG NAME (S) (DOSE STRENGTH)	INACTIVE INGREDIENTS/ EXCIPIENTS	DOSAGE FORM	DISEASE APPLICATION
Proventil® HFA (Schering Corporation, USA)	Albuterol sulfate (120 µg per actuation)	HFA-134a, ethanol, and oleic acid	Suspension	Bronchospasm
Ventolin® HFA (GlaxoSmithKline, USA)	Albuterol sulfate (120 µg per actuation)	HFA-134a	Suspension	Bronchospasm
Xopenex HFA™ (Sepracor Inc., USA)	Levalbuterol tartrate (59 µg per actuation)	HFA-134a, dehydrated alcohol, and oleic acid	Suspension	Bronchospasm
Bevespi Aerosphere® (AstraZeneca Pharmaceuticals LP, USA)	Glycopyrrolate/formoterol fumarate (9 µg/4.8 µg per actuation)	HFA-134a and porous particles (composed of DSPC and calcium chloride)	Co-suspension	COPD
Breztri Aerosphere™ (AstraZeneca Pharmaceuticals LP, USA)	Budesonide/glycopyrrolate/formoterol fumarate (182 µg/10.4 µg/5.5 µg per actuation)	HFA-134a and porous particles (composed of DSPC and calcium chloride)	Co-suspension	COPD

Abbreviations: COPD, chronic obstructive pulmonary disease; DSPC, 1,2-distearoyl-sn-glycero-3-phosphocholine; HFA 134a, hydrofluoroalkane 134a, i.e., 1,1,1,2-tetrafluoroethane; HFA 227, hydrofluoroalkane 227, i.e., 1,1,1,2,3,3,3-heptafluoropropane; NF, national formulary; USP, United States Pharmacopeia.

TABLE 7.4   List of Currently Marketed (FDA-Approved) Soft Mist Inhaler (SMI) Products

PRODUCT NAME (MANUFACTURER)	DRUG NAME (S) (DOSE STRENGTH)	INACTIVE INGREDIENTS/ EXCIPIENTS	DOSAGE FORM	DISEASE APPLICATION
Combivent® Respimat® (Boehringer Ingelheim Pharmaceuticals, Inc., USA)	Ipratropium bromide monohydrate (20 µg/ actuation) and albuterol sulfate (120 µg/actuation)	Water for injection, benzalkonium chloride, edetate disodium, and hydrochloric acid	Solution	COPD
Spiriva® Respimat® (Boehringer Ingelheim Pharmaceuticals, Inc., USA)	Tiotropium bromide (1.25 or 2.5 µg/ actuation)	Water for injection, edetate disodium, benzalkonium chloride, and hydrochloric acid	Solution	Bronchospasm associated with COPD and asthma
Stiolto® Respimat® (Boehringer Ingelheim Pharmaceuticals, Inc., USA)	Tiotropium bromide/ olodaterol (2.5/2.5 µg/ actuation)	Water for injection, benzalkonium chloride, edetate disodium, and hydrochloric acid	Solution	COPD
Stiverdi® Respimat® (Boehringer Ingelheim Pharmaceuticals, Inc., USA)	Olodaterol hydrochloride (2.5 µg/ actuation)	Water for injection, benzalkonium chloride, edetate disodium, and anhydrous citric acid	Solution	COPD, chronic bronchitis, and emphysema

Abbreviation: COPD, chronic obstructive pulmonary disease.

of magnesium stearate along with lactose. The addition of magnesium stearate provides moisture resistance and improves the stability of the formulation (152).

DPI devices are generally classified into three categories based on the dose metering system: unit-dose, multi-unit-dose, and multidose, also called powder reservoir. Table 7.5 lists the currently available DPI products, their formulation compositions, and their therapeutic applications. A unit-dose DPI device is a capsule-based device consisting of a pre-metered formulation packaged in a hard capsule (e.g., Handihaler® and Podhaler™) or a prefilled cartridge (e.g., Dreamboat®). On device activation, the capsule is pierced, and the vibrating capsule dispenses the powder formulation. The mechanisms have been reviewed in detail (8, 26) The Aerolizer® (Novartis Pharmaceuticals Corporation, USA) (Figure 7.5A), HandiHaler® (Boehringer Ingelheim International GmbH, Germany) (Figure 7.5B), Neohaler® (Novartis Pharmaceuticals Corporation, USA), and Podhaler™ (Novartis Pharmaceuticals Corporation, USA), are examples of single-dose DPI products.

A multi-unit-dose DPI device consists of a blister foil strip with pre-metered doses of the powder formulation. On device actuation, the blister is punctured mechanically and releases the dose. The Diskus® (GlaxoSmithKline, USA) (Figure 7.5C), Ellipta® (GlaxoSmithKline, USA), Diskhaler (GlaxoSmithKline, USA), and Afrezza® (MannKind Corporation, USA) are examples of multi-unit-dose DPI devices.

A multidose (powder reservoir) DPI device consists of a powder reservoir from which a fixed amount of powder is metered into a dosing receptacle for each dose. The most common powder reservoir devices include the Turbuhaler® (AstraZeneca Pharmaceuticals LP, USA) (Figure 7.5D), Twisthaler® (Schering Corporation, USA), RespiClick® (Teva Pharmaceutical Industries Ltd., Israel), Flexhaler® (AstraZeneca AB, Sweden), Digihaler® (Teva Pharmaceutical Industries Ltd., Israel), Diskus® (GlaxoSmithKline, USA), and Pressair® (Forest Laboratories Inc., USA).

Two examples of FDA-approved inhalable dry powder biologics acting systemically are Afrezza® and Exubera®, both insulin therapies. Afrezza®, developed by MannKind (USA), is a rapid-acting inhaled insulin, which helps to control blood glucose in adults with diabetes. Afrezza® is composed of a dry

TABLE 7.5 Currently Marketed (FDA-Approved) Dry Powder Inhaler Products

PRODUCT NAME (MANUFACTURER)	DEVICE NAME (TYPE, AIRFLOW RESISTANCE (KPA$^{0.5}$ L/MIN))	DRUG NAME (S), DOSE STRENGTH	INACTIVE INGREDIENTS/ EXCIPIENTS	DISEASE APPLICATION
Asmanex® Twisthaler® (Schering Corporation, USA)	Twisthaler® (multidose, 0.04)	Mometasone furoate, 110 µg or 220 µg	Anhydrous lactose	Asthma
Flovent® Diskus® (GlaxoSmithKline, USA)	Diskus® (multi-unit dose, 0.027)	Fluticasone propionate, 50 µg, 100 µg, or 250 µg	Lactose monohydrate	Asthma
ArmonAir® RespiClick® (Teva Pharmaceutical Industries Ltd., Israel)	RespiClick® (multidose)	Fluticasone propionate, 55 µg, 113 µg, or 232 µg	Lactose monohydrate	Asthma
Pulmicort® Flexhaler® (AstraZeneca AB, Sweden)	Flexhaler® (multidose)	Budesonide 90 µg or 180 µg	Lactose monohydrate	Asthma
Pulmicort® Turbohaler® (AstraZeneca AB, Sweden)	Turbohaler® (multidose)	Budesonide 200 µg	None	Asthma
Arnuity® Ellipta® (GlaxoSmithKline, USA)	Ellipta® (multi-unit dose, 0.027)	Fluticasone furoate, 100 µg or 200 µg	Lactose monohydrate	Asthma
ProAir® RespiClick® (Teva Pharmaceutical Industries Ltd., Israel)	RespiClick® (multidose)	Albuterol sulfate, 117 µg	Lactose monohydrate	Bronchospasm
ProAir® Digihaler® (Teva Pharmaceutical Industries Ltd., Israel)	Digihaler® (multidose)	Albuterol sulfate, 117 µg	Lactose monohydrate	Bronchospasm
Serevent® Diskus® (GlaxoSmithKline, USA)	Diskus® (multidose, 0.027)	Salmeterol xinafoate, 72.5 µg	Lactose monohydrate	Asthma and bronchospasm associated with COPD, emphysema, and chronic bronchitis
Seebri™ Neohaler® (Novartis Pharmaceuticals Corporation, USA)	Neohaler™ (unit-dose, 0.02)	Glycopyrrolate, 15.6 µg	Lactose monohydrate, magnesium stearate	COPD

(Continued)

TABLE 7.5 (Continued)   Currently Marketed (FDA-Approved) Dry Powder Inhaler Products

PRODUCT NAME (MANUFACTURER)	DEVICE NAME (TYPE, AIRFLOW RESISTANCE (KPA$^{0.5}$ L/MIN))	DRUG NAME (S), DOSE STRENGTH	INACTIVE INGREDIENTS/ EXCIPIENTS	DISEASE APPLICATION
Spiriva® HandiHaler® (Boehringer Ingelheim International GmbH, Germany)	HandiHaler® (unit-dose, 0.058)	Tiotropium bromide, 22.5 µg	Lactose monohydrate	Bronchospasm associated with COPD
Arcapta™ Neohaler™ (Novartis Pharmaceuticals Corporation, USA)	Neohaler™ (unit-dose, 0.02)	Indacatero, 75 µg	Lactose monohydrate	COPD, chronic bronchitis, and emphysema
Tudorza® Pressair® (Forest Laboratories Inc., USA)	Pressair® (multidose, 0.031)	Aclidinium bromide, 400 µg	Lactose monohydrate	COPD
Incruse® Ellipta® (GlaxoSmithKline, USA)	Ellipta® (multi-unit dose, 0.027)	Umeclidinium bromide, 74.2 µg	Lactose monohydrate, magnesium stearate	COPD
Tobi® Podhaler™ (Novartis Pharmaceuticals Corporation, USA)	Podhaler™ (unit- dose, 0.025)	Tobramycin, 28 mg	DSPC, calcium chloride, sulfuric acid	Cystic fibrosis
Bronchitol® (Pharmaxis Ltd, Australia)	High resistance Osmohaler™ (unit-dose, 0.036)	Spray-dried mannitol, 40 mg	None	Cystic fibrosis
Aridol® (Pharmaxis Ltd, Australia)	Low resistance Osmohaler™ (unit-dose, 0.021)	Spray-dried mannitol, 40 mg and graduated doses of 0 mg, 5 mg, 10 mg, 20 mg, and 40 mg per kit	None	Assessment of bronchial hyperresponsiveness
Airduo® Digihaler® (Teva Pharmaceutical Industries Ltd., Israel)	Digihaler® (multidose)	Combination of fluticasone propionate/salmeterol xinafoate, 55 µg/14 µg, 113 µg/14 µg, or 232 µg/14 µg	Lactose monohydrate	Asthma
AirDuo™ RespiClick® (Teva Pharmaceutical Industries Ltd., Israel)	RespiClick® (multidose)	Combination of fluticasone propionate/salmeterol xinafoate, 55 µg/14 µg, 113 µg/14 µg, or 232 µg/14 µg	Lactose monohydrate	Asthma
Advair Diskus® (GlaxoSmithKline, USA)	Diskus® (multi-unit dose)	Combination of fluticasone propionate/salmeterol xinafoate, 100 µg/50 µg, 250 µg/50 µg, or 500 µg/50 µg	Lactose	Asthma and COPD

(Continued)

TABLE 7.5 (Continued)   Currently Marketed (FDA-Approved) Dry Powder Inhaler Products

PRODUCT NAME (MANUFACTURER)	DEVICE NAME (TYPE, AIRFLOW RESISTANCE (KPA$^{0.5}$ L/MIN))	DRUG NAME (S), DOSE STRENGTH	INACTIVE INGREDIENTS/ EXCIPIENTS	DISEASE APPLICATION
Generic Advair Diskus® (Hikma Pharmaceuticals, UK)	Vectura Open-Inhale-Close (OIC) device (multidose)	Combination of fluticasone propionate/ salmeterol xinafoate, 100 µg/50 µg or 250 µg/50 µg	Lactose monohydrate	Asthma and COPD
Breo® Ellipta® (GlaxoSmithKline, USA)	Ellipta® (multi-unit dose, 0.027)	Combination of fluticasone furoate/ vilanterol, 100 µg/25 µg or 200 µg/25 µg	Lactose monohydrate, magnesium stearate	Asthma and COPD
Anoro® Ellipta® (GlaxoSmithKline, USA)	Ellipta® (multi-unit dose, 0.027)	Combination of umeclidinium/vilanterol, 62.5 µg/25 µg	Lactose monohydrate, magnesium stearate	COPD
Trelegy® Ellipta® (GlaxoSmithKline, USA)	Ellipta® (multi-unit dose, 0.027)	Combination of fluticasone furoate/ umeclidinium/vilanterol, 100 µg/62.5 µg/25 µg	Lactose monohydrate, magnesium stearate	COPD
Utibron® Neohaler® (Novartis Pharmaceuticals Corporation, USA)	Neohaler™ (unit-dose, 0.02)	Combination of indacaterol/ glycopyrrolate, 27.5 µg/15.6 µg	Lactose monohydrate, magnesium stearate	COPD
Duaklir® Pressair® (AstraZeneca AB, Sweden)	Pressair® (multidose, 0.031)	Combination of aclidinium bromide/ formoterol fumarate, 400 µg/12 µg	Lactose monohydrate	COPD
Relenza® Rotadisk (GlaxoSmithKline, USA)	Diskhaler (multi-unit dose, 0.032)	Zanamivir, 5 mg	Lactose monohydrate	Influenza
Adasuve™ (Alexza Pharmaceuticals, USA)	Staccato® (single-use, 0.025)	Loxapine, 10 mg, single-unit pack	None	Schizophrenia or bipolar I disorder
Afrezza® (MannKind Corporation, USA)	Dreamboat™ (multi-unit dose, 0.093)	Recombinant human insulin, 0.35 mg, 0.7 mg, or 1 mg	FDKP, polysorbate 80	Diabetes mellitus types 1 and 2

Abbreviations: COPD, chronic obstructive pulmonary disease; DSPC, 1,2-distearoyl-sn-glycero-3-phosphocholine; FDKP, fumaryl diketopiperazine; SABA, short-acting β$_2$ agonist

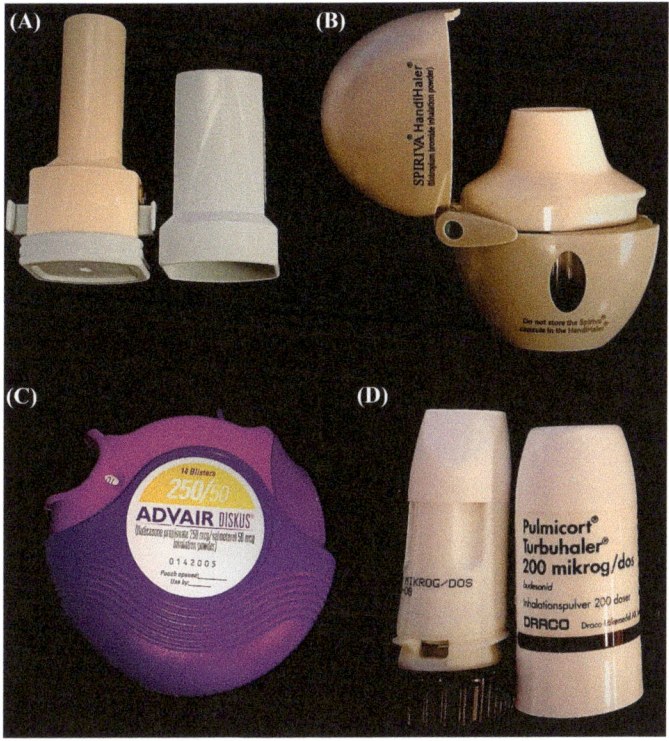

FIGURE 7.5   Examples of dry powder inhaler (DPI) devices. (A) Aerolizer® (low resistance, single-dose inhaler), (B) Handihaler® (high resistance, single-dose inhaler), (C) Diskus® (medium resistance, multi-unit-dose inhaler), and (D) Turbuhaler® (medium/high resistance, multidose inhaler).

powder formulation of recombinant human insulin, fumaryl diketopiperazine (FDKP), an inert excipient, and polysorbate 80. Exubera®, developed by Pfizer, was on the market for around 1 year. It was a rapid-acting insulin dry powder formulation for oral inhalation delivered through an active-blister device containing a 1- or 3-mg dose of insulin with mannitol as stabilizer agent, but due to poor patient acceptance, the company decided to remove it from the market.

7.7 TECHNIQUES TO PRODUCE INHALABLE DRY POWDER FORMULATIONS

Formulations including biologicals as APIs have shown an increase in stability when they are in solid-state rather than liquid formulations, making DPI's most preferred formulations to deliver small biological molecules by lung administration (153). Many biopharmaceuticals have been micronized to produce solid-state powders, mainly by lyophilization. These products, however, are primarily delivered parenterally by the subcutaneous or intramuscular route after being reconstituted; examples include PEG-Intron® and Glucagen® (154). Although freeze drying is a well-established process for preparing solid-state formulations, this technique is not able to control someparticle characteristics that are important for enhancing lung deposition, FPF, and respirable fraction (RF) of the powder. Since inhalable particles must have special characteristics to exert a desirable effect, it is challenging for scientists to make optimal particles without altering the original structure or effect of the API. The aerodynamic diameter, along with other features of the particles, plays a key role in the deposition of aerosols in the lungs; therefore, it is important

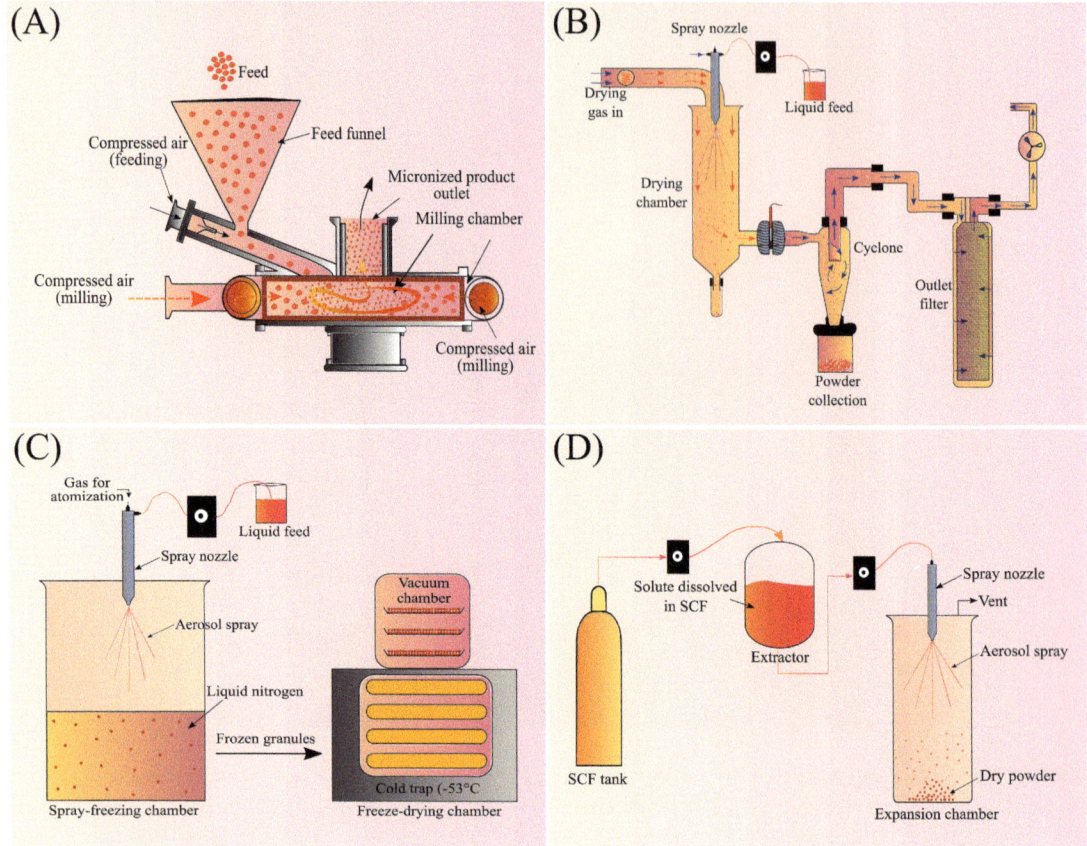

FIGURE 7.6   Particle engineering techniques to develop inhaled dry powder particles. (A) Air jet milling, (B) spray-freeze drying, (C) supercritical fluid technique, and (D) spray drying.

to engineer the particles using the right technique. In this section, some of the most common techniques (Figure 7.6.) used to develop inhaled particles are discussed and compared in Table 7.6. Several technologies are used in creating dry powder formulations (9, 151, 155). Air jet milling and spray drying are the manufacturing techniques used in currently marketed DPI products. Supercritical fluid technology, spray-freeze drying, and Particle Replication in Non-wetting Templates (PRINT) technologies are other unique technologies that are used in research but have not yet been utilized in commercially available marketed products.

7.7.1 Air Jet Milling

Milling is a traditional method of drug powder micronization. Air jet milling (Figure 7.6A) is the most common milling technique used for the preparation of inhalable dry powders. This process involves micronization by interparticle collision and attrition. Two opposing jets of air streams bring the particles into contact, develop fractures, and break them into smaller particles. The resulting particles are collected by a cyclone depending on the aerodynamic diameter (156). In general, milling produces amorphous particles with different charges, which tend to cause adhesion and cohesion.

Recently, Marudamuthu, Bhandary (157) produced an inhalable dry powder formulation of CSP7 (acetate counterion), a caveolin-1-fragment peptide, by micronization using air jet milling. The synthesized particles had an MMAD lower than 5 μm with an RF of 84.5%. Also, their findings showed that local

TABLE 7.6 Comparison of the Techniques Used to Generate Particles Used in Dry Powder Inhaler Formulations

TECHNIQUE	ADVANTAGES	DISADVANTAGES/LIMITATIONS/CHALLENGES	PARTICLE/POWDER CHARACTERISTICS
Air jet milling	• Relatively easy procedure • Fast • Cost-effective • Scalable • A particle size reduction process • Commercially used in most currently marketed DPI pharmaceutical products • Used for many years by the pharmaceutical industry • Can produce solid-state microparticles or nanoparticles (Nanojet milling)	• Can be messy • Not a particle engineering design process • Lack of control on particle size, shape, morphology, surface properties, and electrostatic charge • Produces irregularly shaped solid particles, which can lead to high interparticulate interactions and decreased aerosol dispersion • Produces highly charged and cohesive powders • High energy input may promote chemical degradation • Often introduces surface "hot spots" where unintended loss in crystallinity occurs • Limited to small–molecular weight drugs • Physical mixtures can phase separate and lose content uniformity with time	• Generally crystalline • Irregularly shaped particles • Surface "hot spots" • Cohesive powders • Poor powder flow properties that often require the use of large carrier particles physically mixed with the smaller jet-milled drug particles
Spray drying (SD)	• Relatively fast • High throughput • Scalable • A particle engineering design process • A powder manufacturing process • Good control of solid-state particle morphology, size, density, size distribution, surface roughness, and composition • Can be used for drug encapsulation and taste-masking • Suitable for solution, suspension, colloidal dispersions, and emulsions • Suitable for aqueous or non-aqueous systems • Used for many years by the pharmaceutical industry	• Not suitable for thermosensitive materials and materials sensitive to air or oxygen • Multiple parts involved in the setup	• Crystalline, partially crystalline, liquid crystalline, or amorphous solid particles • Fine powder • Improved aerosolization

(Continued)

TABLE 7.6 (Continued)   Comparison of the Techniques Used to Generate Particles Used in Dry Powder Inhaler Formulations

TECHNIQUE	ADVANTAGES	DISADVANTAGES/LIMITATIONS/CHALLENGES	PARTICLE/POWDER CHARACTERISTICS
Spray-freeze drying (SFD)	• Fast freezing • Particle engineering design	• Two-step process (freezing, lyophilization), time-consuming • High cost and requires liquid nitrogen • Fragile particles • Complex and energy-intensive process	• Can be amorphous, partially crystalline, or crystalline • Spherical shape • Tend to be large and porous particles having low density and smooth surface • High surface area
Supercritical fluid (SCF)	• Fast process, scalable, and aseptic drying • Good control over particle size and shape • Monodisperse particle size possible (i.e., no particle size distribution in the powder)	• Limited to drugs soluble in supercritical fluids • Specialized setup • Very expensive • Very specialized • Not used often by the pharmaceutical industry	• Usually amorphous • Spherical and smooth surface • Monodisperse powder with one particle size
Particle Replication In Non-wetting Templates (PRINT)	• Excellent control over particle size, shape, and composition • Monodisperse particle size possible • Preserves chemical structure and bioactivity of biopharmaceuticals • Suitable for fabrication of therapeutic small molecules, proteins, and nucleic acids	• Multi-step process • Very specialized • Not easily scalable to medium or large scale • Premanufactured template with precise surface properties and precise size properties needed before particles can be created • Not used often by the pharmaceutical industry	• Monodisperse powder with one particle size • Smooth particles

delivery of peptide dry powder was as efficacious as an intraperitoneal injection in reducing bleomycin-induced pulmonary fibrosis at a dose about 30 times lower than that used for intraperitoneal injection. In another more recent study using the same peptide fragment of caveolin-1, Zhang, Qian (158) micronized free excipient by jet milling to a respirable particle size of 1.58 μm, 93.3% of FPF. They found a significant reduction in the collagen of lung fibrosis induced-mice model after peptide inhalation.

7.7.2 Spray Drying (SD)

Spray drying is a well-established particle engineering technique used for the solid particle formation and drying process (159). Spray drying has primarily been used in formulating small-molecule drugs with low solubility; however, it is increasingly being applied to produce dry powders of large biomolecules and biopharmaceuticals (160–163). The spray drying (Figure 7.6B) process involves the transformation of a liquid feed (a solution, suspension, or emulsion) containing the API, with or without excipients, into a solid dry powder in a single step by passing an atomized spray of fine droplets through a high-temperature gaseous medium. Spray drying produces a fine powder with better aerosolization compared with a dry cake produced by a freeze drying technique. It is for this reason that spray drying is a ubiquitous technique to produce powders of micro/nano size in many fields, including pharmaceuticals, food, and cosmetics. Spray drying of pharmaceuticals has become a popular dry powder formulation approach because it allows rational design of particle properties. Manipulation of particle size, surface morphology, density, and internal structure of the dry powder particles can be achieved by controlling and tailoring feed stock and spray drying parameters such as the feed solution concentration, liquid feed rate, inlet air temperature, surface tension, flow of atomizing, and particle residence time (153, 164). Most of the spray-dried powders are in an amorphous state, which makes the product less stable (165). Further, spray drying of macromolecules presents challenges such as thermal stress during the drying process, and high shear stress in the nozzle might result in degradation (166).

7.7.3 Spray Freeze Drying (SFD)

Spray freeze drying is a relatively new technique, which combines spraying and freeze drying (Figure 7.6C). The solution is fed through a spraying nozzle of different diameters into a cryogenic liquid such as nitrogen for fast freezing and instantaneous particle formation. There are three main steps for producing dry powder particles using SFD: the first is the feed solution breaking down into droplets, the second is direct contact with cryogenic liquid producing frozen droplets due to the liquid's low boiling point, and the third is lyophilization to obtain a solid-state particle powder (164, 167, 168). However, this technique is not often used due to its high cost, difficulty, long processing time, and possible safety concerns. Ye et al. (2017) (169) prepared clarithromycin liposomal powder formulations by an ultrasonic SFD method using mannitol (15% w/v) and sucrose (5% w/v) as cryoprotectants. The produced powders had micron-size spherical particles with a rough porous surface texture and an FPF of 53.78%. Lavanya, Preethi (170) used the SFD technique to produce bromelain dry powder particles with MMAD from 2.97 to 3.33 μm. They concluded that this technique is well suited for producing protein powder with desirable particles for delivery through the pulmonary route.

7.7.4 Supercritical Fluid (SCF)

The use of fluids, either gas or liquids, at temperatures and pressures above their critical points is one of the recently leading alternatives for producing dry powders (171, 172). The superfluid exists as a single phase with several advantages; it has lower viscosity than the solutes, which facilitates mass transfer, it is highly compressible, and it has higher density (173). For pharmaceutical applications, the most commonly used supercritical fluid is CO_2 because it is non-expensive, non-toxic, and non-flammable. The technique a role position in the particle engineering of high-value, high-potency, and sensitive drugs. There are several variants of this technology, differing in their principles, and only a few are used for particle engineering in pulmonary drug delivery (153, 164). The solution is first rapidly depressurized by expanding it through a nozzle (Figure 7.6D). This leads to lower solubility of the solute in the SCF due to change in density. Next, precipitation occurs due to a high degree of supersaturation, which produces a high nucleation rate, limiting crystal growth and thus synthesizing small and homogeneous particles (174). Control of parameters in the process, such as temperature and pressure, can induce changes in particle size and crystal formation (175).

The yield and efficiency of producing dry powders with supercritical fluid are based on correct pressure, temperature, and the correct solvent selection during formulation. One of the main drawbacks of using this technology is the poor solubility of polar solutes in SCF using CO_2, limiting the application to small hydrophilic molecules. SCFs are remarkably good solvents for lipophilic compounds such as cholesterol or tocopherol but poor solvents for hydrophilic proteins (176). With recent advances in this technology, there has been an increase in protein dry powder formulation using CO_2 as SCF, assisted by atomization for the enhanced mixing of CO_2 with a liquid solution containing the protein, with a carrier usually being needed as well (177). Hong, Yun (178) fabricated a dry powder of parathyroid hormone (PTH1–34)–loaded chitosan oligosaccharide composite microparticles using SCF-assisted atomization with a narrow size range from 1 to 5 μm and an FPF of 63.51%, maintaining the structure and stability of the protein after the process.

7.7.5 Particle Replication in Non-wetting Templates (PRINT)

PRINT is a top-down particle fabrication technique developed by Liquidia Technologies Inc. In this technique, a mixture of API and excipient(s) is pressed into micro molds. PRINT technology is one way to achieve nanomedicine pulmonary drug delivery (155). The dry powder particles produced using PRINT technology show exactly defined and reproducible particle size, shape, and surface functionality. Rahhal, Fromen (179) developed an inhalable dry powder formulation of butyrylcholinesterase, a model enzyme, using PRINT technology. The produced particles are cylindrical in shape with an MMAD of 2.77 μm. In more recent work, Sato, Tabata (180) developed inhalable calcitonin-loaded poly (lactic-*co*-glycolic acid) (PLGA) –based microparticles using PRINT technology. The produced particles were well separated and spherical in shape with a median diameter of 3.6 μm. The particles showed a SPAN value of 0.6, indicating the uniform size distribution of the particles.

7.8 CHARACTERIZATION AND ANALYTICAL TECHNIQUES

Comprehensive physicochemical characterization is essential for pulmonary drug delivery systems and in particular, for dry powder inhalers (181–183). A successful inhalation aerosol therapy depends on a combination of factors, including physicochemical properties of the formulation (powder or liquid); properties of particles; formulation; respiratory flow rate; design of delivery devices; drug–carrier adhesion; and the physical mechanisms used to aerosolize, deaggregate, disperse, and deposit the drug powders in the deep lungs (184–186). The effective dispersion of the particles from the formulation to form aerosols depends on fundamental properties of particles, including surface properties (morphology, surface area), density, particle size and size distribution, hygroscopicity, electrostatic charge, and adhesion/cohesion forces (184, 187). Thus, the analysis of these properties is crucial, as they affect the final product's stability, functional characteristics, storage, release, and bioavailability. This section presents a general overview of typical characterizations of aerosols and the standard analytical methods (there are others) that are usually applied.

In powder formulations, the morphology, surface area, and interactions of particles are essential properties that should be measured. The surface morphology affects the cohesive/adhesive properties and hence, the aggregation and de-aggregation processes (188). The presence of surface asperities affects the contact area and interaction forces between particles (184). Capillary forces, mechanical interlocking, electrostatics, and van der Waals forces are the key interaction forces. Capillary forces result from water or moisture and inadequate drying processes, leading to solid bridging at the particle surfaces via crystallization/recrystallization phenomena (186). Mechanical interlocking is the main mechanism preventing particle dispersion due to surface roughness, affecting the contact area and interaction forces between particles. For example, particles with corrugated surfaces improve dispersibility by reducing the attractive forces between individual particles (184). Porous particles have recently attracted attention for pulmonary deposition, as they show improved dispersibility due to the low particle density (187). In general, the interparticulate forces can be modulated by optimizing the morphology to improve deposition in the lungs. The contact area and forces should be adjusted to an extent that provides enough stability and adhesion between drug and carrier but at the same time, allows separation upon inhalation (188). The surface area of particles in a powder is measured using the inverse gas chromatography (IGC) technique, which measures the volume of gas adsorbed to the powder surface at a given pressure (184, 188). The atomic force microscopy (AFM)technique allows spray-dried particles to be visualized in three dimensions (188–190). Other microscopic techniques, such as confocal laser scanning microscopy (CLSM), scanning electron microscopy (SEM) (190–192), field emission SEM (FESEM), and transmission electron microscopy (TEM) (190), are used to analyze the morphology of the particles in a powder.

Particle size and distribution are fundamental properties, as they directly affect particle deposition in the lungs (188). The techniques used to measure the particle size and distribution are classified as inertial methods, light-scattering methods, and imaging methods (188). Light-scattering and imaging methods help to characterize raw materials (drug particles or excipient particles alone) (188). In comparison, cascade impaction is mainly used to assess the performance parameters of the formulation, such as FPF, rather than the raw materials (188). The most commonly used aerodynamic particle size measuring devices in pharmaceutical aerosols are impactors (Figure 7.7): such as the liquid impingers, including the multi-stage liquid impinger (MSLI) (193), the electrical low-pressure impactor (194), the Andersen cascade impactor (ACI), and the next generation impactor (NGI) (193, 195). After each run, the impactor is disassembled, and the mass of particles deposited on each stage is measured. In the laser diffractometer technique (188,

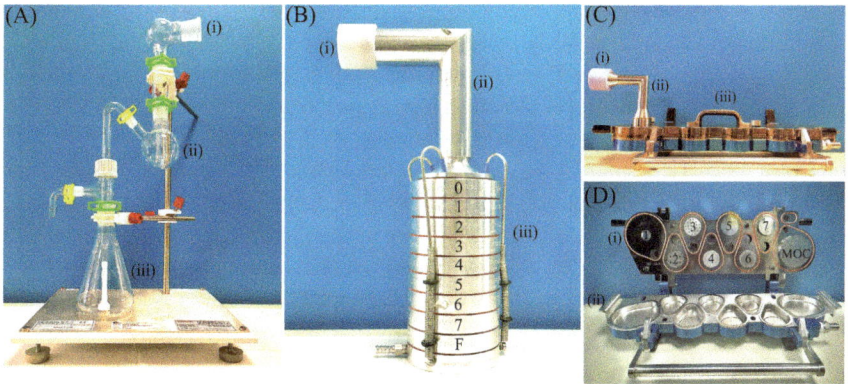

FIGURE 7.7 Various aerosol inertial impactors and their components. (A) Twin stage impinger (TSI): (i) throat, (ii) upper impingement chamber, (iii) lower impingement chamber; (B) Andersen cascade impactor (ACI): (i) mouthpiece adaptor, (ii) induction port, (iii) impactor with stages 0–7 and stage F; (C) next generation impactor (NGI) (closed view): (i) mouthpiece adaptor, (ii) induction port, (iii) impactor; (D) NGI (open view): (i) lid with stages 1 to 7 and micro-orifice collector (MOC), and inter-stage passageways, (ii) cup tray with impaction cups.

196), a laser beam is passed through the sample, which diffracts at different angles according to the particle size. A computer algorithm interprets the diffraction pattern and calculates the size distribution (188). Imaging analysis in pharmaceutical development is usually performed using different types of microscopy by taking and analyzing digital images of particle samples to assess the dimension and particle size data (188, 197–199). Examples of microscopic techniques are light microscopy and electron microscopy, which includes TEM, SEM, and AFM techniques (200).

In powder formulations, the powder's ability to move from one place to another is called the flow property, which is essential to evaluate. It depends on numerous factors that include particle size distribution, particle shape, chemical composition, moisture, and temperature (201). Parameters measured to evaluate flow properties are bulk density (202), tapped density, Carr's compressibility index, Hausner ratio, and the angle of repose (203). Density is a term used to describe the mass/volume ratio; it is an essential property of dry powder formulation that influences aerosolization and deposition. Hausner ratio (HR), and the compressibility index (CI) are measures of the propensity of a powder to consolidate (204).

Low moisture content is a critical quality attribute of a dry powder formulation. The moisture uptake and loss due to relative humidity changes lead to local dissolution and recrystallization (188). Moreover, the FPF of a powder decreases with increasing relative humidity of the dispersing air (187); thus, aggregation through solid bridge formation adversely affects aerosol generation and lung deposition (115). The moisture content is commonly determined by Karl Fischer titration (KFT) or thermogravimetric analysis (TGA) (205–209). Additionally, dynamic vapor sorption (DVS) measures the quantity and the rate of water vapor absorption by a material as a function of relative humidity and temperature.

Another property to determine is the status of the material in terms of crystallinity and polymorphism. Crystalline materials are more ordered and have lower free energies than non-crystalline materials (amorphous), which lack long-range order; upon processing, such as rapid cooling of fluid, it is possible to generate an amorphous solid (188). Due to the differences in the energy states and the range of molecular arrangement, the physicochemical properties also differ, influencing behaviors such as charging and particle interaction. Materials with higher crystallinity and polymorphic purity have low surface energy and electrostatic charge, which results in reduced agglomeration and particle interactions and hence, better aerosolization. The analytical methods to characterize polymorphs include X-ray powder diffraction (XRPD), thermal analysis, and microscopy. XRPD is used to identify crystalline material and provide information on unit cell dimensions (210). Amorphous regions of the samples produce a broad peak, whereas crystalline regions have sharp peaks.

Thermal analysis includes different techniques such as TGA, differential scanning calorimetry (DSC), isothermal microcalorimetry (IMC), and hot-stage microscopy (HSM). TGA is used to measure the amount and rate of change in a material's weight as a function of temperature in a controlled atmosphere (211). DSC monitors heat effects associated with phase transitions and chemical reactions as a function of temperature. It detects phase transitions such as melting point (T_m), heat capacity (C_p), recrystallization time of nanocarriers, and glass transition temperature (T_g) (190, 212). IMC is widely used to determine the amorphicity of a dry powder sample using a thermal activity monitor (TAM) (213–215). IMC is capable of detecting as little as 1% of amorphous content in a sample powder. The measurement is based on the same principle as DSC; i.e., the heat effects associated with the recrystallization are proportional to the amorphicity of the sample (216). HSM combines the best microscopy and thermal analysis properties to enable the characterization of materials' physical properties as a function of temperature. Some of these characteristics include melting point, melting range, morphology studies, amorphous/crystalline form characterization, and polymorphism (217–219).

Moreover, it is crucial to evaluate the chemical nature, interactions, molecular mobility, and drug structures of formulated aerosols. Chemical imaging (220), also called Raman mapping, combines confocal microscopy with Raman spectroscopy simultaneously *in situ*, as described in detail for the chemical imaging and molecular fingerprinting of dry powder inhalation formulations (42–44, 221–223). Chemical imaging enables assessment of the distribution of components within a formulation to determine the homogeneity and solid state of drug substances and excipients, and to characterize contaminations and impurities (200). Vibrational spectroscopy, i.e., Fourier-transformed-infrared spectroscopy (FTIR) (224, 225), and Raman spectroscopy (225) are two complementary analytical techniques that provide "molecular fingerprints" for dry powder inhalation formulations. Raman spectroscopy has been described in detail (226). FTIR provides spectral data regarding any change in a compound molecule's functional group characteristics during formulation processing and after the pharmaceutical process (227, 228). FTIR measurements depend on changes in the dipole moment (asymmetric moieties producing IR spectral bands), while Raman looks at changes in a molecular bond's polarizability (229). Raman spectroscopy is the most beneficial tool to characterize polymorphic forms (200) and powder homogeneity (230). There is a potential change of macromolecules' conformations during the pharmaceutical process due to formulations using excipients and process conditions such as high temperature. In the case of macromolecule-based drugs, it is crucial to check any change in the conformation and the secondary structure after formulation, as this change may affect the bioactivity. FTIR, circular dichroism (CD), and nuclear magnetic resonance (NMR) are mainly applied for this purpose. NMR spectroscopy is a powerful tool in structural characterization; it can determine how all the atoms of a particular molecule are interconnected. It also reflects the chemical nature and molecular mobility of individual components (190, 231). CD spectroscopy is a technique for studying protein structure through numerous algorithms to estimate the secondary structure composition from the CD spectra (232).

In vitro dissolution testing is a standardized quality control tool used to evaluate batch-to-batch consistency, to differentiate immediate and controlled release formulations, and to approximate *in vivo* release profiles. However, there is no accepted standardized method for inhaled particles, although many dissolution methods for testing aerosols have been developed. Various *in vitro* dissolution methods using the paddle over disk apparatus, flow-through cell apparatus, dialysis bag, Franz diffusion cell, Transwell®, Floata-lyzer®, and Dissolv*It* system have been developed and applied to evaluate the drug release characteristics of the inhaled dry powder, even though they are limited in mimicking the *in vivo* conditions (233).

7.9 INNOVATIONS IN MITOCHONDRIAL TARGETED THERAPEUTICS IN LUNG DISEASES

Mitochondria are essential for energy production in eukaryotic cells. However, more recently, it has become clear that the disruption of mitochondrial function also plays an important role in the development of multiple human diseases and/or can contribute to disease progression. Indeed, mitochondrial dysfunction plays a key role in the development of a number of pulmonary vascular diseases, including PH (234), pulmonary endothelial dysfunction (235), ALI (236), asthma (237), COPD (238), and pulmonary fibrosis (239). Thus, delivering therapeutic molecules to the mitochondria for the treatment of these diseases could have significant clinical benefit. However, a significant limitation related to mitochondrial drug targeting is the rigorous control of molecular transport into and out of the mitochondrion itself. For example, the outer mitochondrial membrane (OMM) only allows molecules with a very small molecular weight to pass through. Macromolecules, such as proteins, can only pass into the mitochondrion via a specialized protein import machinery that comprises a number of transport proteins imbedded in the outer and inner mitochondrial membranes. Each of these TOMs (translocase of the outer membranes) and TIMs (translocase of the inner membrane) is responsible for the transport of specific ligands (240–243). A further complexity is introduced through the need to specifically target the protein to the mitochondrion. This occurs through the presence of mitochondrial targeting sequences (MTS) within each protein (244, 245). Thus, the development of systems capable of delivering cargo specifically to the mitochondria is technically challenging. Three major issues need to be overcome to produce an optimized mitochondrial targeted therapy: 1) the therapeutic agent may need to be encapsulated in an appropriate nanocarrier; 2) the drug needs to be internalized by the correct cell(s) and within the diseased organ/tissue; and 3) precise intracellular trafficking needs to occur to ensure that the drug is targeted specifically to the mitochondria. Using these criteria, a number of systems capable of specifically targeting the mitochondria have been reported (235, 241, 242), but these are still being refined.

Mitochondrial-based therapies can be broadly considered within three categories, as proposed by Agrawal and Mabalirajan (246). These are 1) enhancing mitochondrial ROS scavenging; 2) modulation of cellular signaling pathways to modify mitochondrial metabolism; and 3) mitotherapy using exogenous healthy mitochondria to replace damaged mitochondria (246). The current status of these platforms will be briefly discussed in the following subsections.

7.9.1 Enhanced Mitochondrial ROS Scavenging

MitoQ is the prototypical mitochondria-targeted form of CoQ10, which is an important component of the electron transport chain (ETC) first reported by Murphy and Smith (247). When conjugated to a lipophilic triphenylphosphonium cation group, MitoQ is efficiently targeted to the mitochondria. MitoQ has been utilized as a therapy in a number of lung diseases, showing good efficacy in animal models. For example, MitoQ attenuates the inflammation, mucus hypersecretion, and oxidative stress induced by cigarette smoke in mice (248) and the sepsis-induced ALI in the cecal ligation and puncture (CLP) model (249). MitoQ has also been shown to decrease the migration and proliferation of microvascular endothelial cells isolated from the lungs of rats with PAH induced by Sugen and chronic hypoxia (250, 251). It has also been suggested that MitoQ could be a potential treatment for COVID-19 infections by alleviating the cytokine storm and restoring T cell function (252). Another potential antioxidant therapy that has shown great promise is the Szeto and Schiller (SS) peptides, which are targeted to the inner mitochondrial membrane (IMM). SS peptides are tetrapeptides that contain an alternating aromatic–cationic motif and are capable of scavenging a number of ROS species. Despite being water soluble, SS peptides are highly cell permeable and have been shown to be taken up by a number of different cell types, including endothelial cells (253–258). SS peptides appear to become concentrated on the IMM rather than in the mitochondrial matrix (259, 260). Recently, a second generation of the SS peptide was produced, based on SS-31 (D-Arg-2′6′-dimethylTyr-Lys-Phe-NH$_2$) (260), in which the strong antioxidant Tiron was introduced (261). This peptide, T-SSP, was shown to be efficiently taken up by human lung microvascular cells and to be capable of inhibiting inflammasome activation during lipopolysaccharide (LPS) exposure (261). T-SSP was also shown to prevent sepsis-mediated ALI (261).

7.9.2 Modification of Mitochondrial Metabolism

A number of agents have been employed to reprogram mitochondrial function. This is especially critical in PAH, where impaired mitochondrial function in pulmonary arterial smooth muscle cells (PASMC) (262–264) and pulmonary arterial endothelial cells (PAEC) (265–268) creates a Warburg effect that results in a survival advantage (264, 268). In PAEC, the loss of mitochondrial function has been linked to the disruption of β-oxidation secondary to attenuation of the carnitine shuttle (269). To this end, L-carnitine therapy has been investigated in both early forms of pulmonary vascular disease associated with increased pulmonary blood flow (PBF) and pressure in neonatal lambs (270) and in advanced PAH induced by monocrotaline exposure in adult rats (271). In both cases, L-carnitine therapy restored mitochondrial function. In the case of the neonatal sheep, it restored nitric oxide (NO) signaling and endothelial function (270), and in the rat, it prevented the development of PAH (271). More importantly, in the rat studies, this was achieved using an inhalational delivery system to specifically target the lung (271). β-oxidation is also regulated through peroxisome proliferator activated receptor (PPAR)-γ signaling (272), and the thiazolidinedione (TZD) rosiglitazone has been shown to preserve β-oxidation and mitochondrial function as well as NO signaling and pulmonary endothelial function (272, 273). However, there is significant controversy regarding the use of TZDs, as some clinical trials have suggested deleterious effects on heart function that may be class related. It is possible that utilizing inhalational delivery could limit the potential for off-target effects. Archer and Michelakis have utilized the pyruvate dehydrogenase kinase (PDK) inhibitor dichloroacetate to target the mitochondria and prevent the Warburg switch and PAH in rodent models (274–277). Michelakis has also shown that dichloroacetate therapy reduces the progression of PAH in humans (278). Stimulators of mitochondrial biogenesis have also been investigated through the use of resveratrol or L-arginine supplementation. These have been shown to attenuate asthma in animal models (279, 280), and L-arginine preserves endothelial function in lambs with increased PBF and pressure (267, 281). The diabetic drug metformin also has positive effects on allergic asthma (282). An inhalable derivative of metformin has also been developed (283), which could allow more targeted lung delivery, but its efficacy in treating asthma has yet to be evaluated.

Molecular strategies for treating mitochondrial dysfunction are also being evaluated. Of specific interest are the microRNAs (miRs). These are a class of small, endogenous RNAs that are 21–25 nucleotides in length. miRs play an important regulatory role in cells by targeting specific mRNAs for degradation or translation repression (284). Thus, miRs can exert large-scale effects on cellular function. A number of miRs have been shown to affect mitochondrial function: these include miR-106a, which inhibits IL-10 levels and is involved in asthma progression (285), and miR181a/b, which influence mitochondrial biogenesis and quality control, respiratory chain assembly, and mitochondrial antioxidant levels (286). The Let-7 (lethal-7) miR has also been implicated in asthma pathogenesis (287–289). In addition, miR-149 and miR-761 can modulate mitochondrial function by increasing mitochondrial biogenesis (290, 291), while miR-761 (292) and miR-30 (293) modulate mitochondrial network dynamics, which can result in changes in mitochondrial bioenergetics (294). miR-183 has been shown to inhibit bioenergetics by targeting IDH2 (295), while miR-130/301 downregulates PPARγ expression (296), which can indirectly regulate mitochondrial function through disruption of β-oxidation (297). Nevertheless, increasing our knowledge regarding the complex interplay between different miRNAs and their associated genes will be essential to unlocking the therapeutic potential to modify various mitochondrial pathways, including bioenergetics, biogenesis, oxidative stress, mitophagy, and even cell death (298).

7.9.3 Mitotherapy

It is now possible to utilize mitochondrial transfer to replace dysfunctional mitochondria. There are several methods that have been developed to accomplish this (299, 300). Although this technology is still in an early phase of development, there have been some significant achievements. For example, mesenchymal stem cells (MSCs) have been shown to transfer mitochondria to attenuate ARDS phenotypes in a mouse ALI model (301). Pluripotent stem cell–derived MSCs have also been shown to attenuate lung damage in cigarette smoking–induced COPD through mitochondrial transfer (302). Mesenchymal stromal cells–derived extracellular vesicles (MSC EVs) are being investigated as a cell-free therapy for ARDS, and it has been shown that the presence of mitochondria is critical for EV ability to reduce lung injury and restore mitochondrial respiration in precision-cut lung slices exposed to ARDS patient plasma or LPS (301). In addition, MSCs have been shown to promote an anti-inflammatory and highly phagocytic macrophage phenotype through EV-mediated mitochondrial transfer (303). These changes in macrophage phenotype require enhanced macrophage oxidative phosphorylation (303). Further, murine AMs treated with MSC-derived EVs have been shown to ameliorate lung injury *in vivo* (303). Bone marrow–derived stromal cells (BMSCs) also protect against ALI by restoring alveolar bioenergetics via mitochondrial transfer (304). However, a number of issues still remain to be resolved before mitochondrial transfer is in clinical use. These include successful retention of enough MSC-injured sites, determining the optimal dose of MSC used, and developing protocols to measure mitochondrial donor efficiency (246). The evaluation of safety and therapeutic efficacy of MSC in treating lung disease is ongoing.

7.10 CONCLUSIONS

Pulmonary delivery of drugs has been an important route of drug administration for the treatment of respiratory disorders for hundreds of years. Over the past two decades, pulmonary drug delivery has expanded into the treatment of systemic diseases. Understanding the anatomy and physiology of respiratory system and factors affecting the therapeutic effectiveness of drugs delivered by the pulmonary route provides a platform for a better understanding of new drug targets, aerosol deposition and therapeutic effect of inhaled pharmaceuticals.

REFERENCES

1. Rau, J. L. "The Inhalation of Drugs: Advantages and Problems." *Respiratory Care* 50, no. 3 (2005): 367–82.
2. Stein, S. W., and C. G. Thiel. "The History of Therapeutic Aerosols: A Chronological Review." *Journal of Aerosol Medicine & Pulmonary Drug Delivery* 30, no. 1 (2017): 20–41.
3. Gandevia, B. "Historical Review of the Use of Parasympatholytic Agents in the Treatment of Respiratory Disorders." *Postgraduate Medical Journal* 51, no. 7(Suppl.) (1975): 13–20.
4. Chapter, Murphy A. 7. "Drug Delivery to the Lungs." In *Asthma in Focus*, edited by A. Murphy, 113–32. London: Pharmaceutical Press/Royal Pharmaceutical Society of Great Britain Publishing, 2007.
5. Eedara, B. B., I. G. Tucker, and S. C. Das. "In Vitro Dissolution Testing of Respirable Size Anti-Tubercular Drug Particles Using a Small Volume Dissolution Apparatus." *International Journal of Pharmacy* 559 (2019): 235–44.
6. Eedara, B. B., W. Alabsi, D. Encinas-Basurto, R. Polt, J. G. Ledford, and H. M. Mansour. "Inhalation Delivery for the Treatment and Prevention of COVID-19 Infection." *Pharmaceutics* 13, no. 7 (2021): 1077.
7. Yıldız-Peköz, A., and C. Ehrhardt. "Advances in Pulmonary Drug Delivery." *Pharmaceutics* 12, no. 10 (2020): 911.
8. Mansour, H. M., P. B. Myrdal, U. Younis, P. Muralidharan, A. M. Hillery, and D. J. Hayes. "Book Chapter 11: Pulmonary Drug Delivery." In *Drug Delivery: Fundamentals & Applications*, edited by A. M. Hillery, J. Swarbrick, and K. Park, 249–77. London: CRC Press Press/Taylor & Francis, Inc., 2016.
9. Hickey, A. J., and H. M. Mansour. Chapter 5. "Delivery of Drugs by the Pulmonary Route." In *Modern Pharmaceutics. Drugs and the Pharmaceutical Sciences*. 5th ed, edited by A. T. Florence, and J. Siepmann Series 2, 191–219. New York: Taylor and Francis, Inc, 2009.
10. Labiris, N. R., and M. B. Dolovich. "Pulmonary Drug Delivery. Part I: Physiological Factors Affecting Therapeutic Effectiveness of Aerosolized Medications." *British Journal of Clinical Pharmacology* 56, no. 6 (2003): 588–99.
11. Al-Tabakha, M. M. "Future Prospect of Insulin Inhalation for Diabetic Patients: The Case of Afrezza Versus Exubera." *Journal of Controlled Release* 215 (2015): 25–38.
12. Person, A., and M. L. Mintz. "Anatomy and Physiology of the Respiratory Tract." In *Disorders of the Respiratory Tract: Common Challenges in Primary Care*, edited by M. L. Mintz, 11–5. Totowa, NJ: Humana Press, 2006.
13. El-Hashash, A. *Brief Overview of the Human Respiratory System Structure and Development. Lung Stem Cell Behavior*, 1–3. Cham: Springer International Publishing, 2018.
14. Verma, R. K., M. Ibrahim, and L. Garcia-Contreras. "Lung Anatomy and Physiology and Their Implications for Pulmonary Drug Delivery." *Pulmonary Drug Delivery* (2015): 1–18.
15. Aung, H. H., A. Sivakumar, S. K. Gholami, S. P. Venkateswaran, B. Gorain, and Shadab. Chapter 1. "An Overview of the Anatomy and Physiology of the Lung." In *Nanotechnology-Based Targeted Drug Delivery Systems for Lung Cancer*, edited by P. Kesharwani, 1–20. Boston, MA: Academic Press, 2019.
16. Brand-Saberi, B. E. M., and T. Schäfer. "Trachea: Anatomy and Physiology." *Thoracic Surgery Clinics* 24, no. 1 (2014): 1–5.
17. Mansour, H. M., D. Droopad, and J. G. Ledford. "Book Chapter 20: Overview of Lung Surfactant and Respiratory Distress Syndrome." In *Inhalation Aerosols: Physical and Biological Basis for Therapy, Lung Biology in Health and Diseases*. 3rd ed, edited by A. J. Hickey, and H. M. Mansour, 323–6. London: CRC Press Press/Taylor & Francis, Inc, 2019.

18. Barbosa, M. T., M. Morais-Almeida, C. S. Sousa, and J. Bousquet. "The "Big Five" Lung Diseases in CoViD-19 Pandemic - A Google Trends Analysis." *Pulmonology* 27, no. 1 (2021): 71–2.
19. Forum of International Respiratory Societies. *The Global Impact of Respiratory Disease.* 2nd ed. Sheffield: European Respiratory Society, 2017.
20. WHO. *Global Tuberculosis Report 2020.* Geneva: World Health Organization, 2020. Report No.: Licence: CC BY-NC-SA 3.0 IGO.
21. WHO. *WHO Report on Cancer: Setting Priorities, Investing Wisely and Providing Care for All.* Geneva: World Health Organization, 2020. Report No.: Licence: CC BY-NC-SA 3.0 IGO.
22. Ohashi, Y., S. Motojima, T. Fukuda, and S. Makino. "Airway Hyperresponsiveness, Increased Intracellular Spaces of Bronchial Epithelium, and Increased Infiltration of Eosinophils and Lymphocytes in Bronchial Mucosa in Asthma." *American Review of Respiratory Disease* 145, no. 6 (1992): 1469–76.
23. Nakamura, Y., J. Tamaoki, H. Nagase, M. Yamaguchi, T. Horiguchi, S. Hozawa, M. Ichinose, T. Iwanaga, R. Kondo, M. Nagata, A. Yokoyama, Y. Tohda, and Japanese Society of Allergology. "Japanese Guidelines for Adult Asthma 2020." *Allergology International* 69, no. 4 (2020): 519–48.
24. Barjaktarevic, I. Z., and A. P. Milstone. "Nebulized Therapies in COPD: Past, Present, and the Future." *International Journal of Chronic Obstructive Pulmonary Disease* 15 (2020): 1665–77.
25. Xu, Y., A. Thakur, Y. Zhang, and C. Foged. "Inhaled RNA Therapeutics for Obstructive Airway Diseases: Recent Advances and Future Prospects." *Pharmaceutics* 13, no. 2 (2021): 177.
26. Muralidharan, P., D. J. Hayes, and H. M. Mansour. "Dry Powder Inhalers in COPD, Lung Inflammation, and Pulmonary Infections." *Expert Opinion on Drug Delivery* 12, no. 6 (2015): 947–62.
27. Keshavjee, S., and P. E. Farmer. "Tuberculosis, Drug Resistance, and the History of Modern Medicine." *New England Journal of Medicine* 367, no. 10 (2012): 931–6.
28. WHO. *Global Tuberculosis Report 2017.* Geneva: World Health Organization, 2017.
29. Rangnekar, B., M. A. M. Momin, B. B. Eedara, S. Sinha, and S. C. Das. "Bedaquiline Containing Triple Combination Powder for Inhalation to Treat Drug-Resistant Tuberculosis." *International Journal of Pharmacy* 570 (2019): 118689.
30. Hickey, A. J., A. Misra, and P. B. Fourie. "Dry Powder Antibiotic Aerosol Product Development: Inhaled Therapy for Tuberculosis." *Journal of Pharmaceutical Sciences* 102, no. 11 (2013): 3900–7.
31. Momin, M. A. M., B. Rangnekar, S. Sinha, C. Y. Cheung, G. M. Cook, and S. C. Das. "Inhalable Dry Powder of Bedaquiline for Pulmonary Tuberculosis: In Vitro Physicochemical Characterization, Antimicrobial Activity and Safety Studies." *Pharmaceutics* 11, no. 10 (2019): 1–17.
32. Park, C. W., D. J. Hayes, and H. M. Mansour. "Pulmonary Inhalation Aerosols for Targeted Antibiotics Drug Delivery." Invited paper. *European Pharmaceutical Review* 16, no. 1 (2011): 32–6.
33. Hallal, A., S. M. Cohn, N. Namias, F. Habib, G. Baracco, R. J. Manning, B. Crookes, and C. I. Schulman. "Aerosolized Tobramycin in the Treatment of Ventilator-Associated Pneumonia: A Pilot Study." *Surgical Infections* 8, no. 1 (2007): 73–82.
34. Lu, Q., J. Yang, Z. Liu, C. Gutierrez, G. Aymard, J. J. Rouby, and Nebulized Antibiotics Study Group. "Nebulized Ceftazidime and Amikacin in Ventilator-Associated Pneumonia Caused by Pseudomonas aeruginosa." *American Journal of Respiratory & Critical Care Medicine* 184, no. 1 (2011): 106–15.
35. Hayes, D. J., H. M. Mansour, S. Kirkby, and A. B. Phillips. "Rapid Acute Onset of Bronchiolitis Obliterans Syndrome in a Lung Transplant Recipient After Respiratory Syncytial Virus Infection." *Transplant Infectious Disease* 14, no. 5 (2012): 548–50.
36. Eiland, L. S. "Respiratory Syncytial Virus: Diagnosis, Treatment and Prevention." *Journal of Pediatric Pharmacology & Therapeutics* 14, no. 2 (2009): 75–85.
37. Chen, Y., Q. Liu, and D. Guo. "Emerging Coronaviruses: Genome Structure, Replication, and Pathogenesis." *Journal of Medical Virology* 92, no. 4 (2020): 418–23.
38. Ganesh, B., T. Rajakumar, M. Malathi, N. Manikandan, J. Nagaraj, A. Santhakumar, et al. "Epidemiology and Pathobiology of SARS-CoV-2 (COVID-19) in Comparison with SARS, MERS: An Updated Overview of Current Knowledge and Future Perspectives." *Clinical Epidemiology and Global Health* 10 (2021): 100694.
39. Mitchell, J. P., A. Berlinski, S. Canisius, D. Cipolla, M. B. Dolovich, I. Gonda, G. Hochhaus, N. Kadrichu, S. Lyapustina, H. M. Mansour, C. Darquenne, A. R. Clark, M. Newhouse, S. Ehrmann, R. Humphries, and H. Boushey. "Urgent Appeal from International Society for Aerosols in Medicine (ISAM) During COVID-19: Clinical Decision Makers and Governmental Agencies Should Consider the Inhaled Route of Administration: A Statement from the ISAM Regulatory and Standardization Issues Networking Group." *Journal of Aerosol Medicine & Pulmonary Drug Delivery* 33, no. 4 (2020): 235–8.
40. Hayden, F. G., L. V. Gubareva, A. S. Monto, T. C. Klein, M. J. Elliot, J. M. Hammond, S. J. Sharp, M. J. Ossi, and Zanamivir Family Study Group. "Inhaled Zanamivir for the Prevention of Influenza in Families. Zanamivir Family Study Group." *New England Journal of Medicine* 343, no. 18 (2000): 1282–9.

41. Li, L., R. Avery, M. Budev, S. Mossad, and L. Danziger-Isakov. "Oral Versus Inhaled Ribavirin Therapy for Respiratory Syncytial Virus Infection After Lung Transplantation." *Journal of Heart & Lung Transplantation* 31, no. 8 (2012): 839–44.

42. Duan, J., F. G. Vogt, X. Li, D. J. Hayes, and H. M. Mansour. "Design, Characterization, and Aerosolization of Organic Solution Advanced Spray-Dried Moxifloxacin and Ofloxacin Dipalmitoylphosphatidylcholine (DPPC) Microparticulate/Nanoparticulate Powders for Pulmonary Inhalation Aerosol Delivery." *International Journal of Nanomedicine* 8 (2013): 3489–505.

43. Park, C. W., X. Li, F. G. Vogt, D. Hayes, Jr., J. B. Zwischenberger, E. S. Park, and H. M. Mansour. "Advanced Spray-Dried Design, Physicochemical Characterization, and Aerosol Dispersion Performance of Vancomycin and Clarithromycin Multifunctional Controlled Release Particles for Targeted Respiratory Delivery as Dry Powder Inhalation Aerosols." *International Journal of Pharmacy* 455, no. 1–2 (2013): 374–92.

44. Li, X., F. G. Vogt, D. J. Hayes, and H. M. Mansour. "Design, Characterization, and Aerosol Dispersion Performance Modeling of Advanced Co-Spray Dried Antibiotics with Mannitol as Respirable Microparticles/Nanoparticles for Targeted Pulmonary Delivery as Dry Powder Inhalers." *Journal of Pharmaceutical Sciences* 103, no. 9 (2014): 2937–49.

45. Li, X., F. G. Vogt, D. J. Hayes, and H. M. Mansour. "Physicochemical Characterization and Aerosol Dispersion Performance of Organic Solution Advanced Spray-Dried Microparticulate/Nanoparticulate Antibiotic Dry Powders of Tobramycin and Azithromycin for Pulmonary Inhalation Aerosol Delivery." *European Journal of Pharmaceutical Sciences* 52 (2014): 191–205.

46. Ridolfi, L., O. Bertetto, A. Santo, E. Naglieri, M. Lopez, F. Recchia, P. Lissoni, M. Galliano, F. Testore, C. Porta, M. Maglie, M. Dall'agata, L. Fumagalli, and R. Ridolfi. "Chemotherapy with or Without Low-Dose Interleukin-2 in Advanced Non-Small Cell Lung Cancer: Results from a phase III Randomized Multicentric Trial." *International Journal of Oncology* 39, no. 4 (2011): 1011–7.

47. Meenach, S. A., K. W. Anderson, J. Zach Hilt, R. C. McGarry, and H. M. Mansour. "Characterization and Aerosol Dispersion Performance of Advanced Spray-Dried Chemotherapeutic Pegylated Phospholipid Particles for Dry Powder Inhalation Delivery in Lung Cancer." *European Journal of Pharmaceutical Sciences* 49, no. 4 (2013): 699–711.

48. Meenach, S. A., K. W. Anderson, J. Z. Hilt, R. C. McGarry, and H. M. Mansour. "High-Performing Dry Powder Inhalers of Paclitaxel DPPC/DPPG Lung Surfactant-Mimic Multifunctional Particles in Lung Cancer: Physicochemical Characterization, In Vitro Aerosol Dispersion, and Cellular Studies." *AAPS PharmSciTech* 15, no. 6 (2014): 1574–87.

49. Hayes, D., Jr., M. O. Harhay, W. S. Cherikh, D. C. Chambers, K. K. Khush, E. Hsich, L. Potena, A. Sadavarte, T. P. Singh, A. Zuckermann, J. Stehlik, and International Society for Heart and Lung Transplantation. "The International Thoracic Organ Transplant Registry of the International Society for Heart and Lung Transplantation: Twenty-Third Pediatric Lung Transplantation Report –2020; Focus on Deceased Donor Characteristics." *Journal of Heart & Lung Transplantation* 39, no. 10 (2020): 1038–49.

50. Chambers, D. C., A. Zuckermann, W. S. Cherikh, M. O. Harhay, D. Hayes, Jr., E. Hsich, K. K. Khush, L. Potena, A. Sadavarte, T. P. Singh, J. Stehlik, and International Society for Heart and Lung Transplantation. "The International Thoracic Organ Transplant Registry of the International Society for Heart and Lung Transplantation: 37th Adult Lung Transplantation Report –2020; Focus on Deceased Donor Characteristics." *Journal of Heart & Lung Transplantation* 39, no. 10 (2020): 1016–27.

51. Verleden, G. M., A. R. Glanville, E. D. Lease, A. J. Fisher, F. Calabrese, P. A. Corris, C. R. Ensor, J. Gottlieb, R. R. Hachem, V. Lama, T. Martinu, D. A. H. Neil, L. G. Singer, G. Snell, and R. Vos. "Chronic Lung Allograft Dysfunction: Definition, Diagnostic Criteria, and Approaches to treatment-A Consensus Report from the Pulmonary Council of the ISHLT." *Journal of Heart & Lung Transplantation* 38, no. 5 (2019): 493–503.

52. Todd, J. L., M. L. Neely, H. Kopetskie, M. L. Sever, J. Kirchner, C. W. Frankel, L. D. Snyder, E. N. Pavlisko, T. Martinu, W. Tsuang, M. Y. Shino, N. Williams, M. A. Robien, L. G. Singer, M. Budev, P. D. Shah, J. M. Reynolds, S. M. Palmer, J. A. Belperio, and S. S. Weigt. "Risk Factors for Acute Rejection in the First Year After Lung Transplant. A Multicenter Study." *American Journal of Respiratory & Critical Care Medicine* 202, no. 4 (2020): 576–85.

53. Keenan, R. J., A. J. Duncan, S. A. Yousem, M. Zenati, M. Schaper, R. D. Dowling, Y. Alarie, G. J. Burckart, and B. P. Griffith. "Improved Immunosuppression with Aerosolized Cyclosporine in Experimental Pulmonary Transplantation." *Transplantation* 53, no. 1 (1992): 20–5.

54. O'Riordan, T. G., A. Iacono, R. J. Keenan, S. R. Duncan, G. J. Burckart, B. P. Griffith, and G. C. Smaldone. "Delivery and Distribution of Aerosolized Cyclosporine in Lung Allograft Recipients." *American Journal of Respiratory & Critical Care Medicine* 151, no. 2 (1995): 516–21.

55. Iacono, A. T., R. J. Keenan, S. R. Duncan, G. C. Smaldone, J. H. Dauber, I. L. Paradis, N. P. Ohori, W. F. Grgurich, G. J. Burckart, A. Zeevi, E. Delgado, T. G. O'Riordan, M. M. Zendarsky, S. A. Yousem, and B. P. Griffith. "Aerosolized Cyclosporine in Lung Recipients with Refractory Chronic Rejection." *American Journal of Respiratory & Critical Care Medicine* 153, no. 4 (1996): 1451–5.

56. Burckart, G. J., G. C. Smaldone, M. A. Eldon, R. Venkataramanan, J. Dauber, A. Zeevi, K. McCurry, T. P. McKaveney, T. E. Corcoran, B. P. Griffith, and A. T. Iacono. "Lung Deposition and Pharmacokinetics of Cyclosporine After Aerosolization in Lung Transplant Patients." *Pharmaceutical Research* 20, no. 2 (2003): 252–6.

57. Iacono, A., T. Corcoran, B. Griffith, W. Grgurich, D. Smith, A. Zeevi, G. C. Smaldone, K. R. McCurry, B. A. Johnson, and J. H. Dauber. "Aerosol Cyclosporin Therapy in Lung Transplant Recipients with Bronchiolitis Obliterans." *European Respiratory Journal* 23, no. 3 (2004): 384–90.

58. Behr, J., G. Zimmermann, R. Baumgartner, H. Leuchte, C. Neurohr, P. Brand, C. Herpich, K. Sommerer, J. Seitz, G. Menges, S. Tillmanns, M. Keller, and Munich Lung Transplant Group. "Lung Deposition of a Liposomal Cyclosporine A Inhalation Solution in Patients After Lung Transplantation." *Journal of Aerosol Medicine & Pulmonary Drug Delivery* 22, no. 2 (2009): 121–30.

59. Corcoran, T., R. Niven, W. Verret, S. Dilly, and B. Johnson. "Lung Deposition and Pharmacokinetics of Nebulized Cyclosporine in Lung Transplant Patients." *Journal of Aerosol Medicine & Pulmonary Drug Delivery* 27, no. 3 (2014): 178–84.

60. Deuse, T., F. Blankenberg, M. Haddad, H. Reichenspurner, N. Phillips, R. C. Robbins, and S. Schrepfer. "Mechanisms Behind Local Immunosuppression Using Inhaled Tacrolimus in Preclinical Models of Lung Transplantation." *American Journal of Respiratory Cell & Molecular Biology* 43, no. 4 (2010): 403–12.

61. Hayes, D., J. Zwischenberger, and H. Mansour, eds. "Aerosolized Tacrolimus: A Case Report in a Lung Transplant Recipient." In Transplantation Proceedings. Elsevier, 2010.

62. Groves, S., M. Galazka, B. Johnson, T. Corcoran, A. Verceles, E. Britt, N. Todd, B. Griffith, G. C. Smaldone, and A. Iacono. "Inhaled Cyclosporine and Pulmonary Function in Lung Transplant Recipients." *Journal of Aerosol Medicine & Pulmonary Drug Delivery* 23, no. 1 (2010): 31–9.

63. Wu, X., D. J. Hayes, J. B. Zwischenberger, R. J. Kuhn, and H. M. Mansour. "Design and Physicochemical Characterization of Advanced Spray-Dried Tacrolimus Multifunctional Particles for Inhalation." *Drug Design, Development, & Therapy* 7 (2013): 59–72.

64. Wu, X., W. Zhang, D. Hayes, Jr., and H. M. Mansour. "Physicochemical Characterization and Aerosol Dispersion Performance of Organic Solution Advanced Spray-Dried Cyclosporine A Multifunctional Particles for Dry Powder Inhalation Aerosol Delivery." *International Journal of Nanomedicine* 8 (2013): 1269–83.

65. Moore, C., J. Pilewski, K. Robinson, M. Morrell, C. Gries, A. Zeevi, J. F. McDyer, and C. R. Ensor. "Effect of Aerosolized Antipseudomonals on Pseudomonas Recurrence and Bronchiolitis Obliterans Syndrome After Lung Transplantation." *Journal of Heart & Lung Transplantation* 35, no. 4 (2016): S124–SS5.

66. Beyer, J., C. Weyer, W. Siegert, G. Barzen, G. Risse, S. Schwartz, and W. Siegert. "Use of Amphotericin B Aerosols for the Prevention of Pulmonary Aspergillosis." *Infection* 22, no. 2 (1994): 143–8.

67. Calvo, V., J. M. Borro, P. Morales, A. Morcillo, R. Vicente, V. Tarrazona, and F. París. "Antifungal Prophylaxis During the Early Postoperative Period of Lung Transplantation." *Chest* 115, no. 5 (1999): 1301–4.

68. Palmer, S. M., R. H. Drew, J. D. Whitehouse, V. F. Tapson, R. D. Davis, R. R. McConnell, S. S. Kanj, and J. R. Perfect. "Safety of Aerosolized Amphotericin B Lipid Complex In Lung Transplant recipients12." *Transplantation* 72, no. 3 (2001): 545–8.

69. Monforte, Vc, A. Roman, J. Gavalda, C. Bravo, L. Tenorio, A. Ferrer, A. Ferrer, J. Maestre, and F. Morell. "Nebulized Amphotericin B Prophylaxis for Aspergillus Infection in Lung Transplantation: Study of Risk Factors." *Journal of Heart & Lung Transplantation* 20, no. 12 (2001): 1274–81.

70. Marra, F., N. Partovi, K. M. Wasan, E. H. Kwong, M. H. Ensom, S. M. Cassidy, G. Fradet, and R. D. Levy. "Amphotericin B Disposition After Aerosol Inhalation in Lung Transplant Recipients." *Annals of Pharmacotherapy* 36, no. 1 (2002): 46–51.

71. Drew, R. H., E. D. Ashley, D. K. Benjamin Jr., R. D. Davis, S. M. Palmer, and J. R. Perfect. "Comparative Safety of Amphotericin B Lipid Complex and Amphotericin B Deoxycholate as Aerosolized Antifungal Prophylaxis in Lung-Transplant Recipients." *Transplantation* 77, no. 2 (2004): 232–7.

72. Corcoran, T., R. Venkataramanan, K. Mihelc, A. Marcinkowski, J. Ou, B. McCook, L. Weber, M. E. Carey, D. L. Paterson, J. M. Pilewski, K. R. McCurry, and S. Husain. "Aerosol Deposition of Lipid Complex Amphotericin-B (Abelcet) in Lung Transplant Recipients." *American Journal of Transplantation* 6, no. 11 (2006): 2765–73.

73. Monforte, V., P. Ussetti, R. López, J. Gavaldà, C. Bravo, A. de Pablo, L. Pou, A. Pahissa, F. Morell, and A. Román. "Nebulized Liposomal Amphotericin B Prophylaxis for Aspergillus Infection in Lung Transplantation: Pharmacokinetics and Safety." *Journal of Heart & Lung Transplantation* 28, no. 2 (2009): 170–5.

74. Nathan, S. D., D. J. Ross, P. Zakowski, R. M. Kass, and S. K. Koerner. "Utility of Inhaled Pentamidine Prophylaxis in Lung Transplant Recipients." *Chest* 105, no. 2 (1994): 417–20.

75. Hayes Jr., D., B. S. Murphy, T. W. Mullett, and D. J. Feola. "Aerosolized Vancomycin for the Treatment of MRSA After Lung Transplantation." *Respirology* 15, no. 1 (2010): 184–6.

76. Kim, V., and G. J. Criner. "Chronic Bronchitis and Chronic Obstructive Pulmonary Disease." *American Journal of Respiratory & Critical Care Medicine* 187, no. 3 (2013): 228–37.

77. Widysanto, A., and G. Mathew. "Chronic Bronchitis Treasure Island (FL): StatPearls Publishing." 2019. https://www.ncbi.nlm.nih.gov/books/NBK482437/.

78. Cant, N., N. Pollock, and R. C. Ford. "CFTR Structure and Cystic Fibrosis." *International Journal of Biochemistry & Cell Biology* 52 (2014): 15–25.

79. Spencer, H., and A. Jaffe. "Newer Therapies for Cystic Fibrosis." *Current Paediatrics* 13, no. 4 (2003): 259–63.

80. Habib, A.-R. R., M. Kajbafzadeh, S. Desai, C. L. Yang, K. Skolnik, and B. S. Quon. "A Systematic Review of the Clinical Efficacy and Safety of CFTR Modulators in Cystic Fibrosis." *Scientific Report* 9, no. 1 (2019): 7234.

81. Harman, K., R. Dobra, and J. C. Davies. "Disease-Modifying Drug Therapy in Cystic Fibrosis." *Paediatric Respiratory Reviews* 26 (2018): 7–9.

82. Balfour-Lynn, I. M., and J. A. King. "CFTR Modulator Therapies: Effect on Life Expectancy in People with Cystic Fibrosis." *Paediatric Respiratory Reviews* (2020).

83. Mather, N. L., A. D. Padmakumar, R. Milton, and A. B. Lumb. "Emphysema, Lung Volume Reduction and Anaesthesia." *Trends in Anaesthesia & Critical Care* 2, no. 4 (2012): 166–73.

84. Edgar, R. G., M. Patel, S. Bayliss, D. Crossley, E. Sapey, and A. M. Turner. "Treatment of Lung Disease in alpha-1 Antitrypsin Deficiency: A Systematic Review." *International Journal of Chronic Obstructive Pulmonary Disease* 12 (2017): 1295–308.

85. Kradin, R. L.. Chapter 5."Diseases of the Airways." In *Understanding Pulmonary Pathology*, edited by R. L. Kradin, 59–94. Boston, MA: Academic Press, 2017.

86. Chapter, Benca J."Bronchospasm." In *Complications in Anesthesia*. 2nd ed, edited by J. L. Atlee vol. 46, 189–92. Philadelphia, PA: W.B. Saunders, 2007.

87. Spagnolo, P., T. M. Maher, and L. Richeldi. "Idiopathic Pulmonary Fibrosis: Recent Advances on Pharmacological Therapy." *Pharmacology & Therapeutics* 152 (2015): 18–27.

88. King, T. E., Jr., K. K. Brown, G. Raghu, R. M. du Bois, D. A. Lynch, F. Martinez, D. Valeyre, I. Leconte, A. Morganti, S. Roux, and J. Behr. "BUILD-3: A Randomized, Controlled Trial of Bosentan in Idiopathic Pulmonary Fibrosis." *American Journal of Respiratory & Critical Care Medicine* 184, no. 1 (2011): 92–9.

89. Muralidharan, P., D. J. Hayes, and H. M. Mansour. "Book Chapter." In *Inhalation Aerosols: Physical and Biological Basis for Therapy. Lung Biology in Health and Diseases*. 3rd ed, edited by A. J. Hickey, and H. M. Mansour vol. 18: Pulmonary Fibrosis, 303–12. London: CRC Press Press/Taylor & Francis, 2019.

90. Kleniewska, P., and R. Pawliczak. "The Participation of Oxidative Stress in the Pathogenesis of Bronchial Asthma." *Biomedicine & Pharmacotherapy* 94 (2017): 100–8.

91. Jeenakeri, R., and M. Drayton. "Management of Respiratory Distress Syndrome." *Paediatrics & Child Health* 19, no. 4 (2009): 158–64.

92. Hart, R., and E. Black. "Acute Respiratory Distress Syndrome." *Anaesthesia & Intensive Care Medicine* 20, no. 11 (2019): 658–62.

93. Ruopp, N. F., and H. W. Farber. "The New World Symposium on Pulmonary Hypertension Guidelines." *Circulation* 140, no. 14 (2019): 1134–6.

94. Lisa, J. R.-J., and V. M. Vallerie. "Pulmonary Hypertension: Types and Treatments." *Current Cardiology Reviews* 11, no. 1 (2015): 73–9.

95. Ryan, J. J., T. Thenappan, N. Luo, T. Ha, A. R. Patel, S. Rich, and S. L. Archer. "The WHO Classification of Pulmonary Hypertension: A Case-Based Imaging Compendium." *Pulmonary Circulation* 2, no. 1 (2012): 107–21.

96. Hensley, M. K., A. Levine, M. T. Gladwin, and Y.-C. Lai. "Emerging Therapeutics in Pulmonary Hypertension." *American Journal of Physiology. Lung Cellular & Molecular Physiology* 314, no. 5 (2018): L769–LL81.

97. Gessler, T. "Inhalation of Repurposed Drugs to Treat Pulmonary Hypertension." *Advanced Drug Delivery Reviews* 133 (2018): 34–44.

98. Acosta, M. F., D. J. Hayes, J. R. Fineman, J. X.-J. Yuan, S. M. Black, and H. M. Mansour. "Book Chapter 19: Therapeutics in Pulmonary Hypertension." In *Inhalation Aerosols: Physical and Biological Basis for Therapy, Lung Biology in Health and Diseases*. 3rd ed, edited by A. J. Hickey, and H. M. Mansour, 313–22. London: CRC Press Press/Taylor & Francis, 2019.

99. Mansour, H. M. "Inhaled Medical Aerosols by Nebulizer Delivery in Pulmonary Hypertension." *Pulmonary Circulation* 8, no. 4 (2018): 1–2 (2045894018809084).

100. Chrystyn, H., and C. Niederlaender. "The Genuair® Inhaler: A Novel, Multidose Dry Powder Inhaler." *International Journal of Clinical Practice* 66, no. 3 (2012): 309–17.

101. Darquenne, C. "Deposition Mechanisms." *Journal of Aerosol Medicine & Pulmonary Drug Delivery* 33, no. 4 (2020): 181–5.

102. Patton, J. S., and P. R. Byron. "Inhaling Medicines: Delivering Drugs to the Body Through the Lungs." *Nature Reviews. Drug Discovery* 6, no. 1 (2007): 67–74.

103. Kolanjiyil, A. V., and C. Kleinstreuer. "Computational Analysis of Aerosol-Dynamics in a Human Whole-Lung Airway Model." *Journal of Aerosol Science* 114 (2017): 301–16.

104. Carvalho, T. C., J. I. Peters, and R. O. Williams III. "Influence of Particle Size on Regional Lung Deposition–What Evidence Is There?." *International Journal of Pharmacy* 406, no. 1–2 (2011): 1–10.

105. Darquenne, C. "Aerosol Deposition in Health and Disease." *Journal of Aerosol Medicine & Pulmonary Drug Delivery* 25, no. 3 (2012): 140–7.

106. Cheng, Y. S. "Mechanisms of Pharmaceutical Aerosol Deposition in the Respiratory Tract." *AAPS PharmSciTech* 15, no. 3 (2014): 630–40.

107. Zhou, Y., and Y.-S. Cheng. "Technology. Particle Deposition in a Cast of Human Tracheobronchial Airways." *Aerosol Science* 39, no. 6 (2005): 492–500.

108. Li, Z., C. Kleinstreuer, and Z. Zhang. "Particle Deposition in the Human Tracheobronchial Airways Due to Transient Inspiratory Flow Patterns." *Journal of Aerosol Science* 38, no. 6 (2007): 625–44.

109. Kim, C. S., and S. Hu. "Regional Deposition of Inhaled Particles in Human Lungs: Comparison Between Men and Women." *Journal of Applied Physiology* 84, no. 6 (1998): 1834–44.

110. Zhang, Z. "Kleinstreuer CJJocp." *Airflow Structures & Nano-Particle Deposition in a Human Upper Airway Model.* 198, no. 1 (2004): 178–210.

111. Xi, J., X. Si, and W. J. P. Longest. "Electrostatic Charge Effects on Pharmaceutical Aerosol Deposition in Human Nasal–Laryngeal Airways" 6, no. 1 (2014): 26–35.

112. Liang, W., H. W. Pan, D. Vllasaliu, and J. K. Lam. "Pulmonary Delivery of Biological Drugs." *Pharmaceutics* 12, no. 11 (2020): 1025.

113. Hickey, A. J., and H. M. Mansour. *Inhalation Aerosols: Physical and Biological Basis for Therapy.* CRC press, 2019.

114. Pritchard, J. *Particle Growth in the Airways and the Influence of Airflow. A New Concept in Inhalation Therapy Bussum: Medicom,* 3–24. 1987.

115. Crowder, T. M., J. A. Rosati, J. D. Schroeter, A. J. Hickey, and T. B. Martonen. "Fundamental Effects of Particle Morphology on Lung Delivery: Predictions of Stokes' Law and the Particular Relevance to Dry Powder Inhaler Formulation and Development." *Pharmaceutical Research* 19, no. 3 (2002): 239–45.

116. Newman, S. P. "Drug Delivery to the Lungs: Challenges and Opportunities." *Therapeutic Delivery* 8, no. 8 (2017): 647–61.

117. Arora, D., J. Peart, and P. Byron. "USA Market 1990–2005: Products and Instructions for Use." In *Respiratory Drug Delivery,* edited by R. Dalby, P. Byron, J. Peart, J. Suman, and S. Farr, 955–9. River Grove, IL: Davis Healthcare International, 2006.

118. Patton, J. S., J. D. Brain, L. A. Davies, J. Fiegel, M. Gumbleton, K.-J. Kim, M. Sakagami, R. Vanbever, and C. Ehrhardt. "The Particle Has Landed—Characterizing the Fate of Inhaled Pharmaceuticals." *Journal of Aerosol Medicine & Pulmonary Drug Delivery* 23, no. Suppl.2 (2010): S-71-S–S-87.

119. Ganesan, S., A. T. Comstock, and U. S. Sajjan. "Barrier Function of Airway Tract Epithelium." *Tissue Barriers* 1, no. 4 (2013): e24997.

120. Brown, J. S., K. L. Zeman, and W. D. Bennett. "Ultrafine Particle Deposition and Clearance in the Healthy and Obstructed Lung." *American Journal of Respiratory & Critical Care Medicine* 166, no. 9 (2002): 1240–7.

121. Nagre, N., X. Cong, A. C. Pearson, and X. Zhao. "Alveolar Macrophage Phagocytosis and Bacteria Clearance in Mice." *JoVE* 145, no. 145 (2019): e59088.

122. Clua, P., M. Tomokiyo, F. Raya Tonetti, M. Islam, V. García Castillo, G. Marcial, S. Salva, S. Alvarez, H. Takahashi, S. Kurata, H. Kitazawa, and J. Villena. "The Role of Alveolar Macrophages in the Improved Protection Against Respiratory Syncytial Virus and Pneumococcal Superinfection Induced by the Peptidoglycan of Lactobacillus rhamnosus CRL1505." *Cells* 9, no. 7 (2020): 1653.

123. Broug-Holub, E., G. B. Toews, J. F. Van Iwaarden, R. M. Strieter, S. L. Kunkel, R. Paine, and T. J. Standiford. "Alveolar Macrophages Are Required for Protective Pulmonary Defenses in Murine Klebsiella pneumonia: Elimination of Alveolar Macrophages Increases Neutrophil Recruitment but Decreases Bacterial Clearance and Survival." *Infection & Immunity* 65, no. 4 (1997): 1139–46.

124. Olsson, B., E. Bondesson, L. Borgström, S. Edsbäcker, S. Eirefelt, K. Ekelund et al. *Pulmonary Drug Metabolism, Clearance, and Absorption. Controlled Pulmonary Drug Delivery,* 21–50. New York: Springer, 2011.

125. Mejías, J. C., and K. Roy. "In-Vitro and In-Vivo Characterization of a Multi-Stage Enzyme-Responsive Nanoparticle-in-Microgel Pulmonary Drug Delivery System." *Journal of Controlled Release* 316 (2019): 393–403.

126. Thakur, A. K., D. K. Chellappan, K. Dua, M. Mehta, S. Satija, and I. Singh. "Patented Therapeutic Drug Delivery Strategies for Targeting Pulmonary Diseases." *Expert Opinion on Therapeutic Patents* 30, no. 5 (2020): 375–87.

127. Newman, S. P. "Delivering Drugs to the Lungs: The History of Repurposing in the Treatment of Respiratory Diseases." *Advanced Drug Delivery Reviews* 133 (2018): 5–18.

128. Anderson, P. J. "History of Aerosol Therapy: Liquid Nebulization to MDIs to DPIs." *Respiratory Care* 50, no. 9 (2005): 1139–50.

129. Sorino, C., S. Negri, A. Spanevello, D. Visca, and N. Scichilone. "Inhalation Therapy Devices for the Treatment of Obstructive Lung Diseases: The History of Inhalers Towards the Ideal Inhaler." *European Journal of Internal Medicine* 75 (2020): 15–8.

130. Hertel, S. P., G. Winter, and W. Friess. "Protein Stability in Pulmonary Drug Delivery via Nebulization." *Advanced Drug Delivery Reviews* 93 (2015): 79–94.

131. Zhou, Q., S. S. Y. Leung, P. Tang, T. Parumasivam, Z. H. Loh, and H.-K. Chan. "Inhaled Formulations and Pulmonary Drug Delivery Systems for Respiratory Infections." *Advanced Drug Delivery Reviews* 85 (2015): 83–99.

132. Park, C. W., H. M. Mansour, and D. Hayes. "Pulmonary Inhalation Aerosols for Targeted Antibiotics Drug Delivery." *European Pharmaceutical Review* 16, no. 1 (2011): 32–6.

133. Deshmukh, R., N. Bandyopadhyay, S. N. Abed, S. Bandopadhyay, Y. Pal, and P. K. Deb. Chapter 3."Strategies for Pulmonary Delivery of Drugs." In *Drug Delivery Systems*, edited by R. K. Tekade, 85–129. Boston, MA: Academic Press, 2020.

134. Watts, A. B., J. T. McConville, and R. O. Williams III. "Current Therapies and Technological Advances in Aqueous Aerosol Drug Delivery." *Drug Development & Industrial Pharmacy* 34, no. 9 (2008): 913–22.

135. Ghazanfari, T., A. M. Elhissi, Z. Ding, and K. M. Taylor. "The Influence of Fluid Physicochemical Properties on Vibrating-Mesh Nebulization." *International Journal of Pharmacy* 339, no. 1–2 (2007): 103–11.

136. Ari, A. "Jet, Ultrasonic, and Mesh Nebulizers: An Evaluation of Nebulizers for Better Clinical Outcomes." *Eurasian Journal of Pulmonology* 16, no. 1 (2014): 1–7.

137. Singh, N., P. Yadav, P. Gaur, M. Gaur, and A. B. Yadav. "Protein Stability and Functional Activity During Nebulization: A Comparative Study of Three Nebulizer!." bioRxiv (2020).

138. Dolovich, M. A. "Influence of Inspiratory Flow Rate, Particle Size, and Airway Caliber on Aerosolized Drug Delivery to the Lung." *Respiratory Care* 45, no. 6 (2000): 597.

139. Vallorz, E., P. Sheth, and P. Myrdal. "Pressurized Metered Dose Inhaler Technology: Manufacturing." *AAPS PharmSciTech* 20, no. 5 (2019): 177.

140. Myrdal, P. B., P. Sheth, and S. W. Stein. "Advances in Metered Dose Inhaler Technology: Formulation Development." *AAPS PharmSciTech* 15, no. 2 (2014): 434–55.

141. Bailey, M. M., and C. J. Berkland. "Nanoparticle Formulations in Pulmonary Drug Delivery." *Medicinal Research Reviews* 29, no. 1 (2009): 196–212.

142. Huang, Z., H. Wu, B. Yang, L. Chen, Y. Huang, G. Quan, C. Zhu, X. Li, X. Pan, and C. Wu. "Anhydrous Reverse Micelle Nanoparticles: New Strategy to Overcome Sedimentation Instability of Peptide-Containing Pressurized Metered-Dose Inhalers." *Drug Delivery* 24, no. 1 (2017): 527–38.

143. Welin-Berger, K., and B. Bergenståhl. "Inhibition of Ostwald Ripening in Local Anesthetic Emulsions by Using Hydrophobic Excipients in the Disperse Phase." *International Journal of Pharmacy* 200, no. 2 (2000): 249–60.

144. Hatley, R. H., J. Parker, J. N. Pritchard, and D. von Hollen. "Variability in Delivered Dose from Pressurized Metered-Dose Inhaler Formulations due to a Delay Between Shake and Fire." *Journal of Aerosol Medicine & Pulmonary Drug Delivery* 30, no. 1 (2017): 71–9.

145. Della Bella, A., E. Salomi, F. Buttini, and R. Bettini. "The Role of the Solid State and Physical Properties of the Carrier in Adhesive Mixtures for Lung Delivery." *Expert Opinion on Drug Delivery* 15, no. 7 (2018): 665–74.

146. Hou, S., J. Wu, X. Li, and H. Shu. "Practical, Regulatory and Clinical Considerations for Development of Inhalation Drug Products." *Asian Journal of Pharmaceutical Sciences* 10, no. 6 (2015): 490–500.

147. Dieter Hochrainer, H. H., Christoph Kreher, Luigi Scaffidi, Michael Spallek, and Herbert Wachtel. "Comparison of the Aerosol Velocity and Spray Duration of Respimat® Soft Mist™ Inhaler and Pressurized Metered Dose Inhalers." *Journal of Aerosol Medicine* 18, no. 3 (2005): 273–82.

148. Mansour, H. M., P. B. Myrdal, U. Younis, P. Muralidharan, and D. Hayes Jr. *Book Chapter 12: Pulmonary Drug Delivery*. Drug Delivery & Targeting; CRC Press Taylor & Francis, Inc., 2015.

149. *Dry Powder Inhaler Devices Device Pipeline study 2019: Analysis of Devices Under Development, Companies, Developments and Outlook*. Dublin, 2019. Report No.: 4806784.
150. Moon, C., H. D. C. Smyth, A. B. Watts, and R. O. Williams, 3rd. "Delivery Technologies for Orally Inhaled Products: An Update." *AAPS PharmSciTech* 20, no. 3 (2019): 117.
151. Hickey, A. J., and H. M. Mansour. Chapter 43. "Formulation Challenges of Powders for the Delivery of Small Molecular Weight Molecules as Aerosols." In *Modified-Release Drug Delivery Technology. Drugs and the Pharmaceutical Sciences*. 2nd ed, edited by M. J. Rathbone, J. Hadgraft, M. S. Roberts, and M. Lane Series 2, 573–602. New York: Informa Healthcare, 2008.
152. Guchardi, R., M. Frei, E. John, and J. S. Kaerger. "Influence of Fine Lactose and Magnesium Stearate on Low Dose Dry Powder Inhaler Formulations." *International Journal of Pharmacy* 348, no. 1 (2008): 10–7.
153. Chow, A. H., H. H. Tong, P. Chattopadhyay, and B. Y. Shekunov. "Particle Engineering for Pulmonary Drug Delivery." *Pharmaceutical Research* 24, no. 3 (2007): 411–37.
154. Ameri, M., and Y.-F. Maa. "Spray Drying of Biopharmaceuticals: Stability and Process Considerations." *Drying Technology* 24, no. 6 (2006): 763–8.
155. Mansour, H. M., Y. S. Rhee, and X. Wu. "Nanomedicine in Pulmonary Delivery." *International Journal of Nanomedicine* 4, no. Dec. (2009): 299–319.
156. Chamayou, A., and J. A. Dodds. Chapter 8. "Air Jet Milling." In *Handbook of Powder Technology, Particle Breakage*, edited by D. Salman, M. Ghadiri, and J. Hounslow vol. 12, 421–35. Amsterdam: Elsevier BV, 2007.
157. Marudamuthu, A. S., Y. P. Bhandary, L. Fan, V. Radhakrishnan, B. MacKenzie, E. Maier, S. K. Shetty, M. R. Nagaraja, V. Gopu, N. Tiwari, Y. Zhang, A. B. Watts, R. O. Williams, G. J. Criner, S. Bolla, N. Marchetti, S. Idell, and S. Shetty. "Caveolin-1–derived Peptide Limits Development of Pulmonary Fibrosis." *Science Translational Medicine* 11, no. 522 (2019).
158. Zhang, M.-Z., D.-H. Qian, J.-C. Xu, W. Yao, Y. Fan, and C.-Z. Wang. "Statins May Be Beneficial for Patients with Pulmonary Hypertension Secondary to Lung Diseases." *Journal of Thoracic Disease* 9, no. 8 (2017): 2437.
159. Eedara, B. B., W. Alabsi, D. Encinas-Basurto, R. Polt, and H. M. Mansour. "Spray-Dried Inhalable Powder Formulations of Therapeutic Proteins and Peptides." *AAPS PharmSciTech* 22, no. 5 (2021): 185.
160. Lee, G. *Spray-Drying of Proteins. Rational Design of Stable Protein Formulations*, 135–58. Cham: Springer, 2002.
161. Haggag, Y. A., and A. M. Faheem. "Evaluation of Nano Spray Drying as a Method for Drying and Formulation of Therapeutic Peptides and Proteins." *Frontiers in Pharmacology* 6 (2015): 1–5.
162. Sarabandi, K., P. Gharehbeglou, and S. M. Jafari. "Spray-Drying Encapsulation of Protein Hydrolysates and Bioactive Peptides: Opportunities and Challenges." *Drying Technology* 38, no. 5–6 (2020): 577–95.
163. Irngartinger, M., V. Camuglia, M. Damm, J. Goede, and H. Frijlink. "Pulmonary Delivery of Therapeutic Peptides via Dry Powder Inhalation: Effects of Micronisation and Manufacturing." *European Journal of Pharmaceutics & Biopharmaceutics* 58, no. 1 (2004): 7–14.
164. Shoyele, S. A., and S. Cawthorne. "Particle Engineering Techniques for Inhaled Biopharmaceuticals." *Advanced Drug Delivery Reviews* 58, no. 9 (2006): 1009–29.
165. Maa, Y.-F., H. R. Costantino, P.-A. Nguyen, and C. C. Hsu. "The Effect of Operating and Formulation Variables on the Morphology of Spray-Dried Protein Particles." *Pharmaceutical Development & Technology* 2, no. 3 (1997): 213–23.
166. Healy, A. M., M. I. Amaro, K. J. Paluch, and L. Tajber. "Dry Powders for Oral Inhalation Free of Lactose Carrier Particles." *Advanced Drug Delivery Reviews* 75 (2014): 32–52.
167. Ishwarya, S. P., C. Anandharamakrishnan, and A. G. Stapley. "Spray-Freeze-Drying: A Novel Process for the Drying of Foods and Bioproducts." *Trends in Food Science & Technology* 41, no. 2 (2015): 161–81.
168. Vishali, D., J. Monisha, S. Sivakamasundari, J. Moses, and C. Anandharamakrishnan. "Spray Freeze Drying: Emerging Applications in Drug Delivery." *Journal of Controlled Release* 300 (2019): 93–101.
169. Ye, T., J. Yu, Q. Luo, S. Wang, and H.-K. Chan. "Inhalable Clarithromycin Liposomal Dry Powders Using Ultrasonic Spray Freeze Drying." *Powder Technology* 305 (2017): 63–70.
170. Lavanya, M., R. Preethi, J. Moses, and C. Anandharamakrishnan. "Production of Bromelain Aerosols Using Spray-Freeze-Drying Technique for Pulmonary Supplementation." *Drying Technology* (2020): 1–13.
171. Davies, O. R., A. L. Lewis, M. J. Whitaker, H. Tai, K. M. Shakesheff, and S. M. Howdle. "Applications of Supercritical CO2 in the Fabrication of Polymer Systems for Drug Delivery and Tissue Engineering." *Advanced Drug Delivery Reviews* 60, no. 3 (2008): 373–87.
172. Girotra, P., S. K. Singh, and K. Nagpal. "Supercritical Fluid Technology: A Promising Approach in Pharmaceutical Research." *Pharmaceutical Development & Technology* 18, no. 1 (2013): 22–38.
173. Kankala, R. K., Y. S. Zhang, S. B. Wang, C. H. Lee, and A. Z. Chen. "Supercritical Fluid Technology: An Emphasis on Drug Delivery and Related Biomedical Applications." *Advanced Healthcare Materials* 6, no. 16 (2017): 1700433.

174. Chakravarty, P., A. Famili, K. Nagapudi, and M. A. Al-Sayah. "Using Supercritical Fluid Technology as a Green Alternative During the Preparation of Drug Delivery Systems." *Pharmaceutics* 11, no. 12 (2019): 629.

175. Knez, Ž., M. Pantić, D. Cör, Z. Novak, and M. K. Hrnčič. "Are Supercritical Fluids Solvents for the Future?." *Chemical Engineering & Processing-Process Intensification* 141 (2019): 107532.

176. Jovanović, N., A. Bouchard, G. W. Hofland, G.-J. Witkamp, D. J. Crommelin, and W. Jiskoot. "Stabilization of Proteins in Dry Powder Formulations Using Supercritical Fluid Technology." *Pharmaceutical Research* 21, no. 11 (2004): 1955–69.

177. Aguiar-Ricardo, A. "Building Dry Powder Formulations Using Supercritical CO2 Spray Drying." *Current Opinion in Green & Sustainable Chemistry* 5 (2017): 12–6.

178. Hong, D.-X., Y.-L. Yun, Y.-X. Guan, and S.-J. Yao. "Preparation of Micrometric Powders of Parathyroid Hormone (PTH1–34)-Loaded Chitosan Oligosaccharide by Supercritical Fluid Assisted Atomization." *International Journal of Pharmacy* 545, no. 1–2 (2018): 389–94.

179. Rahhal, T. B., C. A. Fromen, E. M. Wilson, M. P. Kai, T. W. Shen, J. C. Luft, and J. M. DeSimone. "Pulmonary Delivery of Butyrylcholinesterase as a Model Protein to the Lung." *Molecular Pharmaceutics* 13, no. 5 (2016): 1626–35.

180. Sato, H., A. Tabata, T. Moritani, T. Morinaga, T. Mizumoto, Y. Seto, and S. Onoue. "Design and Characterizations of Inhalable Poly (Lactic-co-Glycolic Acid) Microspheres Prepared by the Fine Droplet Drying Process for a Sustained Effect of Salmon Calcitonin." *Molecules* 25, no. 6 (2020): 1311.

181. Hickey, A. J., H. M. Mansour, M. J. Telko, Z. Xu, H. D. C. Smyth, T. Mulder, R. McLean, J. Langridge, and D. Papadopoulos. "Physical Characterization of Component Particles Included in Dry Powder Inhalers. I. Strategy Review and Static Characteristics." *Journal of Pharmaceutical Sciences* 96, no. 5 (2007): 1282–301.

182. Muralidharan, P., M. Acosta, D. J. Hayes, S. M. Black, and H. M. Mansour. "Solid-State Physicochemical Characterization & Microscopy of Particles in Dry Powder Inhalers." *Inhalation* 10, no. 2 (2016): 20–6.

183. Wu, X., X. Li, and H. M. Mansour. "Surface Analytical Techniques in Solid-State Particle Characterization: Implications for Predicting Performance in Dry Powder Inhalers." Invited paper. *KONA Powder & Particle Journal* 28 (2010): 3–19.

184. Islam, N., and M. J. Cleary. "Developing an Efficient and Reliable Dry Powder Inhaler for Pulmonary Drug Delivery--A Review for Multidisciplinary Researchers." *Medical Engineering & Physics* 34, no. 4 (2012): 409–27.

185. Islam, N., and E. Gladki. "Dry Powder Inhalers (DPIs): A Review of Device Reliability and Innovation." *International Journal of Pharmacy* 360, no. 1–2 (2008): 1–11.

186. Momin, M. A. M., I. G. Tucker, and S. C. Das. "High Dose Dry Powder Inhalers to Overcome the Challenges of Tuberculosis Treatment." *International Journal of Pharmacy* 550, no. 1–2 (2018): 398–417.

187. Chew, N. Y., and H. K. Chan. "The Role of Particle Properties in Pharmaceutical Powder Inhalation Formulations." *Journal of Aerosol Medicine* 15, no. 3 (2002): 325–30.

188. Telko, M. J., and A. J. Hickey. "Dry Powder Inhaler Formulation." *Respiratory Care* 50, no. 9 (2005): 1209–27.

189. Eedara, B., D. Encinas-Basurto, W. Alabsi, R. Polt, and H. Mansour. "Applications of Surface Analytical Techniques in Characterization of Dry Powder Formulations." *Inhalation* (2021): 1–9.

190. Arpagaus, C., A. Collenberg, D. Rütti, E. Assadpour, and S. M. Jafari. "Nano Spray Drying for Encapsulation of Pharmaceuticals." *International Journal of Pharmacy* 546, no. 1–2 (2018): 194–214.

191. Leamy, H. "Charge Collection Scanning Electron Microscopy." *Journal of Applied Physics* 53, no. 6 (1982): R51–R80.

192. Suga, M., S. Asahina, Y. Sakuda, H. Kazumori, H. Nishiyama, T. Nokuo, V. Alfredsson, T. Kjellman, S. M. Stevens, H. S. Cho, M. Cho, L. Han, S. Che, M. W. Anderson, F. Schüth, H. Deng, O. M. Yaghi, Z. Liu, H. Y. Jeong, A. Stein, K. Sakamoto, R. Ryoo, and O. Terasaki. "Recent Progress in Scanning Electron Microscopy for the Characterization of Fine Structural Details of Nano Materials." *Progress in Solid State Chemistry* 42, no. 1–2 (2014): 1–21.

193. Taki, M., C. Marriott, X.-M. Zeng, and G. P. Martin. "Aerodynamic Deposition of Combination Dry Powder Inhaler Formulations In Vitro: A Comparison of Three Impactors." *International Journal of Pharmacy* 388, no. 1–2 (2010): 40–51.

194. Chapter, Ali M."Pulmonary Drug Delivery." In *Handbook of Non-Invasive Drug Delivery Systems*, edited by V. S. Kulkarni vol. 9, 209–46. Boston, MA: William Andrew Publishing, 2010.

195. Yoshida, H., A. Kuwana, H. Shibata, K.-i. Izutsu, and Y. Goda. "Comparison of Aerodynamic Particle Size Distribution Between a Next Generation Impactor and a Cascade Impactor at a Range of Flow Rates." *AAPS PharmSciTech* 18, no. 3 (2017): 646–53.

196. Song, X., J. Hu, S. Zhan, R. Zhang, and W. Tan. "Effects of Temperature and Humidity on Laser Diffraction Measurements to Jet Nebulizer and Comparison with NGI." *AAPS PharmSciTech* 17, no. 2 (2016): 380–8.

197. Eedara, B. B., B. Rangnekar, C. Doyle, A. Cavallaro, and S. C. Das. "The Influence of Surface Active l-Leucine and 1,2-Dipalmitoyl-sn-Glycero-3-Phosphatidylcholine (DPPC) in the Improvement of Aerosolization of Pyrazinamide and Moxifloxacin Co-Spray Dried Powders." *International Journal of Pharmacy* 542, no. 1–2 (2018): 72–81.

198. Eedara, B. B., B. Rangnekar, S. Sinha, C. Doyle, A. Cavallaro, and S. C. Das. "Development and Characterization of High Payload Combination Dry Powders of Anti-Tubercular Drugs for Treating Pulmonary Tuberculosis." *European Journal of Pharmaceutical Sciences* 118 (2018): 216–26.

199. Eedara, B. B., I. G. Tucker, and S. C. Das. "Phospholipid-Based Pyrazinamide Spray-Dried Inhalable Powders for Treating Tuberculosis." *International Journal of Pharmacy* 506, no. 1 (2016): 174–83.

200. Haefele, T. F., and K. Paulus. "Confocal Raman Microscopy in Pharmaceutical Development." In *Confocal Raman Microscopy*, edited by J. Toporski, T. Dieing, and O. Hollricher, 381–419. Cham: Springer, 2018.

201. Raval, N., R. Maheshwari, D. Kalyane, S. R. Youngren-Ortiz, M. B. Chougule, and R. K. Tekade. Chapter 10. "Importance of Physicochemical Characterization of Nanoparticles in Pharmaceutical Product Development." In *Basic Fundamentals of Drug Delivery*, edited by R. K. Tekade, 369–400. Boston, MA: Academic Press, 2019.

202. Deb, P. K., S. N. Abed, A. M. Y. Jaber, and R. K. Tekade. "Particulate Level Properties and Its Implications on Product Performance and Processing." In *Dosage Form Design Parameters*, 155–220. Amsterdam: Elsevier, 2018.

203. Mosgoeller, W., R. Prassl, and A. Zimmer. "Chapter Seventeen: Nanoparticle-Mediated Treatment of Pulmonary Arterial Hypertension." In *Methods Enzymol*, edited by N. Düzgüneş vol. 508, 325–54. Boston, MA: Academic Press, 2012.

204. Amidon, G. E., P. J. Meyer, and D. M. Mudie. Chapter 10. "Particle, Powder, and Compact Characterization." In *Developing Solid Oral Dosage Forms*. 2nd ed, edited by Y. Qiu, Y. Chen, G. G. Z. Zhang, L. Yu, and R. V. Mantri, 271–93. Boston, MA: Academic Press, 2017.

205. Connors, K. A. "The Karl Fischer Titration of Water." *Drug Development & Industrial Pharmacy* 14, no. 14 (1988): 1891–903.

206. MacLeod, S. K. "Moisture Determination Using Karl Fischer Titrations." *Analytical Chemistry* 63, no. 10 (1991): 557A–66A.

207. Margreth, M., R. Schlink, and A. Steinbach. "Water Determination by Karl Fischer Titration." In *Pharmaceutical Sciences Encyclopedia: Drug Discovery, Development, and Manufacturing*, edited by S. Grad, 1–34. Hoboken, NJ: Wiley, 2010.

208. Ronkart, S. N., M. Paquot, C. Fougnies, C. Deroanne, J.-C. Van Herck, and C. Blecker. "Determination of Total Water Content in Inulin Using the Volumetric Karl Fischer Titration." *Talanta* 70, no. 5 (2006): 1006–10.

209. Schöffski, K. "New Karl Fischer Reagents for the Water Determination in Food." *Food Control* 12, no. 7 (2001): 427–9.

210. Louër, D. "Powder X-Ray Diffraction, Applications." In *Encyclopedia of Spectroscopy and Spectrometry*. 3rd ed, edited by J. C. Lindon, G. E. Tranter, and D. W. Koppenaal, 723–31. Oxford: Academic Press, 2017.

211. Finkelstein, D. M. *A Beginner's Guide to Structural Equation Modeling*. Taylor & Francis, 2005.

212. Schick, C. "Differential Scanning Calorimetry (DSC) of Semicrystalline Polymers." *Analytical & Bioanalytical Chemistry* 395, no. 6 (2009): 1589.

213. Liu, J., D. R. Rigsbee, C. Stotz, and M. J. Pikal. "Dynamics of Pharmaceutical Amorphous Solids: The Study of Enthalpy Relaxation by Isothermal Microcalorimetry." *Journal of Pharmaceutical Sciences* 91, no. 8 (2002): 1853–62.

214. Rehman, M., B. Y. Shekunov, P. York, D. Lechuga-Ballesteros, D. P. Miller, T. Tan, and P. Colthorpe. "Optimisation of Powders for Pulmonary Delivery Using Supercritical Fluid Technology." *European Journal of Pharmaceutical Sciences* 22, no. 1 (2004): 1–17.

215. D'Sa, D. J., D. Lechuga-Ballesteros, and H.-K. Chan. "Isothermal Microcalorimetry of Pressurized Systems II: Effect of Excipient and Water Ingress on Formulation Stability of Amorphous Glycopyrrolate." *Pharmaceutical Research* 32, no. 2 (2015): 714–22.

216. Lehto, V.-P., M. Tenho, K. Vähä-Heikkilä, P. Harjunen, M. Päällysaho, J. Välisaari, P. Niemelä, and K. Järvinen. "The Comparison of Seven Different Methods to Quantify the Amorphous Content of Spray Dried Lactose." *Powder Technology* 167, no. 2 (2006): 85–93.

217. Kumar, A., P. Singh, and A. Nanda. "Hot Stage Microscopy and Its Applications in Pharmaceutical Characterization." *Applied Microscopy* 50, no. 1 (2020): 1–11.

218. Panna, W., P. Wyszomirski, and P. Kohut. "Application of Hot-Stage Microscopy to Evaluating Sample Morphology Changes on Heating." *Journal of Thermal Analysis & Calorimetry* 125, no. 3 (2016): 1053–9.

219. Stieger, N., M. Aucamp, S. W. Zhang, and M. De Villiers. "Hot-Stage Optical Microscopy as an Analytical Tool to Understand Solid-State Changes in Pharmaceutical Materials." *American Pharmaceutical Review* 15 (2012): 32–6.

220. Park, C. W., Y. S. Rhee, F. Vogt, D. J. Hayes, J. B. Zwischenberger, P. P. DeLuca et al. "Advances in Microscopy and Complementary Imaging Techniques to Assess the Fate of Drugs Ex-Vivo in Respiratory Drug Delivery." Invited paper. *Advanced Drug Delivery Reviews* 64, no. 4 (2011): 344–56.

221. Alabsi, W., F. A. Al-Obeidi, R. Polt, and H. M. Mansour. "Organic Solution Advanced Spray-Dried Microparticulate/Nanoparticulate Dry Powders of Lactomorphin for Respiratory Delivery: Physicochemical Characterization, In Vitro Aerosol Dispersion, and Cellular Studies." *Pharmaceutics* 13, no. 1 (2021): Article 26.

222. Li, X., F. Vogt, D. J. Hayes, and H. Mansour. "Design, Characterization, and Aerosol Dispersion Performance Modeling of Advanced Spray-Dried Microparticulate/Nanoparticulate Mannitol Powders for Targeted Pulmonary Delivery as Dry Powder Inhalers." *Journal of Aerosol Medicine & Pulmonary Drug Delivery* 27, no. 2 (2014): 81–93.

223. Muralidharan, P., D. J. Hayes, S. M. Black, and H. M. Mansour. "Microparticulate/Nanoparticulate Powders of a Novel Nrf2 Activator and an Aerosol Performance Enhancer for Pulmonary Delivery Targeting the Lung Nrf2/Keap-1 Pathway." *Molecular Systems Design & Engineering* 1, no. 1 (2016): 48–65.

224. Gomez, A. I., M. F. Acosta, P. Muralidharan, J. X. Yuan, S. M. Black, D. J. Hayes, and H. M. Mansour. "Advanced Spray Dried Proliposomes of Amphotericin B Lung Surfactant-Mimic Phospholipid Microparticles/Nanoparticles as Dry Powder Inhalers for Targeted Pulmonary Drug Delivery." *Pulmonary Pharmacology & Therapeutics* 64 (2020): 101975.

225. Muralidharan, P., B. A. Jones, G. Allaway, S. S. Biswal, and H. M. Mansour. "Llaway G, Biswal SS, Mansour HM. Design and Development of Innovative Microparticulate/Nanoparticulate Inhalable Dry Powders of a Novel Synthetic Trifluorinated Chalcone Derivative and Nrf2 Agonist." *Scientfic Reports* 10, no. 1 (2020): 19771.

226. Mansour, H. M., and A. J. Hickey. "Raman Characterization and Chemical Imaging of Biocolloidal Self-Assemblies, Drug Delivery Systems, and Pulmonary Inhalation Aerosols: A Review." *AAPS PharmSciTech* 8, no. 4 (2007): E99.

227. Glassford, S. E., B. Byrne, and S. G. Kazarian. "Recent Applications of ATR FTIR Spectroscopy and Imaging to Proteins." *Biochimica & Biophysica Acta (BBA): Proteins & Proteomics* 12, no. 1834 (2013): 2849–58.

228. Lee, L. C., C.-Y. Liong, and A. A. Jemain. "A Contemporary Review on Data Preprocessing (DP) Practice Strategy in ATR-FTIR Spectrum." *Chemometrics & Intelligent Laboratory Systems* 163 (2017): 64–75.

229. Butler, H. J., L. Ashton, B. Bird, G. Cinque, K. Curtis, J. Dorney, K. Esmonde-White, N. J. Fullwood, B. Gardner, P. L. Martin-Hirsch, M. J. Walsh, M. R. McAinsh, N. Stone, and F. L. Martin. "Using Raman Spectroscopy to Characterize Biological Materials." *Nature Protocols* 11, no. 4 (2016): 664–87.

230. Chapter Four, Damodaran K. "Recent NMR Studies of Ionic Liquids." In *Annual Reports on NMR Spectroscopy*, edited by G. A. Webb vol. 88, 215–44. Boston, MA: Academic Press, 2016.

231. Eedara, B. B., I. G. Tucker, Z. D. Zujovic, T. Rades, J. R. Price, and S. C. Das. "Crystalline Adduct of Moxifloxacin with Trans-Cinnamic Acid to Reduce the Aqueous Solubility and Dissolution Rate for Improved Residence Time in the Lungs." *European Journal of Pharmaceutical Sciences* 136 (2019): 104961.

232. Johnson, W. C. "Analyzing Protein Circular Dichroism Spectra for Accurate Secondary Structures." *Proteins: Structure, Function, & Bioinformatics* 35, no. 3 (1999): 307–12.

233. Eedara, B. B., I. G. Tucker, and S. C. Das. "A STELLA Simulation Model for In Vitro Dissolution Testing of Respirable Size Particles" *Scientific Report* 9, no. 1 (2019): 18522.

234. Freund-Michel, V., N. Khoyrattee, J. P. Savineau, B. Muller, and C. Guibert. "Mitochondria: Roles in Pulmonary Hypertension." *International Journal of Biochemistry & Cell Biology* 55 (2014): 93–7.

235. Aggarwal, S., C. M. Gross, S. Sharma, J. R. Fineman, and S. M. Black. "Reactive Oxygen Species in Pulmonary Vascular Remodeling." *Comprehensive Physiology* 3, no. 3 (2013): 1011–34.

236. Ten, V. S., and V. Ratner. "Mitochondrial Bioenergetics and Pulmonary Dysfunction: Current Progress and Future Directions." *Paediatric Respiratory Reviews* 34 (2020): 37–45.

237. Mabalirajan, U., and B. Ghosh. "Mitochondrial Dysfunction in Metabolic Syndrome and Asthma." *Journal of Allergy* 2013 (2013): 340476.

238. Ryter, S. W., I. O. Rosas, C. A. Owen, F. J. Martinez, M. E. Choi, C. G. Lee, J. A. Elias, and A. M. K. Choi. "Mitochondrial Dysfunction as a Pathogenic Mediator of Chronic Obstructive Pulmonary Disease and Idiopathic Pulmonary Fibrosis." *Annals of the American Thoracic Society* 15, no. Suppl 4 (2018): S266–SS72.

239. Larson-Casey, J. L., C. He, and A. B. Carter. "Mitochondrial Quality Control in Pulmonary Fibrosis." *Redox Biology* 33 (2020): 101426.

240. Gupta, A., and T. Becker. "Mechanisms and Pathways of Mitochondrial Outer Membrane Protein Biogenesis." *Biochimica & Biophysica Acta: Bioenergetics* 1862, no. 1 (2021): 148323.

241. Hoogenraad, N. J., and M. T. Ryan. "Translocation of Proteins into Mitochondria." *IUBMB Life* 51, no. 6 (2001): 345–50.

242. Endo, T., and H. Sakaue. "Multifaceted Roles of Porin in Mitochondrial Protein and Lipid Transport." *Biochemical Society Transactions* 47, no. 5 (2019): 1269–77.

243. Pfanner, N., and M. Meijer. "The Tom and Tim Machine." *Current Biology* 7, no. 2 (1997): R100–R3.

244. Kim, S., H. Y. Nam, J. Lee, and J. Seo. "Mitochondrion-Targeting Peptides and Peptidomimetics: Recent Progress and Design Principles." *Biochemistry* 59, no. 3 (2020): 270–84.

245. Popov, L. D. "Mitochondrial Peptides-Appropriate Options for Therapeutic Exploitation." *Cell & Tissue Research* 377, no. 2 (2019): 161–5.

246. Agrawal, A., and U. Mabalirajan. "Rejuvenating Cellular Respiration for Optimizing Respiratory Function: Targeting Mitochondria." *American Journal of Physiology. Lung Cellular & Molecular Physiology* 310, no. 2 (2016): L103–L13.

247. Murphy, M. P., and R. A. Smith. "Drug Delivery to Mitochondria: The Key to Mitochondrial Medicine." *Advanced Drug Delivery Reviews* 41, no. 2 (2000): 235–50.

248. Yang, D., D. Xu, T. Wang, Z. Yuan, L. Liu, Y. Shen, and F. Wen. "Mitoquinone Ameliorates Cigarette Smoke-Induced Airway Inflammation and Mucus Hypersecretion in Mice." *International Immunopharmacology* 90 (2021): 107149.

249. Li, R., T. Ren, and J. Zeng. "Mitochondrial Coenzyme Q Protects Sepsis-Induced Acute Lung Injury by Activating PI3K/Akt/GSK-3beta/mTOR Pathway in Rats." *BioMed Research International* 2019 (2019): 5240898.

250. Suresh, K., L. Servinsky, H. Jiang, Z. Bigham, J. Zaldumbide, J. C. Huetsch, C. Kliment, M. G. Acoba, B. J. Kirsch, S. M. Claypool, A. Le, M. Damarla, and L. A. Shimoda. "Regulation of Mitochondrial Fragmentation in Microvascular Endothelial Cells Isolated from the SU5416/Hypoxia Model of Pulmonary Arterial Hypertension." *American Journal of Physiology. Lung Cellular & Molecular Physiology* 317, no. 5 (2019): L639–LL52.

251. Suresh, K., L. Servinsky, H. Jiang, Z. Bigham, X. Yun, C. Kliment, J. Huetsch, M. Damarla, and L. A. Shimoda. "Reactive Oxygen Species Induced Ca(2+) Influx via TRPV4 and Microvascular Endothelial Dysfunction in the SU5416/Hypoxia Model of Pulmonary Arterial Hypertension." *American Journal of Physiology. Lung Cellular & Molecular Physiology* 314, no. 5 (2018): L893–L907.

252. Ouyang, L., and J. Gong. "Mitochondrial-Targeted Ubiquinone: A Potential Treatment for COVID-19." *Medical Hypotheses* 144 (2020): 110161.

253. Szeto, H. H. "Cell-Permeable, Mitochondrial-Targeted, Peptide Antioxidants." *AAPS Journal* 8, no. 2 (2006): E277–E83.

254. Szeto, H. H. "Mitochondria-Targeted Peptide Antioxidants: Novel Neuroprotective Agents." *AAPS Journal* 8, no. 3 (2006): E521–E31.

255. Szeto, H. H., and P. W. Schiller. "Novel Therapies Targeting Inner Mitochondrial Membrane--From Discovery to Clinical Development." *Pharmaceutical Research* 28, no. 11 (2011): 2669–79.

256. Szeto, H. H. "Mitochondria-Targeted Cytoprotective Peptides for Ischemia-Reperfusion Injury." *Antioxidants & Redox Signaling* 10, no. 3 (2008): 601–19.

257. Szeto, H. H. "Development of Mitochondria-Targeted Aromatic-Cationic Peptides for Neurodegenerative Diseases." *Annals of the New York Academy of Sciences* 1147 (2008): 112–21.

258. Szeto, H. H., and A. V. Birk. "Serendipity and the Discovery of Novel Compounds That Restore Mitochondrial Plasticity." *Clinical Pharmacology & Therapeutics* 96, no. 6 (2014): 672–83.

259. Zhao, K., G. M. Zhao, D. Wu, Y. Soong, A. V. Birk, P. W. Schiller, and H. H. Szeto. "Cell-Permeable Peptide Antioxidants Targeted to Inner Mitochondrial Membrane Inhibit Mitochondrial Swelling, Oxidative Cell Death, and Reperfusion Injury." *Journal of Biological Chemistry* 279, no. 33 (2004): 34682–90.

260. Zhao, K., G. Luo, S. Giannelli, and H. H. Szeto. "Mitochondria-Targeted Peptide Prevents Mitochondrial Depolarization and Apoptosis Induced by Tert-Butyl Hydroperoxide in Neuronal Cell Lines." *Biochemistry & Pharmacology* 70, no. 12 (2005): 1796–806.

261. Wang, H., X. Sun, Q. Lu, E. A. Zemskov, M. Yegambaram, X. Wu, T. Wang, H. Tang, and S. M. Black. "The Mitochondrial Redistribution of eNOS Is Involved in Lipopolysaccharide Induced Inflammasome Activation During Acute Lung Injury." *Redox Biology* 41 (2021): 101878.

262. Archer, S. L., G. Marsboom, G. H. Kim, H. J. Zhang, P. T. Toth, E. C. Svensson, J. R. Dyck, M. Gomberg-Maitland, B. Thébaud, A. N. Husain, N. Cipriani, and J. Rehman. "Epigenetic Attenuation of Mitochondrial Superoxide Dismutase 2 in Pulmonary Arterial Hypertension: A Basis for Excessive Cell Proliferation and a New Therapeutic Target." *Circulation* 121, no. 24 (2010): 2661–71.

263. Rehman, J., and S. L. Archer. "A Proposed Mitochondrial-Metabolic Mechanism for Initiation and Maintenance of Pulmonary Arterial Hypertension in Fawn-Hooded Rats: The Warburg Model of Pulmonary Arterial Hypertension." *Advances in Experimental Medicine & Biology* 661 (2010): 171–85.

264. Rafikov, R., X. Sun, O. Rafikova, M. Louise Meadows, A. A. Desai, Z. Khalpey, J. X. Yuan, J. R. Fineman, and S. M. Black. "Complex I Dysfunction Underlies the Glycolytic Switch in Pulmonary Hypertensive Smooth Muscle Cells." *Redox Biology* 6 (2015): 278–86.

265. Masri, F. A., W. Xu, S. A. Comhair, K. Asosingh, M. Koo, A. Vasanji, J. Drazba, B. Anand-Apte, and S. C. Erzurum. "Hyperproliferative Apoptosis-Resistant Endothelial Cells in Idiopathic Pulmonary Arterial Hypertension." *American Journal of Physiology. Lung Cellular & Molecular Physiology* 293, no. 3 (2007): L548–L54.

266. Xu, W., T. Koeck, A. R. Lara, D. Neumann, F. P. DiFilippo, M. Koo, A. J. Janocha, F. A. Masri, A. C. Arroliga, C. Jennings, R. A. Dweik, R. M. Tuder, D. J. Stuehr, and S. C. Erzurum. "Alterations of Cellular Bioenergetics in Pulmonary Artery Endothelial Cells." *Proceedings of the National Academy of Sciences of the United States of America* 104, no. 4 (2007): 1342–7.

267. Sun, X., S. Sharma, S. Fratz, S. Kumar, R. Rafikov, S. Aggarwal, O. Rafikova, Q. Lu, T. Burns, S. Dasarathy, J. Wright, C. Schreiber, M. Radman, J. R. Fineman, and S. M. Black. "Disruption of Endothelial Cell Mitochondrial Bioenergetics in Lambs with Increased Pulmonary Blood Flow." *Antioxidants & Redox Signaling* 18, no. 14 (2013): 1739–52.

268. Sun, X., S. Kumar, S. Sharma, S. Aggarwal, Q. Lu, C. Gross, O. Rafikova, S. G. Lee, S. Dasarathy, Y. Hou, M. L. Meadows, W. Han, Y. Su, J. R. Fineman, and S. M. Black. "Endothelin-1 Induces a Glycolytic Switch in Pulmonary Arterial Endothelial Cells via the Mitochondrial Translocation of Endothelial Nitric Oxide Synthase." *American Journal of Respiratory Cell & Molecular Biology* 50, no. 6 (2014): 1084–95.

269. Sharma, S., N. Sud, D. A. Wiseman, A. L. Carter, S. Kumar, Y. Hou, T. Rau, J. Wilham, C. Harmon, P. Oishi, J. R. Fineman, and S. M. Black. "Altered Carnitine Homeostasis Is Associated with Decreased Mitochondrial Function and Altered Nitric Oxide Signaling in Lambs with Pulmonary Hypertension." *American Journal of Physiology. Lung Cellular & Molecular Physiology* 294, no. 1 (2008): L46–L56.

270. Sharma, S., A. Aramburo, R. Rafikov, X. Sun, S. Kumar, P. E. Oishi, S. A. Datar, G. Raff, K. Xoinis, G. Kalkan, S. Fratz, J. R. Fineman, and S. M. Black. "L-Carnitine Preserves Endothelial Function in a Lamb Model of Increased Pulmonary Blood Flow." *Pediatric Research* 74, no. 1 (2013): 39–47.

271. Acosta, M. F., P. Muralidharan, M. D. Abrahamson, C. L. Grijalva, M. Carver, H. Tang, C. Klinger, J. R. Fineman, S. M. Black, and H. M. Mansour. "Comparison of L-Carnitine and L-Carnitine HCL Salt for Targeted Lung Treatment of Pulmonary Hypertension (PH) as Inhalation Aerosols: Design, Comprehensive Characterization, In Vitro 2D/3D Cell Cultures, and In Vivo MCT-Rat Model of PH." *Pulmonary Pharmacology & Therapeutics* 65 (2021): 101998.

272. Sharma, S., X. Sun, R. Rafikov, S. Kumar, Y. Hou, P. E. Oishi, S. A. Datar, G. Raff, J. R. Fineman, and S. M. Black. "PPAR-Gamma Regulates Carnitine Homeostasis and Mitochondrial Function in a Lamb Model of Increased Pulmonary Blood Flow." *PLOS ONE* 7, no. 9 (2012): e41555.

273. Oishi, P. E., S. Sharma, S. A. Datar, S. Kumar, S. Aggarwal, Q. Lu, G. Raff, A. Azakie, J. H. Hsu, E. Sajti, S. Fratz, S. M. Black, and J. R. Fineman. "Rosiglitazone Preserves Pulmonary Vascular Function in Lambs with Increased Pulmonary Blood Flow." *Pediatric Research* 73, no. 1 (2013): 54–61.

274. Bonnet, S., S. L. Archer, J. Allalunis-Turner, A. Haromy, C. Beaulieu, R. Thompson, C. T. Lee, G. D. Lopaschuk, L. Puttagunta, S. Bonnet, G. Harry, K. Hashimoto, C. J. Porter, M. A. Andrade, B. Thebaud, and E. D. Michelakis. "A Mitochondria-K+ Channel Axis Is Suppressed in Cancer and Its Normalization Promotes Apoptosis and Inhibits Cancer Growth." *Cancer Cell* 11, no. 1 (2007): 37–51.

275. Archer, S. L., Y. H. Fang, J. J. Ryan, and L. Piao. "Metabolism and Bioenergetics in the Right Ventricle and Pulmonary Vasculature in Pulmonary Hypertension." *Pulmonary Circulation* 3, no. 1 (2013): 144–52.

276. Michelakis, E. D., M. S. McMurtry, X. C. Wu, J. R. Dyck, R. Moudgil, T. A. Hopkins, G. D. Lopaschuk, L. Puttagunta, R. Waite, and S. L. Archer. "Dichloroacetate, a Metabolic Modulator, Prevents and Reverses Chronic Hypoxic Pulmonary Hypertension in Rats: Role of Increased Expression and Activity of Voltage-Gated Potassium Channels." *Circulation* 105, no. 2 (2002): 244–50.

277. Michelakis, E. D., J. R. Dyck, M. S. McMurtry, S. Wang, X. C. Wu, R. Moudgil, K. Hashimoto, L. Puttagunta, and S. L. Archer. "Gene Transfer and Metabolic Modulators as New Therapies for Pulmonary Hypertension. Increasing Expression and Activity of Potassium Channels in Rat and Human Models." *Advances in Experimental Medicine & Biology* 502 (2001): 401–18.

278. Michelakis, E. D., V. Gurtu, L. Webster, G. Barnes, G. Watson, L. Howard, J. Cupitt, I. Paterson, R. B. Thompson, K. Chow, D. P. O'Regan, L. Zhao, J. Wharton, D. G. Kiely, A. Kinnaird, A. E. Boukouris, C. White, J. Nagendran, D. H. Freed, S. J. Wort, J. S. R. Gibbs, and M. R. Wilkins. "Inhibition of Pyruvate Dehydrogenase Kinase Improves Pulmonary Arterial Hypertension in Genetically Susceptible Patients." *Science Translational Medicine* 9, no. 413 (2017): 1–12.

279. Aich, J., U. Mabalirajan, T. Ahmad, K. Khanna, R. Rehman, A. Agrawal, and B. Ghosh. "Resveratrol Attenuates Experimental Allergic Asthma in Mice by Restoring Inositol Polyphosphate 4 Phosphatase (INPP4A)." *International Immunopharmacology* 14, no. 4 (2012): 438–43.

280. Mabalirajan, U., T. Ahmad, G. D. Leishangthem, A. K. Dinda, A. Agrawal, and B. Ghosh. "L-Arginine Reduces Mitochondrial Dysfunction and Airway Injury in Murine Allergic Airway Inflammation." *International Immunopharmacology* 10, no. 12 (2010): 1514–9.

281. Sun, X., S. Fratz, S. Sharma, Y. Hou, R. Rafikov, S. Kumar, I. Rehmani, J. Tian, A. Smith, C. Schreiber, J. Reiser, S. Naumann, S. Haag, J. Hess, J. D. Catravas, C. Patterson, J. R. Fineman, and S. M. Black. "C-Terminus of Heat Shock protein 70-Interacting Protein-Dependent GTP Cyclohydrolase I Degradation in Lambs with Increased Pulmonary Blood Flow." *American Journal of Respiratory Cell & Molecular Biology* 45, no. 1 (2011): 163–71.

282. Calixto, M. C., L. Lintomen, D. M. Andre, L. O. Leiria, D. Ferreira, C. Lellis-Santos, G. F. Anhê, S. Bordin, R. G. Landgraf, and E. Antunes. "Metformin Attenuates the Exacerbation of the Allergic Eosinophilic Inflammation in High Fat-Diet-Induced Obesity in Mice." *PLOS ONE* 8, no. 10 (2013): e76786.

283. Acosta, M. F., M. D. Abrahamson, D. Encinas-Basurto, J. R. Fineman, S. M. Black, and H. M. Mansour. "Inhalable Nanoparticles/Microparticles of an AMPK and Nrf2 Activator for Targeted Pulmonary Drug Delivery as Dry Powder Inhalers." *AAPS Journal* 23, no. 1 (2020): 2.

284. Lewis, B. P., I. H. Shih, M. W. Jones-Rhoades, D. P. Bartel, and C. B. Burge. "Prediction of Mammalian microRNA Targets." *Cell* 115, no. 7 (2003): 787–98.

285. Sharma, A., M. Kumar, T. Ahmad, U. Mabalirajan, J. Aich, A. Agrawal, and B. Ghosh. "Antagonism of mmu-mir-106a Attenuates Asthma Features in Allergic Murine Model." *Journal of Applied Physiology* 113, no. 3 (2012): 459–64.

286. Indrieri, A., S. Carrella, A. Romano, A. Spaziano, E. Marrocco, E. Fernandez-Vizarra, S. Barbato, M. Pizzo, Y. Ezhova, F. M. Golia, L. Ciampi, R. Tammaro, J. Henao-Mejia, A. Williams, R. A. Flavell, E. De Leonibus, M. Zeviani, E. M. Surace, S. Banfi, and B. Franco. "miR-181a/b Downregulation Exerts a Protective Action on Mitochondrial Disease Models." *EMBO Molecular Medicine* 11, no. 5 (2019): 1–16.

287. Kumar, M., T. Ahmad, A. Sharma, U. Mabalirajan, A. Kulshreshtha, A. Agrawal et al. "Let-7 microRNA-Mediated Regulation of IL-13 and Allergic Airway Inflammation." *Journal of Allergy & Clinical Immunology* 128, no. 5: (2011): 1077-85, e1–e10.

288. Kumar, M., U. Mabalirajan, A. Agrawal, and B. Ghosh. "Proinflammatory Role of let-7 miRNAs in Experimental Asthma?." *Journal of Biological Chemistry* 285, no. 48 (2010): le19: author reply le20.

289. Polikepahad, S., J. M. Knight, A. O. Naghavi, T. Oplt, C. J. Creighton, C. Shaw, A. L. Benham, J. Kim, B. Soibam, R. A. Harris, C. Coarfa, A. Zariff, A. Milosavljevic, L. M. Batts, F. Kheradmand, P. H. Gunaratne, and D. B. Corry. "Proinflammatory Role for let-7 MicroRNAs in Experimental Asthma." *Journal of Biological Chemistry* 285, no. 39 (2010): 30139–49.

290. Mohamed, J. S., A. Hajira, P. S. Pardo, and A. M. Boriek. "MicroRNA-149 Inhibits PARP-2 and Promotes Mitochondrial Biogenesis via SIRT-1/PGC-1alpha Network in Skeletal Muscle." *Diabetes* 63, no. 5 (2014): 1546–59.

291. Xu, Y., C. Zhao, X. Sun, Z. Liu, and J. Zhang. "MicroRNA-761 Regulates Mitochondrial Biogenesis in Mouse Skeletal Muscle in Response to Exercise." *Biochemical & Biophysical Research Communications* 467, no. 1 (2015): 103–8.

292. Long, B., K. Wang, N. Li, I. Murtaza, J. Y. Xiao, Y. Y. Fan, C. Y. Liu, W. H. Li, Z. Cheng, and P. Li. "miR-761 Regulates the Mitochondrial Network by Targeting Mitochondrial Fission Factor." *Free Radical Biology & Medicine* 65 (2013): 371–9.

293. Li, J., S. Donath, Y. Li, D. Qin, B. S. Prabhakar, and P. Li. "miR-30 Regulates Mitochondrial Fission Through Targeting p53 and the Dynamin-Related protein-1 Pathway." *PLOS Genetics* 6, no. 1 (2010): e1000795.

294. Rahman, M. H., and K. Suk. "Mitochondrial Dynamics and Bioenergetic Alteration During Inflammatory Activation of Astrocytes." *Frontiers in Aging Neuroscience* 12 (2020): 614410.

295. Tanaka, H., T. Sasayama, K. Tanaka, S. Nakamizo, M. Nishihara, K. Mizukawa, M. Kohta, J. Koyama, S. Miyake, M. Taniguchi, K. Hosoda, and E. Kohmura. "MicroRNA-183 Upregulates HIF-1Alpha by Targeting Isocitrate Dehydrogenase 2 (IDH2) in Glioma Cells." *Journal of Neuro-Oncology* 111, no. 3 (2013): 273–83.

296. Bertero, T., Annis S. LY, A. Hale, B. Bhat, R. Saggar, R. Saggar, W. D. Wallace, D. J. Ross, S. O. Vargas, B. B. Graham, R. Kumar, S. M. Black, S. Fratz, J. R. Fineman, J. D. West, K. J. Haley, A. B. Waxman, B. N. Chau, K. A. Cottrill, S. Y. Chan, and S. Y. Chan. "Systems-Level Regulation of microRNA Networks by miR-130/301 Promotes Pulmonary Hypertension." *Journal of Clinical Investigation* 124, no. 8 (2014 Aug.): 3514–28.

297. Sharma, S., J. Barton, R. Rafikov, S. Aggarwal, H. C. Kuo, P. E. Oishi, S. A. Datar, J. R. Fineman, and S. M. Black. "Chronic Inhibition of PPAR-Gamma Signaling Induces Endothelial Dysfunction in the Juvenile Lamb." *Pulmonary Pharmacology & Therapeutics* 26, no. 2 (2013): 271–80.

298. Indrieri, A., S. Carrella, P. Carotenuto, S. Banfi, and B. Franco. "The Pervasive Role of the mir-181 Family in Development, Neurodegeneration, and Cancer." *International Journal of Molecular Sciences* 21, no. 6 (2020): 1–25.

299. Fu, A. "Mitotherapy as a Novel Therapeutic Strategy for Mitochondrial Diseases." *Current Molecular Pharmacology* 13, no. 1 (2020): 41–9.

300. Nakamura, Y., J. H. Park, and K. Hayakawa. "Therapeutic Use of Extracellular Mitochondria in CNS Injury and Disease." *Experimental Neurology* 324 (2020): 113114.

301. Silva, J. D., Y. Su, C. S. Calfee, K. L. Delucchi, D. Weiss, D. F. McAuley et al. "MSC Extracellular Vesicles Rescue Mitochondrial Dysfunction and Improve Barrier Integrity in Clinically Relevant Models of ARDS." *European Respiratory Journal* 58, no. 1 (2020): 1–18.

302. Li, X., Y. Zhang, S. C. Yeung, Y. Liang, X. Liang, Y. Ding, M. S. Ip, H. F. Tse, J. C. Mak, and Q. Lian. "Mitochondrial Transfer of Induced Pluripotent Stem Cell-Derived Mesenchymal Stem Cells to Airway Epithelial Cells Attenuates Cigarette Smoke-Induced Damage." *American Journal of Respiratory Cell & Molecular Biology* 51, no. 3 (2014): 455–65.

303. Morrison, T. J., M. V. Jackson, E. K. Cunningham, A. Kissenpfennig, D. F. McAuley, C. M. O'Kane, and A. D. Krasnodembskaya. "Mesenchymal Stromal Cells Modulate Macrophages in Clinically Relevant Lung Injury Models by Extracellular Vesicle Mitochondrial Transfer." *American Journal of Respiratory & Critical Care Medicine* 196, no. 10 (2017): 1275–86.

304. Islam, M. N., S. R. Das, M. T. Emin, M. Wei, L. Sun, K. Westphalen, D. J. Rowlands, S. K. Quadri, S. Bhattacharya, and J. Bhattacharya. "Mitochondrial Transfer from Bone-Marrow-Derived Stromal Cells to Pulmonary Alveoli Protects Against Acute Lung Injury." *Nature Medicine* 18, no. 5 (2012): 759–65.

Cardiovascular Drug Delivery

8

Jingyan Han, Jena B. Goodman, Mo Zhang, and Zhaoyuan Li

Contents

8.1 INTRODUCTION

The cardiovascular system consisting of the heart and all blood vessels is responsible for the flow of blood, nutrients, oxygen and other gases, and hormones to and from tissues and cells, thus being the center of vitality in the body. Any problem that arises within this system is known as cardiovascular disease (CVD). Despite significant improvements in cardiovascular mortality over the past several decades as a result of significant advances in prevention, diagnosis, and treatment, CVD continues to represent the dominant cause of death among the most prevalent chronic diseases, remaining both a public health concern and growing global challenge. The most up-to-date statistics released by the American Heart Association indicate that in 2017, the overall prevalence of CVD was 485.6 million cases, an increase of 28.5% compared with 2007. Disturbingly, 17.8 million deaths were attributed to CVD globally which was

DOI: 10.1201/9781003092773-9

a 21.1% increase over the past 10 years. (Virani et al., 2020) The estimated annual direct costs of CVD in the United States in 2014–2015 almost doubled since 1996 (103.5 billion in 1996–1997, 213.8 billion in 2014–2015). These facts and statistics clearly underscore the urgent need for innovative therapeutic strategies for CVD. Notwithstanding this steady increase in CVD prevalence, the cardiovascular drug pipeline has been stagnant over the past two decades. With the remarkable advent of systems-based scientific approaches (e.g., functional genomics, proteomics, chemi-informatics), never before has so much information been generated pertaining to causal mechanisms driving CVD and potential new therapeutic targets. Unfortunately, these scientific advances have not stimulated drug development with fewer candidates in the cardiovascular research pipeline – for example, the cardiovascular drug development decreased ~4.57% from 1990–1999 to 2000–2007 contrasting with other therapeutic areas (Pammolli, Magazzini, & Riccaboni, 2011). This adverted trend has been attributed to the complex and costly pathway for drug development as well as the high cost of conducting cardiovascular outcome trials. But inefficient translation from promising candidates into effective therapies is the key issue thwarting the development of novel CVD treatments.

Innovative drug delivery systems (DDS) may provide new and unique treatment opportunities for CVD by transcending the shortcomings of current available therapies or facilitating the translation from novel candidates to approved drugs. DDS are defined as a formulation or device that enables a therapeutic substance to selectively reach its site of action and release in a controlled manner. Although there is no specific DDS approved for the diagnosis or treatment of CVD, several clinical trials have demonstrated the potential of DDS to overcome disadvantages of systemic drug administration, and improve cardiovascular outcomes (Cicha et al., 2018). Current medications for CVD are almost exclusively small molecules and administrated orally for chronic therapeutics such as statins, beta-blockers, and aspirin. However, there are many new biologics such as insoluble proteins, unstable genetic materials, and small molecules with poor kinetic or distribution patterns, which hold great potential therapeutic value in the battle against CVD, but they cannot exert their efficacy and sometimes may lead to deleterious side effects if they are administrated systemically and cannot be effectively delivered and released at diseased sites. This challenge has been part of the driving force to develop specific drug delivery systems that can target the cardiovascular system and diseases, achieving maximal efficacy while minimizing systemic toxicity. The DDS were first intensively researched in the oncology therapeutic area and successfully facilitated the conversion of non-druglike candidates into approved chemotherapeutics, improving mortality rates for oncology patients (Wolfram et al., 2015). For instance, liposomal encapsulation, polyethylene glycol (PEG) modification, and monoclonal antibody or fusion proteins targeted to cell surface receptors are well-established tools with reduced systemic toxicity compared to amphotericin B, doxorubicin, and cytosine arabinose (e.g., Doxil®, Abraxane®, AmBisome®). Fusion proteins (e.g., interleukin-2/diphtheria toxin fusion) and various cell surface-specific monoclonal antibodies (e.g., Rituxan, Berxaar) have proven to be successful strategies for chemotherapy (Sawyers, 2004). Research evaluating DDS efficacy in the cardiovascular system is still in its infancy. To date, there is no approved nanomedicine for CVD treatments. Having said that, a growing number of preclinical and clinical studies give credence to the idea that sophisticated drug delivery systems/devices can improve the pharmacokinetic properties of the current cardiovascular drugs by facilitating delivery and disease-site specificity.

This chapter first briefly introduces the physiology of the cardiovascular system, the major cardiovascular diseases, and currently available treatments with a focus on myocardial infarction and atherosclerosis, which are the primary causes of CVD (Figure 8.1). Building on this information, this chapter next summarizes the cardiovascular DDS that have been developed to (1) improve the pharmacokinetic and pharmacodynamics properties of currently existing cardiovascular drugs; (2) increase delivery payloads (drugs, genetic materials, stem cells) to the specific disease sites of heart and blood vessels; (3) ameliorate pathogenic processes that drive cardiovascular diseases (high lipid levels, oxidative stress, endothelial dysfunction, inflammation, and thrombosis), highlighting how these new drug delivery systems provide new perspectives in the treatment of CVD (Figure 8.2).

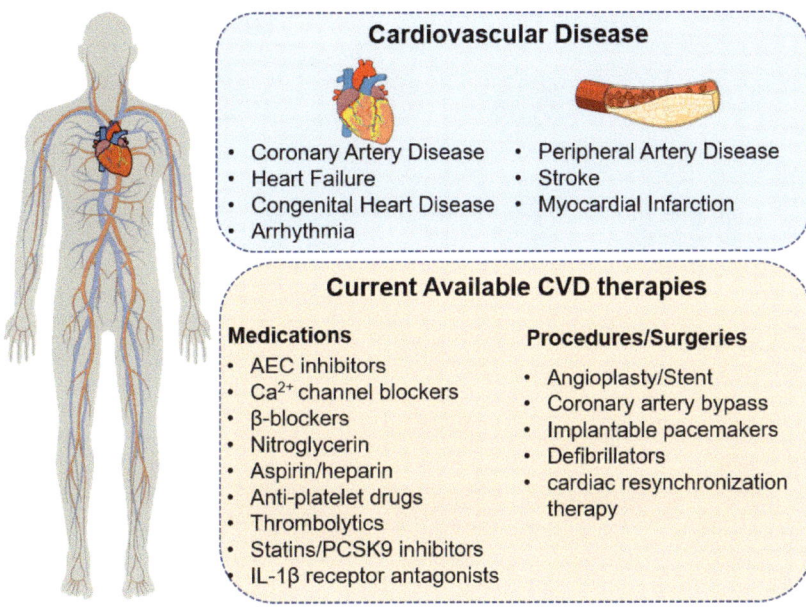

FIGURE 8.1   The cardiovascular system, main cardiovascular diseases, and currently available CVD therapies.

8.2 CARDIOVASCULAR SYSTEM AND DISEASES

8.2.1 Heart

8.2.1.1 Heart: Anatomy, Physiology, and Cell Biology

The heart was first described as a three-chambered organ by the Greek philosopher Aristotle in the fourth century (BC). Aristotle deduced that the heart was the most important organ in the body, with its continuous activity and unique durability, noting the heart's resistance to injury (Pagel, 1970). Nowadays, we know the heart consists of four chambers: two upper chambers called the left atrium and right atrium, and two lower chambers known as the left and right ventricles. The heart acts like a dual-chambered pump that circulates blood through the blood vessels by repeated, rhythmic contractions. One movement of blood during one heartbeat is called a cardiac cycle. The sequence of the cardiac cycle is as follows: (1) de-oxygenated blood returning to the heart enters the right atrium, which is then pumped through the tricuspid valve into the right ventricle; (2) the right ventricle pushes the blood into the lungs via the pulmonary artery, where it becomes oxygenated; (3) oxygenated blood returns and enters the left atrium of the heart via the pulmonary vein; (4) ultimately, oxygenated blood passes through the mitral valve into the left ventricle, where it is forcefully extruded through the aorta supplying oxygen to tissues throughout the body. The cardiac cycle (full contraction and relaxation) occurs more than 100,000 times a day in an adult human. The speed and intensity of contractions can be modulated to cope with physiological and pathological challenges (i.e., exercise, hypertension).

The heart is composed of three layers of tissue: the outer epicardium, the middle myocardium, and the inner endocardium. The epicardium is a thin layer of connective tissue and fat that protects and nourishes the myocardium, playing a key role in the development, homeostasis, and regeneration of the heart after injury such as ischemic myocardial infarction (MI) (Simoes & Riley, 2018; von Gise & Pu, 2012). The myocardium is highly muscular tissue primarily composed of cardiomyocytes (~80% volume

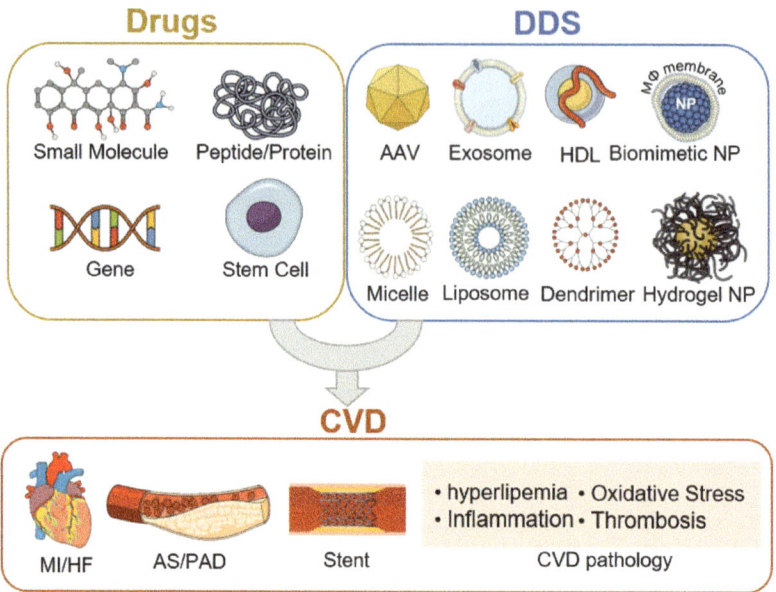

FIGURE 8.2   Drug delivery systems targeting the cardiovascular system and diseases. Np: nanoparticle, CVD: cardiovascular disease, MI: myocardial infarction, HF: heart failure, AS: atherosclerosis, PAD: peripheral artery disease.

of adult heart), generating the contractile force necessary to supply distant tissues with oxygenated blood (Braunwald 1971, Suppl:3–Suppl:8). The endocardium is the smooth endothelial inner lining of heart chambers and valves. Although the endocardium occupies only a small proportion, it is an essential component with several key functions: first, its smooth surface allows blood to flow freely avoiding the adherence of blood cells and platelets to the heart wall, preventing damage and clotting. Second, it supports the subendocardial layer where the Purkinje fibers reside, facilitating coordinated transmission of contractile pulses to the heart muscle. Finally, the transition from endocardial endothelium to mesenchyme (EndMT) – the process of transforming differentiated endothelial cells into developmentally pliable menschemymal cells – forms the valve progenitor cells necessary to build the heart valves and is thus critical to the embryonic development of the heart. However, the aberrant activation of this developmental program in the adult heart contributes to the pathogenesis of heart diseases, such as cardiac fibrosis and ischemic myocardial infarction. Therefore, similar to the epicardium, the endocardium is vital in heart development and disease, and is emerging as a new therapeutic target for heart diseases (Pinto et al., 2016; von Gise & Pu, 2012).

As the most abundant cardiac cells, cardiomyocytes are highly specialized cells with the ability to contract or pace spontaneously (Naqvi, Li, Yahiro, Graham, & Husain, 2009). Each cardiomyocyte is surrounded by a cell membrane called the sarcolemma and within the cell, contains highly organized contractile machinery composed of actin (thin filaments), myosin (thick filaments), and regulatory proteins (troponin and tropomyosin), imperative for proper cardiac function. To meet the high energy demand of the heart beating, cardiomyocytes are full of mitochondria (~30% cell volume), which are the primary source of energy (adenosine triphosphate (ATP)) generation, through a process called oxidative phosphorylation. Mitochondria are strategically positioned between the myofibrils and underneath the sarcolemma to ensure highly efficient delivery of ATP crucial for myocyte contraction, metabolism, and ion homeostasis (Peter, Bjerke, & Leinwand, 2016). These hard-working cardiomyocytes are terminally differentiated cells with limited regeneration and repair capacities. Therefore, sustained stressors (i.e., ischemia, hypertension, elevated lipid and glucose levels) can cause cell damage or even death. Impaired cardiomyocyte function is a hallmark of cardiac pathology including heart failure, myocardial infarction, and ischemia/reperfusion (Chiong et al., 2011).

8.2.1.2 Heart Disease and Current Treatments

Heart disease refers to any disorder of the heart, including coronary artery disease, heart rhythm problems, and congenital heart defects that you are born with. Although "heart disease" and "cardiovascular disease" (CVD) are often used interchangeably, the difference between CVD and heart disease is that CVD includes the pathological function of both the blood vessels and the heart. For instance, peripheral artery disease is a typical CVD, which is a narrowing of the peripheral arteries in the leg, arm, and head. Like coronary artery disease, it is caused by atherosclerosis. In this section, we will summarize the major types of heart diseases that affect heart function and corresponding treatments.

8.2.1.2.1 Coronary Artery Disease

Coronary artery disease (CAD) is the most common type of heart disease, causing 365,914 deaths in 2017. Approximately 18.2 million adult Americans suffer from CAD (~6.7%) – 2 out of 10 CAD deaths occur in adults under 65. CAD is a narrowing or blockage of coronary arteries, usually caused by the accumulation of cholesterol and fatty deposits on the walls of blood vessels, called atherosclerosis, that is the major cause of CVD and will be discussed in the following section. A narrowed or blocked coronary artery restricts blood flow to the heart muscle, and the resulting ischemia can damage or even cause the partial death of the heart. This condition is called a heart attack or myocardial infarction (MI). Depending on the location and degree of the affected myocardium, the coronary artery blockage can severely affect the heart's ability to pump blood or heartbeat. Therefore, the goal of current treatment methods, including medications, surgery, and implantable devices, is to promptly restore blood flow to the damaged myocardium and limit permanent damage. For instance, beta-blockers can reduce the heart's demand for oxygen; nitroglycerin can help blood flow into cardiomyocytes; aspirin and heparin are blood-thinning drugs that can help maintain blood flow through narrowed arteries; antiplatelet drugs and thrombolytics function to prevent new clots and dissolve existing blood clots; angiotensin-converting enzyme inhibitors can reduce the levels of angiotensin II, thereby dilating blood vessels and reducing vascular resistance. There are many surgical procedures that can restore the blood flow. The most noteworthy are (1) coronary angioplasty and stent placement. These procedures use a catheter with a special balloon to open the blocked coronary artery and place a stent coated with slow-release drugs to help keep the artery open; (2) coronary artery bypass surgery, which involves suturing a vein or artery outside the blocked or narrowed coronary artery to allow blood to flow to the heart and bypass the narrowed section. In addition to restoring blood flow, repair and replacement of the damaged heart tissue and even the entire heart is now a reality, such as heart valve repair or replacement, surgery to obtain healthy muscle from the patient's back or abdomen (cardiopasty), or heart transplant.

8.2.1.2.2 Heart Failure

Between 2013 and 2016, heart failure (HF) affected approximately 6.2 million American adults, and as the population ages, the prevalence continues to rise over time. HF is a progressive disease caused by any structural or functional changes in the heart, characterized by the impaired ventricular filling or blood ejection. There are two types of HF: preserved ejection fraction and reduced ejection fraction. By evaluating the development and progression of the disease, HF can also be divided into four stages: Stages A to D, assigned to those who have a high risk of HF but do not have structural heart disease (Stage A), structural heart disease but without signs or symptoms of HF (Stage B), structural heart disease with prior or current symptoms of HF (Stage C), and refractory HF requiring specialized intervention (Stage D). First-line drug therapy for patients with reduced ejection fraction includes angiotensin-converting enzyme (ACE) inhibitors and beta blockers, which have been shown to reduce morbidity and mortality (McMurray et al., 2014). For patients with severe HF, implanting a left ventricular assist device to help maintain the heart's pumping ability, or performing a heart transplant is the main choice for HF treatment.

8.2.1.2.3 Congenital Heart Disease

Congenital heart disease (CHD) occurs at birth. It comes from abnormal heart development during embryogenesis and affects the structure and function of the heart. CHD is the most common congenital malformation in newborns, accounting for about 10% of live births worldwide (Hoffman, Kaplan, & Liberthson, 2004). CHDs can be mild, such as small holes in the heart, or severe, such as missing or deformed parts of the heart. So far, at least 18 different types of CHDs have been identified, most of which are serious and require one or more operations to repair the heart. Unfortunately, there is no cure for this disease; infants may have life-long complications and are at a higher risk of CVD, stroke, and heart failure (Sokolov & Martsinkevich, 2018; Wang et al., 2019). Although surgery and heart transplantation are the main treatments for CHDs, medications may still be needed to treat the symptoms such as helping strengthen the heart muscle, lowering blood pressure, and removing extra fluid.

8.2.1.2.4 Arrhythmia

Arrhythmia is defined as a problem with the heat rate or rhythm. The heart beats too fast (tachycardia), too slowly (bradycardia), or irregularly (fibrillation). The atria and ventricles work together, alternatively contracting and relaxing, pumping blood through the heart. The heart rhythm is normally controlled by a natural pacemaker (sinus node) located in the right atrium. Electrical impulses are generated in the pacemakers to contract the atria muscles and start the heartbeat. When these electrical impulses travel to the artrio-ventricular node and ventricular muscles, they enable the ventricles to fill with blood and contract. In a healthy heart, this process usually goes smoothly, resulting in a normal regular resting heart rate of 60 to 100 beats per minute; depending on physical activity, the heart can beat faster (for example, during exercise) to provide the tissues with more oxygen-rich blood, and a slower heartbeat is normal during sleep or deep relaxation. However, if the change is too large or due to heart damage/abnormal electrical signals, it can be fatal and require immediate treatment. There are a variety of drugs that can be used to treat arrhythmia, mainly including calcium channel blockers and beta-blockers, as well as anticoagulants to reduce the risk of thrombosis.

The concept of using implantable devices to normalize heart rhythm has been a reality for patients for 50 years: these devices include implantable pacemakers, cardiovascular defibrillators, cardiac resynchronization therapy, or combination devices, which have become standards to improve the quality of patient care (Cohen & Klein, 2002; Hoffmann et al., 2006; Mirowski et al., 1980).

8.2.2 Vascular System

8.2.2.1 Physiology of the Vascular System

The vascular system consists of the vessels that carry blood and lymph through the body. Arteries and arterioles bring oxygen-rich blood and nutrients from the heart to the organs and tissues; venules and veins carry deoxygenated blood back to the heart; capillaries are responsible for the exchange of gases and nutrients between blood and tissues; the lymph vessels carry lymphatic fluid, and this system protects and controls the fluid in the body through filtering and draining lymph away from each region of the body.

Blood vessels, except the smallest ones, are composed of three layers: the tunica interna (innermost layer), tunica media (middle layer), and adventitia (outer layer). The tunica interna is only a single layer of endothelial cells called endothelium as a smooth lining of the vessel wall in direct contact with the blood; the tunica media takes up most of the arterial vessel wall and is composed of smooth muscle cells and extracellular matrix, controlling vascular contraction and relaxation; the tunica externa consists mainly of connective tissues, protecting the blood vessels and affixing them to surrounding tissues.

8.2.2.2 Vascular Diseases and Current Therapies

As mentioned in Section 8.2.1, CVD refers to any problem that may arise within the heart and blood vessels, including coronary artery disease, cerebrovascular disease, peripheral artery disease, heart disease, and many others (Benjamin et al., 2018). Impaired cardiac function caused by heart attacks and strokes is usually an acute event mainly caused by a blockage of blood flow to the heart and brain. Atherosclerosis is the main underlying cause of CVD. In this chapter we will briefly articulate the pathophysiology of atherosclerosis, along with the aforementioned vascular diseases, and the current treatment strategies.

8.2.2.2.1 *Atherosclerosis: The Underlying Cause of Cardiovascular Disease*

Atherosclerosis is a type of thickening and hardening of the arteries. It is caused by the buildup of plaques (fatty deposits) inside the lining of the artery wall, which are made up of necrotic cores, calcified regions, modified lipids, and different types of cells (Insull, 2009). Over time, the plaques can narrow the channel within the artery, thus reducing or even blocking blood flow to the heart and other tissues, and causing myocardial infarction, heart failure, stroke, and claudication (Herrington, Lacey, Sherliker, Armitage, & Lewington, 2016).

The plaque buildup is a gradual and lifelong process: it starts with aortic fatty streaks consisting of cholesterol, white blood cells, and other cellular matter that are observed in early childhood or even in one-day-old neonates (Milei et al., 2008). This fatty streak by itself does not cause symptoms of cardiovascular disease, but it can evolve into fibrous plaques, and some of the plaques are vulnerable to rupture, causing thrombosis or stenosis. The extent of plaques is increased with age. They can cover about 20% to 60% of the coronary artery surface by the age of 60 (Eggen & Solberg, 1968). The process of lesion development is believed to be the same regardless of sex, race/ethnicity, and geographic location, but will be accelerated in patients with such risk factors as diabetes mellitus, hypertension, metabolic disorders, and smoking (Herrington et al., 2016; Mcgill et al., 1968).

Currently, there is a consensus view that atherosclerosis is a chronic inflammatory disease of arteries involving multiple cell types (Taleb, 2016). The raised plasma levels of low-density lipoprotein (LDL) cholesterol are of primary importance in atherogenesis. By passively diffusing through endothelial junctions, LDLs are retained in the subendothelial space of the vessel wall, where they are subjected to modifications such as oxidation, proteolysis, and phospholipolysis by enzymes secreted from activated intimal cells. The current hypothesis is that these modified-LDL products likely mimic pathogen- or damage-associated molecular patterns (PAMPs or DAMPs), triggering low-grade inflammation, thereby initiating the atherosclerotic process (Pentikainen, Oorni, Ala-Korpela, & Kovanen, 2000). By contrast, high-density lipoprotein (HDL) protects against atherosclerosis, at least in part by removing excess cholesterol from peripheral tissues, as well as preventing lipoprotein oxidation (Boren & Williams, 2016; Schwenke & Carew, 1989).

Another important initiating event in atherogenesis is vascular endothelial cell activation/dysfunction, which is characterized by the compromised barrier integrity, reduced vasodilation, proinflammatory and prothrombic states in response to pro-atherogenic factors, such as low shear stress and disturbed blood flow, hypercholesterolemia, and hyperglycemia (Sitia et al., 2010; Gimbrone & Garcia-Cardena, 2016). Endothelial cell dysfunction is the earliest detectable change in the course of lesion development; as such, it has been widely used as a reliable marker for subclinical atherosclerosis as well as predicting future cardiovascular events in patients. Early identification and reversal of endothelial cell dysfunction are viewed as attractive targets for the prevention and treatment of cardiovascular disease (Hamburg & Vita, 2006; Stary, 2000). The exact molecular mechanism that underlies lesion formation is complex and not completely deciphered, but several key pathogenic events have been well defined: (1) endothelial cell dysfunction facilitates lipoprotein retention in the subendothelial matrix; (2) circulating monocytes are selectively recruited into the intima, where they differentiate into macrophages and take up oxidized LDL to become foam cells; (3) cytokines and growth factors are released from activated endothelial cells, meanwhile macrophages induce smooth muscle cell proliferation and migration into intima; (4) smooth muscle cells liberate chemokines and chemoattracts, recruiting more inflammatory cells into the arterial wall; (5) migratory smooth muscle cells secrete proteoglycans, collagen, and elastic fibers into the extracellular space to build a fibroatheroma which is a fibrous cap over the lipid-rich necrotic cores and just under the endothelium. The early fibroatheroma severs as a "protective barrier" between platelets in the blood stream and prothrombotic material in lesions (Gimbrone & Garcia-Cardena, 2016; Moore, Sheedy, & Fisher, 2013; Newby & Zaltsman, 1999). Fibroatheromas alone may obstruct blood flow and cause stable angina pectoris, but rarely cause acute vascular disease or sudden cardiac death (Eggen & Solberg, 1968; Stary, 1999).

Alternatively, an advanced, thin-fibrous cap atheroma, known as a "vulnerable plaque", has the potential to rupture at the lesion edges under stress conditions, causing acute coronary thrombosis and myocardial infarction (Casscells, Naghavi, & Willerson, 2003; Little, 1990). These potentially fatal lesions occur primarily in persons aged ≥55 years or in young adults with a high risk of CVD (Virmani, Burke, Kolodgie, & Farb, 2002). There are several factors that determine the vulnerability of plaques, including the size and consistency of the plaque core, the thickness and collagen content of the fibrous cap, and inflammation within the plaque. Exposure to high hemodynamic shear stress may also contribute to cap rupture (Falk, Shah, & Fuster, 1995). Although the underlying mechanisms are not fully understood, increased inflammatory cells, and loss of smooth muscle cells from the fibrous cap along with degradation of collagen-rich cap matrix, have been strongly implicated in plaque rupture (Boyle, Weissberg, & Bennett, 2002; Kolodgie et al., 2001). Infiltrated macrophage foam cells likely secrete proteolytic enzymes including plasminogen activators, cathepsins, and matrix metalloproteinases, which together can degrade virtually all components of the extracellular matrix (Gough, Gomez, Wille, & Raines, 2006; Vanderwal, Becker, Vanderloos, & Das, 1994). With plaque rupture, highly thrombogenic materials (collagen, lipid core, and apoptotic microparticles containing tissue factors) are exposed to blood, attracting and activating platelets, initiating the coagulation cascade, thereby leading to the formation of platelet thrombus. The formed blood clot inside blood vessels may restrict blood flow within the heart, leading to heart tissue damage and a myocardial infarction (Fernandezortiz et al. 1994, 1562–1569).

Given the aforementioned pathogenic mechanisms implicated in atherosclerosis, the therapies to date have largely been focused on drugs that lower blood lipids, such as statins or the recently approved proprotein convertase subtilisin/kexin type 9 (PCSK9) inhibitors (alirocumab and evolocumab), suppress systemic inflammation like IL-1β receptor antagonist (anakinra)/the soluble decoy receptor (rilonacept)/monocloncal antibodies(canakinumab and gevokizumab), or control high blood pressure with angiotensin-converting enzyme (ACE) inhibitors, β-blockers, calcium channel blockers, α-blockers, and nervous system inhibitors (Stern & Lebowitz, 2010). Primary percutaneous coronary intervention (PCI) currently is the primary reperfusion strategy to open up the occluded vessels, improving blood flow to the heart, reducing the myocardial infarction rate. Thrombolytic medicines (e.g., streptokinase, urokinase, or tissue plasminogen activators) that can break up or dissolve platelet thrombus in blood vessels are approved for the emergency treatment of stroke and heart attack. Even with these established drugs and unprecedented progress in primary and secondary prevention, CVD remains the leading cause of death and illness across the world, and recent epidemiological studies indicate the decline in population mortality is slowing down with increases in some groups (Sidney et al., 2016; Stein, Gennuso, Ugboaja, & Remington, 2017). Compared with the high burden of CVD, drug development pipelines have been stagnant, underscoring the need for new therapeutic strategies and approaches (Van Norman, 2017).

8.2.3 Drug Delivery Systems Targeting the Cardiovascular System

In this section, we discuss the use of drug delivery systems for treating cardiovascular disease. Briefly, DDS have the potential to (1) improve the pharmacokinetic and pharmacodynamics properties of currently existing cardiovascular drugs; (2) deliver payloads (pharmacological agents, genetic materials, stem cells) to the specific disease sites of the heart and blood vessels; (3) improve the pathogenesis of cardiovascular disease (high lipid levels, oxidative stress, endothelial dysfunction, inflammation, and thrombosis). We will start with an overview of the background and highlight the challenges and implications of the drug delivery systems. The representative examples will be discussed with respect to their advantages and limitations.

8.2.3.1 Drug Delivery Systems/Devices Improve the Pharmacokinetic and Pharmacodynamics, and Refine Targeting of Existing Cardiovascular Drugs

The first DDS in cardiovascular nanomedicine were designed to improve the pharmacokinetic and pharmacodynamic properties of existing cardiovascular drugs. For example, lipid-based nanocarriers were adopted to solve solubility issue with carvedilol that is β-adrenergic receptor blocker (Virmani et al., 2002), and the liposomal formation of prostaglandin E-1 (Liprostin™) significantly improve the drug dynamics and therapeutic index of various ailments including occlusive disease, peripheral vascular disorders, and arthritis (Bulbake, Doppalapudi, Kommineni, & Khan, 2017). Similarly, dendrimeric formulations enhance the aqueous solubility of candesartan, a clinically approved angiotensin receptor blocker with poor solubility (Erturk, Gurbuz, & Tulu, 2017). A nanomedicine-based formulation loaded with omega-3 polyunsaturated fatty acids (ω-3 PUFAs), well-known dietary factors with beneficial properties for the prevention of CVDs, was tested in the clinical setting and showed significant improvement in bioavailability (Serini, Cassano, Trombino, & Calviello, 2019). A dual polymer system (Aerosil200 combined with polxamer407 and polyvinylpyrrolidone) was recently reported to improve the solubility, dissolution, and stability of Coenzyme Q10, which is an essential mitochondrial enzyme in cellular energy processes in cardiac cells, and thus expected to improve bioavailability and effectiveness in CVD treatments (Choi, Park, & Park, 2019).

Considering CVD is a chronic disease, the delivery systems that provide sustained and controlled release of cardiovascular drugs to the diseased sites have broad prospects for CVD management and have been intensively investigated (Park, 2014). In a recent study demonstrated in a mouse model of restenosis, applying elastin-like recombinant hydrogel to damaged carotid arteries can prolong the release of the embedded Kv1.3 channel blocker PAR-1, which can reduce the proliferation and migration of smooth muscle cells, thus inhibiting the development of carotid artery intimal hyperplasia after ligation (Moreno-Estar et al., 2020). A new biocompatible microcapsule fabricated through microfluidics was recently reported by Dinh et al. (2020) It also exhibits high drug-loading efficiency, and the encapsulated vascular endothelial growth actor (VEGF) and platelet-derived growth factor (PDGF) were continuously released up to 30 days, resulting in blood vessel regeneration and a reduction in the rat heart myocardial infarction size (Dinh et al., 2020, 2756–2764).

In addition to improving bioavailability and reducing systemic toxicity, DDS also facilitate the effective delivery of payload drugs to the diseased sites (Attia, Anton, Wallyn, Omran, & Vandamme, 2019). It is well known that in the case of inflammation/hypoxia – typical pathologic conditions associated with atherosclerotic lesions and myocardial infarction – the barrier integrity of the vascular endothelium is disturbed, being more permeable than in the healthy state, so it can selectively enhance permeation to macromolecules or DDS; meanwhile, the absence of normal lymphatic drainage in lesions contributes to the retention of the drug/DDS. This phenomenon is called enhanced permeation and retention (EPR), which was discovered by Maeda et al. in the 1980s, and quickly became the golden standard in the design of passive targeting DDS to tumors (Matsumura & Maeda, 1986). EPR is also widely applied in devising DDS for the cardiovascular system (Geelen, Paulis, Coolen, Nicolay, & Strijkers, 2013; Lukyanov, Hartner, & Torchilin, 2004). With the ability to be functionalized with different classes of targeting moieties (e.g., antibody, peptides, nucleic acids, aptamers), DDS can be selectively delivered to pathological areas (Kamaly, Xiao, Valencia, Radovic-Moreno, & Farokhzad, 2012; Wang et al., 2014). This active targeting strategy has also been widely employed to improve drug delivery efficiency to the cardiovascular system, while limiting systemic side effects. In this section, we summarize the biomaterials and nanotechnology used to deliver drugs to the heart and vascular system.

8.2.3.2 Current Drug Delivery Systems Alleviate Cardiac Dysfunction Associated with CVD

As mentioned in the previous sections, myocardial infarction (MI) and congestive heart failure (CHF) have been defined as a global pandemic, affecting at least 26 million people worldwide and becoming a huge public medical burden (Benjamin et al., 2018). The most effective treatment for end-stage CHF is heart transplantation, which is a highly invasive and complex surgical procedure and greatly limited by the availability of heart donors. At least in preclinical studies, HF gene or regenerative therapies that are used to correct key molecule defects or enable cardiac regeneration and functional restoration have demonstrated great potential. By facilitating the delivery of DNA/RNA, stem cells, and regenerative factors to diseased cardiomyocytes, cardiac-directed delivery technology such as engineered or natural nanocarriers, hydrogels, and viral vectors have become essential for successful gene and regenerative therapies. The main cardiac-directed DDS are summarized as follows.

8.2.3.2.1 DDS Targeted to Heart: Viral Gene Transfer

The efficiency of gene transfer is the primary obstacle limiting the clinical success of gene therapy. With very few exceptions, when administrated in an extracellular milieu, naked nucleic acids are very poorly internalized by the target cells, and gene transfer must be facilitated by using physical tools (e.g., electroporation, high-pressure injection) or delivery systems including chemical (cationic lipids, polymers) and viral vectors. Of these tools, viral vectors have been the main delivery system for genetic materials *in vivo*. There are five classes of viruses that are used in more than 50% of human gene therapy clinical trials, including members of the retro-viridae family (gammaretroviruses and lentiviruses), adenoviruses, adeno-associated viruses (AAVs), and herpesviruses. Despite the difference in virus type, all the engineered viral vectors available for gene therapy are generated using the same principles: (1) delete the majority of genes encoding viral proteins from the viral genome, especially those with potential pathogenicity; (2) retain viral genome sequences required for viral packing and replication; (3) express viral proteins required for viral replication within the virus-producing cells. These essential viral proteins can be expressed from genes encoded by transiently transfected plasmids, by a previously engineered cellular genome, or by a helper virus simultaneously infecting the packaging cells.

In the context of gene therapy for heart failure, recombinant AAVs (rAAVs) have emerged as the most valuable gene transfer agent due to their efficiency and safety in transducing both dividing and nondividing cells (Pleger et al., 2013). The engineered AAV is a nonpathogenic, nonenveloped DNA virus, containing a linear single-stranded genome from 4.6 to 4.9 kb, without *cap* and *rep* genes encoding alternatively spliced capsid (*cap*) proteins and multifunctional replication (*rep*) proteins, so it needs to be coinfected with helper viruses for viral replication. Compared with other viral vectors, rAAV is very suitable for HF gene therapy due to its low immunogenicity, long-term cardiac expression duration (>24 months), and preferential cardiomyocyte transduction with different stereotypes (e.g., systemic application of rAAV9 in rodent models transduced both the heart and the extracardiac tissues). But they also have some disadvantages, including the low packaging capacity, relative low titer production, and the presence of human anti-AAV antibodies, all of which may limit the efficacy of cardiovascular gene transfer. Nevertheless, rAAV is currently considered to be the most effective gene delivery system. Combined with a clinically favorable physical delivery route, those rAAVs that show the highest affinity for the targeted cardiac cell type, or contain cardiac-targeted expression cassette could be used as a safe and effective delivery system for HF gene therapy in humans. In support of this view, recent studies on clinical trials and animal models of HF have shown that AAV vector can facilitate the gene transfer to the heart and can prevent or even reverse cardiac tissue damage. For instance, the SERC-LVAD trial, which is part of an AAV1/SERCA2a cardiac gene therapy trial program, reported that in adult chronic heart failure patients, a single intracoronary infusion of 1×10^{13} viral particles of DNA-resistant AAV1 carrying the sarcoplasmic reticulum calcium ATPase gene (SERCA2a) was well tolerated. Importantly, during the three-year follow-up, the results of five patients confirmed that viral DNA had been delivered to the failing human heart (Lyon et al., n.d.). While in different mouse models with cardiac dysfunction, the intravenous application of rAAV9 harboring the cardiac beneficial genes (e.g., LAMP2B (Manso et al., 2020), p110α (Prakoso et al., 2020), Tafzzin (Wang, Suya et al., 2020), or restoring calcium sensor protein (Katz et al., 2020)) resulted in homogeneous cardiac expression confined to cardiomyocytes, and significant functional recovery, providing a proof-of-concept for the effectiveness of gene therapy for heart failure.

8.2.3.2.2 DDS Targeted to the Heart: Nanomaterials

Although in animal and clinical studies, virus-mediated gene therapy has shown encouraging prospects in reversing the cardiac function of a failing heart, the path to clinical reality has been arduous because of the inherent challenges and limitations associated with viruses. For a long time, researchers have been exploring nanomaterials as an alternative approach to delivering genetic materials and other bioactive agents to the heart. Compared with viral vectors, nanomaterials hold some advantages, including advanced active targeting strategies, mild immune response, and non-pathogenicity. However, the low transduction efficiency, the possible aggregation in the blood, and short-term expression significantly limit their applications in the treatment of heart disease (Yan, Quan, & Feng, 2019). So far, even in animal models, nanoparticle-mediated gene transfer systems have rarely been studied. Zhang et al. reported that magnetic nanobeads can promote the targeted delivery of the VEGF165 gene to the infarcted rat heart by chemically coupling with adenoviral vectors. The study found strong expression of VEGF165 gene carried by virus detected together with improved cardiac functions (Zhang et al., 2012b). Similarly, VEGF gene directly loaded in poly(D-L-lactide-co-glycolide) PLGA nanoparticles (Yi, Wu, & Jia, 2006) or complexed with graphene oxide in methacrylated gelatin hydrogel (Paul et al., 2014) was also shown to increase capillary density and reduce the scar area four weeks or seven days after local injection into infarcted myocardium of rabbit or rat models, respectively. These preclinical studies suggest such a possibility of nanoparticle-mediated gene therapy for HF, but obviously there are still significant obstacles on the path to clinical reality as aforementioned.

In addition to delivering genetic materials, nanocarriers can also deliver therapeutic small molecules, peptides, and proteins to the myocardium. But most of these delivery systems are locally injected to infarcted tissues in order to achieve high delivery efficacy and therapeutic effect. For example, the biodegradable and biocompatible chitosan-alginate nanoparticles loaded with recombinant placental-induced growth factor were injected into the peri-infarct myocardium area of rats 15 minutes after infarction induction; this local application improved blood flow in the infarction border zone, decreased scar area, and preserved left ventricular function eight weeks after the injection of nanomedicine. Similar cardiac-protective effects were observed when other growth factors that were loaded into different types of nanocarriers were injected intramyocardially, such as insulin-like growth factor complexed 60 mm-sized PLGA nanoparticles (Chang et al., 2013), hybrid nanoparticles constructed with a Pluronic F-127 co-polymer shell, and a lecithin core encapsulating human rVEGF that underwent temperature-dependent gelation, stabilizing the localization of core/shell nanoparticle at the ischemic area (Oh et al., 2010). Targeting cardiac-specific markers that are upregulated under ischemic conditions is another strategy for the heart-specific delivery of therapeutic agents, and allows systemic drug administration. Proof-of-concept studies have shown that after intravenous injection, the liposomes conjugated with CRPPR peptide (Zhang et al., 2012a), or cationic polymers decorated with ischemic myocardium target peptides (Won, McGinn, Lee, Bull, & Kim, 2013) efficiently accumulated in damaged myocardium. In view of the massive upregulation of P-selectin in ischemic heart tissue, the intravenous injection of anti-P-selectin-conjugated liposomes containing VEGF can significantly improve cardiac function, vascular structure, and density (Scott et al., 2009). Recently, the nanocarriers co-functionalized with different targeting ligands have been designed as a new synergistic strategy to improve the addressability of the infarcted myocardium. Co-modified liposomes consisting of red cell membrane (RCM) and the peptides TAT and PCM were formulated, which can effectively target cardiomyocytes and exhibit prolonged retention time in the heart (Liu et al., 2020b). Dual peptide functionalized acetylated-dextran-based nanoparticles can sequentially target macrophages via linTT1 and myocytes via atrial natriuretic peptide during myocardial infarction (Torrieri et al., 2020).

8.2.3.2.3 DDS Targeted to the Heart: Biomaterials for the Delivery of Stem Cells

Stem cells are defined by their ability to self-renew and differentiate into one or more other cell types, and have been intensively studied – over 200 clinical trials have been conducted in the past 2 decades – as a means to replace the damaged or lost myocardium, thereby promoting the tissue repair process. Cells can be delivered into the heart using several established modes, including intravenous delivery, epicardial or trans-endocardial injection, and intracoronary infusion via catheter (Banerjee, Bolli, & Hare, 2018; Golpanian, Wolf, Hatzistergos, & Hare, 2016). However, cell survival and engraftment after transplantation pose major challenges for stem cell therapy. Recently, biomaterials (such as hydrogels) have been introduced as an effective stem cell delivery system, which can increase their survival rate and improve myocardial repair after being injected into the infarct site (Alagarsamy, Yan, Srivastava, Desiderio, & Dhingra, 2019). These hydrophilic polymer networks can be generated from either native extracellular matrix (ECM) components or synthetic polymers, or they can be used in combination (Lee & Kim, 2018). They swell upon absorption of biological fluids and act as soft and elastic scaffolds that mimic the microenvironment of heart tissues. Naturally derived polymers such as chitosan, collagen, gelatin, fibrin, alginate, and other decellularized tissues exhibit excellent biocompatibility and biodegradability and have been extensively studied *in vivo*, rendering them the main polymer sources of injectable hydrogel for cardiac regeneration (Hasan et al., 2015; Pena et al., 2018). However, the utility of this DDS in stem cell therapy is compromised by batch-to-batch variability, weak mechanical strength, and risk of inflammation (Han et al., 2019). In contrast, synthetic hydrogels are easier to manufacture and scale up with consistency with tunable material properties (Guo & Ma, 2014). Three types of synthetic polymers have been used for hydrogels in cardiac tissue regeneration: (1) poly (N-isopropylacrylamide) is a temperature-sensitive polymer that can be readily functionalized for use in tissue engineering applications, but its difficulty in degradation and the poor biological activity of encapsulated stem cells severely weaken the therapeutic efficacy *in vivo* (Cui, Lee, Pauken, & Vernon, 2011), (2) polycaprolactone (PCL) and its derivatives have excellent thermal stability, load-bearing capacity, and adjustable mechanical and elastic strength comparable to native cardiac extracellular matrix. However, they must be used in combination with other hydrophilic or electroactive polymers to improve their water solubility and electric conductivity, which is essential for stem cell attachment and cell-to-cell communication (Piao et al., 2007; Siddiqui, Asawa, Birru, Baadhe, & Rao, 2018; Spearman et al., 2015), (3) self-assembling peptide-based nanostructures are an important and promising type of injectable hydrogel in myocardial repair, because these assemblies offer several advantages such as biocompatibility, biodegradability, nontoxicity, and ease of incorporating functional and bioactive motifs or growth factors and other nutrients that mimic the microenvironment of cardiac extracellular matrix (Yuan, He, Lv, & Luo, 2014). For example, it is reported that synthesized folic acid modified peptide hydrogel can improve the survival and differentiation of induced pluripotent stem cell (iPSC) into functional cardiomyocytes in an *in vivo* mouse model of myocardial infarction, thereby reducing infarct size and severity of fibrosis (Li et al., 2018). Combining the ideal properties of hydrogels based on natural and synthetic polymers, hybrid hydrogels have emerged as a more suitable choice for cardiac repair, which can better mimic natural tissues and overcome inherent challenges in cardiac tissue engineering (Sheffield, Meyers, Johnson, & Rajachar, 2018). A recent study demonstrated that a hybrid hydrogel (oxidized alginate/2-aminopyridine-5-thiocarboxamide/tetraaniline) successfully delivered adipose-derived stem cells to the infarction site of the heart in an MI rat model and improved the infarction area and related pathogenic factors (Liang et al., 2019).

8.2.3.2.4 *Extracellular Vesicle-Based Drug Delivery System Targeting the Heart*
Extracellular vesicles (EV) refer to membrane vesicles produced and secreted by most mammalian cells when activated or under stress. They include the submicron-size microparticles (MPs) and nanometer-size exosomes, which carry RNAs, proteins, and lipids from their parent cells and deliver these contents to other target cells, thereby mediating the cell-to-cell communication (Raposo & Stoorvogel, 2013). All EV components including their native cargo, surface proteins, and membranes can be independently engineered for various applications (Kao & Papoutsakis, 2019). These desirable features of EVs make them an excellent manipulative drug delivery system with high target specificity. (Kao & Papoutsakis, 2019, 89–98).

Two methods have been developed for cargo loading into EVs: endogenous and exogenous. Endogenous loading refers to the overexpression of protein or RNA in EV-producing cells by the transfection of plasmid DNA or RNA, while exogenous loading requires electroporation for RNA or drug loading. The loading capacities of cargo molecules are determined by the type of EVs and characteristics of cargoes. Specifically, small RNAs or small interfering RNAs can be easily loaded into exosomes with electroporation, but linear or plasmid DNA can only be carried by micron-scaled microparticles (MP) (Lamichhane, Raiker, & Jay, 2015). Due to their higher cargo capacity, MPs are more suitable EVs for loading significant amounts of large-size cargo molecules such as a DNA plasmid. The surface modification of EVs is the main strategy to achieve higher delivery efficiency and specificity to target cells and tissues. In addition to the natural target specificity of certain EVs – for example, integrin α-4 and β-4 expressed on EVs derived from endothelial progenitors can target endothelial cells – engineered EVs via expression proteins or peptides on the surface can enhance target specificity. This strategy has been widely employed in developing EV-based drug delivery systems targeting tumor cells and brain tissue *in vivo* (Alvarez-Erviti et al., 2011; Ohno et al., 2013; Tian et al., 2014).

Among EVs, exosomes have been intensively studied due to their potential application in drug delivery, tissue regeneration, and diagnosis of diseases. Although the study of cardiac exosomes is still in its infancy compared with tumor exosomes, a large amount of *in vitro* and *in vivo* evidence supports the suggestion that natural and engineered exosomes have potent therapeutic effects against heart disease. For example, when incubated with cardiac fibroblast-conditioned medium, cardiomyocytes showed changes in impulse contraction, which were associated with altered expression of Na+ and inward rectifying -K+ channels (Pedrotty, Klinger, Kirkton, & Bursac, 2009). The potential for targeting exosomes to specific cells was further implicated in a recent study where researchers found exosomes derived from mesenchymal stem cells can confer cardio-protection and regeneration in target cardiac cells (Ozaki Tan, Floriano, Nicastro, Emanueli, & Catapano, 2020). Lastly, exosomal microRNAs such as miR-21, miR126, and miR210 have prevented myocardial ischemia through promoting cardiac angiogenesis and vascular regeneration, thus resulting in increased blood flow to the ischemic myocardium (Moghiman et al., n.d.). With a better understanding of molecular mechanisms driving the target cell recognition and cardio-protection, engineered exosomes have emerged to achieve higher targeting efficacy and therapeutic effect for heart disease. For instance, macrophage migration inhibitory factor (MIF) is a proinflammatory cytokine that plays a critical role in regulating cell homeostasis. A recent study investigated the cardioprotective effects of exosomes secreted in bone marrow mesenchymal stem cells overexpressing MIF in a rat model of myocardial infarction. Injecting the isolated MIF-overexpressing exosomes intramuscularly into the peri-infarct area of the rat heart was followed by enhanced cardiac function due to a reduction in cardiac remodeling, oxidative stress, and cardiomyocyte apoptosis (Liu et al., 2020). Despite formidable success, exosome-based regenerative therapy is hindered by the complexity of contents and lack of targeting mechanisms. To overcome these limitations, many attempts, some successful, have been made to develop targeted regenerative exosomes for the myocardium. For example, fusing the therapeutic proteins (e.g., autophagy regulatory protein Lamp2b) with ischemic myocardium-targeting peptide (IMTP) (Wang et al., 2018) or cardiac-targeting peptide (CTP) with glycosylation sequence (Kim et al., 2018) promoted the accumulation of these engineered exosomes in the mouse myocardium. These engineered exosomes with improved specificity and efficiency in targeting the myocardium elicit significant therapeutic effects as reflected by the reduction of inflammation and apoptosis, enhanced angiogenesis, decreased infarct size, and restored cardiac function (Vandergriff et al., 2018; Wang et al., 2018).

More and more studies have suggested that EVs could replace most cell therapies and can be engineered to effectively deliver a wide range of therapeutic agents to targeted tissues. Not surprisingly, the designer exosomes are becoming a new frontier in the treatment of cardiovascular disease.

8.2.3.3 Drug Delivery Systems Used to Improve Vascular Function in Atherosclerosis

As mentioned in the previous section, atherosclerosis is the main cause of cardiovascular disease. Plaque deposits can block blood flow, cause a heart attack or stroke, and can also be ruptured, leading to thrombosis. In order to better combat atherosclerotic cardiovascular disease, new methods for early diagnosis and novel targeted therapies are needed. DDS have become an important tool for targeted drug delivery, which can minimize systemic side effects and enhance the positioning and efficacy of drugs in atherosclerotic and thrombotic lesions. So far, liposomes and biomimetic nanocarriers have come to the forefront of nanosystem-based drug delivery systems that target damaged arterial vessels and lesions.

8.2.3.3.1 Liposomes and Lipid-Based Nanoparticles Targeting the Arterial Vessels and Atherosclerosis
Liposomes are specialized delivery vehicles that improve the safety profile, pharmacokinetics, and biodistributions of encapsulated therapeutic reagents by helping to solubilize highly lipophilic compounds,

shielding them from plasma degradation and immune system check, and reducing systemic exposure. Lipid nanoparticles are liposome-like structures especially geared towards encapsulating a broad variety of genetic materials. Nevertheless, both are lipid nano-formulations and are considered to be excellent drug delivery vehicles with great clinical translational potential.

Inflamed endothelium lining the arterial wall has become an important therapeutic target because it represents an early pathogenic event that triggers leukocyte infiltration and consequent atherogenesis process. With the activation of endothelial cells, cell adhesion molecules such as vascular cell adhesion molecule 1 (VCAM-1) and intracellular cell adhesion molecule 1 (ICAM-1) generally are upregulated and can be used for targeted therapy. For example, recently, Kheradmandi et al. (Kheradmandi, Ackers, Burdick, Malgor, & Farnoud, n.d.) reported that VCAM-1 functionalized liposomes were able to specifically target inflammatory endothelial cells and showed no cytotoxicity toward leukocytes and endothelial cells, implicating these VCAM-1-functionalized liposomes as a potential drug delivery system targeting diseased vasculature and atherosclerosis lesions. Another study demonstrated that injectable liposomes encapsulating fluocinolone acetonide, a corticosteroid, were accumulated in atherosclerotic lesions of ApoE$^{-/-}$ mice, and exerted anti-atherosclerotic effects four weeks after administration (Fernandez-Ruiz, 2020).

Cationic lipid particles have been shown to be effective in enhancing transfection both by increasing the rate of internalization and by enhancing the escape of nucleic acids from lysosomal or endosomal compartments. On the other hand, cationic lipid particles have disadvantages such as a tendency to aggregate and increase cytotoxicity (Zakirov et al., 2020). A multifunctional lipid particle developed by Kheirolomoom et al. was used to deliver antiatherogenic reagent (anti-miR712) to inflamed pro-atherosclerotic arterial regions without significant off-target effects in gene expression or particle-induced toxicity. This lipid particle is composed of an aqueous core of nucleic acids complexed with cationic lipids and a neutral lipid-based outer leaflet that was decorated with targeting peptide for VCAM1 (VHPK). With this combined strategy, the toxicity of nanoparticle is minimized, the stability of anti-miR712 is preserved, and loading efficiency and therapeutic efficacy are maximized.

8.2.3.3.2 Biomimetic Nanoparticles Targeting to Atherosclerotic Lesions
Lipoproteins are endogenous nanoparticles that can be engineered to be used as drug delivery systems or nanocarriers for contrast agents (Kornmueller, Vidakovic, & Prassl, 2019). As the smallest class of lipoproteins and the main anti-atherosclerotic factor, high-density lipoproteins (HDL) can be synthesized as nascent nano-discs or spherical nanoparticles to carry various substances including drugs, nuclei acids, and signal-emitting molecules to target tissues such as arterial atherosclerotic lesions. These cargos can be embedded either in the amphiphilic lipid layer of nanodiscs or loaded in the oily inner core of spherical particles. Within the lipid microenvironment of rHDL particles, a huge number of drugs can be loaded and transported in plasma, which are shielded from rapid degradation and immune attack. To achieve efficient delivery of the drugs to the target site, rHDL can be devised to resist against phospholipases by replacing ester bonds with non-hydolyzable ether bonds, or by using saturated long acyl chain lipids for the synthesis of rHDL to increase lipophilicity and resistance to oxidation. Compared with other drug delivery systems such as liposomes or polymeric nanoparticles, rHDL possesses several advantages (Lacko, Sabnis, Nagarajan, & McConathy, 2015), including: (1) as endogenous HDL mimics, they are highly biocompatible and have inherent targeting properties – can be recognized by specific cell surface receptors of targeted cells such as class B scavenger receptors that mediate HDL binding and cellular uptake; (2) they are extremely small and have the ability to penetrate into tissues to some extent, in particular to atherosclerotic lesions via the leaky vasculature; through this mechanism, rHDL particles can be retained in the plaque microenvironment for longer time periods. Considerable effort has been made in controlling the size of rHDL particles, a feature essential for the delivery of payload to the cytoplasm and avoidance of sequestration by the endosomal system (Kornmueller et al., 2019). Shaish et al. were the first to show an accumulation of radiolabeled rHDL in atherosclerotic lesions of the aortic arch in ApoE$^{-/-}$ mice (Shaish, Keren, Chouraqui, Levkovitz, & Harats, 2001). Furthermore, *in vivo* experiments in the mouse models of atherosclerosis revealed an accumulation of nanocrystalline rHDL in the vessel walls and in

macrophages of atherosclerotic plaques (Cormode et al., 2008). HDL-AuNPs was shown to deliver cholesterol-modified DNA into human cells (McMahon et al., 2011). AuNP core functionalized rHDL were also successful in the delivery of therapeutic short interference RNA (siRNA) (McMahon, Plebanek, & Thaxton, 2016). Duivenvoorden et al. have recently developed statin-loaded rHDL particles to deliver simvastatin to atherosclerotic plaques to inhibit inflammation by direct targeting of macrophages in ApoE$^{-/-}$ mice (Duivenvoorden et al., 2014). In addition, Zhang et al. reported that tanshinone IIA, a vasoactive cardioprotective drug, was loaded in discoidal and spherical rHDL particles, and delivered to foam cells in atherosclerotic lesions, and they both showed strong anti-atherogenic efficacies in New Zealand white rabbits of atherosclerosis animal models. Importantly, in a phase I clinical trial, CER-001 – an rHDL consisting of recombinant human apoA-I and phospholipids – was shown to accumulate in arterial wall and plaques after a single infusion (3 mg/kg of body weight) in patients (Chauvierre & Letourneur, 2015). In view of recent successful delivery of rHDL-based drug into atherosclerotic lesions, these small nanoparticles might play a big role in cardiovascular medicine. Through early detection, imaging, and intervention of lesions in the early stages, they can make early diagnosis and targeted therapy a clinical reality.

In addition to rHDL, new biomimetic nanoparticles have also appeared. For example, Boada et al. (Boada et al., 2020) recently developed a new type of biomimetic nanoparticle that was synthesized using membrane proteins extracted from activated macrophages. After seven consecutive days of intravenous injection in ApoE$^{-/-}$ mice, rapamycin – the cargo loaded in these nanoparticles was delivered to the vessel wall and macrophages in plaque, and specifically reduced arterial inflammation. This study provides proof-of-concept that leukocyte-derived biomimetic nanoparticles could be employed for targeted therapy in atherosclerotic cardiovascular disease.

8.2.3.3.3 Nanoparticles Coated on Stents

The use of stents to keep narrowed arteries open has proven to be beneficial to patients suffering from cardiac ischemia, even though in-stent restenosis and thrombosis may develop as a consequence of abnormal cell growth into the vessel lumen, leading to treatment failure. In order to overcome these limitations of stent technology, intensive research efforts have focused on designing new or improving existing stents. Since the advent of bare metal stents in the 1990s, these designs have been continuously improved through the use of new materials and stent coatings. The overarching goal is to control biocompatibility, degradation rate, and protein absorption and allow rapid re-reendothelialization. To overcome the main shortcomings of coated stents, drug-eluting stents (DES) have been developed to reduce the tissue hyperplasia and in-stent restenosis by eluting antiproliferative substances. Achieving the optimal drug release kinetics and drug loading capacity is the most important challenge faced by drug-eluting stents. To overcome this obstacle, different physical and chemical methods have been used to modify the surface of stents. Coating the stent with nanoparticle-based chemotherapeutics is a recent approach for synergy of passive coating and targeted drug delivery (Bartorelli et al., 1999; Kollum et al., 2005). For example, silica-based magnetic nanoparticles and carbon nanotubes are used as nanoparticulate systems to control drug release kinetics (Martin et al., 2005). In addition, Zhao et al. (Desai, Trieu, Yao, Labao, & Soon-Shiong, 2004) developed a novel coating method using sirolimus-loaded poly DL lactide (PDLLA) nanoparticles; this coating was applied to a 3D-printed PLLA biodegradables stent and resulted in a selective inhibition of smooth muscle cell proliferation (Zhao et al., 2018). Another example showing the role of nanoparticles in stents is nitric oxide-eluting bioresorbable stents. The NO-releasing nanoparticles are incorporated in the bioresorbable polymeric coating layer and scaffold.

Nanoparticle-based DDS for anti-restenosis drugs have been in clinical studies, such as paclitaxel-loaded albumin nanoparticles in SNAPIST-I/SNAPIST-III clinical trials. The albumin-coated nanoparticles permit receptor-mediated uptake of paclitaxel into endothelial cells through gp60 receptors activating caveolin-1 (Desai et al., 2004). In the SNAPIST-I study, patients received a single dose of paclitaxel-loaded nanoparticles administered via intracoronary catheter, immediately following percutaneous transluminal coronary angioplasty/stenting or balloon angioplasty. Systemic treatment was well tolerated at doses below 70 mg/m^2 with no significant adverse effects. This clinical study established the safety and optimal dosing of intravenous paclitaxel-nanoparticles to reduce in-stent restenosis in de novo native coronary artery lesions, thus providing an alternative delivery strategy that could be used with any bare metal stent to inhibit restenosis at low cost.

8.2.3.4 Nanomedicine Targeting to Pathological Processes of Cardiovascular Diseases

In the previous section, the drug delivery systems that directly target the heart and vascular system were summarized. Many nanomedicines have been developed to alleviate the pathological processes leading to cardiovascular disease, which will be discussed in this section.

8.2.3.4.1 Nanomedicines Targeting Hyperlipidemia

Hyperlipidemia is a most important independent risk factor for atherosclerosis and cardiovascular disease. Cholesterol, especially low-density lipoprotein cholesterol (LDL-C), levels are usually elevated in hyperlipidemia and represent the primary therapeutic target. Statins are the first-line drugs against heart disease, which effectively reduce the elevated LDL-C by inhibiting 3-hydroxy-3-methylglutaryl coenzyme A (HMG-CoA) reductase. However, due to their poor aqueous solubility and bioavailability when administered by the oral route, high doses of statins are required, which unfortunately are associated with adverse side effects. DDS have shown to enhance the therapeutic potential of statins through improving their pharmacokinetics and bioavailability. Specifically, using a nanoparticle-mediated pitavastatin delivery system targeting vascular endothelial cells, Oda et al. reported improvement in collateral arterial circulation in an exercise-induced rabbit model of chronic hind limb ischemia, a platform potentially beneficial for treating severe organ ischemia (Oda et al., 2010). The oral administration of simvastatin-loaded nanostructured lipid carriers – a combination of solid and liquid lipids – in mice demonstrated a five-fold increase in bioavailability compared with naked simvastatin suspension (Tiwari & Pathak, 2011). Pitavastatin-nanoparticle formulation was shown to be superior to pitvastatin alone for the treatment of pulmonary artery hypertension (Liu et al., 2017).

In addition to improving the therapeutic potential of statin, nanocarriers have also been used to develop new cholesterol-lowing therapies. Pro-protein convertase substilisin/kexin type 9 (PCSK9) protein – an endogenous regulator of LDL receptors in the liver – is a key player in plasma cholesterol metabolism and has been proven to be a new target for treating hypercholesterolemia (Peterson, Fong, & Young, 2008). Therapeutic silencing of PCSK9 preserves LDL receptors in the liver, thereby reducing LDL plasma levels and conferring protection against atherosclerosis (Muro & Muzykantov, 2005). In various preclinical animal models, PCSK9 siRNA encapsulated in lipid nanoparticles reduced the expression of PCSK9 in the liver and lowered the plasma concentration of LDL, while retaining the anti-atherosclerotic HDL and liver triglycerides (Frank-Kamenetsky et al., 2008). Another example of nanocarrier-mediated cholesterol reduction therapy is targeting ApoB, which is the apolipoprotein of LDL and is required for LDL assembly in the liver. Independent studies demonstrated that the systemic injection of lipid nanocarriers containing ApoB-specific siRNA successfully down-regulated ApoB protein in liver, and decreased cholesterol and LDL plasma levels (Zimmermann et al., 2006).

8.2.3.4.2 Nanomedicines Targeting Vascular Oxidative Stress

As mentioned in the previous section, oxidative stress is an important pathogenic factor of atherosclerosis and myocardial ischemia/reperfusion injury, so it has long been the therapeutic target. However, unfortunately, clinical trials of antioxidants have failed to show benefits for patients with cardiovascular diseases, and even show harmful effects in some cases. It is believed that this inefficiency is at least partially due to their poor stability, short half-life in plasma, and insufficient diffusion in cells when administered by conventional delivery modes (Pechanova & Simko, 2009; Steinhubl, 2008).

At least in many preclinical models of CVD, natural polyphenols (such as resveratrol, guercetin, curcumin) have been proven to be effective antioxidants by reducing ROS generation or enhancing the endogenous antioxidant enzymatic defense system, but their low bioavailability and different kinetic restrictions greatly limit their clinical applications. Substantial evidence has demonstrated that polyphenol-loaded nanoparticles exhibited great improvement in *in vivo* absorption, duration of action, and relative bio-availability (Pechanova, Olga, Dayar, & Cebova, 2020). For example, Cheng et al. (2019) reported that dual-shell polymeric nanoparticles, multistage continuous targeted drug delivery carrier (MCTD)-NPs delivered resveratrol specifically to the mitochondria of ischemic cardiomyocytes, increased the distribution of resveratrol in the ischemic myocardium, and reduced infarct size in myocardial ischemia/reperfusion injury in rats.

Coenzyme Q10 (CoQ10) is another highly investigated antioxidant molecule for CVD management. As an essential component of the mitochondrial electron transport chain, CoQ10 is responsible for different functions, including acting as an antioxidant. Independent studies demonstrated CoQ10 encapsulated in liposomes exhibited protective effects on isolated rat hearts after ischemia/reperfusion, on ischemic rabbit heart after coronary artery occlusion. The cardioprotective effects have been attributed to its antioxidant and membrane-stabilizing properties (Verma, Hartner, Thakkar, Levchenko, & Torchilin, 2007; Niibori, Yokoyama, Crestanello, & Whitman, 1998).

Recently, new nanoparticles have been employed to load reactive antioxidants or they themselves exhibit antioxidant effects. As an example of the latter situation, Kim et al. (2012, 11039–11043) developed a PEGylated ceria nanoparticle that demonstrated protective effects against ROS-induced cell death *in vitro*, as well as reduction in infarct volumes and the rate of ischemic cell death *in vivo*. Selenium-mesoporous silica nanocomposites are stable and give sustained release of cargo. Recent studies have shown that it can serve as a new drug delivery platform for synaptic acid in the cardiovascular system.

8.2.3.4.3 Nanomedicines Targeting Vascular Inflammation

Inflammation is the unified mechanism driving atherosclerosis, myocardial ischemia, and reperfusion injury. Therefore, anti-inflammatory therapies have been intensively researched and have recently achieved great success. The CANTOS trial showed that the systemic application of canakinumab (an interleukin (IL)-1β neutralizing monoclonal antibody) to directly reduce inflammation can reduce the incidence of cardiovascular events. In order to further improve the therapeutic effect, different strategies have been developed through nanoparticle engineering systems that target drugs to different inflammatory pathways including the recruitment of monocyte into the arterial wall or atherosclerotic lesions, the latter of which was discussed in a previous section. Therefore, this section will outline nanocarriers that target anti-inflammatory drugs to monocytes and their interactions with endothelial cells. The monocyte CCR2 receptor for chemokine plays an important role in the extravasation and transmigration of monocyte into the subendothelial space of the arterial wall, which is an early triggering event of atherogenesis. The blood, bone marrow, and spleen are the critical reservoirs of monocytes, where nanocarriers are mainly present after systemic injection and can interact with monocytes (Swirski et al., 2009). Accordingly, several nanocarriers have been reported to target the circulating monocytes and can be potentially used for drug delivery systems for CVD treatments. Leuschner et al. (2011) first reported that optimized lipid-based nanomaterials carrying CCR2-silencing short interfering RNA can precisely target monocytes resident in bone marrow and spleen after intravenous injection in mice, and efficiently degrade CCR2 mRNA thereby inhibiting the accumulation of the proinflammatory monocyte into atherosclerotic lesions. Using the same lipid nanocarriers, both CCR2 siRNA and a magnetic resonance image (MRI) sensor were targeted to CCR2 expressing monocytes in ApoE$^{-/-}$ mice, resulting in reduced myocardial infarction that was visualized by MRI imaging (Majmudar et al., 2013). Recently, Decuzzi et al. (2021) reported that the co-delivery of anti-miR 155 and sialic acid-coated baicalein nanorods enabled efficient targeting of macrophages and significantly reduced inflammatory factors after systemic administration; this co-delivery system also allows anti-miR155 to accumulate in atherosclerotic lesions due to prolonged blood circulation time.

Interfering in the interaction of monocytes with endothelial cells is another important modality to curb monocyte infiltration and consequent proatherogenic process. For instance, liposomes coupled with a specific peptide against VCAM-1 that is upregulated on the surface of activated endothelial cells can be directed to the inflamed vascular endothelium, where they release CCR2 antagonist on site to prevent monocyte transmigration (Calin et al., 2015). Alternatively, nanocarriers targeting endothelial cell inflammation could have beneficial effects on atherosclerosis through delivering multiple siRNAs to simultaneously silence key genes responsible for monocyte recruitment. For example, polymer nanocarriers synthesized from epoxide-modified low-molecular-weight polyethyleneimine showed a preference for targeting endothelial cells *in vivo*, and could successfully silence five genes simultaneously even at low doses, thus limiting possible side effects and enhancing therapeutic efficacy (Dahlman et al., 2014).

Glucocorticoid treatment is another important anti-inflammatory approach to CVD management. Glucocorticoids are potent anti-inflammatory steroid hormones; however their receptors are present on all cells which can potentially cause harmful side effects (such as insulin resistance, glaucoma, osteoporosis) with systemic delivery, thus limiting their long-term administration to CVD patients. To overcome this disadvantage, liposomal formulations have been developed to enhance therapeutic efficacy while reducing side effects. For example, compared to free dexamethasone (DXM), DXM encapsulated in 200 nm of liposome can be efficiently taken up by macrophages and exhibit a superior effect on the reduction of lesional burden at a ten-fold lower dosage (55 versus 550 µg/kg of body weight) in atherogenic mice (Chono, Tauchi, Deguchi, & Morimoto, 2005).

Recently, Gao et al. (2020) reported a new biomimetic drug delivery system in which the ROS-responsive nanoparticles were coated with macrophage membrane. The macrophage membrane can enable the NPs to escape clearance by the reticuloendothelial system and target delivery to inflammatory sites, while the ROS-responsive component confers specific drug release due to the high local levels of ROS. Accordingly, this novel macrophage biomimetic drug delivery system has demonstrated high targeting efficiency for atherosclerotic lesions in mice, and effective inhibition of local inflammation by sequestering inflammatory factors. Therefore, this system has broad prospects for the treatment of chronic inflammatory diseases.

8.2.3.4.4 Nanomedicines Targeting Thrombosis

Thrombus formation on ruptured atherosclerotic plaques or arterial erosions frequently causes acute coronary syndromes that include various clinical scenarios from angina to ST-segment elevation myocardial infarction (STEMI). For the long-term treatment of patients with cardiovascular disease, currently available anti-thrombotic therapies (e.g., streptokinase, urokinase, or tissue plasminogen activator – rtPA) are usually insufficient to prevent acute thrombotic events and the deterioration of atherosclerosis. Due to their short half-life in circulation after systemic injection, high dosages are required to achieve the therapeutic effect, which have the potential to cause fatal side effects such as intracranial hemorrhage, which greatly limit their clinical applications (Rauch et al., 2001). Different nanosystem-based strategies have been used to protect the anti-thrombotic drugs from inactivation during the circulation process by concentrating them into the thrombus. Therefore, the accomplishments of nanomedicine in thrombolytic diseases include improving blood half-life, enhancing thrombolytic effect at lower doses, accelerating blood flow recovery, and reducing the risk of systemic bleeding. Overall, three modalities are currently being tested for the targeted delivery of anti-thrombotic drugs in preclinical models: (1) non-targeted nanocarriers; (2) nanoparticles incorporated with active targeting moiety on the surface; (3) nano delivery vehicles, the targeting and drug release of which are controlled by internal or external stimuli such as magnetic field, ultrasound, temperature, and pH (Zenych, Fournier, & Chauvierre, 2020).

Studies have shown that positive and neutral liposomes themselves can efficiently concentrate in regions of myocardial infarction (Geelen, Paulis, Coolen, Nicolay, & Strijkers, 2013); therefore, streptokinase or rtPA encapsulated into liposomes exhibits prolonged circulation time and superior fibrinolytic activity compared to free drugs (Leach, Patterson, & O'Rear, 2004). To overcome the disadvantages associated with liposomes (e.g., limited circulation stability and the risk of premature drug release), other types of nanocarriers have been developed such as water-soluble double emulsion polymer with PVA and PEG nanoparticles, or urokinase-loaded chitosan nanoparticle, which facilitate thrombolysis and reduce bleeding complications (Leach et al., 2004; Jin, Zhang, Sun, Zhang, & Zhang, 2013).

To enhance the accumulation of nanocarriers in thrombus, RGD peptide (arginine-glycine-aspartic acid) has been used to functionalize their surface, which is targeted to GPIIb/IIIa receptor expressed at the surface of the activated platelets in thrombi. With this modification, the targeted liposomes loaded with either streptokinase or rtPA showed increased thrombus accumulation and thrombolytic activity compared to non-targeted carriers (Vaidya, Agrawal, & Vyas, 2011; Absar, Nahar, Kwon, & Ahsan, 2013). In addition, von Willebrand factors (vWF) are highly expressed in thrombus and have relatively higher binding affinity to gelatin. Kawata et al. (2012) developed gelatin-based nanoparticles that are loaded with rtPA and monteplase, together with Zn^{2+} ions. In a swine model of acute myocardial infarction, this nanomedicine elicited effective therapeutic effects. Another promising approach for thrombolytic drug delivery is magnetic drug targeting, which can enhance imaging-guided delivery and therapeutic effects. For example, magnetic nanoparticles coated with polyacrylic acid (PAA) (Ma et al., 2009) or poly(aniline-co-N-[1-monobutyric acid]aniline) (Yang et al., 2012) are covalently conjugated with rtPA. After systemic administration, these drug-loaded magnetic nanoparticles gather in the thrombus under the guidance of a magnetic field, and then dissolve the clot, thereby improving blood flow recovery.

REFERENCES

Absar, S., K. Nahar, Y. M. Kwon, and F. Ahsan. "Thrombus-Targeted Nanocarrier Attenuates Bleeding Complications Associated with Conventional Thrombolytic Therapy." *Pharmaceutical Research* 30, no. 6 (2013): 1663–76. doi:10.1007/s11095-013-1011-x.

Alagarsamy, K. N., W. Yan, A. Srivastava, V. Desiderio, and S. Dhingra. "Application of Injectable Hydrogels for Cardiac Stem Cell Therapy and Tissue Engineering." *Reviews in Cardiovascular Medicine* 20, no. 4 (2019): 221–30. doi:10.31083/j.rcm.2019.04.534.

Alvarez-Erviti, L., Y. Seow, H. Yin, C. Betts, S. Lakhal, and M. J. A. Wood. "Delivery of siRNA to the Mouse Brain by Systemic Injection of Targeted Exosomes." *Nature Biotechnology* 29, no. 4 (2011): 341–U179. doi:10.1038/nbt.1807.

Attia, M. F., N. Anton, J. Wallyn, Z. Omran, and T. F. Vandamme. "An Overview of Active and Passive Targeting Strategies to Improve the Nanocarriers Efficiency to Tumour Sites." *Journal of Pharmacy & Pharmacology* 71, no. 8 (2019): 1185–98. doi:10.1111/jphp.13098.

Banerjee, M. N., R. Bolli, and J. M. Hare. "Clinical Studies of Cell Therapy in Cardiovascular Medicine Recent Developments and Future Directions." *Circulation Research* 123, no. 2 (2018): 266–87. doi:10.1161/CIRCRESAHA.118.311217.

Bartorelli, A. L., F. Fabbiocchi, A. Loaldi, P. Montorsi, S. Galli, D. Trabattoni, … D. Antoniucci. "Clinical and Angiographic Evaluation of the CARBOSTENT: A New Cellular Design Carbofilm Coated Coronary Stent." *American Journal of Cardiology* 84, no. 6A (1999): 109P.

Benjamin, E. J., S. S. Virani, C. W. Callaway, A. M. Chamberlain, A. R. Chang, S. Cheng, S. E. Chiuve, M. Cushman, F. N. Delling, R. Deo, S. D. de Ferranti, J. F. Ferguson, M. Fornage, C. Gillespie, C. R. Isasi, M. C. Jiménez, L. C. Jordan, S. E. Judd, D. Lackland, J. H. Lichtman, L. Lisabeth, S. Liu, C. T. Longenecker, P. L. Lutsey, J. S. Mackey, D. B. Matchar, K. Matsushita, M. E. Mussolino, K. Nasir, M. O'Flaherty, L. P. Palaniappan, A. Pandey, D. K. Pandey, M. J. Reeves, M. D. Ritchey, C. J. Rodriguez, G. A. Roth, W. D. Rosamond, U. K. A. Sampson, G. M. Satou, S. H. Shah, N. L. Spartano, D. L. Tirschwell, C. W. Tsao, J. H. Voeks, J. Z. Willey, J. T. Wilkins, J. H. Wu, H. M. Alger, S. S. Wong, P. Muntner, and American Heart Association Council on Epidemiology and Prevention Statistics Committee and Stroke Statistics Subcommittee. "Heart Disease and Stroke statistics-2018 Update: A Report from the American Heart Association." *Circulation* 137, no. 12 (2018): E67–EE492. doi:10.1161/CIR.0000000000000558.

Boada, C., A. Zinger, C. Tsao, P. Zhao, J. O. Martinez, K. Hartman, T. Naoi, R. Sukhoveshin, M. Sushnitha, R. Molinaro, B. Trachtenberg, J. P. Cooke, and E. Tasciotti. "Rapamycin-Loaded Biomimetic Nanoparticles Reverse Vascular Inflammation." *Circulation Research* 126, no. 1 (2020): 25–37. doi:10.1161/CIRCRESAHA.119.315185.

Boren, J., and K. J. Williams. "The Central Role of Arterial Retention of Cholesterol-Rich Apolipoprotein-B-Containing Lipoproteins in the Pathogenesis of Atherosclerosis: A Triumph of Simplicity." *Current Opinion in Lipidology* 27, no. 5 (2016): 473–8. doi:10.1097/MOL.0000000000000330.

Boyle, J. J., P. L. Weissberg, and M. R. Bennett. "Human Macrophage-Induced Vascular Smooth Muscle Cell Apoptosis Requires NO Enhancement of Fas/Fas-L Interactions." *Arteriosclerosis, Thrombosis & Vascular Biology* 22, no. 10 (2002): 1624–30. doi:10.1161/01.ATV.0000033517.48444.1A.

Bulbake, U., S. Doppalapudi, N. Kommineni, and W. Khan. "Liposomal Formulations in Clinical Use: An Updated Review." *Pharmaceutics* 9, no. 2 (2017): 12. doi:10.3390/pharmaceutics9020012.

Calin, M., D. Stan, M. Schlesinger, V. Simion, M. Deleanu, C. A. Constantinescu, A. M. Gan, M. M. Pirvulescu, E. Butoi, I. Manduteanu, M. Bota, M. Enachescu, L. Borsig, G. Bendas, and M. Simionescu. "VCAM-1 Directed Target-Sensitive Liposomes Carrying CCR2 Antagonists Bind to Activated Endothelium and Reduce Adhesion and Transmigration of Monocytes." *European Journal of Pharmaceutics & Biopharmaceutics* 89 (2015): 18–29. doi:10.1016/j.ejpb.2014.11.016.

Casscells, W., M. Naghavi, and J. T. Willerson. "Vulnerable Atherosclerotic Plaque: A Multifocal Disease." *Circulation* 107, no. 16 (2003): 2072–5. doi:10.1161/01.CIR.0000069329.70061.68.

Chang, M., Y. Yang, C. Chang, A. C. L. Tang, W. Liao, F. Cheng, C. S. Yeh, J. J. Lai, P. S. Stayton, and P. C. H. Hsieh. "Functionalized Nanoparticles Provide Early Cardioprotection After Acute Myocardial Infarction." *Journal of Controlled Release* 170, no. 2 (2013): 287–94. doi:10.1016/j.jconrel.2013.04.022.

Chauvierre, C., and D. Letourneur. "The European Project NanoAthero to Fight Cardiovascular Diseases Using Nanotechnologies." *Nanomedicine* 10, no. 22 (2015): 3391–400. doi:10.2217/nnm.15.170.

Cheng, Y., D. Liu, C. Zhang, H. Cui, M. Liu, B. Zhang, Q. B. Mei, Z. F. Lu, and S. Zhou. "Mitochondria-Targeted Antioxidant Delivery for Precise Treatment of Myocardial Ischemia-Reperfusion Injury Through a Multistage Continuous Targeted Strategy." *Nanomedicine-Nanotechnology, Biology & Medicine* 16 (2019): 236–49. doi:10.1016/j.nano.2018.12.014.

Chiong, M., Z. V. Wang, Z. Pedrozo, D. J. Cao, R. Troncoso, M. Ibacache, A. Criollo, A. Nemchenko, J. A. Hill, and S. Lavandero. "Cardiomyocyte Death: Mechanisms and Translational Implications." *Cell Death & Disease* 2 (2011): e244. doi:10.1038/cddis.2011.130.

Choi, J., J. Park, and J. Park. "Design of Coenzyme Q10 Solid Dispersion for Improved Solubilization and Stability." *International Journal of Pharmaceutics* 572 (2019): 118832. doi:10.1016/j.ijpharm.2019.118832.

Chono, S., Y. Tauchi, Y. Deguchi, and K. Morimoto. "Efficient Drug Delivery to Atherosclerotic Lesions and the Antiatherosclerotic Effect by Dexamethasone Incorporated into Liposomes in Atherogenic Mice." *Journal of Drug Targeting* 13, no. 4 (2005): 267–76. doi:10.1080/10611860500159030.

Cicha, I., C. Chauvierre, I. Texier, C. Cabella, J. M. Metselaar, J. Szebeni, L. Dézsi, C. Alexiou, F. Rouzet, G. Storm, E. Stroes, D. Bruce, N. MacRitchie, P. Maffia, and D. Letourneur. "From Design to the Clinic: Practical Guidelines for Translating Cardiovascular Nanomedicine." *Cardiovascular Research* 114, no. 13 (2018): 1714–27. doi:10.1093/cvr/cvy219.

Cohen, T., and J. Klein. "Cardiac Resynchronization Therapy for Treatment of Chronic Heart Failure." *Journal of Invasive Cardiology* 14, no. 1 (2002): 48–53.

Cormode, D. P., T. Skajaa, M. M. van Schooneveld, R. Koole, P. Jarzyna, M. E. Lobatto, C. Calcagno, A. Barazza, R. E. Gordon, P. Zanzonico, E. A. Fisher, Z. A. Fayad, and W. J. M. Mulder. "Nanocrystal Core High-Density Lipoproteins: A Multimodality Contrast Agent Platform." *Nano Letters* 8, no. 11 (2008): 3715–23. doi:10.1021/nl801958b.

Cui, Z., B. H. Lee, C. Pauken, and B. L. Vernon. "Degradation, Cytotoxicity, and Biocompatibility of NIPAAm-Based Thermosensitive, Injectable, and Bioresorbable Polymer Hydrogels." *Journal of Biomedical Materials Research: Part A* 98A, no. 2 (2011): 159–66. doi:10.1002/jbm.a.33093.

Dahlman, J. E., C. Barnes, O. F. Khan, A. Thiriot, S. Jhunjunwala, T. E. Shaw, Y. Xing, H. B. Sager, G. Sahay, L. Speciner, A. Bader, R. L. Bogorad, H. Yin, T. Racie, Y. Dong, S. Jiang, D. Seedorf, A. Dave, K. S. Sandu, M. J. Webber, T. Novobrantseva, V. M. Ruda, A. K. R. Lytton-Jean, C. G. Levins, B. Kalish, D. K. Mudge, M. Perez, L. Abezgauz, P. Dutta, L. Smith, K. Charisse, M. W. Kieran, K. Fitzgerald, M. Nahrendorf, D. Danino, R. M. Tuder, U. H. von Andrian, A. Akinc, A. Schroeder, D. Panigrahy, V. Kotelianski, R. Langer, and D. G. erson. "In Vivo Endothelial siRNA Delivery Using Polymeric Nanoparticles with Low Molecular Weight." *Nature Nanotechnology* 9, no. 8 (2014): 648–55. doi:10.1038/NNANO.2014.84.

Decuzzi, P., D. Peer, D. Di Mascolo, A. L. Palange, P. N. Manghnani, S. M. Moghimi, Z. S. Farhangrazi, K. A. Howard, D. Rosenblum, T. Liang, Z. Chen, Z. Wang, J. J. Zhu, Z. Gu, N. Korin, D. Letourneur, C. Chauvierre, R. van der Meel, F. Kiessling, and T. Lammers. "Roadmap on Nanomedicine." *Nanotechnology* 32, no. 1 (2021): 012001. doi:10.1088/1361-6528/abaadb.

Desai, N., V. Trieu, R. Yao, E. Labao, and P. Soon-Shiong. "Increased Endothelial Transcytosis of Nanoparticle Albumin Bound Paclitaxel (ABI-007) by gp60-Receptors: A Pathway Inhibited by Taxol." *Breast Cancer Research & Treatment* 88, no. Suppl.65 (2004).

Dinh, N., M. Kukumberg, A. Nguyen, H. Keramati, S. Guo, D. Phan, N. B. Ja'Afar, E. Birgersson, H. L. Leo, R. Y. Huang, T. Kofidis, A. J. Rufaihah, and C. Chen. "Functional Reservoir Microcapsules Generatedviamicrofluidic Fabrication for Long-Term Cardiovascular Therapeutics." *Lab on a Chip* 20, no. 15 (2020): 2756–64. doi:10.1039/d0lc00296h.

Duivenvoorden, R., J. Tang, D. P. Cormode, A. J. Mieszawska, D. Izquierdo-Garcia, C. Ozcan, M. J. Otten, N. Zaidi, M. E. Lobatto, S. M. van Rijs, B. Priem, E. L. Kuan, C. Martel, B. Hewing, H. Sager, M. Nahrendorf,

G. J. Randolph, E. S. G. Stroes , V. Fuster, E. A. Fisher, Z. A. Fayad, and W. J. M. Mulder. "A Statin-Loaded Reconstituted High-Density Lipoprotein Nanoparticle Inhibits Atherosclerotic Plaque Inflammation (vol 5, Pg 3065, 2014)." *Nature Communications* 5, no. 1 (2014): 3531. doi:10.1038/ncomms4531.

Eggen, D. A., and L. A. Solberg. "Variation of Atherosclerosis with Age." *Laboratory Investigation* 18, no. 5 (1968): 571–9.

Erturk, A. S., M. U. Gurbuz, and M. Tulu. "The Effect of PAMAM Dendrimer Concentration, Generation Size and Surface Functional Group on the Aqueous Solubility of Candesartan Cilexetil." *Pharmaceutical Development & Technology* 22, no. 1 (2017): 111–21. doi:10.1080/10837450.2016.1219372.

Falk, E., P. K. Shah, and V. Fuster. "Coronary Plaque Disruption." *Circulation* 92, no. 3 (1995): 657–71. doi:10.1161/01. CIR.92.3.657.

Fernandez-Ruiz, I. "Macrophage Mimetics to Target Atherosclerosis." *Nature Reviews. Cardiology* 17, no. 8 (2020): 454. doi:10.1038/s41569-020-0404-x.

Frank-Kamenetsky, M., A. Grefhorst, N. N. Anderson, T. S. Racie, B. Bramlage, A. Akinc, D. Butler, K. Charisse, R. Dorkin, Y. Fan, C. Gamba-Vitalo, P. Hadwiger, M. Jayaraman, M. John, K. N. Jayaprakash, M. Maier, L. Nechev, K. G. Rajeev, T. Read, I. Röhl, J. Soutschek, P. Tan, J. Wong, G. Wang, T. Zimmermann, A. de Fougerolles, H. P. Vornlocher, R. Langer, D. G. Anderson, M. Manoharan, V. Koteliansky, J. D. Horton, and K. Fitzgerald. "Therapeutic RNAi Targeting PCSK9 Acutely Lowers Plasma Cholesterol in Rodents and LDL Cholesterol in Nonhuman Primates." *Proceedings of the National Academy of Sciences of the United States of America* 105, no. 33 (2008): 11915–20. doi:10.1073/pnas.0805434105.

Gao, C., Q. Huang, C. Liu, C. H. T. Kwong, L. Yue, J. Wan, S. M. Y. Lee, and R. Wang. "Treatment of Atherosclerosis by Macrophage-Biomimetic Nanoparticles via Targeted Pharmacotherapy and Sequestration of Proinflammatory Cytokines." *Nature Communications* 11, no. 1 (2020). doi:10.1038/s41467-020-16439-7.

Geelen, T., L. E. Paulis, B. F. Coolen, K. Nicolay, and G. J. Strijkers. "Passive Targeting of Lipid-Based Nanoparticles to Mouse Cardiac Ischemia-Reperfusion Injury." *Contrast Media & Molecular Imaging* 8, no. 2 (2013): 117–26. doi:10.1002/cmmi.1501.

Gimbrone, M. A., Jr., and G. Garcia-Cardena. "Endothelial Cell Dysfunction and the Pathobiology of Atherosclerosis." *Circulation Research* 118, no. 4 (2016): 620–36. doi:10.1161/CIRCRESAHA.115.306301.

Golpanian, S., A. Wolf, K. E. Hatzistergos, and J. M. Hare. "Rebuilding the Damaged Heart: Mesenchymal Stem Cells, Cell-Based Therapy, and Engineered Heart Tissue." *Physiological Reviews* 96, no. 3 (2016): 1127–68. doi:10.1152/physrev.00019.2015.

Gough, P. J., I. G. Gomez, P. T. Wille, and E. W. Raines. "Macrophage Expression of Active MMP-9 Induces Acute Plaque Disruption in apoE-Deficient Mice." *Journal of Clinical Investigation* 116, no. 1 (2006): 59–69. doi:10.1172/JCI25074.

Guo, BaoLin, and P. X. Ma. "Synthetic Biodegradable Functional Polymers for Tissue Engineering: A Brief Review." *Science in China-(Chemistry)* 57, no. 4 (2014): 490–500. doi:10.1007/s11426-014-5086-y.

Hamburg, N. M., and J. A. Vita. *Molecular Mechanisms of Atherosclerosis*. Edited by J. Loscalzo. Boca Raton, FL: CRC Press, Dec. 22, 2004.

Han, Y., W. Yang, W. Cui, K. Yang, X. Wang, Y. Chen, L. Deng, Y. Zhao, and W. Jin. "Development of Functional Hydrogels for Heart Failure." *Journal of Materials Chemistry B* 7, no. 10 (2019): 1563–80. doi:10.1039/c8tb02591f.

Hasan, A., A. Khattab, M. A. Islam, K. A. Hweij, J. Zeitouny, R. Waters, M. Sayegh, M. M. Hossain, and A. Paul. "Injectable Hydrogels for Cardiac Tissue Repair After Myocardial Infarction." *Advanced Science* 2, no. 11 (2015): 1500122. doi:10.1002/advs.201500122.

Herrington, W., B. Lacey, P. Sherliker, J. Armitage, and S. Lewington. "Epidemiology of Atherosclerosis and the Potential to Reduce the Global Burden of Atherothrombotic Disease." *Circulation Research* 118, no. 4 (2016): 535–46. doi:10.1161/CIRCRESAHA.115.307611.

Hoffman, J., S. Kaplan, and R. R. Liberthson. "Prevalence of Congenital Heart Disease." *American Heart Journal* 147, no. 3 (2004): 425–39. doi:10.1016/j.ahj.2003.05.003.

Hoffmann, E., N. Sulke, N. Edvardsson, J. Ruiter, T. Lewalter, A. Capucci, A. Schuchert, S. Janko, J. Camm, and Atrial Fibrillation Therapy Trial Investigators, … AFT Trial Investigators. "New Insights into the Initiation of Atrial Fibrillation: A Detailed Intraindividual and Interindividual Analysis of the Spontaneous Onset of Atrial Fibrillation Using New Diagnostic Pacemaker Features." *Circulation* 113, no. 16 (2006): 1933–41. doi:10.1161/CIRCULATIONAHA.105.568568.

Insull, W., Jr. "The Pathology of Atherosclerosis: Plaque Development and Plaque Responses to Medical Treatment." *American Journal of Medicine* 122, no. 1 Suppl. (2009): S3–SS14. doi:10.1016/j.amjmed.2008.10.013.

Jin, H., H. Zhang, M. Sun, B. Zhang, and J. Zhang. "Urokinase-Coated Chitosan Nanoparticles for Thrombolytic Therapy: Preparation and Pharmacodynamics In Vivo." *Journal of Thrombosis & Thrombolysis* 36, no. 4 (2013): 458–68. doi:10.1007/s11239-013-0951-7.

Kamaly, N., Z. Xiao, P. M. Valencia, A. F. Radovic-Moreno, and O. C. Farokhzad. "Targeted Polymeric Therapeutic Nanoparticles: Design, Development and Clinical Translation." *Chemical Society Reviews* 41, no. 7 (2012): 2971–3010. doi:10.1039/c2cs15344k.

Kao, C., and E. T. Papoutsakis. "Extracellular Vesicles: Exosomes, Microparticles, Their Parts, and Their Targets to Enable Their Biomanufacturing and Clinical Applications." *Current Opinion in Biotechnology* 60 (2019): 89–98. doi:10.1016/j.copbio.2019.01.005.

Katz, M. G., S. M. Gubara, Y. Hadas, T. Weber, A. Kumar, E. Eliyahu, C. R. Bridges, and A. S. Fargnoli. "Effects of Genetic Transfection on Calcium Cycling Pathways Mediated by Double-Stranded Adeno-Associated Virus in Postinfarction Remodeling." *Journal of Thoracic & Cardiovascular Surgery* 159, no. 5 (2020): 1809–1819. e3. doi:10.1016/j.jtcvs.2019.08.089.

Kawata, H., Y. Uesugi, T. Soeda, Y. Takemoto, J. Sung, K. Umaki, K. Kato, K. Ogiwara, K. Nogami, K. Ishigami, M. Horii, S. Uemura, M. Shima, Y. Tabata, and Y. Saito. "A New Drug Delivery System for Intravenous Coronary Thrombolysis with Thrombus Targeting and Stealth Activity Recoverable by Ultrasound." *Journal of the American College of Cardiology* 60, no. 24 (2012): 2550–7. doi:10.1016/j.jacc.2012.08.1008.

Kheradmandi, M., I. Ackers, M. M. Burdick, R. Malgor, and A. M. Farnoud (n.d.). "Targeting Dysfunctional Vascular Endothelial Cells Using Immunoliposomes Under Flow Conditions." *Cellular & Molecular Bioengineering* 13, no. 3-1 (2020 May 4): 189–99. doi:10.1007/s12195-020-00616.

Kim, H., N. Yun, D. Mun, J. Kang, S. Lee, H. Park, H. Park, and B. Joung. "Cardiac-Specific Delivery by Cardiac Tissue-Targeting Peptide-Expressing Exosomes." *Biochemical & Biophysical Research Communications* 499, no. 4 (2018): 803–8. doi:10.1016/j.bbrc.2018.03.227.

Kollum, M., A. Farb, R. Schreiber, K. Terfera, A. Arab, A. Geist, J. Haberstroh, S. Wnendt, R. Virmani, and C. Hehrlein. "Particle Debris from a Nanoporous Stent Coating Obscures Potential Antiproliferative Effects of Tacrolimus-Eluting Stents in a Porcine Model of Restenosis." *Catheterization & Cardiovascular Interventions* 64, no. 1 (2005): 85–90. doi:10.1002/ccd.20213.

Kolodgie, F. D., A. P. Burke, A. Farb, H. K. Gold, J. Y. Yuan, J. Narula, A. V. Finn, and R. Virmani. "The Thin-Cap Fibroatheroma: A Type of Vulnerable Plaque: The Major Precursor Lesion to Acute Coronary Syndromes." *Current Opinion in Cardiology* 16, no. 5 (2001): 285–92. doi:10.1097/00001573-200109000-00006.

Kornmueller, K., I. Vidakovic, and R. Prassl. "Artificial High Density Lipoprotein Nanoparticles in Cardiovascular Research." *Molecules* 24, no. 15 (2019): 2829. doi:10.3390/molecules24152829.

Lacko, A. G., N. A. Sabnis, B. Nagarajan, and W. J. McConathy. "HDL as a Drug and Nucleic Acid Delivery Vehicle." *Frontiers in Pharmacology* 6 (2015): 247. doi:10.3389/fphar.2015.00247.

Lamichhane, T. N., R. S. Raiker, and S. M. Jay. "Exogenous DNA Loading into Extracellular Vesicles via Electroporation Is Size-Dependent and Enables Limited Gene Delivery." *Molecular Pharmaceutics* 12, no. 10 (2015): 3650–7. doi:10.1021/acs.molpharmaceut.5b00364.

Leach, J. K., E. Patterson, and E. A. O'Rear. "Encapsulation of a Plasminogen Activator Speeds Reperfusion, Lessens Infarct and Reduces Blood Loss in a Canine Model of Coronary Artery Thrombosis." *Thrombosis & Haemostasis* 91, no. 6 (2004): 1213–8. doi:10.1160/TH03-11-0704.

Lee, J., and H. Kim. "Emerging Properties of Hydrogels in Tissue Engineering." *Journal of Tissue Engineering* 9 (2018): 2041731418768285. doi:10.1177/2041731418768285.

Leuschner, F., P. Dutta, R. Gorbatov, T. I. Novobrantseva, J. S. Donahoe, G. Courties, K. M. Lee, J. I. Kim, J. F. Markmann, B. Marinelli, P. Panizzi, W. W. Lee, Y. Iwamoto, S. Milstein, H. Epstein-Barash, W. Cantley, J. Wong, V. Cortez-Retamozo, A. Newton, K. Love, P. Libby, M. J. Pittet, F. K. Swirski, V. Koteliansky, R. Langer, R. Weissleder, D. G. Anderson, and M. Nahrendorf. "Therapeutic siRNA Silencing in Inflammatory Monocytes in Mice." *Nature Biotechnology* 29, no. 11 (2011): 1005–U73. doi:10.1038/nbt.1989.

Li, H., J. Gao, Y. Shang, Y. Hua, M. Ye, Z. Yang, C. Ou, and M. Chen. "Folic Acid Derived Hydrogel Enhances the Survival and Promotes Therapeutic Efficacy of iPS Cells for Acute Myocardial Infarction." *ACS Applied Materials & Interfaces* 10, no. 29 (2018): 24459–68. doi:10.1021/acsami.8b08659.

Liang, W., J. Chen, L. Li, M. Li, X. Wei, B. Tan, Y. Shang, G. Fan, W. Wang, and W. Liu. "Conductive Hydrogen Sulfide-Releasing Hydrogel Encapsulating ADSCs for Myocardial Infarction Treatment." *ACS Applied Materials & Interfaces* 11, no. 16 (2019): 14619–29. doi:10.1021/acsami.9b01886.

Little, W. C. "Angiographic Assessment of the Culprit Coronary-Artery Lesion Before Acute Myocardial-Infarction." *American Journal of Cardiology* 66, no. 16 (1990): G44–G7. doi:10.1016/0002-9149(90)90395-H.

Liu, H., P. Bao, L. Li, Y. Wang, C. Xu, M. Deng, J. Zhang, and X. Zhao. "Pitavastatin Nanoparticle-Engineered Endothelial Progenitor Cells Repair Injured Vessels." *Scientific Reports* 7, no. 1 (2017): 18067. doi:10.1038/s41598-017-18286-x.

Liu, X., X. Li, W. Zhu, Y. Zhang, Y. Hong, X. Liang, B. Fan, H. Zhao, H. He, and F. Zhang. "Exosomes from Mesenchymal Stem Cells Overexpressing MIF Enhance Myocardial Repair." *Journal of Cellular Physiology* 235, no. 11 (2020a): 8010–22. doi:10.1002/jcp.29456.

Liu, X., L. Zhang, W. Jiang, Z. Yang, Z. Gan, C. Yu, R. Tao, and H. Chen. "In Vitro and In Vivo Evaluation of Liposomes Modified with Polypeptides and Red Cell Membrane as a Novel Drug Delivery System for Myocardium Targeting." *Drug Delivery* 27, no. 1 (2020b): 599–606. doi:10.1080/10717544.2020.1754525.

Lukyanov, A. N., W. C. Hartner, and V. P. Torchilin. "Increased Accumulation of PEG-PE Micelles in the Area of Experimental Myocardial Infarction in Rabbits." *Journal of Controlled Release* 94, no. 1 (2004): 187–93. doi:10.1016/j.jconrel.2003.10.008.

Lyon, A. R., D. Babalis, A. C. Morley-Smith, M. Hedger, A. S. Barrientos, G. Foldes, L. S. Couch, R. A. Chowdhury, K. N. Tzortzis, N. S. Peters, E. A. Rog-Zielinska, H. Y. Yang, S. Welch, C. T. Bowles, S. Rahman Haley, A. R. Bell, A. Rice, T. Sasikaran, N. A. Johnson, E. Falaschetti, J. Parameshwar, C. Lewis, S. Tsui, A. Simon, J. Pepper, J. J. Rudy, K. M. Zsebo, K. T. Macleod, C. M. Terracciano, R. J. Hajjar, N. Banner, and S. E. Harding. "Investigation of the Safety and Feasibility of AAV1/SERCA2a Gene Transfer in Patients with Chronic Heart Failure Supported with a Left Ventricular Assist Device: The SERCA-LVAD TRIAL." *Gene Therapy* 27, no. 7 (2020): 579–90. doi:10.1038/s41434-020-0171.

Ma, Y., S. Wu, T. Wu, Y. Chang, M. Hua, and J. Chen. "Magnetically Targeted Thrombolysis with Recombinant Tissue Plasminogen Activator Bound to Polyacrylic Acid-Coated Nanoparticles." *Biomaterials* 30, no. 19 (2009): 3343–51. doi:10.1016/j.biomaterials.2009.02.034.

Majmudar, M. D., E. J. Keliher, T. Heidt, F. Leuschner, J. Truelove, B. F. Sena, R. Gorbatov, Y. Iwamoto, P. Dutta, G. Wojtkiewicz, G. Courties, M. Sebas, A. Borodovsky, K. Fitzgerald, M. W. Nolte, G. Dickneite, J. W. Chen, D. G. Anderson, F. K. Swirski, R. Weissleder, and M. Nahrendorf. "Monocyte-Directed RNAi Targeting CCR2 Improves Infarct Healing in Atherosclerosis-Prone Mice." *Circulation* 127, no. 20 (2013): 2038. doi:10.1161/CIRCULATIONAHA.112.000116.

Manso, A. M., S. I. Hashem, B. C. Nelson, E. Gault, A. Soto-Hermida, E. Villarruel, J. Bogomolovas, P. J. Bushway, C. Chen, P. Battiprolu, A. Keravala, J. D. Schwartz, G. Shah, Y. Gu, N. D. Dalton, K. Hammond, K. Peterson, P. Saftig, and E. D. Adler. "Systemic AAV9.LAMP2B Injection Reverses Metabolic and Physiologic Multiorgan Dysfunction in a Murine Model of Danon Disease." *Science Translational Medicine* 12, no. 535 (2020): eaax1744. doi:10.1126/scitranslmed.aax1744.

Martin, F., R. Walczak, A. Boiarski, M. Cohen, T. West, C. Cosentino, J. Shapiro, and M. Ferrari. "Tailoring Width of Microfabricated Nanochannels to Solute Size Can Be Used to Control Diffusion Kinetics (vol 102, Pg 123, 2005)." *Journal of Controlled Release* 107, no. 1 (2005): 183. doi:10.1016/j.jconrel.2004.09.033.

Matsumura, Y., and H. Maeda. "A New Concept for Macromolecular Therapeutics in Cancer-Chemotherapy: Mechanism of Tumoritropic Accumulation of Proteins and the Antitumor Agent Smancs." *Cancer Research* 46, no. 12 (1986): 6387–92.

Mcgill, H. C., J. Ariasste, L. M. Carbonell, P. Correa, E. A. Deveyra, S. Donoso, … J. Wainwrig. "General Findings of International Atherosclerosis Project." *Laboratory Investigation* 498, no. 502 (1968);18, no. 5: 498–502. PubMed: 5681193.

McMahon, K. M., R. K. Mutharasan, S. Tripathy, D. Veliceasa, M. Bobeica, D. K. Shumaker, A. J. Luthi, B. T. Helfand, H. Ardehali, C. A. Mirkin, O. Volpert, and C. S. Thaxton. "Biomimetic High Density Lipoprotein Nanoparticles for Nucleic Acid Delivery." *Nano Letters* 11, no. 3 (2011): 1208–14. doi:10.1021/nl1041947.

McMahon, K. M., M. P. Plebanek, and C. S. Thaxton. "Properties of Native High-Density Lipoproteins Inspire Synthesis of Actively Targeted In Vivo siRNA Delivery Vehicles." *Advanced Functional Materials* 26, no. 43 (2016): 7824–35. doi:10.1002/adfm.201602600.

McMurray, J. J. V., M. Packer, A. S. Desai, J. Gong, M. P. Lefkowitz, A. R. Rizkala, J. L. Rouleau, V. C. Shi, S. D. Solomon, K. Swedberg, M. R. Zile, and PARADIGM-HF Investigators and Committees, … PARADIGM-HF Investigators Comm. "Angiotensin-Neprilysin Inhibition Versus Enalapril in Heart Failure." *New England Journal of Medicine* 371, no. 11 (2014): 993–1004. doi:10.1056/NEJMoa1409077.

Milei, J., G. Ottaviani, A. M. Lavezzi, D. R. Grana, I. Stella, and L. Matturri. "Perinatal and Infant Early Atherosclerotic Coronary Lesions." *Canadian Journal of Cardiology* 24, no. 2 (2008): 137–41. doi:10.1016/S0828-282X(08)70570-1.

Mirowski, M., P. R. Reid, M. M. Mower, L. Watkins, V. L. Gott, J. F. Schauble, A. Langer, M. S. Heilman, S. A. Kolenik, R. E. Fischell, and M. L. Weisfeldt. "Termination of Malignant Ventricular Arrhythmias with an Implanted Automatic Defibrillator in Human-Beings." *New England Journal of Medicine* 303, no. 6 (1980): 322–4. doi:10.1056/NEJM198008073030607.

Moghiman, T., B. Barghchi, S. Esmaeili, M. M. Shabestari, S. S. Tabaee, and A. A. Momtazi-Borojeni (n.d.). "Therapeutic Angiogenesis with Exosomal microRNAs: An Effectual Approach for the Treatment of Myocardial Ischemia." *Heart Failure Reviews* 26, no. 1–9 (2021): 205–13. doi:10.1007/s10741-020-10001.

Moore, K. J., F. J. Sheedy, and E. A. Fisher. "Macrophages in Atherosclerosis: A Dynamic Balance." *Nature Reviews. Immunology* 13, no. 10 (2013): 709–21. doi:10.1038/nri3520.

Moreno-Estar, S., S. Serrano, M. Arevalo-Martinez, P. Cidad, J. Ramon Lopez-Lopez, M. Santos, M. Santos, M. T. Pérez-Garcia, and F. Javier Arias. "Elastin-like Recombinamer-based Devices Releasing Kv1.3 Blockers for the Prevention of Intimal Hyperplasia: An in vitro and in vivo Study." *Acta Biomaterialia* 115 (2020): 264–74. doi:10.1016/j.actbio.2020.07.053.

Muro, S., and V. R. Muzykantov. "Targeting of Antioxidant and Anti-Thrombotic Drugs to Endothelial Cell Adhesion Molecules." *Current Pharmaceutical Design* 11, no. 18 (2005): 2383–401.

Naqvi, N., M. Li, E. Yahiro, R. M. Graham, and A. Husain. "Insights into the Characteristics of Mammalian Cardiomyocyte Terminal Differentiation Shown Through the Study of Mice with a Dysfunctional c-kit." *Pediatric Cardiology* 30, no. 5 (2009): 651–8. doi:10.1007/s00246-008-9366-1.

Newby, A. C., and A. B. Zaltsman. "Fibrous Cap Formation or Destruction: The Critical Importance of Vascular Smooth Muscle Cell Proliferation, Migration and Matrix Formation." *Cardiovascular Research* 41, no. 2 (1999): 345–60. doi:10.1016/S0008-6363(98)00286-7.

Niibori, K., H. Yokoyama, J. A. Crestanello, and G. J. R. Whitman. "Acute Administration of Liposomal Coenzyme Q10Increases Myocardial Tissue Levels and Improves Tolerance to Ischemia Reperfusion Injury." *Journal of Surgical Research* 79, no. 2 (1998): 141–5. doi:10.1006/jsre.1998.5411.

Oda, S., R. Nagahama, K. Nakano, T. Matoba, M. Kubo, K. Sunagawa, R. Tominaga, and K. Egashira. "Nanoparticle-Mediated Endothelial Cell-Selective Delivery of Pitavastatin Induces Functional Collateral Arteries (Therapeutic Arteriogenesis) in a Rabbit Model of Chronic Hind Limb Ischemia." *Journal of Vascular Surgery* 52, no. 2 (2010): 412–20. doi:10.1016/j.jvs.2010.03.020.

Oh, K. S., J. Y. Song, S. J. Yoon, Y. Park, D. Kim, and S. H. Yuk. "Temperature-Induced Gel Formation of Core/Shell Nanoparticles for the Regeneration of Ischemic Heart." *Journal of Controlled Release* 146, no. 2 (2010): 207–11. doi:10.1016/j.jconrel.2010.04.014.

Ohno, S., M. Takanashi, K. Sudo, S. Ueda, A. Ishikawa, N. Matsuyama, K. Fujita, T. Mizutani, T. Ohgi, T. Ochiya, N. Gotoh, and M. Kuroda. "Systemically Injected Exosomes Targeted to EGFR Deliver Antitumor MicroRNA to Breast Cancer Cells." *Molecular Therapy* 21, no. 1 (2013): 185–91. doi:10.1038/mt.2012.180.

Ozaki Tan, S. J., J. F. Floriano, L. Nicastro, C. Emanueli, and F. Catapano. "Novel Applications of Mesenchymal Stem Cell-Derived Exosomes for Myocardial Infarction Therapeutics." *Biomolecules* 10, no. 5 (2020): 707. doi:10.3390/biom10050707.

Pagel, W. "Galen and the Usefulness of the Parts of the Body, Translated from the Greek with an Introduction and Commentary by Margaret Tallmadge May, Ithaca, New York, Cornell University Press1968." *Medical History* 2 vols 14, no. 4 (1970): 406–408, pp. xv, 802, $25 (238s). doi:10.1017/S0025727300015878.

Pammolli, F., L. Magazzini, and M. Riccaboni. "The Productivity Crisis in Pharmaceutical R&D." *Nature Reviews. Drug Discovery* 10, no. 6 (2011): 428–38. doi:10.1038/nrd3405.

Park, K. "Controlled Drug Delivery Systems: Past Forward and Future Back." *Journal of Controlled Release* 190 (2014): 3–8. doi:10.1016/j.jconrel.2014.03.054.

Paul, A., A. Hasan, H. Al Kindi, A. K. Gaharwar, V. T. S. Rao, M. Nikkhah, S. R. Shin, D. Krafft, M. R. Dokmeci, D. Shum-Tim, and A. Khademhosseini. "Injectable Graphene Oxide/Hydrogel-Based Angiogenic Gene Delivery System for Vasculogenesis and Cardiac Repair." *ACS Nano* 8, no. 8 (2014): 8050–62. doi:10.1021/nn5020787.

Pechanova, O., E. Dayar, and M. Cebova. "Therapeutic Potential of Polyphenols-Loaded Polymeric Nanoparticles in Cardiovascular System." *Molecules* 25, no. 15 (2020): 3322. doi:10.3390/molecules25153322.

Pechanova, O., and F. Simko. "Chronic Antioxidant Therapy Fails to Ameliorate Hypertension: Potential Mechanisms Behind." *Journal of Hypertension* 27, no. 6 (2009): 32. doi:10.1097/01.hjh.0000358835.25934.5e.

Pedrotty, D. M., R. Y. Klinger, R. D. Kirkton, and N. Bursac. "Cardiac Fibroblast Paracrine Factors Alter Impulse Conduction and Ion Channel Expression of Neonatal Rat Cardiomyocytes." *Cardiovascular Research* 83, no. 4 (2009): 688–97. doi:10.1093/cvr/cvp164.

Pena, B., M. Laughter, S. Jett, T. J. Rowland, M. R. G. Taylor, L. Mestroni, and D. Park. "Injectable Hydrogels for Cardiac Tissue Engineering." *Macromolecular Bioscience* 18, no. 6 (2018). doi:10.1002/mabi.201800079, PubMed: 1800079.

Pentikainen, M. O., K. Oorni, M. Ala-Korpela, and P. T. Kovanen. "Modified LDL-Trigger of Atherosclerosis and Inflammation in the Arterial Intima." *Journal of Internal Medicine* 247, no. 3 (2000): 359–70. doi:10.1046/j.1365-2796.2000.00655.x.

Peter, A. K., M. A. Bjerke, and L. A. Leinwand. "Biology of the Cardiac Myocyte in Heart Disease." *Molecular Biology of the Cell* 27, no. 14 (2016): 2149–60. doi:10.1091/mbc.E16-01-0038.

Peterson, A. S., L. G. Fong, and S. G. Young. "PCSK9 Function and Physiology (vol 49, Pg 1303, 2008)." *Journal of Lipid Research* 49, no. 7 (2008): 1595–9. doi:10.1194/jlr.CX00001-JLR200.

Piao, H., J. Kwon, S. Piao, J. Sohn, Y. Lee, J. Bae, K. K. Hwang, D. W. Kim, O. Jeon, B. S. Kim, Y. B. Park, and M. Cho. "Effects of Cardiac Patches Engineered with Bone Marrow-Derived Mononuclear Cells and

PGCL Scaffolds in a Rat Myocardial Infarction Model." *Biomaterials* 28, no. 4 (2007): 641–9. doi:10.1016/j.biomaterials.2006.09.009.

Pinto, A. R., A. Ilinykh, M. J. Ivey, J. T. Kuwabara, M. L. D'Antoni, R. Debuque, A. Chandran, L. Wang, K. Arora, N. A. Rosenthal, and M. D. Tallquist. "Revisiting Cardiac Cellular Composition." *Circulation Research* 118, no. 3 (2016): 400–9. doi:10.1161/CIRCRESAHA.115.307778.

Pleger, S. T., H. Brinks, J. Ritterhoff, P. Raake, W. J. Koch, H. A. Katus, and P. Most. "Heart Failure Gene Therapy the Path to Clinical Practice." *Circulation Research* 113, no. 6 (2013): 792–809. doi:10.1161/CIRCRESAHA.113.300269.

Prakoso, D., M. J. De Blasio, M. Tate, H. Kiriazis, D. G. Donner, H. Qian, D. Nash, M. Deo, K. L. Weeks, L. J. Parry, P. Gregorevic, J. R. McMullen, and R. H. Ritchie. "Gene Therapy Targeting Cardiac Phosphoinositide 3-Kinase (p110 Alpha) Attenuates Cardiac Remodeling in type 2 Diabetes." *American Journal of Physiology-Heart & Circulatory Physiology* 318, no. 4 (2020): H840–H52. doi:10.1152/ajpheart.00632.2019.

Raposo, G., and W. Stoorvogel. "Extracellular Vesicles: Exosomes, Microvesicles, and Friends." *Journal of Cell Biology* 200, no. 4 (2013): 373–83. doi:10.1083/jcb.201211138.

Rauch, U., J. I. Osende, V. Fuster, J. J. Badimon, Z. Fayad, and J. H. Chesebro. "Thrombus Formation on Atherosclerotic Plaques: Pathogenesis and Clinical Consequences." *Annals of Internal Medicine* 134, no. 3 (2001): 224–38. doi:10.7326/0003-4819-134-3-200102060-00014.

Sawyers, C. "Targeted Cancer Therapy." *Nature* 432, no. 7015 (2004): 294–7. doi:10.1038/nature03095.

Schwenke, D. C., and T. E. Carew. "Initiation of Atherosclerotic Lesions in Cholesterol-Fed rabbits 0.2. Selective Retention of Ldl vs Selective Increases in Ldl Permeability in Susceptible Sites of Arteries." *Arteriosclerosis* 9, no. 6 (1989): 908–18. doi:10.1161/01.ATV.9.6.908.

Scott, R. C., J. M. Rosano, Z. Ivanov, B. Wang, P. L. Chong, A. C. Issekutz, D. L. Crabbe, and M. F. Kiani. "Targeting VEGF-Encapsulated Immunoliposomes to MI Heart Improves Vascularity and Cardiac Function." *FASEB Journal* 23, no. 10 (2009): 3361–7. doi:10.1096/fj.08-127373.

Serini, S., R. Cassano, S. Trombino, and G. Calviello. "Nanomedicine-Based Formulations Containing omega-3 Polyunsaturated Fatty Acids: Potential Application in Cardiovascular and Neoplastic Diseases." *International Journal of Nanomedicine* 14 (2019): 2809–28. doi:10.2147/IJN.S197499.

Shaish, A., G. Keren, P. Chouraqui, H. Levkovitz, and D. Harats. "Imaging of Aortic Atherosclerotic Lesions by I-125-LDL, I-125-Oxidized-LDL, I-125-HDL and I-125-BSA." *Pathobiology* 69, no. 4 (2001): 225–9. doi:10.1159/000055947.

Sheffield, C., K. Meyers, E. Johnson, and R. M. Rajachar. "Application of Composite Hydrogels to Control Physical Properties in Tissue Engineering and Regenerative Medicine." *Gels* 4, no. 2 (2018): 51. doi:10.3390/gels4020051.

Siddiqui, N., S. Asawa, B. Birru, R. Baadhe, and S. Rao. "PCL-Based Composite Scaffold Matrices for Tissue Engineering Applications." *Molecular Biotechnology* 60, no. 7 (2018): 506–32. doi:10.1007/s12033-018-0084-5.

Sidney, S., C. P. Quesenberry, Jr., M. G. Jaffe, M. Sorel, M. N. Nguyen-Huynh, L. H. Kushi, A. S. Go, and J. S. Rana. "Recent Trends in Cardiovascular Mortality in the United States and Public Health Goals." *JAMA Cardiology* 1, no. 5 (2016): 594–9. doi:10.1001/jamacardio.2016.1326.

Simoes, F. C., and P. R. Riley. "The Ontogeny, Activation and Function of the Epicardium During Heart Development and Regeneration." *Development* 145, no. 7 (2018): dev155994. doi:10.1242/dev.155994.

Sitia, S., L. Tomasoni, F. Atzeni, G. Ambrosio, C. Cordiano, A. Catapano, S. Tramontana, F. Perticone, P. Naccarato, P. Camici, E. Picano, L. Cortigiani, M. Bevilacqua, L. Milazzo, D. Cusi, C. Barlassina, P. Sarzi-Puttini, and M. Turiel. "From Endothelial Dysfunction to Atherosclerosis." *Autoimmunity Reviews* 9, no. 12 (2010): 830–4. doi:10.1016/j.autrev.2010.07.016.

Sokolov, A. A., and G. I. Martsinkevich. "Heart Failure in Patients with Preserved Ejection Fraction - Pumping Heart Failure?." *Kardiologiya* 58, no. 6 (2018): 79–84. doi:10.18087/cardio.2018.6.10125.

Spearman, B. S., A. J. Hodge, J. L. Porter, J. G. Hardy, Z. D. Davis, T. Xu, X. Zhang, C. E. Schmidt, M. C. Hamilton, and E. A. Lipke. "Conductive Interpenetrating Networks of Polypyrrole and Polycaprolactone Encourage Electrophysiological Development of Cardiac Cells." *Acta Biomaterialia* 28 (2015): 109–20. doi:10.1016/j.actbio.2015.09.025.

Stary, H. C. *An Atlas of Atherosclerosis Progression and Regression*. Boca Raton, FL: CRC Press Press, 1999.

Stary, H. C. "Natural History and Histological Classification of Atherosclerotic Lesions: An Update." *Arteriosclerosis, Thrombosis & Vascular Biology* 20, no. 5 (2000): 1177–8. doi:10.1161/01.ATV.20.5.1177.

Stein, E. M., K. P. Gennuso, D. C. Ugboaja, and P. L. Remington. "The Epidemic of Despair Among White Americans: Trends in the Leading Causes of Premature Death, 1999–2015." *American Journal of Public Health* 107, no. 10 (2017): 1541–7. doi:10.2105/AJPH.2017.303941.

Steinhubl, S. R. "Why Have Antioxidants Failed in Clinical Trials?." *American Journal of Cardiology* 101, no. 10A (2008): 14D–9D. doi:10.1016/j.amjcard.2008.02.003.

Stern, C. S., and J. Lebowitz. "Latest Drug Developments in the Field of Cardiovascular Disease." *International Journal of Angiology* 19, no. 3 (2010): e100–e5. doi:10.1055/s-0031-1278379.

Swirski, F. K., M. Nahrendorf, M. Etzrodt, M. Wildgruber, V. Cortez-Retamozo, P. Panizzi, J. L. Figueiredo, R. H. Kohler, A. Chudnovskiy, P. Waterman, E. Aikawa, T. R. Mempel, P. Libby, R. Weissleder, and M. J. Pittet. "Identification of Splenic Reservoir Monocytes and Their Deployment to Inflammatory Sites." *Science* 325, no. 5940 (2009): 612–6. doi:10.1126/science.1175202.

Taleb, S. "Inflammation in Atherosclerosis." *Archives of Cardiovascular Diseases* 109, no. 12 (2016): 708–15. doi:10.1016/j.acvd.2016.04.002.

Tian, Y., S. Li, J. Song, T. Ji, M. Zhu, G. J. Anderson, J. Wei, and G. Nie. "A Doxorubicin Delivery Platform Using Engineered Natural Membrane Vesicle Exosomes for Targeted Tumor Therapy." *Biomaterials* 35, no. 7 (2014): 2383–90. doi:10.1016/j.biomaterials.2013.11.083.

Tiwari, R., and K. Pathak. "Nanostructured Lipid Carrier Versus Solid Lipid Nanoparticles of Simvastatin: Comparative Analysis of Characteristics, Pharmacokinetics and Tissue Uptake." *International Journal of Pharmaceutics* 415, no. 1–2 (2011): 232–43. doi:10.1016/j.ijpharm.2011.05.044.

Torrieri, G., F. Fontana, P. Figueiredo, Z. Liu, M. P. A. Ferreira, V. Talman, J. P. Martins, M. Fusciello, K. Moslova, T. Teesalu, V. Cerullo, J. Hirvonen, H. Ruskoaho, V. Balasubramanian, and H. A. Santos. "Dual-Peptide Functionalized Acetalated Dextran-Based Nanoparticles for Sequential Targeting of Macrophages During Myocardial Infarction." *Nanoscale* 12, no. 4 (2020): 2350–8. doi:10.1039/c9nr09934d.

Vaidya, B., G. P. Agrawal, and S. P. Vyas. "Platelets Directed Liposomes for the Delivery of Streptokinase: Development and Characterization." *European Journal of Pharmaceutical Sciences* 44, no. 5 (2011): 589–94. doi:10.1016/j.ejps.2011.10.004.

Van Norman, G. A.. "Overcoming the Declining Trends in Innovation and Investment in Cardiovascular Therapeutics." *JACC: Basic to Translational Science* 2, no. 5 (2017): 613–25. doi:10.1016/j.jacbts.2017.09.002.

Vandergriff, A., K. Huang, D. Shen, S. Hu, M. T. Hensley, T. G. Caranasos, L. Qian, and K. Cheng. "Targeting Regenerative Exosomes to Myocardial Infarction Using Cardiac Homing Peptide." *Theranostics* 8, no. 7 (2018): 1869–78. doi:10.7150/thno.20524.

Vanderwal, A. C., A. E. Becker, C. M. Vanderloos, and P. K. Das. "Site of Intimal Rupture or Erosion of Thrombosed Coronary Atherosclerotic Plaques Is Characterized by an Inflammatory Process Irrespective Of the Dominant Plaque Morphology." *Circulation* 89, no. 1 (1994): 36–44. doi:10.1161/01.CIR.89.1.36.

Verma, D. D., W. C. Hartner, V. Thakkar, T. S. Levchenko, and V. P. Torchilin. "Protective Effect of Coenzyme Q10-Loaded Liposomes on the Myocardium in Rabbits with an Acute Experimental Myocardial Infarction." *Pharmaceutical Research* 24, no. 11 (2007): 2131–7. doi:10.1007/s11095-007-9334-0.

Virani, S. S., A. Alonso, E. J. Benjamin, M. S. Bittencourt, C. W. Callaway, A. P. Carson, A. M. Chamberlain, A. R. Chang, S. Cheng, F. N. Delling, L. Djousse, M. S. V. Elkind, J. F. Ferguson, M. Fornage, S. S. Khan, B. M. Kissela, K. L. Knutson, T. W. Kwan, D. T. Lackland, T. T. Lewis, J. H. Lichtman, C. T. Longenecker, M. S. Loop, P. L. Lutsey, S. S. Martin, K. Matsushita, A. E. Moran, M. E. Mussolino, A. M. Perak, W. D. Rosamond, G. A. Roth, U. K. A. Sampson, G. M. Satou, E. B. Schroeder, S. H. Shah, C. M. Shay, N. L. Spartano, A. Stokes, D. L. Tirschwell, L. B. VanWagner, C. W. Tsao, and American Heart Association Council. "Heart Disease and Stroke Statistics-2020 Update: A Report from the American Heart Association." *Circulation* 141, no. 9 (2020): E139–E596. doi:10.1161/CIR.0000000000000757.

Virmani, R., A. P. Burke, F. D. Kolodgie, and A. Farb. "Vulnerable Plaque: The Pathology of Unstable Coronary Lesions." *Journal of Interventional Cardiology* 15, no. 6 (2002): 439–46. doi:10.1111/j.1540-8183.2002.tb01087.x.

von Gise, A., and W. T. Pu. "Endocardial and Epicardial Epithelial to Mesenchymal Transitions in Heart Development and Disease." *Circulation Research* 110, no. 12 (2012): 1628–45. doi:10.1161/CIRCRESAHA.111.259960.

Wang, S., Y. Li, Y. Xu, Q. Ma, Z. Lin, M. Schlame, V. J. Bezzerides, D. Strathdee, and W. T. Pu. "AAV Gene Therapy Prevents and Reverses Heart Failure in a Murine Knockout Model of Barth Syndrome." *Circulation Research* 126, no. 8 (2020): 1024–39. doi:10.1161/CIRCRESAHA.119.315956.

Wang, T., L. Chen, T. Yang, P. Huang, L. Wang, L. Zhao, S. Zhang, Z. Ye, L. Chen, Z. Zheng, and J. Qin. "Congenital Heart Disease and Risk of Cardiovascular Disease: A Meta-Analysis of Cohort Studies." *Journal of the American Heart Association* 8, no. 10 (2019): e012030. doi:10.1161/JAHA.119.012030.

Wang, X., S. Li, Y. Shi, X. Chuan, J. Li, T. Zhong, H. Zhang, W. Dai, B. He, and Q. Zhang. "The Development of Site-Specific Drug Delivery Nanocarriers Based on Receptor Mediation." *Journal of Controlled Release* 193 (2014): 139–53. doi:10.1016/j.jconrel.2014.05.028.

Wang, X., Y. Chen, Z. Zhao, Q. Meng, Y. Yu, J. Sun, Z. Yang, Y. Chen, J. Li, T. Ma, H. Liu, Z. Li, J. Yang, and Z. Shen. "Engineered Exosomes with Ischemic Myocardium-Targeting Peptide for Targeted Therapy in Myocardial Infarction." *Journal of the American Heart Association* 7, no. 15 (2018): e008737. doi:10.1161/JAHA.118.008737.

Wolfram, J., M. Zhu, Y. Yang, J. Shen, E. Gentile, D. Paolino, M. Fresta, G. Nie, C. Chen, H. Shen, M. Ferrari, and Y. Zhao. "Safety of Nanoparticles in Medicine." *Current Drug Targets* 16, no. 14 (2015): 1671–81. doi:10.2174 /1389450115666140804124808.

Won, Y., A. N. McGinn, M. Lee, D. A. Bull, and S. W. Kim. "Targeted Gene Delivery to Ischemic Myocardium by Homing Peptide-Guided Polymeric Carrier." *Molecular Pharmaceutics* 10, no. 1 (2013): 378–85. doi:10.1021/ mp300500y.

Yan, C., X. Quan, and Y. Feng. "Nanomedicine for Gene Delivery for the Treatment of Cardiovascular Disease." *Current Gene Therapy* 19, no. 1 (2019): 20–30. doi:10.2174/1566523218666181003125308.

Yang, H., M. Hua, K. Lin, S. Wey, R. Tsai, S. Wu, Y. C. Lu, H. L. Liu, T. Wu, and Y. Ma. "Bioconjugation of Recombinant Tissue Plasminogen Activator to Magnetic Nanocarriers for Targeted Thrombolysis." *International Journal of Nanomedicine* 7 (2012): 5159–73. doi:10.2147/IJN.S32939.

Yi, F., H. Wu, and G. L. Jia. "Formulation and Characterization of Poly (D,L-Lactide-Co-Glycolide) Nanoparticle Containing Vascular Endothelial Growth Factor for Gene Delivery." *Journal of Clinical Pharmacy & Therapeutics* 31, no. 1 (2006): 43–8. doi:10.1111/j.1365-2710.2006.00702.x.

Yuan, X., B. He, Z. Lv, and S. Luo. "Fabrication of Self-Assembling Peptide Nanofiber Hydrogels for Myocardial Repair." *RSC Advances* 4, no. 96 (2014): 53801–11. doi:10.1039/c4ra08582e.

Zakirov, F. H., D. Zhang, A. V. Grechko, W. Wu, A. V. Poznyak, and A. N. Orekhov. "Lipid-Based Gene Delivery to Macrophage Mitochondria for Atherosclerosis Therapy." *Pharmacology Research & Perspectives* 8, no. 2 (2020): e00584. doi:10.1002/prp2.584.

Zenych, A., L. Fournier, and C. Chauvierre. "Nanomedicine Progress in Thrombolytic Therapy." *Biomaterials* 258 (2020): 120297. doi:10.1016/j.biomaterials.2020.120297.

Zhang, H., N. Li, P. Sirish, L. Mahakian, E. Ingham, F. Curry, S. Yamada, N. Chiamvimonvat, and K. W. Ferrara. "The Cargo of CRPPR-Conjugated Liposomes Crosses the Intact Murine Cardiac Endothelium." *Journal of Controlled Release* 163, no. 1 (2012a): 10–7. doi:10.1016/j.jconrel.2012.06.038.

Zhang, Y., W. Li, L. Ou, W. Wang, E. Delyagina, C. Lux, H. Sorg, K. Riehemann, G. Steinhoff, and N. Ma. "Targeted Delivery of Human VEGF Gene via Complexes of Magnetic Nanoparticle-Adenoviral Vectors Enhanced Cardiac Regeneration." *PLOS ONE* 7, no. 7 (2012b): e39490. doi:10.1371/journal.pone.0039490.

Zhao, J., Z. Mo, F. Guo, D. Shi, Q. Q. Han, and Q. Liu. "Drug Loaded Nanoparticle Coating on Totally Bioresorbable PLLA Stents to Prevent In-Stent Restenosis." *Journal of Biomedical Materials Research. Part B - Applied Biomaterials* 106, no. 1 (2018): 88–95. doi:10.1002/jbm.b.33794.

Zimmermann, T. S., A. Lee, A. Akinc, B. Bramlage, D. Bumcrot, M. N. Fedoruk, J. Harborth, J. A. Heyes, L. B. Jeffs, M. John, A. D. Judge, K. Lam, K. McClintock, L. V. Nechev, L. R. Palmer, T. Racie, I. Röhl, S. Seiffert, S. Shanmugam, V. Sood, J. Soutschek, I. Toudjarska, A. J. Wheat, E. Yaworski, W. Zedalis, V. Koteliansky, M. Manoharan, H. P. Vornlocher, and I. MacLachlan. "RNAi-Mediated Gene Silencing in Non-Human Primates." *Nature* 441, no. 7089 (2006): 111–4. doi:10.1038/nature04688.

Localizing Therapeutics to the Gastrointestinal System

9

Chunhua Yang and Didier Merlin

Contents

DOI: 10.1201/9781003092773-10

9.1 INTRODUCTION

The gastrointestinal (GI) system is responsible for hydrolyzing complex macromolecules (mostly from food) into small-molecule nutrients and absorbing these nutrients. This process includes four main phases that occur within respective regions of the GI tract: (1) temporal storage and fragmentation (stomach); (2) digestion (stomach and small intestine [SI]); (3) absorption (SI and large intestine); (4) elimination of waste (large intestine).

When seeking to localize therapeutics in different regions of the GI system, it is important to consider physiological variations. For example, it is challenging to restrain therapeutics in the stomach due to the gastric emptying process, and a colon-targeted drug delivery system (DDS) may encounter significant pH and digestive enzyme variations during the drug's transition.[1,2] Despite these obstacles, biomedical scientists have made numerous achievements in GI-targeted drug delivery, some of which may prove especially beneficial for the treatment of regional GI diseases. Oral drug delivery to the regional GI tract can largely avoid biodistribution to the circulation, which is what generally causes systemic side effects.[3] Significant efforts have been made to increase the residence time of drugs inside the stomach, SI (duodenum, jejune, and ileum), and the large intestine (colon and rectum).[4] As the physiological factors that influence oral drug delivery vary significantly in different parts of the GI system, we will explore these drug delivery strategies in an anatomy-orientated manner. While other delivery routes (such as intravenous, intramuscular, subcutaneous, or rectal administration) have also played substantial roles in GI disease treatment, their discussion is beyond the scope of this chapter.

9.2 ANATOMY AND PHYSIOLOGICAL TRAITS OF THE GI SYSTEM

The GI tract has a tubular structure of approximately 9 m in length. An orally administered substance (that starts from the oral cavity) will pass through the esophagus (~0.25 m in length), stomach (~0.3 m in length when empty), SI (~7 m in length), and large intestine (~1.5 m in length). The transit time of ingested therapeutic is one of the crucial factors that affect its regional absorption.[5] Generally, the transition of solid substance through the esophagus is immediate, and the average gastric retention of solid substance at 1, 2, and 4 h is estimated to be 90, 60, and 10%, respectively. Although the SI is the most extended GI segment, it has a medium transition time between 2 and 6 h. Impressively, the large intestine has the longest and most variable transition time, varying from 6 to 70 h[6] (Figure 9.1).

Apart from the lengths and transition times, the pH and ion strength of the stomach and different intestinal segments are noticeably distinct. The stomach secretes acidic gastric fluid with a pH between 1.0 and 2.0 and maintains a pH between 1.5 and 5.0 in fasting and fed states.[7] The ionic strength of gastric fluid is estimated to be in the range of 0.051 to 0.151 M. Small intestinal fluid's pH increases gradually from 6.5 (in the duodenum) to between 7.0 and 8.5 (in the jejunum) and is maintained at ~7.4 in the terminal ileum. The ionic strength of small intestinal fluid is slightly greater than that of the stomach (0.070 to 0.166 M). In the large intestine, the pH drops to 5.7 in the caecum and gradually increases to pH 6.7 in the rectum. As the large intestine absorbs the excessive ions and the intestinal fluid, the ionic strength is reduced to ~0.14 M, a level similar to the stomach.[8]

Enzymes in the GI tract play essential roles in the digestion of proteins, lipids (fats), and carbohydrates. Gastric acid and enzymes, especially peptidases, assist in digesting the proteins in the stomach.[9] The SI fluid combines bile and pancreatic juice secreted from the liver and the pancreas, respectively. Bile juice contains bilirubin and biliverdin that help break down large fat globules into smaller globules; the pancreatic juice then digests the smaller globule with lipase. Pancreatic juice also contains a rich abundance of pancreatic amylase, trypsin, and nuclease, being secreted to the SI, which is the primary absorption site of the digested food.[10,11]

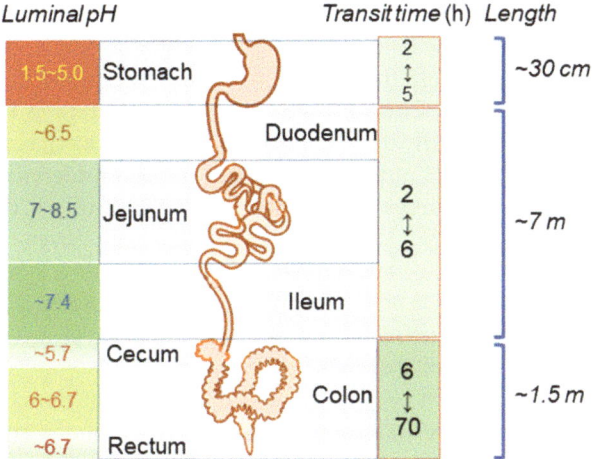

FIGURE 9.1   pH and transition time in the gastrointestinal tract.

Recent discoveries have shown that the GI tract hosts more than 500 gut microbiota species, essential for both digestion and intestinal health. Most of the intestinal microbiome inhabit the anaerobic colon, where they ferment carbohydrates and use them as the primary source of nutrition for themselves and the host.[12,13] The dominant species of colonic microbiota are *Firmicutes*, *Bacteroidetes*, *Proteobacteria*, *Actinobacteria*, and *Fusobacteria*. There are considerable variations in these species' ratio between individuals due to genetic and diet factors.[14,15] In comparison to the colon, small intestinal microbiota presents lesser abundance and diversity. However, researchers found that specific genera such as *Clostridium* and *Lactobacillus* played critical roles in small intestinal lipid metabolism, absorption, and host adaptability to dietary lipid variations.[16] Besides, the microbiome's composition in the SI presents rapid fluctuation in response to the food uptake.

GI mucus is a complex gel-like layer inside the GI tract, lubricating and aiding the passage of food, chyme, and feces through the GI tract. Mucus is mainly made of water and mucins, a group of highly glycosylated proteins that can form an entangled network through disulfide bonds linked with each other.[17,18] GI mucus's mesh-like structure also protects the epithelium from bacterial pathogens, large molecule toxins, pepsin, and other endogenous digestive enzymes. However, it still allows the penetrating of small molecule nutrients. GI mucus is thus a barrier to the delivery of macromolecule drugs, such as polypeptides, proteins, and nucleic acids. The diffusion and penetration behaviors of a formulation through mucus are crucial in determining the bioavailability of orally administered macromolecule drugs.

Challenges for localizing therapeutics to the GI system (via oral drug delivery) are related to factors that affect the stability of susceptible drugs (pH, enzyme, microbiota) and factors that reflect the physiological barriers (gastric emptying, transition time, mucus). From the drug formulation's perspective, these factors can generally be exploited in the regional drug delivery system's design.

9.3 GENERAL STRATEGY FOR GASTROINTESTINAL TARGETED DRUG DELIVERY

9.3.1 pH-Dependent Delivery

A pH-dependent drug delivery system typically involves pH-responsive coating or matrices that release the drug when they reach a suitable environment within the GI system, most often in the lower part of the GI tract.[19] Coating a formulation with a pH-sensitive enteric polymer is particularly beneficial for drugs that are susceptible to degradation by the acidic gastric fluid or by gastric enzymes and for drugs that can irritate the gastric mucosa.[20] Due to the high variability in gastric emptying time and the relatively short transit time of the SI, formulations intended to target the SI must be stable in gastric fluid but readily disintegrated and absorbed upon entering the SI.[6] Intra- and inter-individual variabilities in the pH of the SI tract need to be considered when designing clinical treatment strategies, as these variabilities could impact the release of a drug from a pH-dependent DDS. The first extensively used enteric polymer was shellac, a natural resin secreted by the female lac bug.[21] Since then, various synthetic enteric polymers have been developed, such as methyl acrylate-methacrylic acid copolymers (trade name, Eudragit), cellulose acetate phthalate (CAP), cellulose acetate succinate, hydroxypropyl methylcellulose phthalate, hydroxypropyl methylcellulose acetate succinate, and polyvinyl acetate phthalate (PVAP).

Several enteric polymers have been synthesized specifically for colon-targeting purposes. To make full use of the higher levels of resident bacteria and related enzymes in the colon, compared to the SI, researchers incorporated biodegradable particles in the enteric-coated formulations. Biodegradable polymeric particles, such as poly-lactic acid (PLA) and poly (lactic-co-glycolic acid; PLGA), have been commonly used for the formulation of colon-targeted DDS. These particles can also be embedded in hydrogel matrices (such as alginate or chitosan) that are designed to be specifically degraded by colonic enzymes.[22] Some natural polymers, such as albumin and gelatin, have also been tested for their ability to produce pH-susceptible systems that release antibiotics inside the colon.

9.3.2 Time-Dependent Drug Delivery

Time-dependent drug delivery systems feature a predetermined lag-time with minimum drug release, followed by a rapid and complete drug release on a designated schedule. The theory is to delay the drug release until the system is expected to reach the target in the GI tract. One approach uses erodible devices coated with swellable hydrophilic polymeric layers that are primarily composed of hydrophilic cellulose derivatives, such as hydroxypropyl methylcellulose (HPMC). The utilized coating methods typically include spray-coating and press-coating. The delay time can be generally adjusted by using the appropriate HMPC polymer grade to construct the multilayer coatings. After oral administration, the coated layers are subject to typical time-responsive swelling and dissolution and will thus release the encapsulated drug in a predictable timeframe. Another approach uses a hydrophobic material (such as surface-modified natural wax) as the erodible coating layer(s). In this case, the intestinal fluids gradually disperse the coated hydrophobic layer(s) and trigger drug release after a lag period. Many pH-responsive polymers also degrade in a time-dependent fashion in the GI tract and are thus categorized as an additional type of time-dependent DDS.

9.3.3 Mucoadhesive Formulation

Mucus acts as a dynamic steric barrier for drug delivery due to its continuous secretion and shedding from the GI lumen. A mucoadhesive delivery system (or bioadhesive delivery system) attaches to the mucus or epithelial layer in the lumen to increase its gastrointestinal residence time. This approach requires the use of bioadhesive polymers (such as polyacrylic acid, polycarbophil, polyvinyl alcohol, chitosan, or carboxymethyl cellulose [CMC]) for the construction of the delivery system. These polymers generally contain numerous hydrophilic functional groups (hydroxyl, carboxyl, amide, or sulfate); the polymers swell in the aqueous fluids, the functional groups attach to mucus or the epithelial cell membrane, and the adhesive sites are exposed. Their adhesive abilities are subject to various strong noncovalent forces, including hydrogen bonding, electrostatic, and hydrophobic interactions. An ideal mucoadhesive system should be nontoxic, nonabsorbable, and non-irritating to the GI tract. It also needs to be biocompatible, able to be loaded with macromolecular drugs, biodegradable to release the drugs under the designated physiological condition, and stable during storage (a long shelf time).

Naturally, mucoadhesive systems have the risk of adhering to nonspecific mucosal surfaces upon oral administration. For example, gastric mucoadhesive formulations may bind to the esophagus or SI (which is extensive in length). They may also suffer from quick elimination due to the high mucus turnover rate in the stomach.[2] No gastric mucoadhesive DDS has been successfully developed, as this strategy is not strong enough to resist the propulsive forces of the stomach wall.[4]

Unlike the stomach mucus, which provides strong physical protection, the SI has loose and penetrable mucus that allows easy absorption of small to middle-sized molecules.[23] In this regard, mucoadhesive SI patches can extend the contact time of the mucosa to improve the absorption of the drug.[24] The SI patch can also be engineered to protect the drug from premature release (i.e., during transit in the upper GI tract) by coating it with an enteric material. The ideal target of an SI patch is the proximal region of the duodenum, as digested food boluses are more substantial in this region, and the patch may be easily detached from the luminal surface. However, it is hard to predict where a patch might bind in the highly convoluted lumen of the SI. The release of a drug from an SI patch may be impacted by various factors, including the polymer's composition and adhesive strength and the drug's properties, including the charge, concentration, release rate, and release direction.[25] The efficacy of some drugs with preferential absorption sites other than the proximal region of the duodenum might be affected.

The colon absorbs water from the intestinal fluid, resulting in a colonic mucus that is more viscous than that in the upper GI tract. The higher viscosity of colonic mucus can increase the strength of adhesion between a DDS and the colonic mucus, compared to other GI sections.[26] However, the inner mucus layer, which separates bacteria and pathogens from the epithelium, makes it difficult for large-molecule therapeutics and nano-size formulations to penetrate. Today, mucus-penetrable drug delivery is a very active research field, especially since the global population of colonic disease patients is increasing rapidly by the year.[27] However, although researchers have developed various colonic mucoadhesive biomaterials, the overall efficiency of these biomaterials in promoting the mucus penetration and absorption of a loaded drug remains limited. Data have shown that DDS that rely solely on mucoadhesive function rarely succeed; thus, many DDS employ multifunctional polymers that combine swelling-based, adhesive, time-dependent, and/or pH-dependent delivery mechanisms.

9.3.4 Magnetic Systems

Magnetic targeting, which is accomplished using magnetic carriers whose localizations are guided by an external magnetic field, has emerged as a promising approach for accumulating a drug at target tissues. Given a sufficiently strong magnetic force, a magnetic DDS can be retained in the designated part of the GI tract, despite the forces of contractions and emptying.[28] Compared to noncovalent interaction-based targeting, magnetic targeting offers precise control of the gastric residence time (GRT) and generally does not involve a DDS that requires complicated chemical fabrication.

Although magnetic targeting has been used successfully in a number of animal studies, its clinical translation has been slow. The side effects of long-term exposure of the human body to a strong magnet are not well known, and retained magnetic material may penetrate deeply in the GI mucus to damage the epithelial or mucus layers and induce inflammation. New techniques are needed to minimize such side effects and facilitate the development of a conveniently applicable magnetic field for the precise localization of a DDS. Patient compliance is also a concern when repeated treatments are needed, as this strategy requires that an instrument capable of generating a precisely controllable external magnetic field must stay adjacent to the abdominal region for hours. This would not be suitable for a chronic disease that requires extensive treatment cycles. However, it could be a compelling method to treat lethal GI diseases, such as cancer.[29]

9.4 GASTRO-RETENTIVE DRUG DELIVERY SYSTEM (GRDDS)

The stomach is a muscular organ between the esophagus and SI. Its primary functions are secreting acid and enzymes that digest food, storing ingested food (temporally), mixing it with stomach fluid, and sending the mixture to the SI (gastric emptying). Gastric emptying presents a drastically varied pattern between fed and fasted states.[2,30] Such a nature limits the categories of drugs that can be applied to target the stomach. Conventional formulations can only deliver drugs that are stable and readily absorbed in the acidic gastric tract. As the GRDDS can stay in the gastric region for several hours and significantly increase the GRT of loaded drugs, drugs with low solubilities and narrow absorption windows may be feasible to be delivered to the stomach.[2,31] Nevertheless, those drugs that irritate the gastric mucosa are not suitable for being restrained in the stomach. To date, researchers have developed several formulation strategies to achieve gastric retention (Figure 9.2), including floating (low-density), non-floating (sinking or high-density), mucoadhesive, expandable, superporous hydrogels, and magnetic DDS.

9.4.1 Floating (Low-Density) DDS

The most commonly used GRDDS is the floating system, which includes gas-generating (effervescent) and non-effervescent systems. To work efficiently, a floating DDS requires a high level of fluid in the stomach on which it can float. Thus, a floating system is always co-administered with a certain amount of fluid (i.e., ~200–250 mL).[32]

9.4.1.1 Effervescent Floating Systems

The generation of gas bubbles (usually CO_2) creates the floating ability of the effervescent system. Many effervescent systems are organically composed of gas-generating components (e.g., sodium bicarbonate, citric acid, or tartaric acid) and swellable polymers (e.g., chitosan, sodium alginate, and hydroxypropyl methylcellulose [HPMC]). After oral administration, swellable polymers absorb water in the stomach; thereafter, sodium bicarbonate/citric acid releases a significant amount of carbon dioxide, which causes the formulation to float in the stomach.[32] Some systems also have adhesive and controlled-release properties.[33] Different grades of HPMC polymers (such as K4M or K15M) can be combined to facilitate the formation of a controllable hydrogel, which is then incorporated with the gas-generating agents to enable

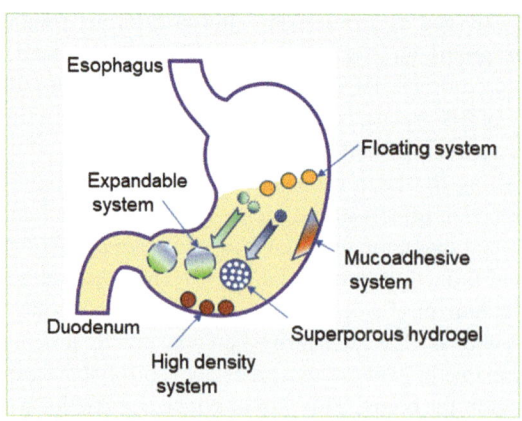

FIGURE 9.2 Different types of gastro-retentive drug system.

controlled drug release. Bilayer or multilayer systems contain matrix-coated layers with formulated units (composed of drugs and excipients) interposed between the layers. This sort of design has been shown to prolong the gastric residence time and increase the bioavailability of the encapsulated drugs.

9.4.1.2 Non-Effervescent Floating System

Non-effervescent floating DDS uses gel-forming or rapidly swellable polymers to create a system with a relatively lower density than the gastric fluid. The system maintains its integrity and traps air when swollen, thereby gaining the ability to float. Rapidly swellable polymeric excipients (including HPMC, polyacrylates, polyvinyl acetate, agar, sodium alginate, polyethylene oxide, and polycarbonates) are often employed to construct non-effervescent floating systems.[34–36] Several distinct approaches have been used to construct such systems, including the fabrication of hollow microspheres, microporous compartments, colloidal gel barriers, or alginate beads.

The non-effervescent floating DDS include *hollow microspheres (HMS)*, which are often designed as multi-unit systems with central hollow spaces inside. Drugs are loaded into the outer polymer shells of the HMS via emulsion-solvent diffusion. In vitro studies showed that HMS could float in an aqueous solution for more than 12 h. In clinical trials, orally administrated HMS were found to be dispersed in the upper part of the stomach and remain there for ~3 hours against peristalsis, suggesting that HMS could be an effective buoyant system for keeping a loaded drug in the stomach. HMS has been used to successfully deliver therapeutics, including rosiglitazone maleate,[37] clindamycin,[38] glipizide,[34,39,40] aspirin,[41,42] griseofulvin,[43] p-nitroaniline,[44] and others.[45,46] Some recently developed HMS has also incorporated mucoadhesive polymers to extend their gastric residence time.[46,47]

Another example, the microporous floating system contains a floatation chamber and drug reservoir (the microporous compartment). The floatation chamber entraps air from the stomach; this lifts the drug reservoir to float atop the gastric fluids,[48] which pass through micropores on the compartment wall and dissolve the drug to enable its continuous release.

The colloidal gel barrier system (CGBS) is a hydrodynamically balanced DDS[49] that incorporates a gel-forming hydrocolloid (e.g., hydroxypropyl cellulose, hydroxyethylcellulose, or HPMC) and a low-density matrix-forming polymer (e.g., polycarbophil, polyacrylate, or polystyrene). In gastric fluid, the hydrocolloid hydrates and forms a colloidal gel barrier around its surface, which keeps the system afloat on the stomach contents. The CGBS encapsulates the drug within its matrix-forming polymer, prolonging GRT and creating a sustained release of the loaded drug.

Isolated initially from Phaeophyceae (brown algae), alginate is a group of natural polymers consisting of linear β-(1–4)-linked d-mannuronic acid and β-(1–4)-linked l-guluronic acid units. Crosslinking sodium alginate solution with an aqueous calcium chloride solution generates calcium alginate, which is a water-insoluble gel-like substance. Spherical calcium alginate (alginate beads) is often made by dropping sodium alginate solution into an aqueous calcium chloride solution,[50] with the dropping speed typically determining the diameter of the spherical calcium alginate. Researchers have also added low-methoxylated pectin to the beads to generate a multiple-unit system. Upon multiple freeze-dry cycles (lyophilization), alginate beads form a porous microstructure that can maintain a floating force for over 12 h. In vivo, these floating beads exhibited a prolonged gastric residence time of more than 5.5 h.[51,52]

9.4.2 High-Density (Sinking) System

In contrast to the floating systems, sinking systems use heavy inert materials to increase the GRT of the formulation. Commonly used heavy inert materials include barium sulfate, iron powder, titanium dioxide, and zinc oxide. A sinking system is prepared by coating or mixing the heavy inert material with the drug, such that the formulation's overall density is significantly greater than that of the regular stomach contents (~1.004 g/cm^3), enabling the sinking system to resist peristalsis. The retention mechanism of a sinking system is commonly believed to be sedimentation, and such systems are expected to target the lowest point of the stomach (at upright posture). Many sinking DDSs have been small enough to fit into the stomach rugae (or folds) near the pyloric region. The rugae/folds can trap dense pellets (~3 g/cm^3) and prevent them from undergoing gastric emptying caused by peristaltic movements of the stomach wall. The main limitation of high-density DDS is that a large amount of drug must be loaded in order to prevent the matrix from becoming progressively lighter as the drug is released.[53] The GI transit time of a sinking system can be extended from an average of 5.8 to 25 h, largely by altering the density rather than the pellet diameter. However, no successful high-density system has yet reached the market.

9.4.3 Expandable Systems

If a drug formulation located in the stomach is larger than the pyloric sphincter (the connection between the stomach and duodenum), it will be retained in the stomach until it is degraded into smaller particles. Researchers thus developed expandable DDSs that are designed to initially be small enough to swallow and pass through the esophagus and thereafter (once they reach the stomach) swell to the point that they cannot be cleared via the pyloric sphincter. As the diameter of the pylorus is ~15 mm (and it never exceeds 19 mm),[54] it is generally accepted that a diameter above 15 mm is suitable for prolonging gastric retention, especially in the fasted state.[4] Caution should be exercised, however, as expandable systems may cause safety issues, such as gastric obstruction, either alone or by accumulation and possible occlusion of the esophagus or pylorus.[30] Thus, rapidly biodegradable polymers should be used when constructing an expandable system.

9.4.4 Superporous Hydrogel

Superporous hydrogel (SPH) was introduced as a category of polymers that differ from conventional hydrogels. SPH has dense concentrations of open porous structures; these form capillary channels that can quickly absorb water and thus switch to the swollen state much faster than traditional hydrogels.[55] The gelation of the traditional hydrogel is a slow process: It typically takes hours for these gels to reach a swollen equilibrium state, leaving them at risk of being evacuated from the stomach. In contrast, SPH systems swell to reach equilibrium within seconds (100 times quicker than traditional hydrogel) and thereby exhibit significantly greater GRT. The first generation of SPH suffered from low mechanical strength, but this limitation was overcome in the development of the second-generation (SPH composites, or SPHCs) and third-generation (SPH hybrids, or SPHHs) platforms, both of which can withstand the pressure of gastric contractions. Third-generation SPHs gained popularity for use in controlled-release systems due to their excellent mechanical properties (strength and elasticity).[2] Notably, however, SPH often uses swellable polymers, such as alginate or cross-linked polymers of CMC sodium, whose mechanical strength may be altered by the acidic pH in the stomach.

9.4.5 Molecular Target

Programmed death-ligand 1 (PD-L1) is one of two ligands (the second being PD-L2) that bind to PD-1, which is a cell-surface receptor that suppresses the immune system and promotes self-tolerance by restraining T cell responses. The PD-L1/PD-1' interaction transmits signals to reduce antigen-specific T cell proliferation in lymph nodes. PD-L1 expression is upregulated in more than 40% of human gastric cancer (GC) upon *Helicobacter pylori* infection, suggesting that PD-L1 could be considered a potential molecular target for drug delivery.[56] The use of a monoclonal antibody against PD-L1 (PD-L1 mAb) is a promising therapy for treating advanced GC, and PD-L1 mAb was found to specifically bind the extracellular domain of PD-L1. A PD-L1 mAb-coated nano-drug formulation recently exhibited potency in delivering the anti-cancer drug doxorubicin, suggesting that PD-L1 is an excellent target for anti-GC drug delivery.[57]

9.5 DELIVERING DRUGS TO THE SMALL INTESTINE

Due to the extensive length of the SI (~7 m) and the complex microstructure (presence of villi, microvilli, and numerous blood vessels) of the duodenum and jejunum regions, the SI has a vast surface area (~200 m²) that effectively absorbs nutrients and drugs. The SI has a shorter and more consistent transit time (~4 h) than the large intestine (6–70 h), making the SI an ideal target for drug delivery.[10,11,58] The delivery of drugs to the SI (including the duodenum, jejune, and ileum) can usually be achieved by pH-dependent, mucoadhesive, and gastro-retentive DDS, and sometimes by cell-mediated DDS.

9.5.1 pH-Responsive Formulations

Most of the current SI-targeting DDS are pH-responsive formulations (coatings or matrices). They are designed for drugs that may become destabilized by gastric fluid and/or irritate the gastric mucosa.[59,60] Enteric coating is widely used to prevent the release of a drug from tablets or capsules in gastric fluid. Such formulations employ pH-responsive polymers, such as polymethacrylates, polymethacrylic acids, polyacrylic acids, or their esters for SI-targeted drug release. These polymers are generally stable in an acidic solution but hydrolyze at a higher pH, such as that of the SI fluid. As a formulation will experience a relatively short transit time in the SI, the rapid degradation (or dissolution) of polymers is required for SI-targeted delivery.[61] The considerable variability in gastric emptying time can also affect drug release. More importantly, significant intra- and inter-individual variability in the pH of the GI tract is a primary factor that needs to be considered when designing an SI-targeted DDS.[62]

9.5.2 Mucoadhesive Polymer

A mucoadhesive polymer can be incorporated into a pH-dependent DDS or applied independently. For drug uptake, a mucoadhesive drug formulation must cross multiple barriers, including the mucus layer and the intestinal epithelium.[63] Nano- to micro-sized formulations may penetrate the SI mucus layer, depending on their surface charge, size, and shape. Usually, drug formulations cross the intestinal epithelium via transcellular transport. In rare cases, such as when cellular tight junctions are compromised in pathological conditions (such as Crohn's disease), drug formulation can be taken up via paracellular transport. It is worth noting that microfold cells (M-cells, representing a type of specialized epithelial cell) are present on gut-associated lymphoid tissues (GALT), where they are mainly localized in Peyer's patches. M-cells play a sentinel role in the intestinal immune system, as they can transport luminal antigens through the follicle-associated epithelium to the underlying immune cells.[64,65] As such, M-cells have become an attractive target for SI-targeted drug delivery.

9.5.3 M-Cell-Mediated Particle Transport

Compared to normal enterocytes, M-cells are covered by a relatively thinner mucus layer and glycocalyx and have a reduced intracellular enzymatic activity.[66] These factors make M-cells an excellent site for drug access and intracellular transport. Following the uptake of a formulation into M-cells, the loaded drugs might be engulfed by macrophages or dendritic cells inside the Peyer's patches (Figure 9.3). This pathway is usually exploited to deliver orally administered vaccines. Alternatively, drug formulations can undergo passive lymphatic transportation; although this route can be beneficial for systemic drug delivery,

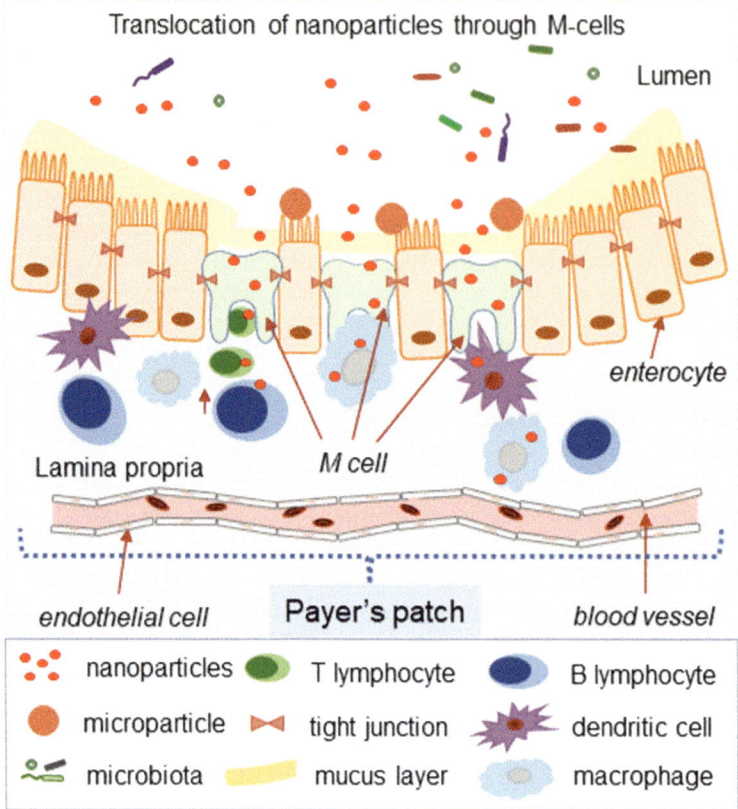

FIGURE 9.3   M-cell-mediated particle transport.

it should be avoided when treating regional SI diseases as it can be associated with severe systemic side effects.

In general, particle size is crucial for M-cell-mediated particle transport. Microparticles >5 μm in diameter are entrapped in Peyer's patches, whereas nanoparticles (<1 μm) are taken up by M-cells and transported through the efferent lymphatics.[67] The hydrophilicity (polarity) of the polymer used to construct the particle also plays a critical role in the M-cell-mediated transportation. M-cells take up hydrophobic or non-ionic nanoparticles more efficiently than hydrophilic or charged nanoparticles.[65] Surface decoration of the nanoparticles can improve the efficiency of targeting M-cells. Inspired by ligand-receptor interactions, researchers have developed surface-modified particles conjugated with mannose-, lectin-, or integrin-based ligands to enable the targeting of Peyer's patches. However, many of the currently employed ligands lack specificity. For example, mannose receptors are also localized on the apical surface of enterocytes,[68] and lectins may interact with the carbohydrate –OH residues in the mucus layer of the intestinal epithelium;[69] to date, only the integrin ligands have shown relatively specific targeting ability in vitro. Future in vivo studies are needed to verify the specificity of integrin ligand-based drug delivery. It should also be noted that several laboratory animal species have a significantly higher density of intestinal Peyer's patches than humans, which often leads to an overestimation of the M-cell-mediated particle transport capacity in humans.[70]

Due to the low proportion of M-cells (~1%) in the intestinal epithelium, the overall absorption of nanoparticles by M-cells is limited. Also, uptake by M-cells can be low because the nanoparticles are not specific to M-cells. Many ongoing studies are focusing on optimizing the composition of nanoparticles to improve their specific targeting of M-cells, as this could significantly reduce the required drug dosage without compromising the efficacy.[64,71]

9.6 COLON-TARGETED DRUG DELIVERY

The oral administration of a colon-targeted formulation has long been considered an attractive alternative to the systemic dosing of proteins or peptides, as the oral route offers better patient compliance than other delivery routes.[72] The physiological traits of the colon, including the proteolytic activity of the colon mucosa, are milder than those of the SI, supporting the concept of macromolecules' oral delivery via colon targeting. More importantly, colon-targeted formulations could enable the local treatment of various colonic disorders, such as ulcerative colitis, Crohn's disease, irritable bowel syndrome, and colon cancer. Colon-targeted delivery offers huge advantages (e.g., reducing doses and preventing side effects) over non-targeted drugs, which often must be applied at a relatively high dose. As a drug delivery site, the colon offers various therapeutic advantages, such as its near-neutral pH and longer transit time than those of the stomach and SI. General strategies such as pH-responsive, time-dependent, or mucoadhesive drug delivery can also be applied for colon-targeted drug delivery, and emerging information on the pathophysiology of colonic diseases can suggest new specific targets for drug delivery, such as transmembrane proteins that can be actively targeted.

9.6.1 Molecular Targets for Cell-Specific Drug Delivery

Colorectal cancer (CRC) cells present significantly different cell-surface receptor and transporter profiles compared to normal or lung cancer cells. For example, CRC overexpresses folic acid (FA) receptors and transporters, and thus FA-coated formulations are expected to exhibit increased uptake by CRC cells. Studies showed that HCT119 and HT29 cells (human CRC), but not A549 cells (lung cancer), could efficiently take up FA-decorated chitosan nanoparticles. Moreover, an FA-decorated chitosan formulation showed excellent tumor growth inhibition and safety in a xenograft CRC mouse model.[73]

Epithelial cell adhesion molecule glycoprotein (EpCAM) is a transmembrane glycoprotein associated with the development and metastasis of colonic adenocarcinoma. Elevated expression of EpCAM is attributable to rapid proliferating of colorectal tumors. In colonic adenocarcinoma, EpCAM also functions in various processes, such as the cell cycle, cell signaling, migration, proliferation, and differentiation.[74,75] EpCAM is thus a therapeutic target for drug delivery, and EpCAM aptamer-functionalized PLGA nanoparticles have been exploited for EpCAM-targeted drug delivery to human colorectal adenocarcinoma cells.[76]

P-selectin (CD62P) is a cancer-associated cell adhesion molecule. It is upregulated in human and murine colon cancer tissues, but not healthy tissues, and thus was proposed as a colon cancer-specific delivery target. The polysaccharide fucoidan is a natural seaweed-derived polymer that exhibits a high affinity for P-selectin. Studies have used fucoidan-decorated layer-by-layer nanoparticles to target the colon cancer region in an animal model.[71,77]

Other emerging CRC-associated molecular targets, such as EGFR and integrin,[75,78,79] have also been tested for their potential as targets for cell-specific drug delivery (Table 9.1). Notably, therapeutics that target colon cancer stem cells (CCSCs) may have an increased chance of eradicating the disease.[80] Accumulating evidence suggests that some populations of CCSCs can be characterized by their specific expression of surface glycoproteins, such as CD44, CD133, CD166, EpCAM, and Lgr5. Targeting one or more of these glycoproteins could offer a practical approach for effectively delivering anticancer drugs to CCSCs. For example, CD44 is the receptor of hyaluronic acid (HA). Thus, formulations with HA-decorated surfaces could potentially target CD44-expressing CCSCs. When a 5-FU-loaded HA-modified liposome formulation (5-FU-lipo-HA) was applied to CD44-expressing HT29 cells and a

TABLE 9.1 Examples of Molecular Targets for Colon-Targeted Drug Delivery

MOLECULAR TARGET	CELL TYPE	DISEASE
Folic acid receptor	Epithelial cells	Colon cancer
EpCAM*	Epithelial cells	Colorectal cancer
P-selectin (CD62P)	Endothelial cells	Colon cancer
EGFR**	Endothelial cells	IBD***; cancer
CD44	Cancer stem cells	Colon cancer
CD98	Lymphocytes (Immune cells)	IBD; colon cancer
PePT1	Epithelial cells	IBD; colon cancer
Integrin	Widespread, fibroblasts, epithelial cells	Cancer

*Epithelial cell adhesion molecule glycoprotein
**Epidermal growth factor receptor
***Inflammatory bowel disease

non-CD44 expressing hepatoma cell line, optimal cell uptake and drug release were seen with HT29 cells while only minimal 5-FU uptake was seen with hepatoma cells.[81]

Pathological analysis of human ulcerative colitis specimens found elevated expression of amino acid transporters, such as CD98, on the surface of colonic epithelial cells. Thus, researchers speculated that CD98 might be targeted for anti-inflammatory drug delivery. This hypothesis was validated using CD98 Fab'-bearing quantum dot (QD)-loaded nanoparticles (Fab'-NPs) in an ex vivo colitis tissue uptake experiment. Fab'-NPs, but not PEG-NPs, were efficiently accumulated at the inflamed tissue due to the overexpression of CD98.[82]

9.6.2 Targeting the Colonic Microbiota

More than 10^{13} commensal microorganisms reside in the intestines of an adult human, and >90% live in the colon. Patients with colonic diseases demonstrate a decrease in microbial diversity and a reduction of about 25% in microbial genes.[15] As the colon has a significantly higher pH (5.5–7.5) than the stomach (pH 1.5–2.0), many pH-sensitive polymeric materials can be used to target a drug to the colon region with the goal of altering the ecosystem of the microbiota.[19,83]

Some novel strategies have harnessed genetically engineered probiotic bacteria as the delivery system. *Lactococcus lactis*, a probiotic strain, was genetically engineered to express interleukin-10 (IL-10) with the goal of restoring colon homeostasis and treating colitis in a mouse model. This platform was also applied to produce an immunomodulatory pathogenic protein (low calcium response V protein); upon its oral delivery to the colonic region of mice, the host colonic immune cells undertook IL-10 secretion, and the colitis was reduced.[84] These probiotics-based NPs are nano-factories that target immune cells to tailor the microbiota structure. The oral administration of probiotics also modifies the microbial ecosystem, triggering the immune response and reshaping the microbiota structure.

Studies have shown that plant-derived exosomal NPs target specific strains of the microbiota. Orally administered ginger-derived lipid nanoparticles (GDLPs) were found to target the Lactobacillaceae in a specific lipid-dependent manner.[85] The delivered GDLPs contained microRNAs that were shown to affect various genes in *Lactobacillus rhamnosus* (LGG). The GDLPs microRNA, mdo-miR7267-3p, mediated targeting of an LGG monooxygenase (ycnE), increased indole-3-carboxaldehyde (I3A), and subsequently induced the production of IL-22, which can improve barrier function and ameliorate colitis in a mouse model. These findings indicated that edible plant-derived NPs might also be used to target specific components of the microbiome to alleviate inflammation.

9.7 CONCLUSIONS AND OUTLOOK

The development of targeted strategies for GI tract-localized delivery has yielded substantial advances in preclinical and clinical studies. Although oral administration is the most favorable delivery route for localizing therapeutics to the GI system, orally delivered drugs must overcome the environmental extremes of the GI tract. Molecular target-guided oral drugs are only effective when the formulation remains stable until it reaches the delivery targets. Various factors, including pH, transit time, enzymes, and microbiota, will affect the stability and targeting efficiency of oral formulations.

To date, many DDSs have been designed with the goal of retaining the drug in the stomach. Due to the fast-emptying process, limited molecular targets, and harsh environment of the stomach, relatively few drugs are suitable for gastric drug delivery. The SI is the primary absorption site for nutrients, as well as for many drug formulations. However, how to prevent the SI uptake of a colon-targeted formation is an active yet challenging research topic. The development of new and effective delivery systems will rely heavily on continued progress in our understanding of GI disease pathophysiology. As the deliverable molecular and cellular targets vary widely between individual patients, molecular targeting-based drug delivery can be considered a personalized drug delivery strategy. No standardized platform can be applied for such delivery tasks. However, the available generalized delivery platforms can be applied for more specific targeting purposes, and molecular targeting-based nanoplatforms can be incorporated as an add-on function in the available systems. For example, specific targeting nanoparticles can be encapsulated in a pH-dependent or mucoadhesive hydrogel to form a so-called "nano-in-micro" system that could prevent premature drug release and increase delivery efficiency. Such an approach can also be used when researchers seek to combine multiple drugs or targeting strategies.

ACKNOWLEDGMENTS

The authors wish to thank the Institute for Biomedical Sciences of Georgia State University, the National Institute of Diabetes and Digestive and Kidney Diseases (RO1-DK-116306 and RO1-DK-107739 to D. Merlin), and the Department of Veterans Affairs (BX002526 to DM) for their support of this chapter. D. Merlin is a recipient of a Senior Research Career Scientist Award from the Department of Veterans Affairs (BX004476).

REFERENCES

1. Zhou, Y., N. Gu, and F. Yang. "In Situ Microbubble-Assisted, Ultrasound-Controlled Release of Superparamagnetic Iron Oxide Nanoparticles from Gastro-Retentive Tablets." *International Journal of Pharmacy* 586 (2020): 119615.
2. Tripathi, J., P. Thapa, R. Maharjan, and S. H. Jeong. "Current State and Future Perspectives on Gastroretentive Drug Delivery Systems." *Pharmaceutics* 11, no. 4 (2019): 193.
3. Naeem, M., J. Bae, M. A. Oshi, M. S. Kim, H. R. Moon, B. L. Lee, E. Im, Y. Jung, and J. W. Yoo. "Colon-Targeted Delivery of Cyclosporine A Using Dual-Functional Eudragit((R)) FS30D/PLGA Nanoparticles Ameliorates Murine Experimental Colitis." *International Journal of Nanomedicine* 13 (2018): 1225–40.
4. Souza, M. P. C., R. M. Sabio, T. C. Ribeiro, A. M. D. Santos, A. B. Meneguin, and M. Chorilli. "Highlighting the Impact of Chitosan on the Development of Gastroretentive Drug Delivery Systems." *International Journal of Biological Macromolecules* 159 (2020): 804–22.

5. Higaki, K., S. Yamashita, and G. L. Amidon. "Time-Dependent Oral Absorption Models." *Journal of Pharmacokinetics & Pharmacodynamics* 28, no. 2 (2001): 109–28.
6. Hua, S. "Advances in Oral Drug Delivery for Regional Targeting in the Gastrointestinal Tract: Influence of Physiological, Pathophysiological and Pharmaceutical Factors." *Frontiers in Pharmacology* 11 (2020): 524.
7. Bratten, J., and M. P. Jones. "New Directions in the Assessment of Gastric Function: Clinical Applications of Physiologic Measurements." *Digestive Diseases* 24, no. 3–4 (2006): 252–9.
8. Ibekwe, V. C., H. M. Fadda, E. L. McConnell, M. K. Khela, D. F. Evans, and A. W. Basit. "Interplay Between Intestinal pH, Transit Time and Feed Status on the In Vivo Performance of pH Responsive Ileo-Colonic Release Systems." *Pharmaceutical Research* 25, no. 8 (2008): 1828–35.
9. Roussel, A., S. Canaan, M. P. Egloff, M. Rivière, L. Dupuis, R. Verger, and C. Cambillau. "Crystal Structure of Human Gastric Lipase and Model of Lysosomal Acid Lipase, Two Lipolytic Enzymes of Medical Interest." *Journal of Biological Chemistry* 274, no. 24 (1999): 16995–7002.
10. Komuro, Y., T. Kondo, S. Hino, T. Morita, and N. Nishimura. "Oral Intake of Slowly Digestible Alpha-Glucan, Isomaltodextrin, Stimulates Glucagon-Like peptide-1 Secretion in the Small Intestine of Rats." *British Journal of Nutrition* 123, no. 6 (2020): 619–26.
11. Lee, S. B., K. W. Lee, J. S. Lee, K. H. Kim, and H. G. Lee. "Impacts of Whey Protein on Starch Digestion in Rumen and Small Intestine of Steers." *Journal of Animal Science & Technology* 61, no. 2 (2019): 98–108.
12. Viennois, E., A. Pujada, J. Sung, C. Yang, A. T. Gewirtz, B. Chassaing, and D. Merlin. "Impact of PepT1 Deletion on Microbiota Composition and Colitis Requires Multiple Generations." *npj Biofilms & Microbiomes* 6, no. 1 (2020): 27.
13. Donaldson, G. P., S. M. Lee, and S. K. Mazmanian. "Gut Biogeography of the Bacterial Microbiota." *Nature Reviews in Microbiology* 14, no. 1 (2016): 20–32.
14. Litvak, Y., M. X. Byndloss, and A. J. Baumler. "Colonocyte Metabolism Shapes the Gut Microbiota." *Science* 362, no. 6418 (2018): eaat9076.
15. Franzosa, E. A., A. Sirota-Madi, J. Avila-Pacheco, N. Fornelos, H. J. Haiser, S. Reinker, T. Vatanen, A. B. Hall, H. Mallick, L. J. McIver, J. S. Sauk, R. G. Wilson, B. W. Stevens, J. M. Scott, K. Pierce, A. A. Deik, K. Bullock, F. Imhann, J. A. Porter, A. Zhernakova, J. Fu, R. K. Weersma, C. Wijmenga, C. B. Clish, H. Vlamakis, C. Huttenhower, and R. J. Xavier. "Gut Microbiome Structure and Metabolic Activity in Inflammatory Bowel Disease." *Nature Microbiology* 4, no. 2 (2019): 293–305.
16. Maslowski, K. M., and C. R. Mackay. "Diet, Gut Microbiota and Immune Responses." *Nature Immunology* 12, no. 1 (2011): 5–9.
17. Shin, W., and H. J. Kim. "Intestinal Barrier Dysfunction Orchestrates the Onset of Inflammatory Host-Microbiome Cross-Talk in a Human Gut Inflammation-On-a-Chip." *Proceedings of the National Academy of Sciences of the United States of America* 115, no. 45 (2018): E10539–E47.
18. Engevik, M. A., A. C. Engevik, K. A. Engevik, J. M. Auchtung, A. L. Chang-Graham, W. Ruan, R. A. Luna, J. M. Hyser, J. K. Spinler, and J. Versalovic. "Mucin-Degrading Microbes Release Monosaccharides That Chemoattract Clostridioides difficile and Facilitate Colonization of the Human Intestinal Mucus Layer." *ACS Infectious Diseases* 7, no. 5 (2021): 1126–42.
19. Ali, H., B. Weigmann, M. F. Neurath, E. M. Collnot, M. Windbergs, and C. M. Lehr. "Budesonide Loaded Nanoparticles with pH-Sensitive Coating for Improved Mucosal Targeting in Mouse Models of Inflammatory Bowel Diseases." *Journal of Controlled Release* 183 (2014): 167–77.
20. Wang, X. Q., and Q. Zhang. "pH-Sensitive Polymeric Nanoparticles to Improve Oral Bioavailability of Peptide/Protein Drugs and Poorly Water-Soluble Drugs." *European Journal of Pharmaceutics & Biopharmaceutics* 82, no. 2 (2012): 219–29.
21. Riedel, A., and C. S. Leopold. "Degradation of Omeprazole Induced by Enteric Polymer Solutions and Aqueous Dispersions: HPLC Investigations." *Drug Development & Industrial Pharmacy* 31, no. 2 (2005): 151–60.
22. Jain, S. K., A. Jain, Y. Gupta, and M. Ahirwar. "Design and Development of Hydrogel Beads for Targeted Drug Delivery to the Colon." *AAPS PharmSciTech* 8, no. 3 (2007): E56.
23. Godugu, C., A. R. Patel, R. Doddapaneni, J. Somagoni, and M. Singh. "Approaches to Improve the Oral Bioavailability and Effects of Novel Anticancer Drugs Berberine and Betulinic Acid." *PLOS ONE* 9, no. 3 (2014): e89919.
24. Banerjee, A., R. Chen, S. Arafin, and S. Mitragotri. "Intestinal Iontophoresis from Mucoadhesive Patches: A Strategy for Oral Delivery." *Journal of Controlled Release* 297 (2019): 71–8.
25. Panigrahi, L., S. Pattnaik, and S. K. Ghosal. "Design and Characterization of Mucoadhesive Buccal Patches of Salbutamol Sulphate." *Acta Poloniae Pharmaceutica* 61, no. 5 (2004): 351–60.
26. Duan, H., S. Lu, C. Gao, X. Bai, H. Qin, Y. Wei, X. Wu, and M. Liu. "Mucoadhesive Microparticulates Based on Polysaccharide for Target Dual Drug Delivery of 5-Aminosalicylic Acid and Curcumin to Inflamed Colon." *Colloids & Surfaces, Part B: Biointerfaces* 145 (2016): 510–9.

27. Varum, F. J., F. Veiga, J. S. Sousa, and A. W. Basit. "Mucoadhesive Platforms for Targeted Delivery to the Colon." *International Journal of Pharmacy* 420, no. 1 (2011): 11–9.

28. Guo, W., D. Li, J. A. Zhu, X. Wei, W. Men, D. Yin, M. Fan, and Y. Xu. "A Magnetic Nanoparticle Stabilized Gas Containing Emulsion for Multimodal Imaging and Triggered Drug Release." *Pharmaceutical Research* 31, no. 6 (2014): 1477–84.

29. Xue, P., J. Bao, L. Zhang, Z. Xu, C. Xu, Y. Zhang, and Y. Kang. "Functional Magnetic Prussian Blue Nanoparticles for Enhanced Gene Transfection and Photothermal Ablation of Tumor Cells." *Journal of Materials Chemistry B* 4, no. 27 (2016): 4717–25.

30. Melocchi, A., M. Uboldi, N. Inverardi, F. Briatico-Vangosa, F. Baldi, S. Pandini, G. Scalet, F. Auricchio, M. Cerea, A. Foppoli, A. Maroni, L. Zema, and A. Gazzaniga. "Expandable Drug Delivery System for Gastric Retention Based on Shape Memory Polymers: Development via 4D Printing and Extrusion." *International Journal of Pharmacy* 571 (2019): 118700.

31. Higaki, K., S. Y. Choe, R. Lobenberg, L. S. Welage, and G. L. Amidon. "Mechanistic Understanding of Time-Dependent Oral Absorption Based on Gastric Motor Activity in Humans." *European Journal of Pharmaceutics & Biopharmaceutics* 70, no. 1 (2008): 313–25.

32. Shishu Gupta, N., N. Aggarwal, and N. Aggarwal. "Bioavailability Enhancement and Targeting of Stomach Tumors Using Gastro-Retentive Floating Drug Delivery System of Curcumin: 'a Technical Note'." *AAPS PharmSciTech* 9, no. 3 (2008): 810–3.

33. Tadros, M. I. "Controlled-Release Effervescent Floating Matrix Tablets of Ciprofloxacin Hydrochloride: Development, Optimization and In Vitro-In Vivo Evaluation in Healthy Human Volunteers." *European Journal of Pharmaceutics & Biopharmaceutics* 74, no. 2 (2010): 332–9.

34. Meka, V. S., S. Pillai, S. R. Dharmalingham, R. Sheshala, and A. Gorajana. "Preparation and In Vitro Characterization of a Non-Effervescent Floating Drug Delivery System for Poorly Soluble Drug, Glipizide." *Acta Poloniae Pharmaceutica* 72, no. 1 (2015): 193–204.

35. Srikanth Meka, V., V. A. Wee Liang, S. R. Dharmalingham, R. Sheshala, and A. Gorajana. "Preparation and In Vitro Characterization of Non-Effervescent Floating Drug Delivery System of Poorly Soluble Drug, Carvedilol Phosphate." *Acta Pharmaceutica* 64, no. 4 (2014): 485–94.

36. Acharya, S., S. Patra, and N. R. Pani. "Optimization of HPMC and Carbopol Concentrations in Non-Effervescent Floating Tablet Through Factorial Design." *Carbohydrate Polymers* 102 (2014): 360–8.

37. Hu, L. D., Q. B. Xing, C. Shang, W. Liu, C. Liu, Z. L. Luo, and H. X. Xu. "Preparation of Rosiglitazone Maleate Sustained-Release Floating Microspheres for Improved Bioavailability." *Pharmazie* 65, no. 7 (2010): 477–80.

38. Mohamed, A. I., O. A. Ahmed, S. Amin, O. A. Elkadi, and M. A. Kassem. "In-Vivo Evaluation of Clindamycin Release from Glyceryl Monooleate-Alginate Microspheres by NIR Spectroscopy." *International Journal of Pharmacy* 494, no. 1 (2015): 127–35.

39. Pandya, N., M. Pandya, and V. H. Bhaskar. "Preparation and In Vitro Characterization of Porous Carrier-Based Glipizide Floating Microspheres for Gastric Delivery." *Journal of Young Pharmacists* 3, no. 2 (2011): 97–104.

40. Gaba, P., S. Singh, M. Gaba, and G. D. Gupta. "Galactomannan Gum Coated Mucoadhesive Microspheres of Glipizide for Treatment of Type 2 Diabetes Mellitus: In Vitro and In Vivo Evaluation." *Saudi Pharmaceutical Journal* 19, no. 3 (2011): 143–52.

41. Zhang, H., L. Z. Hao, J. A. Pan, Q. Gao, J. F. Zhang, R. K. Kankala, S. B. Wang, A. Z. Chen, and H. L. Zhang. "Microfluidic Fabrication of Inhalable Large Porous Microspheres Loaded with H2S-Releasing Aspirin Derivative for Pulmonary Arterial Hypertension Therapy." *Journal of Controlled Release* 329 (2020): 286–98.

42. Shi, Z. D., X. M. Qian, C. Y. Liu, L. Han, K. L. Zhang, L. Y. Chen, J. X. Zhang, P. Y. Pu, X. B. Yuan, C. S. Kang, and Chinese Glioma Cooperative Group (CGCG). "Aspirin-/TMZ-coloaded Microspheres Exert Synergistic Antiglioma Efficacy via Inhibition of Beta-Catenin Transactivation." *CNS Neuroscience & Therapeutics* 19, no. 2 (2013): 98–108.

43. Vojnovic, D., F. Rubessa, M. Bogataj, and A. Mrhar. "Formulation and Evaluation of Vinylpyrrolidone/Vinylacetate Copolymer Microspheres with Griseofulvin." *Journal of Microencapsulation* 10, no. 1 (1993): 89–99.

44. Lu, X., Y. Yang, Y. Zeng, L. Li, and X. Wu. "Rapid and Reliable Determination of p-Nitroaniline in Wastewater by Molecularly Imprinted Fluorescent Polymeric Ionic Liquid Microspheres." *Biosensors & Bioelectronics* 99 (2018): 47–55.

45. Pi, C., T. Feng, J. Liang, H. Liu, D. Huang, C. Zhan, J. Yuan, R. J. Lee, L. Zhao, and Y. Wei. "Polymer Blends Used to Develop Felodipine-Loaded Hollow Microspheres for Improved Oral Bioavailability." *International Journal of Biological Macromolecules* 112 (2018): 1038–47.

46. Huang, Y., Y. Wei, H. Yang, C. Pi, H. Liu, Y. Ye, and L. Zhao. "A 5-Fluorouracil-Loaded Floating Gastroretentive Hollow Microsphere: Development, Pharmacokinetic in Rabbits, and Biodistribution in Tumor-Bearing Mice." *Drug Design, Development & Therapy* 10 (2016): 997–1008.

47. Upadhyay, M. S., and K. Pathak. "Glyceryl Monooleate-Coated Bioadhesive Hollow Microspheres of Riboflavin for Improved Gastroretentivity: Optimization and Pharmacokinetics." *Drug Delivery & Translation Research* 3, no. 3 (2013): 209–23.

48. Zhang, L., J. Xing, X. Wen, J. Chai, S. Wang, and Q. Xiong. "Plasmonic Heating from Indium Nanoparticles on a Floating Microporous Membrane for Enhanced Solar Seawater Desalination." *Nanoscale* 9, no. 35 (2017): 12843–9.

49. Pawar, V. K., S. Kansal, G. Garg, R. Awasthi, D. Singodia, and G. T. Kulkarni. "Gastroretentive Dosage Forms: A Review with Special Emphasis on Floating Drug Delivery Systems." *Drug Delivery* 18, no. 2 (2011): 97–110.

50. Torre, M. L., P. Giunchedi, L. Maggi, R. Stefli, E. O. Machiste, and U. Conte. "Formulation and Characterization of Calcium Alginate Beads Containing Ampicillin." *Pharmaceutical Development & Technology* 3, no. 2 (1998): 193–8.

51. Majumdar, S., G. Krishnatreya, N. Gogoi, D. Thakur, and D. Chowdhury. "Carbon-Dot-Coated Alginate Beads as a Smart Stimuli-Responsive Drug Delivery System." *ACS Applied Materials & Interfaces* 8, no. 50 (2016): 34179–84.

52. Liakos, I., L. Rizzello, I. S. Bayer, P. P. Pompa, R. Cingolani, and A. Athanassiou. "Controlled Antiseptic Release by Alginate Polymer Films and Beads." *Carbohydrate Polymers* 92, no. 1 (2013): 176–83.

53. Rouge, N., E. Allemann, M. Gex-Fabry, L. Balant, E. T. Cole, P. Buri, and E. Doelker. "Comparative Pharmacokinetic Study of a Floating Multiple-Unit Capsule, a High-Density Multiple-Unit Capsule and an Immediate-Release Tablet Containing 25 mg Atenolol." *Pharmaceutica Acta Helvetiae* 73, no. 2 (1998): 81–7.

54. Petrides, C., K. Neofytou, and A. Z. Khan. "Pancreatic Perivascular Epithelioid Cell Tumour Presenting with Upper Gastrointestinal Bleeding." *Case Reports in Oncological Medicine* 2015 (2015): 431215.

55. Omidian, H., J. G. Rocca, and K. Park. "Advances in Superporous Hydrogels." *Journal of Controlled Release* 102, no. 1 (2005): 3–12.

56. Li, H., J. Q. Xia, F. S. Zhu, Z. H. Xi, C. Y. Pan, L. M. Gu, and Y. Z. Tian. "LPS Promotes the Expression of PD-L1 in Gastric Cancer Cells Through NF-KappaB Activation." *Journal of Cellular Biochemistry* 119, no. 12 (2018): 9997–10004.

57. Xu, S., F. Cui, D. Huang, D. Zhang, A. Zhu, X. Sun, Y. Cao, S. Ding, Y. Wang, E. Gao, and F. Zhang. "PD-L1 Monoclonal Antibody-Conjugated Nanoparticles Enhance Drug Delivery Level and Chemotherapy Efficacy in Gastric Cancer Cells." *International Journal of Nanomedicine* 14 (2019): 17–32.

58. Laroui, H., D. Geem, B. Xiao, E. Viennois, P. Rakhya, T. Denning, and D. Merlin. "Targeting Intestinal Inflammation with CD98 siRNA/PEI-Loaded Nanoparticles." *Molecular Therapy* 22, no. 1 (2014): 69–80.

59. AlHajri, L. "Enteric-Coated, Extended-Release and Sustained-Release Formulations of NSAIDs." *Annals of Pharmacotherapy* 51, no. 4 (2017): 354–6.

60. Davies, N. M. "Sustained Release and Enteric Coated NSAIDs: Are They Really GI Safe?." *Journal of Pharmacy & Pharmaceutical Sciences* 2, no. 1 (1999): 5–14.

61. Kamaly, N., B. Yameen, J. Wu, and O. C. Farokhzad. "Degradable Controlled-Release Polymers and Polymeric Nanoparticles: Mechanisms of Controlling Drug Release." *Chemical Reviews* 116, no. 4 (2016): 2602–63.

62. Zhang, Y., E. Viennois, M. Zhang, B. Xiao, M. K. Han, L. Walter, P. Garg, and D. Merlin. "PepT1 Expression Helps Maintain Intestinal Homeostasis by Mediating the Differential Expression of miRNAs Along the Crypt-Villus Axis" *Scientific Report* 6 (2016): 27119.

63. Chen, M. C., F. L. Mi, Z. X. Liao, C. W. Hsiao, K. Sonaje, M. F. Chung, L. W. Hsu, and H. W. Sung. "Recent Advances in Chitosan-Based Nanoparticles for Oral Delivery of Macromolecules." *Advanced Drug Delivery Reviews* 65, no. 6 (2013): 865–79.

64. Batrakova, E. V., H. E. Gendelman, and A. V. Kabanov. "Cell-Mediated Drug Delivery." *Expert Opinion on Drug Delivery* 8, no. 4 (2011): 415–33.

65. Man, A. L., F. Lodi, E. Bertelli, M. Regoli, C. Pin, F. Mulholland, A. R. Satoskar, M. J. Taussig, and C. Nicoletti. "Macrophage Migration Inhibitory Factor Plays a Role in the Regulation of Microfold (M) Cell-Mediated Transport in the Gut." *Journal of Immunology* 181, no. 8 (2008): 5673–80.

66. Man, A. L., M. E. Prieto-Garcia, and C. Nicoletti. "Improving M Cell Mediated Transport Across Mucosal Barriers: Do Certain Bacteria Hold the Keys?" *Immunology* 113, no. 1 (2004): 15–22.

67. Smyth, S. H., S. Feldhaus, U. Schumacher, and K. E. Carr. "Uptake of Inert Microparticles in Normal and Immune Deficient Mice." *International Journal of Pharmacy* 346, no. 1–2 (2008): 109–18.

68. Si, X. Y., D. Merlin, and B. Xiao. "Recent Advances in Orally Administered Cell-Specific Nanotherapeutics for Inflammatory Bowel Disease." *World Journal of Gastroenterology* 22, no. 34 (2016): 7718–26.

69. Liu, M., F. Luo, C. Ding, S. Albeituni, X. Hu, Y. Ma, Y. Cai, L. McNally, M. A. Sanders, D. Jain, G. Kloecker, M. Bousamra, H. G. Zhang, R. M. Higashi, A. N. Lane, T. W. Fan, and J. Yan. "Dectin-1 Activation by a Natural Product Beta-Glucan Converts Immunosuppressive Macrophages into an M1-Like Phenotype." *Journal of Immunology* 195, no. 10 (2015): 5055–65.

70. Kararli, T. T. "Comparison of the Gastrointestinal Anatomy, Physiology, and Biochemistry of Humans and Commonly Used Laboratory Animals." *Biopharmaceutics & Drug Disposition* 16, no. 5 (1995): 351–80.

71. Jin, K., Z. Luo, B. Zhang, and Z. Pang. "Biomimetic Nanoparticles for Inflammation Targeting." *Acta Pharmacologica Sinica B* 8, no. 1 (2018): 23–33.

72. Amidon, S., J. E. Brown, and V. S. Dave. "Colon-Targeted Oral Drug Delivery Systems: Design Trends and Approaches." *AAPS PharmSciTech* 16, no. 4 (2015): 731–41.

73. Soe, Z. C., B. K. Poudel, H. T. Nguyen, R. K. Thapa, W. Ou, M. Gautam, K. Poudel, S. G. Jin, J. H. Jeong, S. K. Ku, H. G. Choi, C. S. Yong, and J. O. Kim. "Folate-Targeted Nanostructured Chitosan/Chondroitin Sulfate Complex Carriers for Enhanced Delivery of Bortezomib to Colorectal Cancer Cells." *Asian Journal of Pharmaceutical Sciences* 14, no. 1 (2019): 40–51.

74. Zhou, F. Q., Y. M. Qi, H. Xu, Q. Y. Wang, X. S. Gao, and H. G. Guo. "Expression of EpCAM and Wnt/ Beta-Catenin in Human Colon Cancer." *Genetics & Molecular Research* 14, no. 2 (2015): 4485–94.

75. Liang, K. H., H. C. Tso, S. H. Hung, I. I. Kuan, J. K. Lai, F. Y. Ke, Y. T. Chuang, I. J. Liu, Y. P. Wang, R. H. Chen, and H. C. Wu. "Extracellular Domain of EpCAM Enhances Tumor Progression Through EGFR Signaling in Colon Cancer Cells." *Cancer Letters* 433 (2018): 165–75.

76. Xie, X., F. Li, H. Zhang, Y. Lu, S. Lian, H. Lin, Y. Gao, and L. Jia. "EpCAM Aptamer-Functionalized Mesoporous Silica Nanoparticles for Efficient Colon Cancer Cell-Targeted Drug Delivery." *European Journal of Pharmaceutical Sciences* 83 (2016): 28–35.

77. Zhang, M., C. Yang, X. Yan et al. "Highly Biocompatible Functionalized Layer-by-Layer Ginger Lipid Nano Vectors Targeting P-Selectin for Delivery of Doxorubicin to Treat Colon Cancer." *Advances in Therapy* 2 (2019). PubMed: 1900129.

78. Bamias, G., T. T. Pizarro, and F. Cominelli. "Pathway-Based Approaches to the Treatment of Inflammatory Bowel Disease." *Translational Research: the Journal of Laboratory & Clinical Medicine* 167, no. 1 (2016): 104–15.

79. Hoshino, A., B. Costa-Silva, T. L. Shen, G. Rodrigues, A. Hashimoto, M. Tesic Mark, H. Molina, S. Kohsaka, A. Di Giannatale, S. Ceder, S. Singh, C. Williams, N. Soplop, K. Uryu, L. Pharmer, T. King, L. Bojmar, A. E. Davies, Y. Ararso, T. Zhang, H. Zhang, J. Hernandez, J. M. Weiss, V. D. Dumont-Cole, K. Kramer, L. H. Wexler, A. Narendran, G. K. Schwartz, J. H. Healey, P. Sandstrom, K. J. Labori, E. H. Kure, P. M. Grandgenett, M. A. Hollingsworth, M. de Sousa, S. Kaur, M. Jain, K. Mallya, S. K. Batra, W. R. Jarnagin, M. S. Brady, O. Fodstad, V. Muller, K. Pantel, A. J. Minn, M. J. Bissell, B. A. Garcia, Y. Kang, V. K. Rajasekhar, C. M. Ghajar, I. Matei, H. Peinado, J. Bromberg, and D. Lyden. "Tumour Exosome Integrins Determine Organotropic Metastasis." *Nature* 527, no. 7578 (2015): 329–35.

80. Fu, C., X. Xiao, H. Xu, W. Lu, and Y. Wang. "Efficacy of Atovaquone on EpCAM(+)CD44(+) HCT-116 Human Colon Cancer Stem Cells Under Hypoxia." *Experimental & Therapeutic Medicine* 20, no. 6 (2020): 286.

81. Mansoori, B., A. Mohammadi, F. Abedi-Gaballu, S. Abbaspour, M. Ghasabi, R. Yekta, S. Shirjang, G. Dehghan, M. R. Hamblin, and B. Baradaran. "Hyaluronic Acid-Decorated Liposomal Nanoparticles for Targeted Delivery of 5-Fluorouracil into HT-29 Colorectal Cancer Cells." *Journal of Cellular Physiology* 235, no. 10 (2020): 6817–30.

82. Xiao, B., Y. Yang, E. Viennois, Y. Zhang, S. Ayyadurai, M. Baker, H. Laroui, and D. Merlin. "Glycoprotein CD98 as a Receptor for Colitis-Targeted Delivery of Nanoparticle." *Journal of Materials Chemistry B* 2, no. 11 (2014): 1499–508.

83. Chassaing, B., and E. Cascales. "Antibacterial Weapons: Targeted Destruction in the Microbiota." *Trends in Microbiology* 26, no. 4 (2018): 329–38.

84. Steidler, L., W. Hans, L. Schotte et al. "Treatment of Murine Colitis by Lactococcus lactis Secreting IL-10." *Science* 289 (2000): 4.

85. Teng, Y., Y. Ren, M. Sayed, X. Hu, C. Lei, A. Kumar, E. Hutchins, J. Mu, Z. Deng, C. Luo, K. Sundaram, M. K. Sriwastva, L. Zhang, M. Hsieh, R. Reiman, B. Haribabu, J. Yan, V. R. Jala, D. M. Miller, K. Van Keuren-Jensen, M. L. Merchant, C. J. McClain, J. W. Park, N. K. Egilmez, and H. G. Zhang. "Plant-Derived Exosomal microRNAs Shape the Gut Microbiota." *Cell Host & Microbe* 24, no. 5 (2018): 637–652 e8.

Targeting Immune Cells and Dysfunction 10

Lara Scheherazade Milane

Contents

10.1 OVERVIEW OF THE INNATE AND ADAPTIVE IMMUNE RESPONSES

The innate and adaptive immune responses work in synergy to defend the host from invading pathogens and dysfunctional cells that could become malignant. The innate immune system is the first response which occurs within minutes to hours of pathogen exposure. The innate immune response includes the anatomical barrier, the physiological response, phagocytosis, and inflammation[1] The skin and mucosa provide important anatomical barriers to pathogens while increased temperature (fever), the low pH of the stomach, and chemical inactivation of pathogens (lysozymes, interferon mediated, and complement mediated) are physiological responses[1] When pattern recognition receptors (PRRs) on immune cells recognize pathogen-associated molecular patterns (PAMPs) or damage-associated molecular patterns (DAMPs), cytokines such as tumor necrosis factor (TNF) and interleukin-6 (IL-6) are released resulting in acute, localized inflammation that attracts phagocytic cells to help eliminate the pathogen or damaged cell[1]

The key functions of the adaptive immune response are to fight and to remember. Generating immunological memory is the basis for immunization.[1] The key cells of the adaptive immune response include T cells, antigen presenting cells (APCs), and B cells.[1] APCs (mainly dendritic cells and some macrophages, to a lesser degree B cells and non-immune cells) express major histocompatibility complex (MHC) molecules for the presentation of endogenous (MHC class I) and exogenous (MHC class II) antigens to T cells.[1] After MHC-bound antigens activate T cell receptors, T cells release signaling cytokines and begin to differentiate into specialized T cells: cytotoxic T cells (CD8+ cells), T helper cells (Th; CD4+ cells), and regulatory T cells (Tregs; CD4+ cells).[1] It is the expansion of cytotoxic T cells that kills target cells while the helper T cells mediate and guide the immune response of additional cells through (1) interferon gamma (IFN-γ) release resulting in a Th1 response that activates macrophages and B cell differentiation, (2) cytokine (IL-4, 5, 13) signaling promoting B cells to produce immunoglobulin E (IgE) antibodies and

DOI: 10.1201/9781003092773-11

the activation of mast cells, and (3) IL-17 signaling which further promotes inflammation.[1] Tregs contribute to resolution.

When B cells are directly activated by antigens (no involvement of APCs), they differentiate into antibody-producing plasma cells and memory B cells.[1] The function of plasma cells is to rapidly produce and spread antibodies against a pathogen, cascading the immune response.[1] The memory B cells are critical to future recognition of the pathogen as these cells continue to express antigen binding receptors.[1] The creation of memory B cells is the principle of vaccination.

There are five types of antibodies that govern antibody-mediated immunity with various tissue expressions, opsonization, and complement interactions (IgM, IgG, IgD, IgA, and IgE). The antibody response is the initial response of the adaptive immune system which is followed by a cell response including activation of cytotoxic T cells, macrophages, natural killer cells, and cytokine signalling.[1]

10.2 IMMUNE DYSFUNCTION

Immune system dysfunction contributes to multiple pathologies, and there are many levels to manipulate immune function for therapeutic outcomes. Stem cell dysfunction and manipulation are the first line of intersection as T cells and B cells are derived from hematopoietic stem cells in the bone marrow.[1] Stem cell dysfunction can result in multiple blood disorders and leukemias. Likewise, dysfunctional lymphatics can result in multiple disorders and lymphomas. However, the most critical aspect of the immune response that contributes to pathologies and is a therapeutic target is the development of chronic inflammation.[2] As illustrated in Figure 10.1,[3] during acute inflammation there is resolution of inflammation and wound healing. As illustrated in Figure 10.2,[3] during chronic inflammation

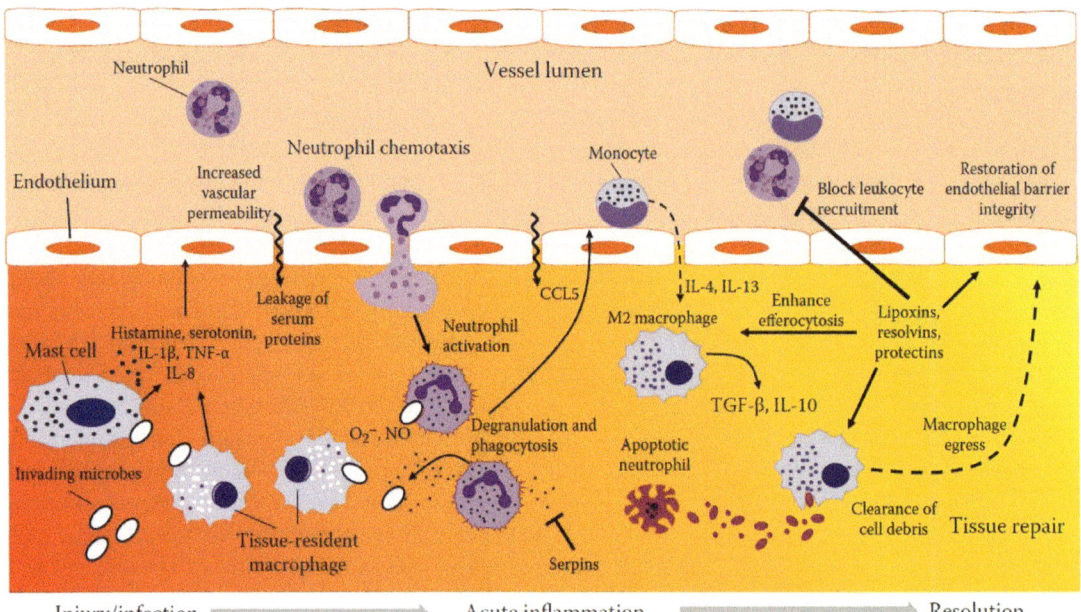

FIGURE 10.1   Acute inflammation. Acute inflammation is marked by the beginning of injury or inflammation which leads to the recruitment, infiltration, and activation of circulating neutrophils which help to remove the pathogen or damaged cells. M2a, M2b, and M2c macrophages are critical to the repair process and the resolution phase. Reprinted with permission from *Fundamentals of Immunology and Inflammation*.[3]

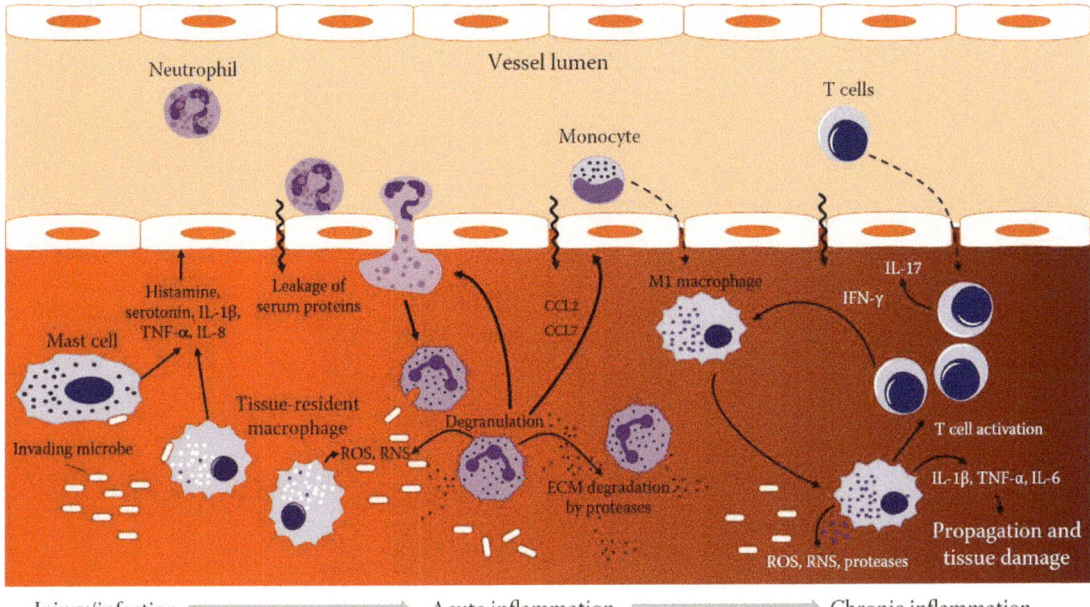

FIGURE 10.2   Chronic inflammation. Chronic inflammation begins with the same processes as acute inflammation but during chronic inflammation there is no resolution phase. Proteases, ROS, T cells, and pro-inflammatory cytokines contribute to tissue damage and sustained inflammation. Reprinted with permission from *Fundamentals of Immunology and Inflammation*[3]

there is no resolution and inflammation drives pathological outcomes. During acute infection, there is injury or infection that triggers phagocytosis by tissue-resident macrophages and the release of cytokines and other signaling factors from mast cells and tissue-resident macrophages.[3] In response to these signals, vascular permeability is increased and there is neutrophil chemotaxis into the tissue.[3] Once neutrophils enter the tissue they are activated and undergo degranulation, releasing proteases, and begin phagocytosis.[3] An important regulator of this response is the level of endogenous serpins (serine protease inhibitors) which inactivate neutrophil proteases if the level is close to inducing tissue damage.[3] Degranulation of neutrophils also leads to the recruitment of circulating monocytes.[3] Local IL-4 and IL-13 cytokines polarize the recruited monocytes into M2a (alternative) macrophages.[3] M2 macrophages are critical to resolution.[4] The different macrophage polarization states are illustrated in Figure 10.3.[4] The polarizing signals as well as the secreted factors and functions are shown. It is important to note that most often macrophages are only referred to as M1 (classical) or M2, but there are actually three different M2 states.[4] M2a macrophages phagocytosis cell debris and apoptotic bodies from surrounding, dying cells.[3,4] Pro-resolving lipid mediators (PRLM) such as resolvins signal M2a macrophages to initiate efferocytosis, the important process of cell debris clearing and exocytosis.[3,4] PRLM are derived from polyunsaturated fatty acids and are produced and released through a series of enzymatic steps that can occur in mononuclear cells (neutrophils and macrophages) or through cell-to-cell interactions (immune-immune or immune-endothelial)[5] The dietary benefit of polyunsaturated fatty acids (from sources such as salmon) is correlated with PRLM synthesis and signaling.[6] M2a macrophages can secrete factors that polarize the M2b state (IL-1R ligands) or the M2c state (IL-10) of macrophages resulting in respective immunoregulation or completion of resolution.[4]

Immune complexes and toll-like receptor (TLR) activation or IL-1R activation can polarize macrophages into an M2b state; M2b (type II) macrophages activate Th2 cells and regulate the immune response.[4] The M2b macrophages can be considered as the decision state or balancing scales of the

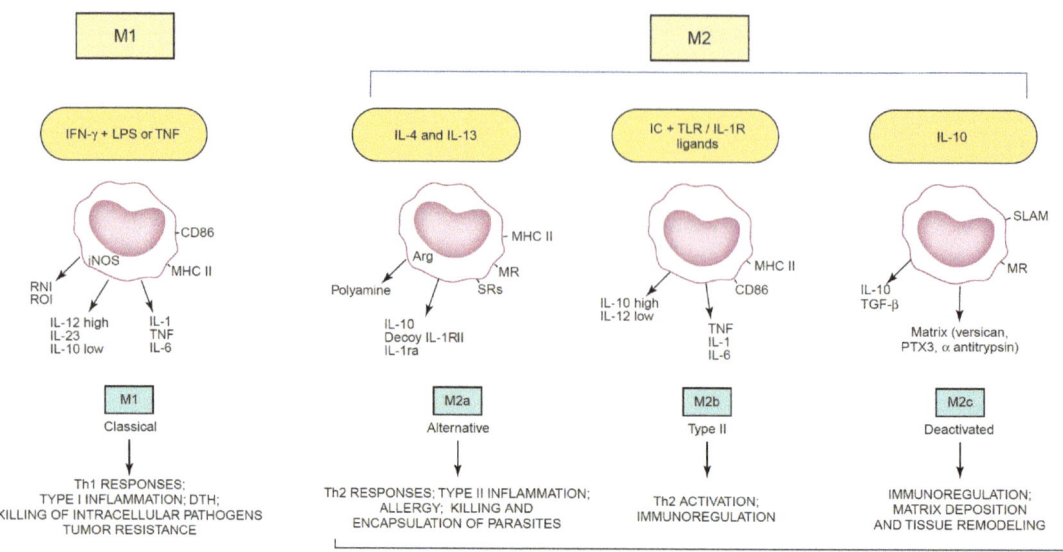

FIGURE 10.3   Macrophage polarization states. Macrophages are polarized in response to local signals. M1 or classical macrophages are polarized in response to IFN-γ and LPS or TNF, and they secrete multiple cytokines including TNF, IL-1, and IL-6. M1 macrophages are known as pro-inflammatory macrophages with anti-tumor activity. M2 macrophages exist in three substates: a, b, and c. M2a macrophages are alternative macrophages that are polarized in response to IL-4 and IL-13 and lead to type II inflammation such as allergy. M2b macrophages are decision point macrophages that can either lead to M1 activation and more of an immune response or M2c activation and resolution of inflammation. M2c macrophages are critical for tissue remodeling and repair. The M2 macrophages are known as anti-inflammatory macrophages with pro-tumor activity. Reprinted with permission from *TRENDS in Immunology*[4]

macrophage spectrum as these macrophages can signal for M1 polarization or M2c polarization and progression of resolution. M2b macrophages can release tumor necrosis factor (TNF) which could lead to M1 polarization.[4] M2b macrophages are also capable of releasing IL-10; IL-10 polarizes macrophages into an M2c (deactivated) state.[4] M2c macrophages function in matrix deposition and tissue remodeling.[4] M2c macrophages mediate the final stage of resolution until the tissue is cleared, repaired, and the endothelial barrier is restored.[3,4] As illustrated in Figure 10.1, the critical steps of the resolution phase are: (1) endogenous serpins, (2) IL-4 and IL-13 M2a macrophage polarization, (3) phagocytosis, (4) pro-resolving lipid mediator synthesis and release promoting M2a mediated efferocytosis, and (5) IL-10 activation of M2c macrophages to repair tissue damage.

As illustrated in Figure 10.2, there is no resolution phase in chronic inflammation.[3] During acute inflammation there is increased reactive oxygen species (ROS), increased reactive nitrogen species (RNS), and degradation of the extracellular matrix by degranulation of infiltrating neutrophils and from tissue-resident macrophages.[3] Monocyte chemoattractants (CCL2 and CCL7) are released to recruit monocytes which are polarized into the M1 state upon entry into the tissue.[3] T cells are recruited, and IL-1β, TNF-α, IL-6, IFN-γ, and IL-17 activate T cells resulting in sustained tissue damage and chronic inflammation.[3] Inflammation is a driver for diseases spanning from atherosclerosis, to multiple sclerosis, and cancer.[2] Targeting immune cells and correcting immune dysfunction is an important approach to the treatment of immune-related pathologies including inflammation-driven disease. Nanomedicine is ideal for the systemic targeting of pathologies as the vasculature of damaged tissue is more permeable than normal vasculature, allowing for non-specific, passive targeting as nanoparticles accumulate to a higher degree in damaged tissue than in normal tissue.

10.3 MACROPHAGE TARGETING AND REPROGRAMMING

M1 macrophage infiltration in synovial joints drives chronic inflammation in rheumatoid arthritis (RA)[7] To resolve inflammation in RA PEGylated (polyethylene glycol) folic acid (FA) modified silver (Ag) nanoparticles (FA-Ag-NP) have demonstrated efficacy and safety in a pre-clinical mouse model of RA.[7] The rationale of this system is that M1 macrophages express a high level of folic acid receptors; decorating the silver nanoparticles with folic acid permits active targeting of M1 macrophages while the PEG enhances stability of the nanoparticles, and the silver acts as the bioactive agent, killing M1 macrophages and inducing M2 macrophage polarization.[7] Treatment with the FA-Ag-NP was compared to treatment with methotrexate (MTX) and methotrexate PEGylated silver nanoparticles (MTX-Ag-NP) as MTX is disease-modifying anti-rheumatic drug (DMARD) commonly used to treat RA.[7] In the collagen-induced RA mouse model, the FA-Ag-NP significantly reduced the arthritis score (degree of paw redness, swelling, inflammation) and paw thickness relative to MTX-Ag-NP, MTX, and saline treated mice[7] The expression level of M1 macrophage markers was reduced; IL-1β in synovial fluid was significantly reduced with FA-Ag-NP treatment relative to all other treatments, and the level of IL-6 and TNF-α was significantly reduced with FA-Ag-NP treatment relative to saline treatment.[7] The medical use of colloidal silver dates back to the late 1800s and the antimicrobial properties are well established.[8] The FA-Ag-NP study in the mouse RA model demonstrated clearance of the Ag-NP by 28 days after administration and no residual toxicity.[7] This system is very promising for reversing M1 inflammation in RA. The use of silver as the bioactive agent is very promising for RA as there is no actual drug in the FA-Ag-NP system which could prove to be a much safer strategy for treating RA than the current DMARDs. This FA-Ag-NP system could also be applied to other pathologies with M1 macrophage-driven inflammation.

Atherosclerosis is the primary contributor to cardiovascular disease which is the leading cause of death in the world.[9] Atherosclerosis is actually a disease caused by transformed macrophages.[9] Intimal macrophages in the vascular wall phagocytosis oxidized low-density lipoproteins and are overloaded and transform into foam cells.[9] Foam cells drive the collection of lipids and eventually these foam cells rupture, the transformed macrophages do not perform efferocytosis, and lipids and cell debris collect in the vascular wall forming a necrotic core with a fibrous cap.[9] When the fibrous cap ruptures, thrombi stick to the cap and continue to collect until a thrombus can induce complete vascular blockage.[9] Researchers at Texas Tech University recently developed foam cell targeting nanoparticles.[9] The CD36 receptor was used as the nanoparticle target and this receptor is a lipid-scavenging receptor overexpressed in intimal macrophages.[9] The group synthesized non-targeted phosphatidylcholine liposomes (lipid nanoparticles) and CD36 receptor targeted phosphatidylcholine liposomes.[9] To target the CD36 receptor, 30 mol% of 1-palmitoyl-2-(4-keto-dodec-3-enedioyl) phosphatidylcholine (KDdiA-PC), a keto acid analogue of 1-palmitoyl-2-linoleoyl-sn-glycero-3-phosphocholine (PLPC), was used in the liposome formulation as KDdiA-PC is a potent ligand for the CD36 receptor.[9] The study demonstrated that the CD36 receptor targeting liposomes actively targeted atherosclerotic lesions in atherosclerotic mice.[9] Although this system effectively targeted foam cells, the study did not include any biologically active agents. The next step would be evaluating the therapeutic efficacy of drug loaded foam cell targeting nanoparticles.[9] This system could prove to be very promising for the treatment of cardiovascular disease which could have tremendous global impact.

The resident macrophages of the central nervous system are called microglia.[10] Microglia are important targets in neurological disease as different polarization states are associated with different pathologies. For example, early state Alzheimer's disease and amyotrophic lateral sclerosis are associated with M2 polarization whereas advanced disease is associated with M1 polarization.[10] Similarly, in multiple sclerosis there is an increased ratio of M1/M2 macrophages and the progressive stage of the disease is associated with M1 polarization whereas remyelination is associated with M2 polarization.[10] Nanomedicines

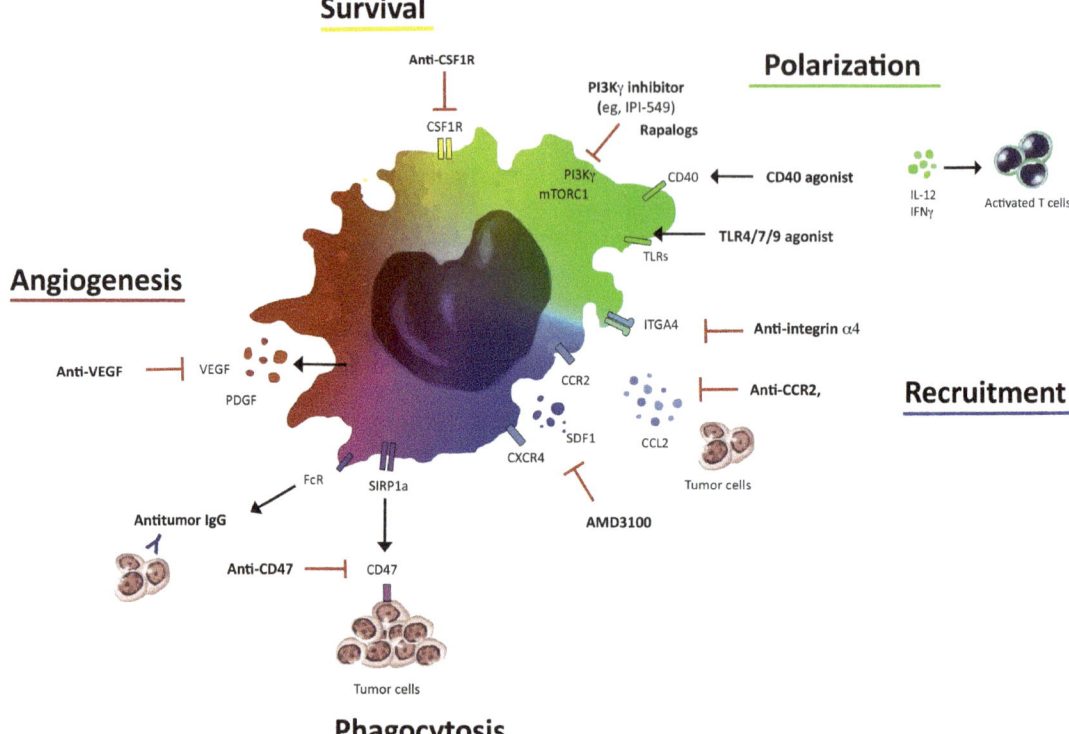

FIGURE 10.4   TAM targeting strategies. The two main strategies for manipulating tumor-associated macrophages for therapeutic outcomes are to either reduce infiltration of circulating myeloid cells or to repolarize the TAMs into M1 macrophages. CSF1R inhibitors suppress TAM survival. PI3Kγ inhibitors, mTOR inhibitors, CD40 agonists, and TLR4, 7, 8, and 9 agonists repolarize TAMS into M1 states. Suppressing monocyte infiltration can be achieved with integrin α4β1 (ITGA4) inhibitors, CCL2 and CCR2 inhibitors, CXCR4 inhibitors, and SDF1 inhibitors. Reprinted with permission from *TRENDS in Immunology*[13]

that repolarize microglia and resolve neuroinflammation are in development and are important to the future of treating neurodegenerative disease.[11]

Macrophages in the solid tumor microenvironment are referred to as either tumor-associated macrophages (TAMs) or cancer-associated macrophages (CAMs) as these macrophages are known to be transformed and contribute to disease progression and aggression.[12,13] TAMs are mostly M2 macrophages that contribute to immune evasion, inflammation, and tumor remodeling.[12,13] There are two therapeutic strategies for reducing TAMS; the first is to reduce myeloid cell recruitment to the tumor and the second is to repolarize TAMS to M1 macrophages that aid in tumor elimination. The strategy for TAM repolarization is that replacing the immunosuppressive, pro-angiogenic, and matrix deposition of TAMS with immunostimulation, antigen presentation, and T cell activation of M1 macrophages will lead to tumor regression. Figure 10.4[13] illustrates some of the common TAM targeting strategies. There are numerous clinical trials and targeting strategies for repolarizing TAMs. Some of the common TAM targets that are used for TAM-specific drug delivery are the folate receptor β, the transferrin receptor, and the mannose receptor CD206.[12,13] A newer approach in clinical trials to preventing the recruitment and accumulation of macrophages in a tumor is to inhibit chemoattractant factors such as chemokine CCL2 (current small molecule and antibody clinical trials), CSF1R (current small molecule and antibody clinical trials), and IL-1β (antibody in clinical trial).[13] Activated chemokine receptors activate integrin receptors to help promote myeloid cell infiltration from the vasculature; the integrins α4β1 and αLβ2 are also being explored as TAM targets.[13]

The chemoattractants activate the phosphoinositide 3-kinase γ (PI3Kγ) pathway in recruited myeloid cells; as such, multiple levels of this pathway as well as the mTOR pathway have been used to target TAMs.[13] The common repolarization strategies for transforming TAMs into M1 macrophages include mTOR and PI3Kγ inhibitors, CD40 agonists, and Toll-like receptor (TLR4, 7, 8, and 9) agonists.[13] Due to the enhanced permeability and retention effect (EPR) in solid tumors, nanomedicine is ideal for reaching the aforementioned TAM targets. The enhanced permeability is due to the leaky vasculature resulting from constant vascular deconstruction, reconstruction, and angiogenesis which makes it easier for nanoparticles to enter a tumor, and the enhanced retention is due to the poor lymphatic drainage which results in prolonged tumor residence of nanoparticles.

10.4 TARGETING AND EXPLOITING T CELL RESPONSES

Chimeric antigen receptor (CAR) T cell therapy is an important approach to treating cancer. CARs are synthetic receptors that are engineered to promote T cell recognition and response to a tumor. CARs are engineered and a patient's own T cells are extracted, transfected to express the CAR, propagated, and injected back into the patient. CAR T cell therapy manipulates the patient's endogenous immune response to recognize, kill, and resolve a tumor. The reason this strategy is so important is that the patient's immune system not only kills cancer cells, it also digests and clears the cellular debris, resolving the tumor without leaving necrotic or apoptotic debris. There are numerous, clinically approved CAR T cell therapies including idecabtagene vicleucel (Abecma®) for treating relapsed or refractory multiple myeloma, brexucabtagene autoleucel (Tecartus™) for treating relapsed or refractory mantle cell lymphoma, lisocabtagene maraleucel (Breyanzi®) for treating relapsed or refractory large B cell lymphoma, tisagenlecleucel (Kymriah™) for treating adults with relapsed or refractory diffuse large B cell lymphoma and young adults with relapsed or refractory acute lymphoblastic leukemia, and axicabtagene ciloleucel (Yescarta™) for treating certain B cell lymphomas.[14] CAR T cell therapies are continually advancing as CAR protein engineering, T cell engineering, and T cell/tumor interactions are optimized.[14]

A second important approach for T cell activation also applies to cancer; immune checkpoint inhibition. Programmed cell death protein 1 (PD-1) is a deactivating receptor that is coupled to the T cell receptor on T cells. When the T cell receptor is bound to an antigen, the T cell cytotoxic response will not occur if the coupled deactivating receptors such as PD-1 are engaged. These immune checkpoint receptors are important for T cells not to illicit responses to healthy self-cells. Tumor cells exploit the immune checkpoint process by overexpressing PD-L1 which binds to the PD-1 receptor and prevents cytotoxic T cell activation even in the presence of T cell receptor antigens. The checkpoint inhibitors include antibodies against PD-1 and PD-L1. Nivolumab (Opdivo®) and pembrolizumab (Keytruda®) are PD-1 inhibitors while atezolizumab, avelumab, and durvalumab are PD-L1 inhibitors.[15] Combining immune checkpoint inhibitors with nanomedicines that have targeting peptides, penetrating peptides, or therapeutic peptides is an approach that is being considering to improve the treatment of glioblastoma.[16]

As illustrated in Figure 10.5[17,18] peptide nano-assemblies are also being developed to improve the delivery and tumor residence of checkpoint inhibitors.[17,18] In this study investigators at the National Center for Nanoscience and Technology in Beijing, China, developed a click reaction-assisted peptide immune checkpoint blockade (CRICB) strategy for improving checkpoint inhibition.[17,18] The investigators combined a PD-L1 targeting peptide (TP) with an azide-tethered assembled peptide (AP) resulting in nanofiber constructs of TP-AP.[17,18] The group compared TP-AP to standard PD-L1 antibody treatment and showed that there was a higher degree of TP-AP accumulation in 4T1 tumor spheroids (Figure 10.5, Panel B), which correlated to higher relative intensity of Cy (Panel C).[17,18] The group compared TP, TP-AP, and low-dose (LD) TP-AP tumor localization in mice from 4 hours until 120 hours and

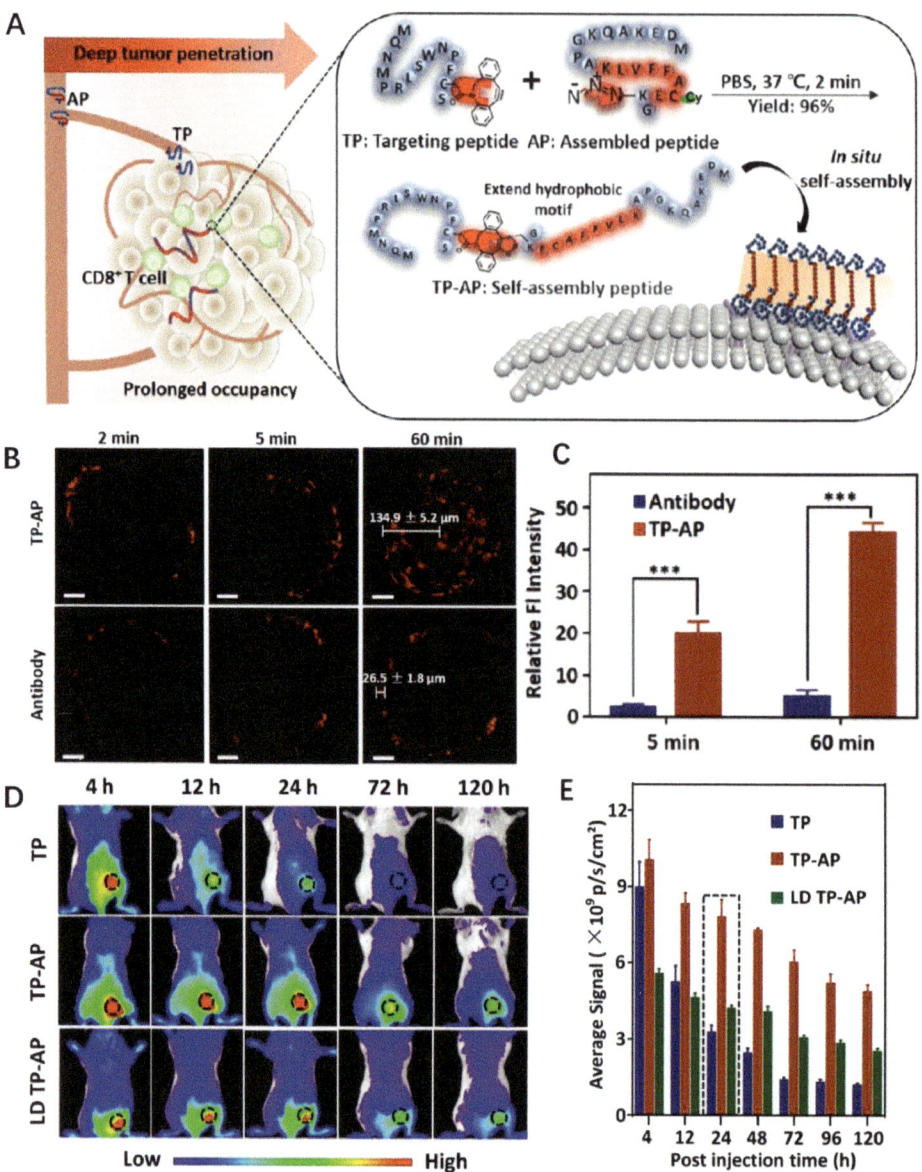

FIGURE 10.5 Peptide nanofiber immune checkpoint inhibition. Improvement in checkpoint inhibition includes this novel peptide approach with increased tumor penetration, residence, and efficacy. The strategy is demonstrated in Panel A; an anti-PD-L1 targeting peptide complexes with an assembly peptide to form nanofibers. As illustrated in Panel B, the TP-AP nanofibers accumulate more than the standard PD-L1 antibody in tumor spheroids and this correlates to relative intensity shown in Panel C. Panel D and E illustrated tumor accumulation over time as compared to the targeting peptide alone (TP) and low-dose (LD) TP-AP. Reprinted with permission from *Applied Materials Today*[17,18]

demonstrated high TP-AP tumor association even after 120 hours (Panel D and E).[17,18] Relative to the antibody, TP-AP was able to transverse the microenvironment of the tumor and was localized up to 150 μm from vessels whereas antibody localization was less than 50 μm from vasculature.[17,18] Importantly, both the TP-AP and low-dose TP-AP significantly reduced tumor volume relative to antibody treatment.[17,18] New and improved strategies for checkpoint inhibition and T cell activation are being developed and will undoubtedly lead to future clinically approved immunotherapies.

10.5 ACTIVATING MEMORY RESPONSES

One of the most important strategies for immune targeting and manipulation is activation of the memory response with vaccines. The critical need and phenomenal capabilities of vaccine development have been demonstrated during the COVID-19 pandemic, which is caused by the SARS-CoV-2 virus.[19] In December of 2019 the first case of COVID-19 was reported in Wuhan, China; by March 11th, 2020, the World Health Organization declared COVID-19 a pandemic.[19] On December 2nd, 2020, Pfizer and BioNTech received the first emergency use authorization in the world for their COVID-19 mRNA BNT162b2 vaccine.[19,20] The rapid speed of vaccine development and approval is truly astounding. By January 10th, 2020, the first RNA genome sequence of SARS-CoV-2 was published.[19,20] This enabled the design and development of molecular therapeutics targeted against the SARS-CoV-2 RNA genome. The first two emergency use vaccines to receive global approval (Pfizer's BNT162b2 and Moderna's mRNA1273) are message RNA (mRNA) vaccines delivered via lipid nanoparticles. The lipid nanoparticles enable the delivery of mRNA; without these drug delivery systems the mRNA would degrade and not elicit an immune response. Both of

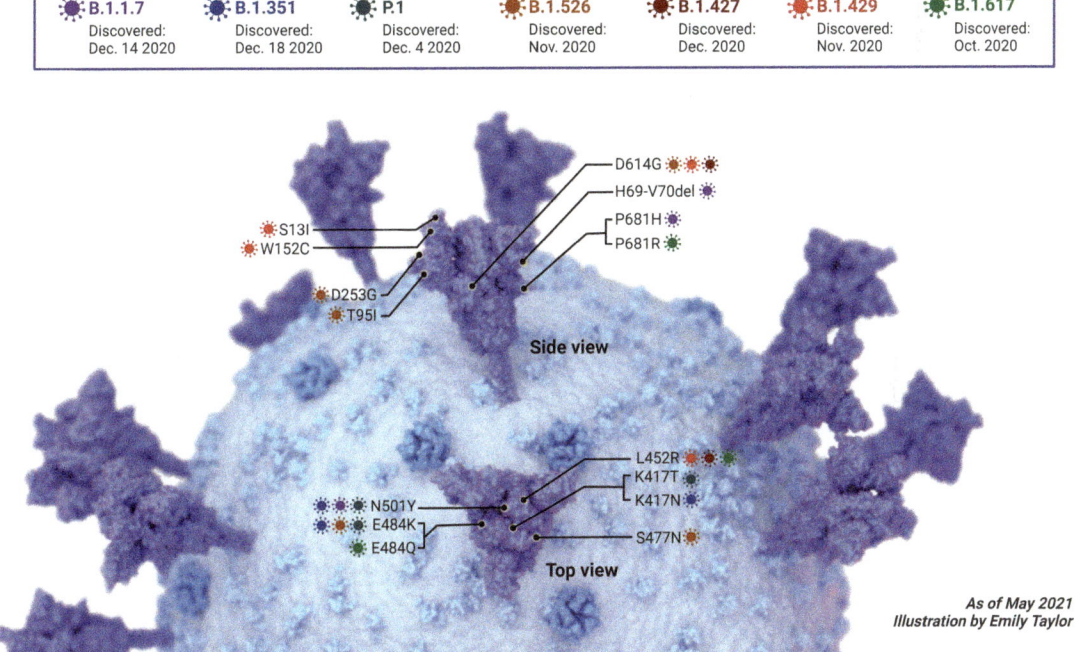

FIGURE 10.6 SARS-CoV-2 variants. The SARS-CoV-2 virus is rapidly and rampantly mutating, and there is concern that variants may develop that evade protection from the current vaccines. The B.1.1.7 variant is known as the United Kingdom variant as it was first discovered in the UK on December 14th, 2020. This variant has 23 mutations with 17 amino acid changes. The B.1.351 is also known as the 501Y.V2 variant and the South African variant; although different from the B.1.1.7, this variant also has 23 mutations and 17 amino acid changes. The P.1 variant is also known as the Brazil variant and this has 35 mutations and 17 amino acid changes. The South African variant is up to 50% more transmissible and the United Kingdom variant is between 43–82% more transmissable.[21] These variants have been shown to have a 1.8× to 86× decrease in neutralization by existing vaccines.[21] By Emily Taylor, reprinted with permission and credited to Biorender.com.

these vaccines encode for the viral spike (entry) protein of the SARS-CoV-2 virus; the spike protein binds to ACE2 receptors in host cells and mediates viral entry.[19,20] The rationale for immunization with these mRNA vaccines is that the mRNA is released from the lipid nanoparticles and host cells ribosomes on the endoplasmic reticulum translate the mRNA into the viral spike proteins. These proteins are replicated after a first inoculation. A second vaccine is required to induce a B cell memory response (mentioned earlier in the chapter).[19,20] Two weeks after the second inoculation patients are presumed to have generated sufficient memory B cells with antigen binding receptors for the SARS-CoV-2 viral spike protein.[19,20] The COVID-19 vaccine development has emphasized how vaccines are one of the most important medical advancements in human history. There are additional approvals and continued development of COVID-19 mRNA vaccines, DNA vaccines, and protein-based vaccines.[19,20] Nanotechnology is enabling many of these vaccines.[19,20] A concern of the current vaccines in development is the efficacy against SARS-CoV-2 variants. As demonstrated in Figure 10.6, the SARS-CoV-2 virus continues to mutate, and this image only demonstrates a few of the many mutants that have been discovered. As new pathogens continue to emerge and threaten global health, there will always be a demand for vaccine development and improvement. Activating the B cell memory response is the most important strategy for immune manipulation that has aided human health. Due to the respiratory transmission of viral particles and aerosols, and the highly transmissible and infectivity of the SARS-CoV-2 virus, the recommendations during the pandemic have been to socially distance and to wear facial masks covering the nose and mouth. Figure 10.7 demonstrates the principles of herd immunity and social distancing. As demonstrated in the illustration, achieving herd immunity without vaccination and only with social distancing and immunity acquired from infection would not be possible. Herd immunity does not stop the existence of a pathogen, it reduces the host propagation and transmission of the pathogen. This is why booster shots and updated vaccines (such as the

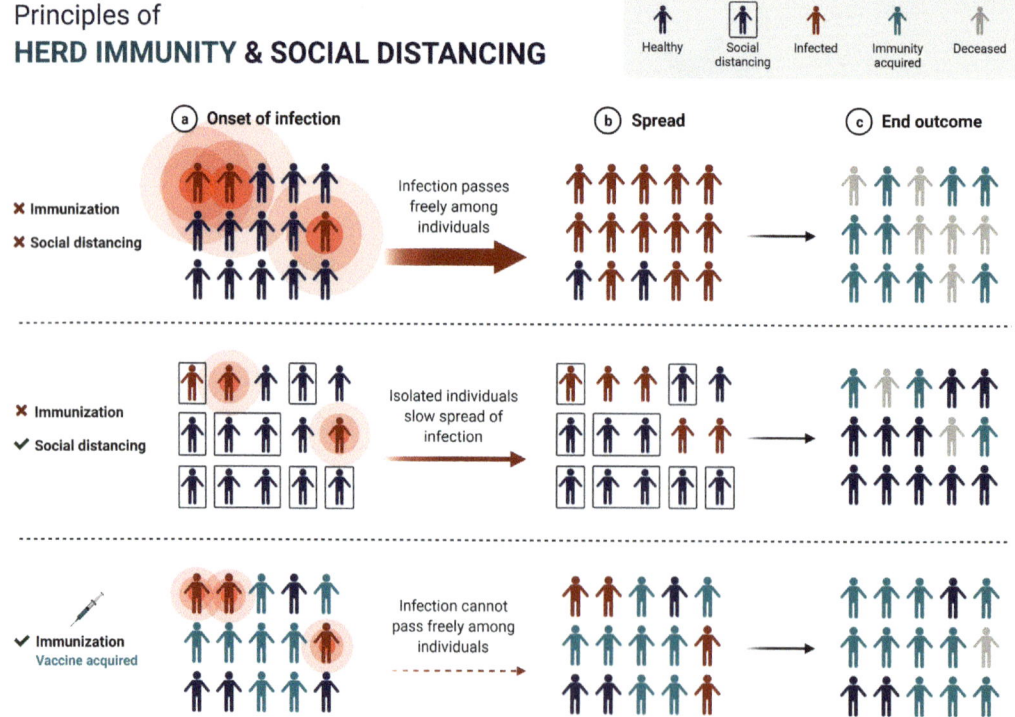

FIGURE 10.7   Vaccine requirement for herd immunity to the SARS-CoV-2 virus. As illustrated, herd immunity to SARS-CoV-2 would not be possible without vaccination as enough of the population could not acquire immunity but social distancing during the COVID-19 pandemic has helped to minimize the spread of the virus. Reprinted with permission and credited to Biorender.com.

seasonal influenza vaccine) are important. Inducing the B cell memory response is critical in pandemic responsiveness, managing the health burden of the seasonal influenza virus, and has been critical in generating herd immunity to polio, tetanus, hepatitis A and B, Rubella, measles, varicella, and diphtheria to name a few. Activating B cell memory responses will continue to be one of the most critical medical tools in global health.

REFERENCES

1. Marshall, J. S., R. Warrington, W. Watson, and H. L. Kim. "An Introduction to Immunology and Immunopathology." *Allergy, Asthma & Clinical Immunology* 14, no. Suppl 2 (2018): 49. doi:10.1186/s13223-018-0278-1.
2. Milane, L., and M. Amiji. *Nanomedicine for Inflammatory Diseases.* Boca Raton, FL: CRC Press, 2017.
3. Woods, M. E. *Nanomedicine for Inflammatory Diseases.* Edited by L. Milane, and M. Amiji. Boca Raton, FL: CRC Press, 2017.
4. Mantovani, A., A. Sica, S. Sozzani, P. Allavena, A. Vecchi, and M. Locati. "The Chemokine System in Diverse Forms of Macrophage Activation and Polarization." *Trends in Immunology* 25, no. 12 (2004): 677–86. doi:10.1016/j.it.2004.09.015.
5. Li, C., X. Wu, S. Liu, D. Shen, J. Zhu, and K. Liu. "Role of Resolvins in the Inflammatory Resolution of Neurological Diseases." *Frontiers in Pharmacology* 11 (2020). doi:10.3389/fphar.2020.00612.
6. Carracedo, M., G. Artiach, H. Arnardottir, and M. Bäck. "The Resolution of Inflammation Through Omega-3 Fatty Acids in Atherosclerosis, Intimal Hyperplasia, and Vascular Calcification." *Seminars in Immunopathology* 41, no. 6 (2019): 757–66. doi:10.1007/s00281-019-00767-y.
7. Yang, Y., L. Guo, Z. Wang, P. Liu, X. Liu, J. Ding, and W. Zhou. "Targeted Silver Nanoparticles for Rheumatoid Arthritis Therapy via Macrophage Apoptosis and re-Polarization." *Biomaterials* 264 (2021): 120390. doi:10.1016/j.biomaterials.2020.120390.
8. Sim, W., R. T. Barnard, M. A. T. Blaskovich, and Z. M. Ziora. "Antimicrobial Silver in Medicinal and Consumer Applications: A Patent Review of the Past Decade." *Antibiotics* 7, no. 4 (2018): 93. doi:10.3390/antibiotics7040093 (2007–2017).
9. Dhanasekara, C. S., J. Zhang, S. Nie, G. Li, Z. Fan, and S. Wang. "Nanoparticles Target Intimal Macrophages in Atherosclerotic Lesions." *Nanomedicine: Nanotechnology, Biology & Medicine* 32 (2021): 102346.
10. Du, L., Y. Zhang, Y. Chen, J. Zhu, Y. Yang, and H. L. Zhang. "Role of Microglia in Neurological Disorders and Their Potentials as a Therapeutic Target." *Molecular Neurobiology* 54, no. 10 (2017): 7567–84. doi:10.1007/s12035-016-0245-0.
11. Zhang, F., Y.-A. Lin, S. Kannan, and R. M. Kannan. "Targeting Specific Cells in the Brain with Nanomedicines for CNS Therapies." *Journal of Controlled Release* 240 (2016): 212–26. doi:10.1016/j.jconrel.2015.12.013.
12. Ngambenjawong, C., H. H. Gustafson, and S. H. Pun. "Progress in Tumor-Associated Macrophage (TAM)-Targeted Therapeutics." *Advanced Drug Delivery Reviews* 114 (2017): 206–21 (2017). doi:10.1016/j.addr.2017.04.010.
13. Pathria, P., T. L. Louis, and J. A. Varner. "Targeting Tumor-Associated Macrophages in Cancer." *Trends in Immunology* 40, no. 4 (2019): 310–27. doi:10.1016/j.it.2019.02.003.
14. Hong, M., J. D. Clubb, and Y. Y. Chen. "Engineering CAR-T Cells for Next-Generation Cancer Therapy." *Cancer Cell* 38, no. 4 (2020): 473–88. doi:10.1016/j.ccell.2020.07.005.
15. Bi, K., M. X. He, Z. Bakouny, A. Kanodia, S. Napolitano, J. Wu, G. Grimaldi, D. A. Braun, M. S. Cuoco, A. Mayorga, L. DelloStritto, G. Bouchard, J. Steinharter, A. K. Tewari, N. I. Vokes, M. Shannon, M. Sun, J. Park, S. L. Chang, B. A. McGregor, R. Haq, T. Denize, S. Signoretti, J. L. Guerriero, S. Vigneau, O. Rozenblatt-Rosen, A. Rotem, A. Regev, T. K. Choueiri, and E. M. Van Allen. "Tumor and Immune Reprogramming During Immunotherapy in Advanced Renal Cell Carcinoma." *Cancer Cell* 39, no. 5, (2021): 649–661, e645. doi:10.1016/j.ccell.2021.02.015.
16. Song, P., X. Zhao, and S. Xiao. "Application Prospect of Peptide-Modified Nano Targeting Drug Delivery System Combined with PD-1/PD-L1 Based Immune Checkpoint Blockade in Glioblastoma." *International Journal of Pharmaceutics* 589 (2020): 119865. doi:10.1016/j.ijpharm.2020.119865.
17. Xiao, W.-Y., Y. Wang, H. W. An, D. Hou, M. Mamuti, M. D. Wang, J. Wang, W. Xu, L. Hu, and H. Wang. "Click Reaction-Assisted Peptide Immune Checkpoint Blockade for Solid Tumor Treatment." *ACS Applied Materials & Interfaces* 12, no. 36 (2020): 40042–51. doi:10.1021/acsami.0c10166.

18. Deng, Z.-W., C.-S. Yuan, T. Wang, X.-G. Chen, and Y. Liu. "Peptide-Based Assemblies as Immune Checkpoint Inhibitor Delivery Systems for Enhanced Immunotherapy." *Applied Materials Today* 23 (2021): 101063.

19. Milane, L., and M. Amiji. "Clinical Approval of Nanotechnology-Based SARS-CoV-2 mRNA Vaccines: Impact on Translational Nanomedicine." *Drug Delivery & Translational Research* (2021). doi:10.1007/s13346-021-00911-y.

20. Kamidani, S., C. A. Rostad, and E. J. Anderson. "COVID-19 Vaccine Development: A Pediatric Perspective." *Current Opinion in Pediatrics* 33, no. 1 (2021): 144–51.

21. Abdool Karim, S. S., T. de Oliveira, and SARS-Co New. "V-2 Variants: Clinical, Public Health, and Vaccine Implications." *New England Journal of Medicine* 384 (2021): 1866–8. doi:10.1056/NEJMc2100362.

SECTION TWO

Overcoming Cellular Barriers

In the simplest terms a diseased cell can be considered as any cell that has deviated from its basal, healthy state of homeostasis and requires restoration of homeostasis. This applies to any pathology, from autosomal recessive cystic fibrosis to multidrug resistant triple negative breast cancer. As molecular therapeutics advance, more precise ways to manipulate cells and elicit highly specific cellular responses are being developed for common (and some less frequent) pathologies. We are truly in the Age of Molecular Therapeutics. This is emphasized by the recent rapid (less than one year) development and emergency use approval of numerous SARS-CoV-2 vaccines around the globe in response to the COVID-19 pandemic. Some of these are the first ever mRNA vaccines directed to manipulate the host cell ribosomes and endoplasmic reticulum to produce copies of the SARS-CoV-2 spike protein for immune recognition and to acquire a memory B cell response. The design of these vaccines was made possible by the rapid sequencing and publication of the viral RNA genome. These mRNA vaccines are enabled by nanotechnology; without nanoparticle protected delivery, the mRNA constructs would degrade rapidly. The rapid development of these vaccines attests to the capabilities and demand for molecular therapeutics. This demand will continue to persist and solutions such as nanomedicine will continue to enable these molecular therapeutics.

Although there are hundreds, if not thousands of important cell and molecular targets, this section focuses on the targets with high promise and significant advances toward clinical translation. The chapters in this section cover molecular and organelle targeting of lysosomes, microtubules, the endoplasmic reticulum, mitochondria, DNA, RNA, and combination organelle targeting. The critical demand for organelle and molecular targeting continues to grow and these chapters discuss the current and translational molecular targeted therapies.

DOI: 10.1201/9781003092773-12

Overcoming the Plasma Membrane

11

Nuno Bernardes and Arsenio M. Fialho

Contents

11.1 INTRODUCTION

The plasma membrane is a major cellular barrier composing the outer boundary of each cell ensuring its protection from the surrounding environment and the stability of its intracellular composition (Zhang et al. 2019). In eukaryotic cells, the active internalization of substances from the extracellular environment, such as nutrients, growth factors, and others, is essential to the proper environment sensing and to maintain their normal physiology (Saric and Freeman 2021). In addition, most drugs intended for therapeutic purposes are designed to target intracellular components of the cell, thus the plasma membrane is a barrier that exogenous compounds need to cross to reach the cytosol, which limits the use of many potential drugs. For small, moderately polar molecules, uptake is achieved by passive diffusion across the plasma membrane. However, for larger, more polar compounds like sugars, amino acids, peptides, or nucleosides, membrane transporters are required (Yang and Hinner 2015). When the molecules or systems are too large to easily cross the plasma membrane, endocytosis is required for them to reach the cytosol. Thus, many strategies have been proposed to overcome this limitation with the development of effective delivery systems using cell-penetrating peptides (CPP), antibodies, dendrimers, and lipid- and polymer-based nanoparticles which ultimately aim at promoting more efficient uptake by the cells (Zhang et al. 2019).

Endocytosis is an energy-dependent cellular process through which the cells internalize such compounds located in their extracellular medium and membrane receptor proteins through the formation of vesicles from their plasma membrane. Here, we will briefly review some plasma membrane properties important for their action as a cellular barrier, and how some endocytic pathways are currently being used for the development of efficient delivery strategies. Finally, we will review the current literature of a bacterial-derived cell penetrating peptide, p28, and how it can be explored to transport new therapeutics through the plasma membrane for selective anti-cancer drug delivery strategies.

11.2 THE PLASMA MEMBRANE COMPOSITION AND FUNCTION

The plasma membrane is composed essentially of proteins and lipids, creating a thin layer of a few nanometers (5–10 nm) (Zhang et al. 2019; Yang and Hinner 2015). The general structure comprising the lipid polar head and the long hydrophobic tail provides the thermodynamic environment for their association as bilayered sheets where the tails are surrounded by the polar heads (Zalba and ten Hagen 2017; Jacobson, Mouritsen, and Anderson 2007). The biochemical differences in the lipid polar heads or the hydrocarbon chains composing the membrane lipids originate different properties such as overall structure, charge, and packing, thus modulating the behavior of the membrane. Overall, three major classes of lipids are the main constituents including glycerophospholipids, sphingolipids, and cholesterol. Regarding the glycerophospholipids these are primarily composed of phospatidylcoline (PC), phosphatidylethanolamine (PE), and phosphatidylserine (PS) (Zhang et al. 2019). Sphingolipids, of which sphingomyelin (SM) is the major representative, contain long fatty acid chains forming solid gel phases, which in turn are fluidized by sterols like cholesterol, the major non-polar lipid of cell membranes (Bernardes and Fialho 2018).

The lipid bilayers forming the plasma membranes of normal non-cancer cells present a lipid asymmetry between the inner and outer leaflets. The outer leaflet contains mainly zwitterionic lipids such as PC and SM while in the inner leaflet phospholipids containing amine ethanolamine (phsphatidylethanolamine, PE) or PS are more prevalent. The maintenance of this asymmetry is an energy-dependent process provided by enzymes such as flipases, scramblases, and translocases (Zalba and ten Hagen 2017; Shevchenko and Simons 2010). The presence of the anionic PS in the inner leaflet confers on it a negative surface charge which influences numerous signaling mechanisms and with PE they stabilize interactions with the cytoskeleton by the amine and serine moieties, limiting the movement within the membrane, contributing to maintaining its curvature and mechanical properties (Nicolson 2014). However, in cancer cells, PS is often found in the outer leaflet which contributes to a negative surface charge in these cells correlating as well with a more acidic pH in their external environment (Ran, Stafford, and Thorpe 2002; Zwaal, Comfurius, and Bevers 2005). In endothelial cells residing in tumor microenvironments, PE was also found exposed in the outer leaflet of the cells (Stafford and Thorpe 2011).

The hydrophobic portions of these lipids are closely related to the uptake of several chemical entities, mainly small lipophilic molecules. These molecules simply diffuse due to their solubility in the hydrophobic region of the phospholipid bilayer where they tend to accumulate at high concentrations through hydrophobic interactions. Indeed, a strategy to promote a more efficient uptake of some drugs may be to anchor moieties that can interact with the hydrophobic tails of the lipid bilayers, as for example anchoring to cholesterol, squalene, and fatty acids (Zhang et al. 2019). Additionally, some drugs can also be delivered as pro-drugs to increase their lipophilicity.

Proteins, the other main constituents of the plasma membrane, also contribute actively to its organization. According to the lipid raft hypothesis, proteins contribute to the membrane lateral organization creating highly dynamic nanodomains enriched in cholesterol, sphingolipids, and glycosylphosphati-dylinositol (GPI)-enriched proteins. These rafts not only influence the structural integrity and organization of this cellular barrier, they also create interfaces that function as signaling hubs for many metabolic processes between the extra- and intracellular space. Furthermore, membrane rafts contribute greatly to the internalization of many drugs and other chemical entities (for a detailed review see (Bernardes and Fialho 2018)), and the proteins there located mediate many receptor-mediated uptake mechanisms.

11.3 PATHWAYS AND MECHANISMS OF ENDOCYTOSIS

Endocytosis is the main mechanism used by most nucleated cells for nutrient uptake and receptor signaling regulation (Saric and Freeman 2021). Multiple endocytic pathways exist to facilitate the internalization of the different exogenous cargo. Although different interpretations exist regarding the role of some pathway-specific characteristic proteins and how they may contribute to the uptake of drugs or nanomedicines, in general endocytic pathways follow similar trends (Wang et al. 2020). First, molecules or nanomedicines establish either non-specific interactions (mainly electrostatic and hydrophobic interactions) or ligand-receptor specific interactions. These interactions result in the engulfment of the transported cargo forming membrane invaginations, a step that Wang et al. (2020) defined as binding and budding. Next, these invaginated buds are pinched off from the membrane, resulting in endocytic vesicles which then fuse creating the early endosomes. Finally, the cargo transported by these endosomes can meet different fates: ligand-receptors may be recycled back to the membrane, the cargo transported by these vesicles can be directed elsewhere in the cell, namely into the *trans*-Golgi network (TGN) to be released from the cell, or ultimately early endosomes can mature to late endosomes and fuse with lysosomes resulting in the degradation of the cargo that could not escape (Yang and Hinner 2015; Zhang et al. 2019; Wang et al. 2020; Khan and Steeg 2021; Rennick, Johnston, and Parton 2021).

In general, according to the proteins involved, endocytosis pathways are divided into phagocytosis and pinocytosis (Wang et al. 2020; Manzanares and Ceña 2020). In phagocytosis the plasma membrane absorbs large particles while in pinocytosis solutes are uptaken. The latter is ubiquitous in almost every eukaryotic cell whereas phagocytosis typically occurs in phagocytes. Pinocytosis can be further divided in clathrin-mediated, caveolae-mediated, clathrin- and caveolae-independent endocytosis, and macropinocytosis. Clathrin and caveolin-1 are structural proteins for the translocation of many ligands and characterize their respective endocytic pathway. However, due to the participation of these pathways in the uptake of other specific ligand-receptor pairs, they are often also classified as receptor-mediated endocytic pathways. A significant difference between them seems to be the diameter of endocytic vesicles formed in each of these pathways. Clathrin-coated vesicles have a greater diameter (~100–120 nm) (Ehrlich et al. 2004) compared to caveolin-coated vesicles (~50 nm in diameter) (Rennick, Johnston, and Parton 2021). This difference can be the reason behind the nature of their endocytosed cargo, while some authors even dispute the involvement of a caveolin-1 mediated endocytic pathway in the uptake of larger cargoes such as nanoparticles. Nevertheless, caveolin-1 appears to be involved in the uptake of bacteria which could be difficult to accommodate in the predicted diameter of the vesicles generated. So, a hypothesis is that caveolar proteins could still be used to facilitate their internalization process without being considered a bona-fide caveolin-mediated endocytosis (Rennick, Johnston, and Parton 2021). Other pathways are now being identified such as the fast endophilin-mediated endocytosis (FEME), a clathrin-independent but dynamin-dependent pathway for ligand-receptor endocytosis, as well as a clathrin-independent carrier (CLIC)/glycosylphosphatidylinositol-anchored protein-enriched early endocytic compartment (GEEC) endocytosis, which is a clathrin- and dynamin-independent pathway. These two pathways are often confused with caveolae-mediated endocytosis since they are also not inhibited by many chemical inhibitors and seem to depend strongly on cholesterol (Wang et al. 2020; Rennick, Johnston, and Parton 2021). Figure 11.1 depicts the different major endocytosis pathways and their fundamental steps.

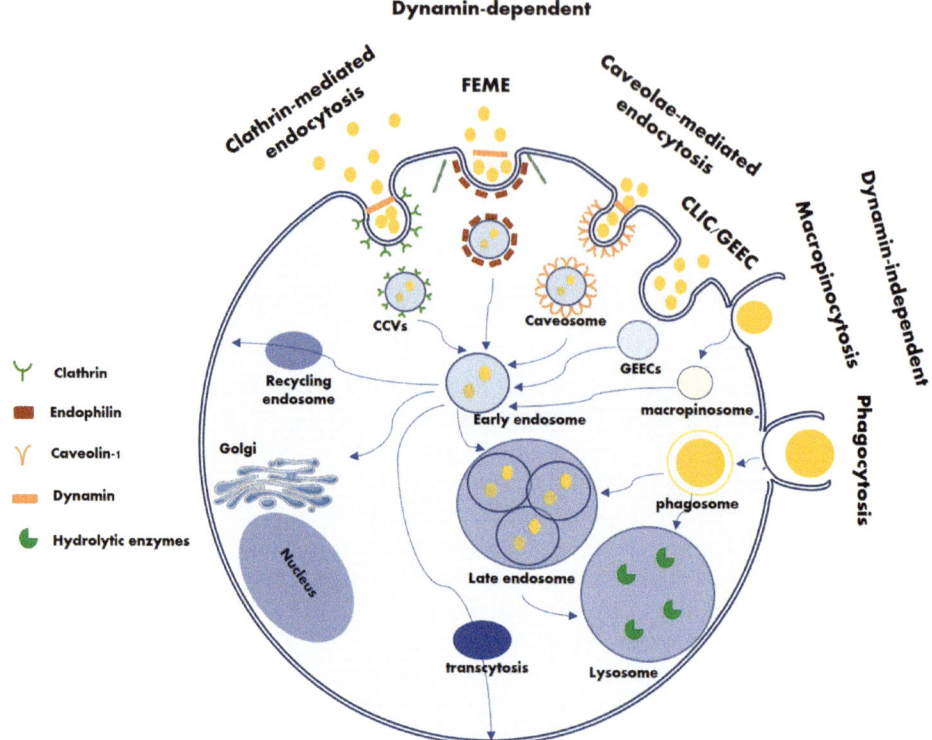

FIGURE 11.1 Schematic overview of endocytic pathways used to deliver biological therapies and nanomedicines. Biomacromolecules or nanocarriers may enter the cells via different endocytosis pathways, including clathrin-mediated endocytosis (CME), caveolae-mediated endocytosis (CavME), clathrin-independent/dynamin-dependent endocytosis (FEME), clathrin-independent/dynamin-independent endocytosis (CLIC/GEEC), micropinocytosis, and phagocytosis. Endocytosed materials follow the same fundamental actions. After interaction with the extracellular components of the cell, they are engulfed in the cell membrane to form invaginations and pinch off the membrane composing the various endocytic vesicles: clathrin-coated vesicles (CCV), caveosomes, GPI-anchored proteins-enriched early endosomal compartments (CLIC/GEEC), macropinosome, and phagosomes. After internalization, these vesicles merge into early endosomes to be sorted, where materials can be sent back to the plasma membrane, to the *trans*-Golgi network for exocytosis or mature into late endosomes to fuse with lyzosomes where materials that have not escaped are then degraded by cleavage enzymes. Some icons of this Figure were obtained from Servier Medical Art by Servier, which is licensed under a Creative Commons Attribution 3.0 Unported License (https://creativecommons.org/licenses/by/3.0/).

11.3.1 Clathrin-Mediated Endocytosis (CME)

The clathrin-dependent pathway for endocytosis (CME) is the best recognized mechanism for the uptake of nutrients like iron (mediated by the transferrin receptor) or cholesterol (mediated by low-density proteins), and epidermal growth factor (EGF) upon binding to its receptor. Indeed, clathrin-coated pits are estimated to account for 0.5–2% of cell surface (Brown and Petersen 1999; Ehrlich et al. 2004). This pathway is triggered by membrane receptor clustering or phosphorylation within the cytoplasmic tail of the receptors, which recruits a number of adaptin proteins and initiates a cascade of low-affinity protein-protein and protein-lipid interactions (in particular phosphatidylinositol 4,5-biphosphate (PtdIns(4,5)P$_2$)). These events lead to the formation of clathrin-coated vesicle pits, which finally scission from the membrane with the help of the GTPase dynamin that squeezes the head of the bud. This highly dynamic mechanism (pits are formed 30–120 s after ligand-receptor recognition (Ehrlich et al. 2004)) then faces different fates once within the cells. The clathrin coat is disassembled and recycled back to the membrane, while the uncoated vesicles now encapsulating the cargoes fuse with endosomes to be sorted. Here, they can be sorted to recycling endosomes and are also transported back to the membrane, mature into multi-vesicular bodies, and enter the TGN, or mature to late endosomes to face fusion with lysosomes to degradation. Thus, CME not only controls nutrient uptake required for cell growth, but also controls receptor signaling by removing these proteins from the membrane as needed, which has also a strong effect in cancer progression and metastasis (Khan and Steeg 2021).

11.3.2 Caveolae-Mediated Endocytosis (CavME)

Caveolae-mediated endocytosis (CavME) is the second-best studied pathway for uptake from the plasma membrane. Additionally, the role of CavME is very relevant in the context of transcytotic trafficking across cells and mechanosensing (Parton and Simons 2007). Caveolae are non-planar lipid rafts which present as flask-shaped membrane invaginations of 60–80 nm, identified by electron microscopy (Rothberg et al. 1992). Contrarily to the highly dynamic nature of clathrin-coated vesicles, caveolae present their shape constantly on the cell surface (Wang et al. 2020). Caveolae are generated by the integral membrane proteins caveolins, mainly caveolin-1 (Cav-1) and the peripheral membrane proteins named cavins. Caveolin-1 is inserted into the inner surface of the membrane bilayer through its cytosolic N-terminal that binds to cholesterol through a specific motif within the caveolin scaffolding domain (CSD, residues 82–101). CavME is triggered by ligand binding to the receptors within these domains, and its budding from the plasma membrane is regulated by Src tyrosine kinases and the serine/threonine phosphatases PP1 and PP2A. As for CME, dynamin is required for the pinching of these vesicles from the plasma membrane. Regarding their intracellular trafficking, caveolae can be utilized for the trans-vascular endothelial cell delivery to tumor tissues since the pathway has been demonstrated to perform trans-endothelial transport in endothelial cells. Within cancer cells, caveolar vesicles then fuse with early endosomes, following the same fate as described for clathrin-coated vesicles. Albumin-bound drugs are a paradigmatic case of the ability of CavME to promote cross-endothelial transport to reach tumor cells (Wang et al. 2020; Yang et al. 2021). Albumin binds to the glycoreceptor 60 in endothelial cells and to the SPARC receptor which is overexpressed in cancer cells. CavME was shown to be responsible for the uptake of the albumin-bound form of paclitaxel (nab-paclitaxel) in pancreatic cancer cells, in which the Cav-1 expression levels were also correlated to cell responsiveness to nab-paclitaxel. Moreover, nab-paclitaxel is currently approved by the FDA for metastatic or relapsed breast cancer. It was also uncovered that negatively charged liposomes were more likely to be endocytosed by CavME. Doxil, a liposomal formulation of doxorubicin (surface charge of –2.6 mV) also approved by the FDA, enters the drug-resistant MCF7/Adr cell line through CavME (Yang et al. 2021).

11.3.3 Clathrin-Independent/Dynamin-Dependent Endocytosis (FEME)

Another pathway for rapid endocytosis of specific transmembrane receptors has been described (Boucrot et al. 2015). This pathway involves the uptake of ligand-receptors and plays an important role for growth factor signaling and cell migration, including G-protein-coupled receptors (β_1-adrenergic dopaminergic and acetylcholine receptors), the IL-2 receptor and growth factors like EGFR, or the hepatocyte growth factor receptor (HGFR). FEME depends on the pre-enrichment of endophilin localized to the leading edge of migrating cells through its SH3 domain which interacts with the membrane receptors described above, stabilizing them and leading to the formation of tubular carriers. Despite being clathrin-independent, FEME is a dynamin-dependent pathway (Boucrot et al. 2015; Rennick, Johnston, and Parton 2021).

11.3.4 Clathrin-Independent/Dynamin-Independent Endocytosis (CLIC/GEEC)

Like FEME, this pathway occurs in the leading edge of migrating cells; however, it is dynamin-independent and is not dependent on a specific ligand-receptor interaction; instead it is a constitutive pathway. Nevertheless, this pathway exhibits a dependence on cholesterol and is involved in the uptake of the hyaluronic acid receptor CD44 and GPI-anchored proteins (GPI-AP) (Sathe et al. 2018; Thottacherry et al. 2018). Flotillin, and the GTPases ARF6, RAC1, and CDC42 lead to the actin-dependent formation of clathrin-independent carriers (CLIC), which further mature into GPI-AP-enriched endosomal compartments (GEEC), followed by the transfer to late endosomes and lysosomes, or to follow a route to the TGN or be recycled back to the membrane as in the other pathways (Howes et al. 2010; Doherty and McMahon 2009).

11.3.5 Macropinocytosis

Macropinocytosis is a clathrin-, caveolae-, and dynamin-independent transient mechanism of endocytosis which may initiate spontaneously or in response to growth factor stimulation. It is formed by the active extension of plasma membrane sheets succeeded by the enclosure of a large volume of the extracellular medium surrounding the cell (Swanson 2008; Kerr and Teasdale 2009; Saric and Freeman 2021).

11.4 STRATEGIES TO IMPROVE DELIVERY OF THERAPIES TO TARGETED CELLS

CME is very important for the development of new therapeutic strategies to overcome the plasma membrane in cancer cells, particularly targeting them via receptor-mediated endocytosis. In exploring these pathways, strategies using receptors that are commonly found overexpressed in the membrane of cancer cells or other cells from the tumor microenvironment have been followed, namely the transferrin receptor (TfR), folate receptor (FR), prostate specific membrane antigen (PSMA), glucose transporters (GLUT), EGFR, and epithelial cell adhesion molecule (Ep-CAM). The conjugation of drugs or drug carriers to ligands recognized by these membrane proteins can significantly increase the uptake of those therapeutics in cancer cells. A few examples are listed below; for more extensive reviews see (Zhang et al. 2019; Wang et al. 2020).

MBP-426 is a liposomal formulation loaded with oxaliplatin and conjugated to Tf. The presence of this ligand strongly promoted the internalization in Tf-overexpressing colon 26 cells both *in vitro* and *in vivo* where results evidenced a superior tumor suppression (Ishida et al. 2001; Suzuki et al. 2008; Wei et al. 2019). A formulation of immunoliposomes loaded with doxorubicin (DOX) functionalized with Fab fragments of the anti-EGFR monoclonal cetuximab has also been reported (anti-EGFR-IL-DOX) (Mamot et al. 2003, 2012). Compared to the formulations lacking the ligand, anti-EGFR-IL-DOX showed a 30-fold increase in cell internalization and a 29-fold increase in effectiveness. This formulation is now in phase II clinical trials in patients with advanced triple negative breast cancer that are positive for EGFR (NCT02833766). The Ep-CAM transmembrane glycoprotein has also been targeted with liposomes with the humanized single-chain Fv antibody fragment 4D5MOCB covalently linked, which increased the specific binding to tumor cells by 10–20-fold (Hussain et al. 2006). The A10 2'-fluoropyrimidine RNA aptamer recognizes specifically the extracellular domain of PSMA prostate cancer cells. This aptamer has been used to surface functionalize docetaxel-encapsulated nanoparticles exhibiting a 3.77-fold increase *in vivo* (Cheng et al. 2007). Another example is the Arg-Gly-Asp (RGD) peptide which has high affinity for the αv-β3 integrin. To overcome the limited intracellular uptake of naked siRNA therapeutics, Schifflers et al. (2003) prepared self-assembled nanoparticles with RGD ligands and improved cellular uptake by six- to eight-fold. In addition, they proved that RGD was truly responsible through a competition assay with free RGD peptide which abrogated the nanoparticles' uptake (Schiffelers et al. 2003, 2004).

In addition to membrane receptors, transporters in the plasma membrane are also being used to deliver therapeutics. To satisfy the nutrient demands of cancer cells, many transporters are up-regulated, thus providing an opportunity to target these cells with the advantage that most transporters are substrate specific and have a site-specific expression in different tissues which also provides selectivity. The conjugation of L-carnitine to PLGA nanoparticles targets the OCTN2 and ATB$^{0,+}$ transporters in Caco-2 cells where these transporters are up-regulated. The uptake was mediated by clathrin- and caveolae-dependent endocytosis (Kou et al. 2017a, b). As well, PLGA nanoparticles decorated with glutamate targeted LAT-1-expressing tumor cells better than undecorated nanoparticles (Li et al. 2017). In addition, membrane transporters also play a very important role in controlling the efflux of substances to the brain. Selective transporters are expressed in the endothelial cells that compose the blood–brain barrier (BBB), such as OCTN2, LAT1, and ChT1. L-carnitine conjugated PLGA nanoparticles targeting OCTN2 also demonstrated an enhanced uptake in hCMEC/DE3 endothelial cells and in T98G glioma cell line (Kou et al. 2018). In C6 glioma cells, LAT1-targeting liposomes conjugated to glutamate and loaded with docetaxel (DTX-TGL) also exhibited an enhanced penetration through the BBB to target the brain cancer cells (Li et al. 2016).

11.5 CELLULAR UPTAKE MEDIATED BY AZURIN/P28

Azurin (128 amino acids, 14 kDa) originating from the bacterium *Pseudomonas aeruginosa* was found to penetrate cancer cells and exert an anticancer activity (Yamada et al. 2002; Punj et al. 2004; Yamada et al. 2004). The first evidence for its anticancer role relied on its ability to enter cells and induce apoptosis in murine J774 macrophages, melanoma, and breast cancer cells through stabilizing the anticancer protein p53 (Punj et al. 2004; Yamada et al. 2004). The uptake of azurin into cells was proven to be temperature-dependent, as it was inhibited at 4°C, and to enter preferentially into cancer cells compared to the normal counterparts. Studies with chemical inhibitors associated with the endocytic pathways described above evidenced that azurin would enter the cells by a mechanism mediated, at least in part, by a receptor-mediated endocytic pathway (Yamada et al. 2005).

A fragment of the protein was identified as the main mediator for the protein uptake, composed of residues 50 to 77, and termed p28. Using a series of truncated constructions of azurin fused to glutathione-S-transferase (GST) or the green fluorescent protein (GFP), Yamada et al. (2005) revealed the capacity of this fragment to act as a vehicle to transport other proteins not capable of entering the cell by themselves, thus acting as a protein transduction domain (PTD). The peptide p28 contains the α-helical structure of azurin as well as a partial β-sheet structure (Yamada et al. 2005).

In relation to normal cells, the content of p28 in cancer cells was found to be about three- to six-fold higher (Taylor et al. 2009). However, the true nature of the mechanism for uptake of p28 into cells is still not completely understood. Contrarily to the cationic CPP, p28 uptake is not dependent on the interaction with negatively charged membrane bound glycosaminoglycans nor does it induce a disruption of the plasma membrane integrity. Moreover, mucin-type O-glycosylation which is frequently encountered differentially expressed in cancer cells was not involved in the entry of p28. However, the same was not true for N-glycosylation (Taylor et al. 2009).

11.5.1 Mechanistic Insight on Azurin/p28 Uptake

Taylor and colleagues (2009) investigated deeply the possible endocytic mechanisms using a combination of chemical inhibitors and co-localization with protein markers by immunocytochemistry.

As observed for azurin, taking into consideration that it is temperature-dependent and a saturable process, it is assumed that it depends, at least in part, on the recognition by a membrane receptor protein, which, however, is still not identified. Further, by looking carefully at the amphipathic structure of p28, they identified the minimal motif comprising the N-terminal 18 residues of the peptide (p18) as controlling the uptake, while the C-terminal 10 residues were more associated with its cytotoxicity once within the cells. The kinetics of both p28 and p18 entry into melanoma cells suggested that p18 would enter the cells about 40% faster than p28; however p28 seemed to accumulate more in the membrane of the cells and higher intensity values for total fluorescence intensity could be observed. The higher V_{max} of p18 in entering the cells, compared to p28, led Taylor et al. to suggest that it might define an amphipathic structure when associated with membrane phospholipids and resemble more the PTD of azurin.

Regarding the mechanism for uptake, neither p28 nor p18 uptake was impaired by chlorpromazine (CPZ) or amiloride which excludes a clathrin-mediated endocytic process or micropinocytosis for these peptides. The depletion of cholesterol with β-mehtylcyclodextran, filipin, or nystatin to disrupt lipid rafts from the membrane and nocodazole which prevents caveolae transport significantly inhibited the penetration of both p18 and p28 (~50 and 60%, respectively) and its co-localization with caveolin-1 upon uptake suggested the involvement of caveolae-mediated endocytic routes (Taylor et al. 2009), which has been observed in cancer cells, but also in endothelial cells (HUVEC) and non-cancer cells like fibroblasts (Yamada et al. 2005; Mehta et al. 2011). However, the lack of effect of wortmannin or staurosporine also suggests that both early endosome formation and dynamin might not play an important role in their endocytosis. Additionally, not all the uptake seems to be dependent on an energy-dependent endocytic process since sodium azide and ouabain (Na^+K^+ ATPase inhibitor) could also inhibit the entry of both p18 and p28 into cancer and non-cancer cells (Taylor et al. 2009).

In our group, using a high-throughput molecular profiling of how an aggressive model of breast cancer responded to azurin, we found that azurin up-regulated apoptosis in the breast cancer cells, but also endocytosis, membrane reorganization, and vesicle-mediate transport. In contrast, genes associated with several cell surface membrane receptors, signal transduction, and biological adhesion were amongst the more down-regulated classes of genes (Bernardes et al. 2014). We also found that azurin and p28 may initiate their action in cancer cells by interacting with lipid raft components, i.e., the ganglioside GM1 leading to its cellular internalization and that silencing of caveolin-1 impaired azurin entry, increasing membrane fluidity and cells' sensitivity to anti-cancer drugs (Bernardes et al. 2016, 2018).

Thus, from these studies, it was suggested that azurin, p18, and p28 might enter the cells through a receptor-mediated mechanism, likely to be localized within caveolae and probably harboring an aberrant N-glycosylation, and were internalized moving to the Golgi, endoplasmic reticulum, and eventually the nucleus, but also through a clathrin-caveolae-independent pathway like CLIC/GEEC referred to above.

11.5.2 Anti-Cancer Activity of Azurin/p28

The higher accumulation of p28 in cancer cells suggests that this peptide could serve as a novel chemotherapeutic, an adjuvant to other drugs, or even as a CPP to transport cargos to accumulate preferentially in cancer cells. Indeed, azurin and p28 have been extensively studied regarding their anti-cancer activities that are not only related to their ability to induce apoptosis through p53. We have demonstrated that azurin has a strong impact on several membrane proteins related to adhesion and receptor-mediated signaling. In breast cancer cells, azurin down-regulates the cell-cell adhesion protein P-cadherin but not the tumor-suppressor E-cadherin, which consequently down-regulates signaling pathways dependent on P-cadherin expression for increased tumor progression and invasion through Matrigel (Bernardes et al. 2013). In lung cancer cells, pre-treating the cells with azurin could also impair the proper EGFR signaling triggered by the natural ligand EGF, relating the changes caused by azurin in the membrane organization with its functional impact on tumor progression (Bernardes et al. 2016). In both models, we could also observe an impact on the protein levels of several integrin subunits, key membrane proteins in the adhesion and migration of tumor cells, which can also be related to the extensive membrane remodeling caused by the azurin/p28 entry in cancer cells. In fact, through atomic force microscopy (AFM), we characterized lung cancer cells treated with azurin and could observe a reduction in the Young's modulus of the plasma membrane after exposition (Bernardes et al. 2016). Overall, we identified the changes in the membrane physiology as another anti-cancer trait of azurin with functional consequences at invasion, capable of attenuating multiple tumorigenic signaling pathways, and improving the response of cancer cells to multiple anti-cancer drugs (Bernardes et al. 2016, 2018). In addition, Yamada et al. (2016) also related p28 with an increase in the sensitivity of cancer cells to multiple chemotherapeutic drugs facilitated through the p53/p21/CDK2 pathway (Yamada, Das Gupta, and Beattie 2016). Thus, there appears to be a role for azurin/p28 in maximizing the activity of chemotherapeutic agents while reducing the side effects related to dose-related toxicity.

The p28 peptide (28 aa) has already completed two phase I clinical trials in cancer patients. In either adult multiple grade IV or pediatric brain tumor patients, p28 induced disease stabilization or even tumor regression while showing no significant toxicity (Warso et al. 2013; Lulla et al. 2016). Thus, FDA granted azurin-p28 the designation as an orphan drug for the treatment of brain tumor glioma.

The C-terminal region of azurin (residues 96-112) was also found to target the ephrin receptors in prostate cancer cells and to inhibit significantly tumor progression by interfering with this proliferative signaling pathway (Chaudhari et al. 2007). Later, this region of the protein was also used as a scaffold to search for small analogues that bind to the ephrin receptors EphA2, EphB2, and EpahB4 (Micewicz et al. 2011). One of those peptides consisting of a linear 15 residues peptide (AzV36) was then conjugated with nicotinic acid forming AzV36-NicL and tested for its ability to radiosensitize Lewis lung carcinoma cells (LCC), significantly increasing the efficacy of radiotherapy *in vivo* compared to each agent alone.

11.5.3 p28 as a Transporter Agent

Related to their enhanced ability to enter in cancer cells, both azurin and p28 have been used as cancer-targeted carriers of several therapies. A fusion of p28 with the HPV16 E7 oncoprotein allowed an effective and controlled delivery to cancer cells both *in vitro* and *in vivo*. The complex elicited a strong immune Th1 cellular response with high levels of interferon-gamma (IFN-γ) and granzyme B secreted which promoted a complete tumor-free maintenance for >60 days (Shahbazi and Bolhassani 2018). p28 has also been combined with the NRC peptide which is an antimicrobial peptide that also displays anti-tumor activity mainly through mitochondrial membrane damage. The fusion of these peptides demonstrated selectivity towards cancer cells with a significant increase in the expression of pro-apoptotic genes by both mitochondria caspase-dependent and -independent pathways (Soleimani et al. 2016). Another protein that induces apoptosis, apoptin, has been linked to p28 by means of a furin cleavage site. The linker could then be cleaved by furin which is present within the tumor microenvironment. The fusion protein increased the activity of apoption when compared to its single administration in breast cancer cells, reinforcing the synergistic potential between the two agents (Noei, Nili-Ahmadabadi, and Soleimani 2019). p28 has also been fused to a photosensitizer domain (EcFbFP) derived from a bacterial blue-light receptor belonging to the family of light-oxygen-voltage proteins, creating azulitox. Upon excitation with blue light, azulitox significantly induced cytotoxicity compared to EcFbFP alone, causing the death of about 90% of the cells correlating directly to the amount of intracellular ROS in lung cancer cells. This study opens new avenues for the study of photosensitizer-based photodynamic therapies with the cell targeting mediated by p28, that may contribute to the reduction in the systemic toxicity observed with other photosensitizers (Raber et al. 2020).

Table 11.1 summarizes the studies where azurin/p28 have been used in combination with chemotherapeutics or biological therapies and the phase I clinical trials where p28 has been studied.

TABLE 11.1 Summary of Combinatorial Treatments with Azurin/p28

PROTEIN/ PEPTIDE	DRUG (CHEMOTHERAPEUTIC/ BIOLOGICAL)	TARGETED PATHWAY/CELL MODEL	REFERENCE
AzV36 (derived from the C-terminal region of azurin)	nicotinic acid (for radiosensitization)	Eph receptor signaling; Lewis lung carcinoma (LCC)	(Micewicz et al. 2011)
p28	n.a.	Multiple solid tumors in adult patients, phase I clinical trial	(Warso et al. 2013)
Azurin	Tyrosine kinase inhibitors (gefitinib, erlotinib)	EGFR signaling; A549 lung cancer cells	(Bernardes et al. 2016)
p28	DNA damaging (doxorubicin, dacarbazine, temozolomide) and antimitotic drugs (paclitaxel and docetaxel)	p53/p21/CDK2 pathway; multiple cancer models	(Yamada, Das Gupta, and Beattie 2016)
p28	n.a.	Non-HDM2-mediated inhibition of p53; pediatric patients with recurrent or progressive central nervous system tumors	(Lulla et al. 2016)
Azurin	DNA damaging (doxorubicin) and antimitotic drug (paclitaxel)	Lipid-raft mediated plasma membrane order; MCF-7 breast cancer cells, HeLa cervical cancer cells, HT-29 colon cancer cells	(Bernardes et al. 2018)
p28	HPV16 E7 antigen	Th1 cellular immune response with increase IFN-γ and granzyme B secretion; CRL-2785 from primary murine lung epithelial cells by co-transformation with HPV16 E6 and E7 and ras oncogenes	(Shahbazi and Bolhassani 2018)
p28	NRC antimicrobial peptide	Apoptosis; breast cancer cell lines	(Noei, Nili-Ahmadabadi, and Soleimani 2019)
p28	Apoptin	Apoptosis; breast cancer cells	(Noei, Nili-Ahmadabadi, and Soleimani 2019)
p28	Photosensitizer EcFbFP	Production of reactive oxygen species (ROS); breast cancer cells	(Raber et al. 2020)

n.a. – not applicable.

11.6 CONCLUSIONS AND FUTURE PERSPECTIVES

The plasma membrane represents a major biological barrier that needs to be crossed efficiently to promote drug bioavailability and efficacy. As we discussed above, several strategies have been explored to increase the efficiency of drugs or nanocarriers either by using pro-drugs with higher lipophilicity, by exploring membrane transporters or receptors to improve cell uptake through ligand-receptor interactions, or by resorting to natural agents with improved capacity to cross the membrane of diseased cells compared to normal cells. However, the increased level of crosstalk between different pathways still requires a more comprehensive understanding of cellular entry and intracellular trafficking for improved design of targeted delivery strategies to harness the biological mechanisms for more efficient delivery. Importantly, an issue not fully addressed here is the endosomal escape that may represent an additional barrier after cellular uptake against the delivery of biomacromolecules or nanocarriers.

Most of the knowledge regarding the mechanism for the uptake of a given molecule or carrier has been obtained with pharmacological inhibition of the endocytic pathways in cell lines. However, it is necessary to keep in mind that most endocytosis inhibitors target more than one pathway, which may introduce a bias in the interpretation of the results. A combination with data obtained by RNA interference or genetic knockdowns of relevant key protein players in each pathway will certainly help in advancing our knowledge of the intricate nature of the pathways. Additionally, the use of fluorescent reporters in fusion with such proteins combined with current super-resolution microscopy technologies and advanced data analysis will certainly help to achieve a visual confirmation of the interactions of endocytosed materials and specific endosome/organelle markers. As well, *in vitro* studies may not reflect entirely the complex nature of endocytosis that occurs *in vivo*. Thus, the use of more relevant cellular models such as organoids and/or patient-derived cells that can be manipulated in vitro may help in filling in the gap between *in vitro* and *in vivo* to improve the efficacy of newly developed therapeutic delivery strategies.

Finally, azurin and its derived peptide p28 may represent a new interesting and distinctive strategy for the development of a new generation of drug carriers with preference to cancer cells. The impact already demonstrated in remodeling the plasma membrane and its influence in endocytosis appears to confirm the interest in these agents. Their ability to increase the efficiency of several chemotherapeutics and biomolecules has been demonstrated by different research groups and across a wide range of cellular panels which contributes to the excitement around their possible use in more advanced drug delivery systems. However, no receptor has been identified yet which might help to further stratify the patients that would benefit the most from such strategies. With the advances observed in the personalized medicine field, understanding the distinct endocytosis pathway(s) utilized by each carrier and the proteins involved would certainly help in defining the clinical biomarkers to offer each patient the delivery strategy that they would benefit the most , thus improving greatly the clinical success of each therapy.

ACKNOWLEDGMENTS

The studies with azurin/p28 realized in our laboratory at the Institute for Bioengineering and Biosciences were financed by the scientific project PTDC/BTM-SAL/30034/2017_LISBOA-01-0145-FEDER-03003 4. Funding received by iBB from the Portuguese Science and Technology Foundation (FCT) (UID/BIO/04565/2020) and the project LA/P/0140/2020 of the Associate Laboratory Institute for Health and Bioeconomy - i4HB.

REFERENCES

Bernardes, Nuno, and Arsenio M. Fialho. "Perturbing the Dynamics and Organization of Cell Membrane Components: A New Paradigm for Cancer-Targeted Therapies." *International Journal of Molecular Sciences* 19, no. 12 (2018). doi:10.3390/ijms19123871.

Bernardes, Nuno, Ana Sofia Ribeiro, Sofia Abreu, Bruna Mota, Rute G. Matos, Cecilia M. Arraiano, Raquel Seruca, Joana Paredes, and Arsenio M. Fialho. "The Bacterial Protein Azurin Impairs Invasion and FAK/Src Signaling in P-Cadherin-Overexpressing Breast Cancer Cell Models." *PLOS ONE* 8, no. 7 (2013). doi:10.1371/journal.pone.0069023.

Bernardes, Nuno, Ana Sofia Ribeiro, Sofia Abreu, André F. Vieira, Laura Carreto, Manuel Santos, Raquel Seruca, Joana Paredes, and Arsenio M. Fialho. "High-Throughput Molecular Profiling of a P-Cadherin Overexpressing Breast Cancer Model Reveals New Targets for the Anti-Cancer Bacterial Protein Azurin." *International Journal of Biochemistry & Cell Biology* 50, no. 1 (2014): 1–9. doi:10.1016/j.biocel.2014.01.023.

Bernardes, Nuno, Sofia Abreu, Filomena A. Carvalho, Fábio Fernandes, Nuno C. Santos, and Arsénio M. Fialho. "Modulation of Membrane Properties of Lung Cancer Cells by Azurin Enhances the Sensitivity to EGFR-Targeted Therapy and Decreased B1 Integrin-Mediated Adhesion." *Cell Cycle* 15, no. 11 (2016): 1415–24. doi:10.1080/15384101.2016.1172147.

Bernardes, Nuno, Ana Rita Garizo, Sandra N. Pinto, Bernardo Caniço, Catarina Perdigão, Fábio Fernandes, and Arsenio M. Fialho. "Azurin Interaction with the Lipid Raft Components Ganglioside GM-1 and Caveolin-1 Increases Membrane Fluidity and Sensitivity to Anti-Cancer Drugs." *Cell Cycle* 17, no. 13 (2018): 1649–66. doi:10.1080/15384101.2018.1489178.

Boucrot, Emmanuel, Antonio P. Ferreira, Leonardo Almeida-Souza, Sylvain Debard, Yvonne Vallis, Gillian Howard, Laetitia Bertot, Nathalie Sauvonnet, and Harvey T. McMahon. "Endophilin Marks and Controls a Clathrin-Independent Endocytic Pathway." *Nature* 517, no. 7535 (2015): 460–65. doi:10.1038/nature14067.

Brown, C. M., and N. O. Petersen. "Free Clathrin Triskelions Are Required for the Stability of Clathrin-Associated Adaptor Protein (AP-2) Coated Pit Nucleation Sites." *Biochemistry & Cell Biology* 77, no. 5 (1999): 439–48.

Chaudhari, Anita, Magdy Mahfouz, Arsenio M. Fialho, Tohru Yamada, Ana Teresa Granja, Yonghua Zhu, Wataru Hashimoto, B. Schlarb-Ridley, W. Cho, T. K. Das Gupta, and A. M. Chakrabarty. "Cupredoxin-Cancer Interrelationship: Azurin Binding with EphB2, Interference in EphB2 Tyrosine Phosphorylation, and Inhibition of Cancer Growth." *Biochemistry* 46, no. 7 (2007): 1799–810. doi:10.1021/bi061661x.

Cheng, Jianjun, Benjamin A. Teply, Ines Sherifi, Josephine Sung, Gaurav Luther, Frank X. Gu, Etgar Levy-Nissenbaum, Aleksandar F. Radovic-Moreno, Robert Langer, and Omid C. Farokhzad. "Formulation of Functionalized PLGA-PEG Nanoparticles for In Vivo Targeted Drug Delivery." *Biomaterials* 28, no. 5 (2007): 869–76. doi:10.1016/j.biomaterials.2006.09.047.

Doherty, Gary J., and Harvey T. McMahon. "Mechanisms of Endocytosis." *Annual Review of Biochemistry* 78 (2009): 857–902. doi:10.1146/annurev.biochem.78.081307.110540.

Ehrlich, Marcelo, Werner Boll, Antoine Van Oijen, Ramesh Hariharan, Kartik Chandran, Max L. Nibert, and Tomas Kirchhausen. "Endocytosis by Random Initiation and Stabilization of Clathrin-Coated Pits." *Cell* 118, no. 5 (2004): 591–605. doi:10.1016/j.cell.2004.08.017.

Howes, Mark T., Matthew Kirkham, James Riches, Katia Cortese, Piers J. Walser, Fiona Simpson, Michelle M. Hill, A. Jones, R. Lundmark, M. R. Lindsay, D. J. Hernandez-Deviez, G. Hadzic, A. McCluskey, R. Bashir, L. Liu, P. Pilch, H. McMahon, P. J. Robinson, J. F. Hancock, S. Mayor, and R. G. Parton. "Clathrin-Independent Carriers Form a High Capacity Endocytic Sorting System at the Leading Edge of Migrating Cells." *Journal of Cell Biology* 190, no. 4 (2010): 675–91. doi:10.1083/jcb.201002119.

Hussain, Sajid, Andreas Plückthun, Theresa M. Allen, and Uwe Zangemeister-Wittke. "Chemosensitization of Carcinoma Cells Using Epithelial Cell Adhesion Molecule-Targeted Liposomal Antisense Against Bcl-2/Bcl-XL." *Molecular Cancer Therapeutics* 5, no. 12 (2006): 3170–80. doi:10.1158/1535-7163.MCT-06-0412.

Ishida, O., K. Maruyama, H. Tanahashi, M. Iwatsuru, K. Sasaki, M. Eriguchi, and H. Yanagie. "Liposomes Bearing Polyethyleneglycol-Coupled Transferrin with Intracellular Targeting Property to the Solid Tumors In Vivo." *Pharmaceutical Research* 18, no. 7 (2001): 1042–48. doi:10.1023/a:1010960900254.

Jacobson, Ken, Ole G. Mouritsen, and Richard G. W. Anderson. "Lipid Rafts: At a Crossroad Between Cell Biology and Physics." *Nature Cell Biology* 9, no. 1 (2007): 7–14. doi:10.1038/ncb0107-7.

Kerr, Markus C., and Rohan D. Teasdale. "Defining Macropinocytosis." *Traffic* 10, no. 4 (2009): 364–71. doi:10.1111/j.1600-0854.2009.00878.x.

Khan, Imran, and Patricia S. Steeg. "Endocytosis: A Pivotal Pathway for Regulating Metastasis." *British Journal of Cancer* 124, no. 1 (2021): 66–75. doi:10.1038/s41416-020-01179-8.

Kou, Longfa, Qing Yao, Mengchi Sun, Chunnuan Wu, Jia Wang, Qiuhua Luo, Gang Wang, Y. Du, Q. Fu, J. Wang, Z. He, V. Ganapathy, and J. Sun. "Cotransporting Ion Is a Trigger for Cellular Endocytosis of Transporter-Targeting Nanoparticles: A Case Study of High-Efficiency SLC22A5 (OCTN2)-Mediated Carnitine-Conjugated Nanoparticles for Oral Delivery of Therapeutic Drugs." *Advanced Healthcare Materials* 6, no. 17 (2017a). doi:10.1002/adhm.201700165.

Kou, Longfa, Qing Yao, Sathish Sivaprakasam, Qiuhua Luo, Yinghua Sun, Qiang Fu, Zhonggui He, Jin Sun, and Vadivel Ganapathy. "Dual Targeting of L-Carnitine-Conjugated Nanoparticles to OCTN2 and ATB(0,+) to Deliver Chemotherapeutic Agents for Colon Cancer Therapy." *Drug Delivery* 24, no. 1 (2017b): 1338–49. doi:10.1080/10717544.2017.1377316.

Kou, Longfa, Yanxian Hou, Qing Yao, Weiling Guo, Gang Wang, Menglin Wang, Qiang Fu, Zhonggui He, Vadivel Ganapathy, and Jin Sun. "L-Carnitine-Conjugated Nanoparticles to Promote Permeation Across Blood-Brain

Barrier and to Target Glioma Cel ls for Drug Delivery via the Novel Organic Cation/Carnitine Transporter OCTN2." *Artificial Cells, Nanomedic ine, & Biotechnology* 46, no. 8 (2018): 1605–16. doi:10.1080/21691401 .2017.1384385.

Li, Lin, Xingsheng Di, Shenwu Zhang, Qiming Kan, Hao Liu, Tianshu Lu, Yongjun Wang, Qiang Fu, Jin Sun, and Zhonggui He. "Large Amino Acid Transporter 1 Mediated Glutamate Modified Docetaxel-Loaded Liposomes for Glioma Targeting." *Colloids & Surfaces, Part B* 141, no. May (2016): 260–67. doi:10.1016/j. colsurfb.2016.01.041.

Li, Lin, Xingsheng Di, Mingrui Wu, Zhisu Sun, Lu Zhong, Yongjun Wang, Qiang Fu, Qiming Kan, Jin Sun, and Zhonggui He. "Targeting Tumor Highly-Expressed LAT1 Transporter with Amino Acid-Modified Nanoparticles: Toward a Novel Active Targeting Strategy in Breast Cancer Therapy." *Nanomedicine : Nanotechnology, Biology, & Medicine* 13, no. 3 (2017): 987–98. doi:10.1016/j.nano.2016.11.012.

Lulla, Rishi R., Stewart Goldman, Tohru Yamada, Craig W. Beattie, Linda Bressler, Michael Pacini, Ian F. Pollack, P. G. Fisher, R. J. Packer, I. J. Dunkel, G. Dhall, S. Wu, A. Onar, J. M. Boyett, and M. Fouladi. "Phase i Trial of P28 (NSC745104), a Non-HDM2-Mediated Peptide Inhibitor of P53 Ubiquitination in Pediatric Patients with Recurrent or Progressive Central Nervous System Tumors: A Pediatric Brain Tumor Consortium Study." *Neuro-Oncology* 18, no. 9 (2016): 1319–25. doi:10.1093/neuonc/now047.

Mamot, Christoph, Daryl C. Drummond, Udo Greiser, Keelung Hong, Dmitri B. Kirpotin, James D. Marks, and John W. Park. "Epidermal Growth Factor Receptor (EGFR)-Targeted Immunoliposomes Mediate Specific and Efficient Drug Delivery to EGFR- and EGFRvIII-Overexpressing Tumor Cells." *Cancer Research* 63, no. 12 (2003): 3154–61.

Mamot, Christoph, Reto Ritschard, Andreas Wicki, Willy Küng, Jan Schuller, Richard Herrmann, and Christoph Rochlitz. "Immunoliposomal Delivery of Doxorubicin Can Overcome Multidrug Resistance Mechanisms in EGFR-Overexpressing Tumor Cells." *Journal of Drug Targeting* 20, no. 5 (2012): 422–32. doi:10.3109/10611 86X.2012.680960.

Manzanares, Darío, and Valentín Ceña. "Endocytosis: The Nanoparticle and Submicron Nanocompounds Gateway into the Cell." *Pharmaceutics* 12, no. 4 (2020): 1–22. doi:10.3390/pharmaceutics12040371.

Mehta, Rajeshwari R., Tohru Yamada, Brad N. Taylor, Konstantin Christov, Marissa L. King, Dibyen Majumdar, Fatima Lekmine, C. Tiruppathi, A. Shilkaitis, L. Bratescu, A. Green, C. W. Beattie, and T. K. Das Gupta. "A Cell Penetrating Peptide Derived from Azurin Inhibits Angiogenesis and Tumor Growth by Inhibiting Phosphorylation of VEGFR-2, FAK and Akt." *Angiogenesis* 14, no. 3 (2011): 355–69. doi:10.1007/ s10456-011-9220-6.

Micewicz, Ewa D., Chun-Ling Jung, Dorthe Schaue, Hai Luong, William H. McBride, and Piotr Ruchala. "Small Azurin Derived Peptide Targets Ephrin Receptors for Radiotherapy." *International Journal of Peptide Research & Therapeutics* 17, no. 3 (2011): 247. doi:10.1007/s10989-011-9265-9.

Nicolson, Garth L. "The Fluid–Mosaic Model of Membrane Structure: Still Relevant to Understanding the Structure, Function and Dynamics of Biological Membranes After More Than 40 Years." *Biochimica & Biophysica Acta (BBA): Reviews on Biomembranes* 1838, no. 6 (2014): 1451–66. doi:10.1016/j.bbamem.2013.10.019.

Noei, Ahmad, Amir Nili-Ahmadabadi, and Meysam Soleimani. "The Enhanced Cytotoxic Effects of the P28-Apoptin Chimeric Protein as A Novel Anti-Cancer Agent on Breast Cancer Cell Lines." *Drug Research* 69, no. 3 (2019): 144–50. doi:10.1055/a-0654-4952.

Parton, Robert G., and Kai Simons. "The Multiple Faces of Caveolae." *Nature Reviews. Molecular Cell Biology* 8, no. 3 (2007): 185–94. doi:10.1038/nrm2122.

Punj, Vasu, Suchita Bhattacharyya, Djenann Saint-Dic, Chenthamarakshan Vasu, Elizabeth A. Cunningham, Jewell Graves, Tohru Yamada, A. I. Constantinou, K. Christov, B. White, G. Li, D. Majumdar, A. M. Chakrabarty, and T. K. Das Gupta. "Bacterial Cupredoxin Azurin as an Inducer of Apoptosis and Regression in Human Breast Cancer." *Oncogene* 23, no. 13 (2004): 2367–78. doi:10.1038/sj.onc.1207376.

Raber, Heinz Fabian, Thomas Heerde, Suzanne Nour El Din, Carolin Flaig, Fabienne Hilgers, Nora Bitzenhofer, Karl Erich Jäger, T. Drepper, K. E. Gottschalk, N. E. Bodenberger, T. Weil, D. H. Kubiczek, and F. Rosenau. "Azulitox-A Pseudomonas aeruginosa P28-Derived Cancer-Cell-Specific Protein Photosensitizer." *Biomacromolecules* 21, no. 12 (2020): 5067–76. doi:10.1021/acs.biomac.0c01216.

Ran, Sophia, Jason H. Stafford, and Philip E. Thorpe. "Increased Exposure of Phosphatidylethanolamine on the Surface of Tumor Blood Vessels." *Cancer Research* 62, no. 4 (2002): 6132–40. https://www.ncbi.nlm.nih.gov /pubmed/12414638.

Rennick, Joshua J., Angus P. R. Johnston, and Robert G. Parton. "Key Principles and Methods for Studying the Endocytosis of Biological and Nanoparticle Therapeutics." *Nature Nanotechnology* 16, no. 3 (2021): 266–76. doi:10.1038/s41565-021-00858-8.

Rothberg, K. G., J. E. Heuser, W. C. Donzell, Y. S. Ying, J. R. Glenney, and R. G. Anderson. "Caveolin, a Protein Component of Caveolae Membrane Coats." *Cell* 68, no. 4 (1992): 673–82. doi:10.1016/0092-8674(92)90143-z.

Saric, Amra, and Spencer A. Freeman. "Endomembrane Tension and Trafficking." *Frontiers in Cell & Developmental Biology* 8, no. Jan. (2021): 1–19. doi:10.3389/fcell.2020.611326.

Sathe, Mugdha, Gayatri Muthukrishnan, James Rae, Andrea Disanza, Mukund Thattai, Giorgio Scita, Robert G. Parton, and Satyajit Mayor. "Small GTPases and BAR Domain ProteinS Regulate Branched Actin Polymerisation for Clathrin and Dynamin-Independent Endocytosis." *Nature Communications* 9, no. 1 (2018): 1835. doi:10.1038/s41467-018-03955-w.

Schiffelers, Raymond M., Gerben A. Koning, Timo L. M. ten Hagen, Marcel H. A. M. Fens, Astrid J. Schraa, P. C. Adriënne, A. Janssen, Robbert J. Kok, Grietje Molema, and Gert Storm. "Anti-Tumor Efficacy of Tumor Vasculature-Targeted Liposomal Doxorubicin." *Journal of Controlled Release* 91, no. 1–2 (2003): 115–22. doi:10.1016/s0168-3659(03)00240-2.

Schiffelers, Raymond M., Aslam Ansari, Jun Xu, Qin Zhou, Qingquan Tang, Gert Storm, Grietje Molema, Patrick Y. Lu, Puthupparampil V. Scaria, and Martin C. Woodle. "Cancer SiRNA Therapy by Tumor Selective Delivery with Ligand-Targeted Sterically Stabilized Nanoparticle." *Nucleic Acids Research* 32, no. 19 (2004): e149. doi:10.1093/nar/gnh140.

Shahbazi, Sepideh, and Azam Bolhassani. "Comparison of Six Cell Penetrating Peptides with Different Properties for In Vitro and In Vivo Delivery of HPV16 E7 Antigen in Therapeutic Vaccines." *International Immunopharmacology* 62, no. Sept. (2018): 170–80. doi:10.1016/j.intimp.2018.07.006.

Shevchenko, Andrej, and Kai Simons. "Lipidomics: Coming to Grips with Lipid Diversity." *Nature Reviews. Molecular Cell Biology* 11, no. 8 (2010): 593–98. doi:10.1038/nrm2934.

Soleimani, Meysam, Hamid Mirmohammad-Sadeghi, Hojjat Sadeghi-Aliabadi, and Ali Jahanian-Najafabadi. "Expression and Purification of Toxic Anti-Breast Cancer P28-NRC Chimeric Protein." *Advanced Biomedical Research* 5 (2016): 70. doi:10.4103/2277-9175.180639.

Stafford, Jason H., and Philip E. Thorpe. "Increased Exposure of Phosphatidylethanolamine on the Surface of Tumor Vascular Endothelium." *Neoplasia* 13, no. 4 (2011): 299–308. doi:10.1593/neo.101366.

Suzuki, Ryo, Tomoko Takizawa, Yasuhiro Kuwata, Mahito Mutoh, Nobuyuki Ishiguro, Naoki Utoguchi, Atsuko Shinohara, Masazumi Eriguchi, Hironobu Yanagie, and Kazuo Maruyama. "Effective Anti-Tumor Activity of Oxaliplatin Encapsulated in Transferrin-PEG-Liposome." *International Journal of Pharmaceutics* 346, no. 1–2 (2008): 143–50. doi:10.1016/j.ijpharm.2007.06.010.

Swanson, Joel A. "Shaping Cups into Phagosomes and Macropinosomes." *Nature Reviews. Molecular Cell Biology* 9, no. 8 (2008): 639–49. doi:10.1038/nrm2447.

Taylor, Brad N., Rajeshwari R. Mehta, Tohru Yamada, Fatima Lekmine, Konstantin Christov, Ananda M. Chakrabarty, Albert Green, L. Bratescu, A. Shilkaitis, C. W. Beattie, and T. K. Das Gupta. "Noncationic Peptides Obtained from Azurin Preferentially Enter Cancer Cells." *Cancer Research* 69, no. 2 (2009): 537–46. doi:10.1158/0008-5472.CAN-08-2932.

Thottacherry, Joseph Jose, Anita Joanna Kosmalska, Amit Kumar, Amit Singh Vishen, Alberto Elosegui-Artola, Susav Pradhan, Sumit Sharma, P. P. Singh, M. C. Guadamillas, N. Chaudhary, R. Vishwakarma, X. Trepat, M. A. Del Pozo, R. G. Parton, M. Rao, P. Pullarkat, P. Roca-Cusachs, and S. Mayor. "Mechanochemical Feedback Control of Dynamin Independent Endocytosis Modulates Membrane Tension in Adherent Cells." *Nature Communications* 9, no. 1 (2018): 4217. doi:10.1038/s41467-018-06738-5.

Wang, Xiaowei, Qiu Yuhan, Mengyan Wang, Conghui Zhang, Tianshu Zhang, Huimin Zhou, Wenxia Zhao, Wuli Zhao, Guimin Xia, and Rongguang Shao. "Endocytosis and Organelle Targeting of Nanomedicines in Cancer Therapy." *International Journal of Nanomedicine* 15 (2020): 9447–67. doi:10.2147/IJN.S274289.

Warso, M. A., J. M. Richards, D. Mehta, K. Christov, C. Schaeffer, L. Rae Bressler, T. Yamada, D. Majumdar, S. A. Kennedy, C. W. Beattie, and T. K. Das Gupta. "A First-in-Class, First-In-human, Phase i Trial of P28, a Non-HDM2-Mediated Peptide Inhibitor of P53 Ubiquitination in Patients with Advanced Solid Tumours." *British Journal of Cancer* 108, no. 5 (2013): 1061–70. doi:10.1038/bjc.2013.74.

Wei, Yaohua, Xiaolei Gu, Liang Cheng, Fenghua Meng, Gert Storm, and Zhiyuan Zhong. "Low-Toxicity Transferrin-Guided Polymersomal Doxorubicin for Potent Chemotherapy of Orthotopic Hepatocellular Carcinoma In Vivo." *Acta Biomaterialia* 92, no. Jul. (2019): 196–204. doi:10.1016/j.actbio.2019.05.034.

Yamada, Tohru, Masatoshi Goto, Vasu Punj, Olga Zaborina, Mei Ling Chen, Kazuhide Kimbara, Dibyen Majumdar, Elizabeth Cunningham, Tapas K. Das Gupta, and Ananda M. Chakrabarty. "Bacterial Redox Protein Azurin, *Tumor Suppressor Protein P53, and Regression of Cancer.*" *Proceedings of the National Academy of Sciences of the United States of America* 99, no. 22 (2002): 14098–103. doi:10.1073/pnas.222539699.

Yamada, Tohru, Yoshinori Hiraoka, Masateru Ikehata, Kazuhide Kimbara, Benjamin S. Avner, Tapas K. Das Gupta, and Ananda M. Chakrabarty. "Apoptosis or Growth Arrest: Modulation of Tumor Suppressor P53's Specificity by Bacterial Redox Protein Azurin." *Proceedings of the National Academy of Sciences of the United States of America* 101, no. 14 (2004): 4770–75. doi:10.1073/pnas.0400899101.

Yamada, Tohru, Arsenio M. Fialho, Vasu Punj, Laura Bratescu, Tapas K. Das Gupta, and Ananda M. Chakrabarty. "Internalization of Bacterial Redox Protein Azurin in Mammalian Cells: Entry Domain and Specificity." *Cellular Microbiology* 7, no. 10 (2005): 1418–31. doi:10.1111/j.1462-5822.2005.00567.x.

Yamada, Tohru, Tapas K. Das Gupta, and Craig W. Beattie. "P28-Mediated Activation of P53 in G2-M Phase of the Cell Cycle Enhances the Efficacy of DNA Damaging and Antimitotic Chemotherapy." *Cancer Research* 76, no. 8 (2016): 2354–65. doi:10.1158/0008-5472.CAN-15-2355.

Yang, Canyu, Bing He, Wenbing Dai, Hua Zhang, Ying Zheng, Xueqing Wang, and Qiang Zhang. "The Role of Caveolin-1 in the Biofate and Efficacy of Anti-Tumor Drugs and Their Nano-Drug Delivery Systems." *Acta Pharmaceutica Sinica B* 11, no. 4 (2021): 961–77. doi:10.1016/j.apsb.2020.11.020.

Yang, Nicole J., and Marlon J. Hinner. "Getting Across the Cell Membrane: An Overview for Small Molecules, Peptides, and ProteinS." In *Site-Specific Protein Labeling. Methods & Protocols* 1266 (2015): 1–267. doi:10.1007/978-1-4939-2272-7.

Zalba, Sara, and Timo L. M. ten Hagen. "Cell Membrane Modulation as Adjuvant in Cancer Therapy." *Cancer Treatment Reviews* 52 (2017): 48–57. doi:10.1016/j.ctrv.2016.10.008.

Zhang, Renshuai, Xiaofei Qin, Fandong Kong, Pengwei Chen, and Guojun Pan. "Improving Cellular Uptake of Therapeutic Entities Through Interaction with Components of Cell Membrane." *Drug Delivery* 26, no. 1 (2019): 328–42. doi:10.1080/10717544.2019.1582730.

Zwaal, R. F. A., P. Comfurius, and E. M. Bevers. "Surface Exposure of Phosphatidylserine in Pathological Cells." *Cellular & Molecular Life Sciences* 62, no. 9 (2005): 971–88. doi:10.1007/s00018-005-4527-3.

Overcoming the Mucus Barrier

12

Janni Støvring Mortensen, Mai Bay Stie,
Stine Harloff-Helleberg, and Hanne Mørck Nielsen

Contents

12.1 MUCUS AS A BARRIER FOR DRUG DELIVERY

Specifically targeting mucosal regions as sites for drug administration continuously gains increasing interest for the delivery of both small molecule drugs and biopharmaceuticals. The main reasons being that (i) in contrast to administration by injection, mucosal drug delivery benefits from generally higher patient acceptance and thus compliance as the discomfort and pain associated with needles are avoided

DOI: 10.1201/9781003092773-14

and (ii) production and storage costs are in most cases lower than for injectables as the strict regulations and higher cost for manufacturing of aseptic drugs are avoided. Further, (iii) the systemic delivery of drugs through the mucosa in, e.g., the nose, lungs, oral cavity, and vagina circumvents the hepatic first pass metabolism, and administration by these mucosal routes are thus beneficial for drugs, which have an undesired turnover in the liver. Therapeutic arguments include that (iv) direct administration to diseased mucosal areas that are therapy targets inevitably increases as well as controls the dose at the target site, (v) it limits unnecessary systemic exposure to the drug, and (vi) eliminates the risk of infections at the injection site. Also, (vii) pharmacological responses can be improved as is the case for some immunizations that not only offer better protection at the mucosal pathogen exposure site, but also represent a safer and more cost-effective alternative to traditional vaccines (Miquel-Clopés et al. 2019, Boegh et al. 2013a).

The efficient systemic delivery of drugs via mucosal routes is, however, limited by the major absorptive biological barrier, i.e., the epithelium, as well as by the mucus barrier, the latter being the focus of this chapter. Even local drug delivery to the tissue at the administration site may be challenged by the presence of mucus. Mucus is a viscoelastic gel that lines the eyes, ears, digestive tract, respiratory tract, and female reproductive tract. It plays an important role in human health as a lubricant that protects the underlying epithelium against physical damage and acts as a selective natural barrier, which limits the entrance of pathogens and other foreign entities into the human body. Accordingly, mucus has proven to be a significant diffusion and interactive barrier for the permeation of drug delivery systems (DDSs) and drugs of both small and large molecular weight (Boegh et al. 2013a, Sigurdsson et al. 2013, Carlson et al. 2018).

Mucus is continuously produced, secreted, and cleared. The turnover time varies by anatomical location and species (Lai et al. 2009a). For example, studies in rats suggest that the turnover time of mucus in the intestine may take hours (Lehr et al. 1991), whereas mucus from the ocular surface is cleared in minutes in humans (Greaves and Wilson 1993). Table 12.1 includes estimated clearance times for mucus at different human anatomical sites. Loss of drug by mucus shedding or washout in addition to significant dilution of drug in the fluid present in and at the surface of the mucus decreases drug concentration at the site of absorption, which consequently impairs drug permeation across the mucosa (Madsen et al. 2013). Thus, penetration into mucus, diffusion within and through mucus, and epithelial drug absorption must be significantly faster than the clearance of mucus to fully circumvent this barrier. To overcome the delivery challenges associated with mucosal administration, innovative DDSs have been engineered to increase mucoadhesion, improve diffusion through, and/or disrupt the mucus barrier to facilitate enhanced drug diffusion through mucus and thus permeation across the epithelial barrier into the systemic circulation or as local treatment of conditions affecting the mucosa.

12.1.1 Mucus Composition and Primary Barrier Properties

In general, mucus is composed mainly of water (90–95%), mucins (1–5%), lipids (1–2%), electrolytes (~1%), and a smaller amount of other proteins, DNA, cells, and cellular debris (Bansil and Turner 2017, Creeth 1978). The specific composition of mucus is complex and depends on, e.g., anatomical origin, species, stimuli from the surroundings, and health state as well as inter-individual variations, which can also be significant (Bansil and Turner 2017). The viscoelastic nature and thus the barrier properties of mucus mainly originate from interactions between mucins. However, ionic strength, pH, and non-mucin compounds present in mucus affect the intermolecular mucin interactions and thus the viscoelastic properties of mucus (Thim et al. 2002, Leal et al. 2017). Mucins are high molecular weight glycoproteins that entangle into the porous network constructing the mucus barrier (Figure 12.1). The protein backbone of mucin is characterized by repeated domains rich in proline, threonine, and serine (PTS-domains) separated by hydrophobic cysteine-rich domains (Boegh et al. 2014, Leal et al. 2017, Bansil and Turner 2006). The PTS domains are heavily glycosylated with mainly O-linked polysaccharides such as sialic acid, galactose, and fucose residues, which gives the hydrophilic nature of the glycoproteins (Larsson et al. 2009, Bansil and Turner 2006). Additionally, terminal fucose and sialic acid residues are often sulfated, which gives mucin a net negative charge (Dekker et al. 1989, Gerken 1993, Brockhausen 2003, Boegh et al. 2014, Bansil and Turner 2006, Leal et al. 2017).

TABLE 12.1 Representation of the Most Abundant MUC Genes Expressed at Various Human Anatomical Mucosae

	SURFACE-BOUND MUCINS	SECRETED MUCINS	CLEARANCE TIME*	DISEASE EXAMPLE(S)	REVIEWED IN
Eyes	MUC1 MUC4 MUC16	MUC5AC	~5 minutes	Glaucoma	(Mantelli and Argüeso 2008, Greaves and Wilson 1993)
Respiratory tract	MUC1 MUC4 MUC16	MUC5AC MUC5B	10–20 minutes	Cystic fibrosis Asthma	(Lillehoj et al. 2013, Ali and Pearson 2007)
Oral cavity	MUC1 MUC16	MUC5B MUC7	Within minutes	Xerostomia	(Dawes 2008, Johansson et al. 2013)
Digestive tract	MUC1 MUC3 MUC4 MUC12 MUC13 MUC16 MUC17	MUC2 (small intestine) MUC5AC MUC5B MUC6 MUC7 (stomach)	Most likely within hours	Crohn's disease Ulcerative colitis	(Lehr et al. 1991, Boegh and Nielsen 2015, Johansson et al. 2013)
Female reproductive tract	MUC1 MUC4 MUC15 MUC16 MUC17	MUC2 MUC5AC MUC5B MUC6 MUC9	Most likely within hours	Bacterial vaginosis	(Gipson 2005, Lai, Wang, Wirtz, et al. 2009, Lacroix et al. 2020)

*Estimated human clearance times are given.

Mucins are produced by specialized goblet or acinar cells and can either be anchored to the underlying epithelial membrane or secreted (Pelaseyed et al. 2014, Guzman-Aranguez and Argüeso 2010, Boegh and Nielsen 2015). Interactions between the membrane-bound and secreted mucins result in a mucin layer adherent to the underlying epithelium. Studies indicate that at least at some anatomic locations, two distinct mucus layers may be present, i.e., an adherent mucus layer tightly connected to the glycocalyx of the mucosal membrane and that covered by an adherent, yet loosely bound layer of mucus (Figure 12.1) (Atuma et al. 2001, Varum et al. 2012). Today, approximately 20 mucin genes have been identified (Boegh and Nielsen 2015). Table 12.1 includes an overview of mucin types and corresponding anatomic location. Several mucin genes may be expressed within a single cell, and the expression of a single mucin gene can result in mucins of different glycoforms due to variability in the glycosylation pattern, which overall provides a heterogeneity and complexity of mucus still not fully elucidated (Round et al. 2007, Taherali et al. 2018). Accordingly, depending on the composition of the polysaccharides, the overall charge of mucin and hence the mucus properties may vary (Boegh et al. 2014). In general, the overall negative charge of mucins increases adhesion to positively charged molecules or DDSs and thus restricts their diffusion through mucus. By inter- and intramolecular entanglement through non-covalent and covalent interactions, e.g., by hydrophobic interactions and disulfide bridges, mucins form a mesh of strands acting as a selective barrier hindering the permeation of drugs and DDSs through the mucus (Figure 12.1) (Boegh and Nielsen 2015). Studies indicate that not only the physicochemical properties, e.g., the charge of a drug or DDS, influence the diffusion through the mucus barrier (interactive barrier), but also that the pore size of the mucus network (steric size-exclusion barrier) influences the diffusion of entities within and through the mucus (Boegh et al. 2015, Boegh and Nielsen 2015). The nature of the entanglement of mucin strands defines the mesh spacing (pore size) of the mucus network, which sets a size threshold for particle diffusion.

In summary, the healthy mucus barrier is a dynamic barrier that protects and regulates exposure of the underlying absorptive epithelium to, e.g., drugs by both a dynamic, a steric, and an interactive barrier.

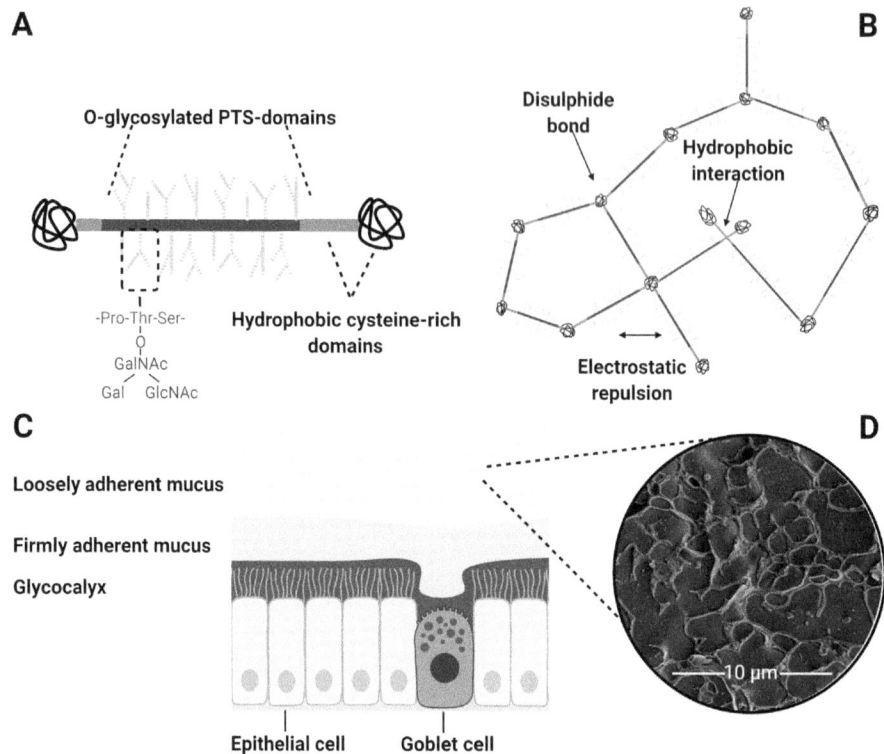

FIGURE 12.1 Simplified illustration of mucin domains (A) and mucin entanglement with representation of different types of interactions (B). Illustration of mucosa with the different mucus layers (C) and scanning electron cryomicroscopy picture of *ex vivo* porcine intestinal mucus (D). Created with Biorender.com.

12.2 DISEASES RELATED TO MUCUS DYSFUNCTION AND IMPACT ON THE BARRIER FUNCTION

As mentioned, the mucus barrier is the first line of defense for the underlying epithelial barrier, protecting against exposure to pathogenic microorganisms, endogenous digestive compounds such as gastric acid and enzymes, and in the gastrointestinal tract also against mechanical stress and shear induced by food intake (Johansson 2014). Consequently, a dysfunctional mucus barrier may severely impact the underlying epithelial barrier, and hence impact drug delivery. This may cause a disease or vice versa be the result of a disease or associated therapies, intake of certain drugs, as well as related to fungal, viral, and bacterial infections. The number of diseases related to or directly leading to mucus dysfunction are many and a few examples thereof will be given in this section.

12.2.1 Respiratory Tract Diseases

The primary defense mechanism in the nose and upper respiratory tract is mucociliary clearance (MCC) as a result of the continuous lateral clearance of mucus (Nawroth et al. 2020). MCC dysfunction is directly related to both chronic and potentially life-threatening as well as less severe diseases. In the nose, naturally occurring MCC is reported to reduce contact time of applied DDS to the absorptive surface, thus decreasing drug absorption (Taherali et al. 2018). In patients suffering from rhinitis or bronchitis however, the nasal mucus is characterized by a decrease in viscoelasticity leading to MCC, due to gravitational forces, directing increased amounts of mucus into the lungs (Taherali et al. 2018), hence impacting the absorption of nasally administered drugs.

Another disease example is cystic fibrosis (CF), an autosomal recessive genetic disease caused by mutations in the cystic fibrosis transmembrane conductance regulator (CFTR) gene (Elborn 2016). The CFTR gene is responsible for the transportation of ions and thus regulation of pH in the epithelial cells of the respiratory tract. Gene mutations result in altered pH, reduced chloride, and hydrogen carbonate ion secretion, leading to excessive mucin cross-linkage by calcium ions as well as mucus dehydration and to a hyper viscoelastic sputum (Ensign et al. 2012, d'Angelo et al. 2014, Mrsny et al. 1996, Lai et al. 2009b, Matthews et al. 1963, Chen et al. 2010, Fahy and Dickey 2010). Consequently, CF mucus is more prone to forming adhesive interactions with drugs and DDSs via hydrophobic and electrostatic interactions together with the formation of hydrogen bonds compared to mucus from healthy individuals (d'Angelo et al. 2014). Moreover, the increased viscoelasticity of mucus and hence decreased mesh size also challenge drug permeation (Duncan et al. 2016).

12.2.2 Digestive Tract Diseases

Saliva plays an important role as a lubricant in the oral cavity supporting chewing, swallowing, and protecting the teeth and underlying oral epithelium (Pedersen et al. 2018). Lack of saliva secretion or compositional changes in, e.g., mucin content can be the consequence of chronic damage to salivary glands, e.g., by radiotherapy used for the treatment of head and neck cancer, or due to Sjogren's syndrome, an autoimmune disease attacking the exocrine glands of the mouth and eyes (Pedersen et al. 2018). Furthermore, dry mouth, also referred to as xerostomia, can occur as a side-effect of medication such as diuretics (Pedersen et al. 2018). The amount and composition of mucins in secreted saliva are important for the mucus layer in the oral cavity, and irregularities can have a detrimental impact on the mucus barrier properties, leading to a higher risk of infections by bacteria and fungi as well as ulcers and oral candidiasis (Pedersen et al. 2018).

Crohn's disease (CD) and ulcerative colitis (UC), two examples of inflammatory bowel diseases (IBDs), are characterized by chronic relapsing intestinal inflammation. In IBDs, the mucus thickness changes and becomes more penetrable for bacteria leading to an increased risk of triggering inflammatory responses (Johansson 2014, Pullan et al. 1994). Normally, glycosylation of mucins protects the protein core against degradation. However, in the case of IBDs the polysaccharide structure of mucins has been reported to be both shorter and/or altered, facilitating degradation of the mucus barrier by bacteria and endogenous enzymes, thereby making the mucus barrier more permeable (Johansson 2014, An et al. 2007, Fu et al. 2011, Larsson et al. 2011, Okumura and Takeda 2017).

12.2.3 Other Mucosal Diseases

Ocular diseases, such as glaucoma, affect mucus properties. In patients suffering from glaucoma, the number of goblet cells is reduced, resulting in decreased mucin concentration, hence thinning of the mucus layer. This contributes to a critical alteration of the tear film that should be considered for topical drug delivery to the eye (Mastropasqua et al. 2019). As is the case for all mucosal sites, bacterial and viral infections can also be associated with altered mucus barrier properties. In bacterial vaginosis, the vaginal mucus has a dysbiotic vaginal flora with depletion of lactobacilli. The depletion of lactobacilli is, amongst others, correlated with decreased lactic acid production, hence increased pH (Lacroix et al. 2020). Consequently, the vaginal mucus is more penetrable to human immunodeficiency virus than a healthy mucosal barrier.

12.3 TARGETING THE MUCUS BARRIER TO IMPROVE DRUG DELIVERY

As previously described, the mucus barrier property profile depends on its physicochemical properties such as pore size, mucin type, viscoelasticity, pH, ionic strength, and charge. Whereas the pore size in general is the most significant limiting factor to nanoparticle diffusion, the overall negative charge, hydrophilicity, and mesh network of mucins do not favor the diffusion of large, cationic, and/or hydrophobic drugs through mucus (Boegh and Nielsen 2015). To overcome the mucus barrier several strategies can be employed with attention to parameters related to the mucin type (e.g., degree and type of mucin glycosylation), mucus thickness and viscosity, and anatomical location of the targeted mucosa (Lock et al. 2018, Kararli 1995, Freire et al. 2011, Sakata and Engelhardt 1981, Karlsson et al. 1997, Johansson et al. 2011, Veerman et al. 2003). Figure 12.2 provides an overview of strategies to overcome the mucus barrier.

Modulating the properties of the diffusing compound or DDS may be sufficient to achieve impactful changes in the delivery of drugs through mucus. Likewise, the barrier properties may be modulated to enhance diffusion.

12.3.1 Size and Shape Strategies

The diffusion behavior of a drug or DDS within and through mucus is directly related to its size due to the mesh network within the mucosal matrix constituting an effective steric barrier (Lai et al. 2009c, Friedl et al. 2013). The mesh spacing dimensions are heterogeneous, and depend on anatomical location, species, and health state (Leal et al. 2017). Overall, diffusion decreases with increasing molecular size and with increasing particle size (Lai et al. 2009c, Friedl et al. 2013). Besides the size of the DDS, also the DDS shape and deformability can be tailored to increase diffusion in mucus (Yu et al. 2018, Garcia-Diaz et al. 2018). Ellipsoids and rod shapes have been shown to display increased diffusion through mucus compared to DDSs with irregular or spherical forms (Yu et al. 2016, 2018). The ellipsoid and rod shape enables rotation-facilitated penetration of mucus in contrast to spherical or irregular-shaped DDSs, where penetration is decreased due to increased steric obstruction or increased interaction with the mucin network (Yu et al. 2016, 2018, Garcia-Diaz et al. 2018). Diffusion through mucus is, however, not only related to the size and shape of the DDS, but depends also on their physicochemical properties, including surface properties (Olmsted et al. 2001, Laffleur et al. 2014).

12.3.2 Surface Modification Strategies

Mucus is not only a steric barrier. The negative charges of the carboxyl and sulfate groups and the cysteine-rich domains of mucin are sites for non-covalent electrostatic and hydrophobic interactions, respectively. Thus, this interactive barrier limits the diffusion of especially drugs and DDSs with cationic and hydrophobic areas (Sigurdsson et al. 2013, Boegh and Nielsen 2015, Boegh et al. 2015). However, the impact of even a dense representation of cationic charges may be diminished if the surface is net neutral as a result of a correspondingly dense representation of negative charges. This is clearly demonstrated by the fact that, e.g., the capsid proteins from the Norwalk (acute nonbacterial gastroenteritis) virus and human papilloma viruses are able to diffuse through mucus as fast as through water, owing to their dense coat of both cationic and anionic moieties (Olmsted et al. 2001). This strategy can minimize both electrostatic and hydrophobic mucus interactions, overall facilitating penetration through mucus (Olmsted et al. 2001, Dünnhaupt et al. 2015a). The strategy designed by Nature to overcome mucus has been tested as a drug delivery approach. Creating a densely charged DDS with cationic and anionic excipients such as, e.g., chitosan or polyallylamine and polyacrylic acid or chondroitin sulfate, respectively, forms a "slippery" DDS

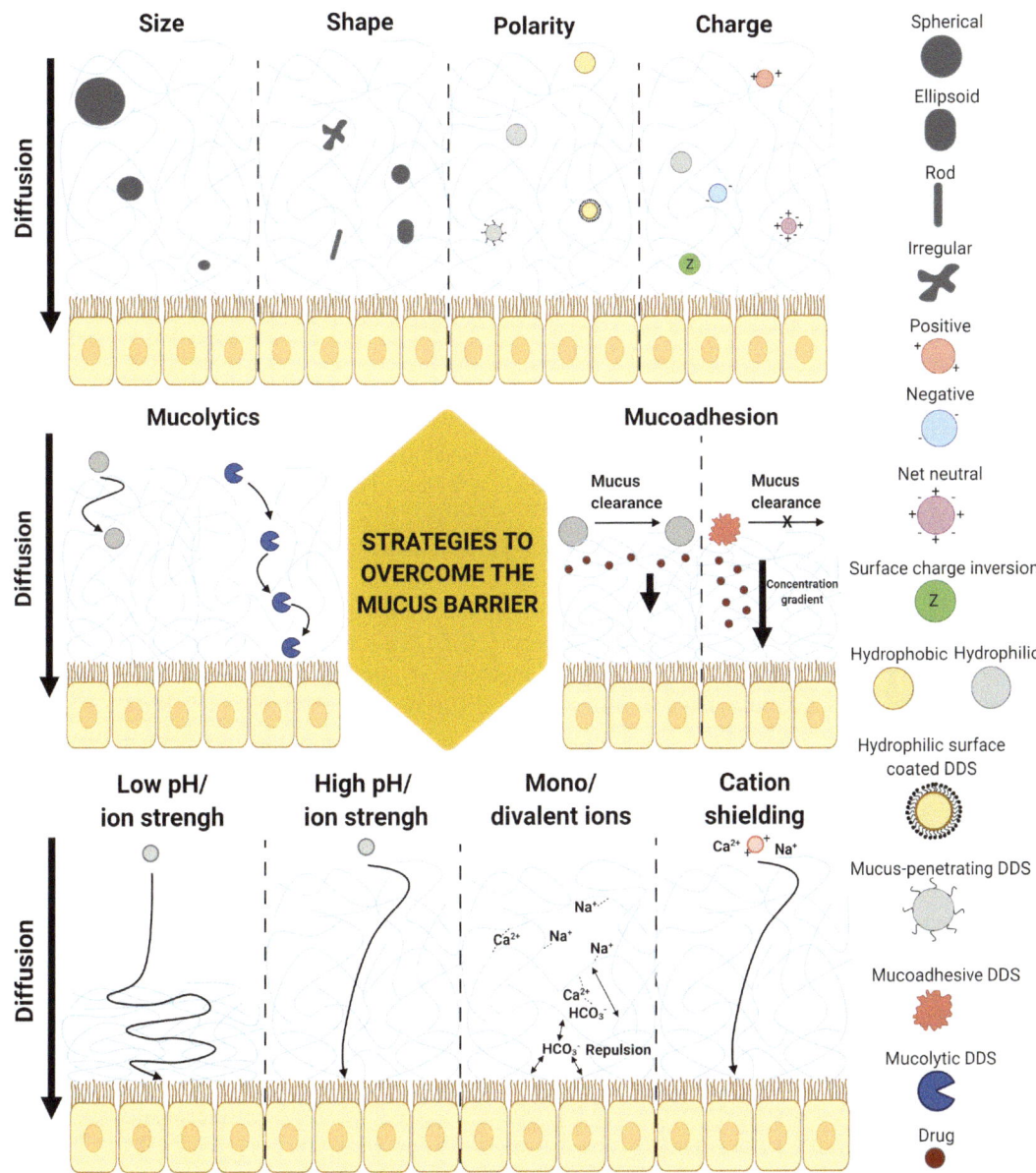

FIGURE 12.2 Overview of different strategies including modifications of drug delivery system (DDS) employed to overcome the mucus barrier. Created with Biorender.com.

and is referred to as the slippery surface strategy. This strategy has led to a two- to three-fold increased diffusion of the combined cationic-anionic DDSs compared to that of the individual cationic or anionic DDSs in intestinal mucus (Laffleur et al. 2014, Pereira de Sousa et al. 2015).

In addition to altering the net surface charge of the DDS to increase diffusivity in mucus, increased hydrophilicity and neutrality also improve penetration into mucus. Mucus-penetrating particles have surfaces modified with different polymers such as poly(ethylene) glycol (PEG), poly(sebacic acid), or ethylene oxide/propylene oxide copolymers to achieve hydrophilic and near neutral particles. This strategy has been reported to increase diffusion in mucus several hundredfold compared to that of the corresponding unmodified particles (Yang et al. 2011, Wang et al. 2008, Huckaby and Lai 2018). Additionally,

PEGylation of particles of 200 nm and larger can facilitate mobilization of particles that otherwise would be immobilized in mucus due to steric obstruction (Lai et al. 2007). The strategy of surface modification with PEG is amongst the most reported strategies to overcome the mucus barrier due to its promising outcomes and is thus seen as a golden standard in engineering mucus-penetrating DDSs applied to all anatomical sites (Huckaby and Lai 2018, Dünnhaupt et al. 2015a, Carlson et al. 2018).

When considering penetration into mucus, anionic DDSs are generally more favorable than cationic DDSs. In contrast, cationic nanoparticles have shown to be more efficiently endocytosed by cells compared to anionic nanoparticles, as the negative charge of the cell membrane attracts cationic DDSs and repulses negatively charged DDSs (des Rieux et al. 2006, Adler and Leong 2010). To address this, one approach is to design a DDS that can change from being slightly anionic to becoming slightly cationic when reaching the epithelial cell barrier. This surface charge (or zeta potential) inversion strategy has been achieved by conjugating nanoparticles with polymers such as carboxymethyl cellulose and chitosan to phosphotyrosine. This leads to the release of phosphate ions from the polymers in the presence of intestinal alkaline phosphatase changing the zeta potential from -8 mV to $+8$ (Perera et al. 2015). Utilization of this strategy is still in its early stages as the *in vivo* effect is yet to be investigated and would likely require a more radical shift in zeta potential than that reported by Perera et al. (Griesser et al. 2019, Prüfert et al. 2020, Perera et al. 2015).

The use of self-nanoemulsifying DDS (SNEDDS), potentially surface-coated, is another approach to increase the penetration of hydrophobic compounds into mucus, as these inherently (in addition to their poor aqueous solubility) have limited diffusivity in mucus due to interactions with the hydrophobic domains of mucins and lipophilic mucus components. SNEDDS are isotropic mixtures of oil, surfactant, and co-surfactant and spontaneously form an o/w nanoemulsion upon mixture with water. The small size (≤ 50 nm) and deformability of SNEDDS promote their diffusion through mucus (Friedl et al. 2013). The selection of excipient as well as the ratio of oil, surfactant, and co-surfactant can tailor the penetration of SNEDDS through mucus (Friedl et al. 2013, Dünnhaupt et al. 2015a).

12.3.3 Exogenous Ion Strategies

The ionic strength and the presence of specific ions are important in maintaining the mucus barrier function (Leal et al. 2017, Lai et al. 2009b). Alteration of the ion concentration, e.g., induced by a DDS or caused by a disease, affects the intermolecular interaction between the mucin strands leading to reorganization of these. This ion-dependency can be exploited by altering the exogenous ion composition and concentration by, e.g., co-formulating DDSs with high concentrations of aqueous cationic buffers. It has been shown, that the addition of 500 mM NaCl or $CaCl_2$ to a 1% (w/w) aqueous porcine gastric mucin (PGM) dispersion increased the diffusion coefficient for positively charged amine-modified polystyrene particles by a factor of 10 compared to the control (Lieleg et al. 2010). This occurred as a result of shielding the particle charge, yet the effect was reduced when decreasing the concentration of PGM (Lieleg et al. 2010).

Additions of exogenous monovalent cations or HCO_3^- are alternative strategies to overcome mucus barriers with high endogenous levels of Ca^{2+}, Na^+, and K^+, as this approach has been reported to increase the fluidity of a mucin dispersion by minimizing the inherent Ca^{2+} cross-linkage to mucin (Crowther et al. 1984). In addition, HCO_3^- was found to chelate Ca^{2+} and reduce the amount of free Ca^{2+} and thereby alter the viscoelastic properties of the mucin dispersion (Elborn 2016, Ermund et al. 2015, Chen et al. 2010). This supports the observation of decreased drug and DDS diffusivity in mucus from CF patients, corresponding to the fact that HCO_3^- levels are decreased leading to increased Ca^{2+}-mediated cross-linking of mucins, promoting dehydration and increased viscoelasticity of CF patient mucus (Elborn 2016, Dawson et al. 2003).

The ionic strength, often also reflected in tonicity, is also known to affect interactions in the mucus. Studies have shown enhanced diffusion of small molecules and nanoparticles through vaginal and colorectal mucus when administered in a hypotonic aqueous formulation as compared to when dosed in an isotonic aqueous formulation. This is explained by increased water flow from the hypotonic area to epithelial cells (Ensign et al. 2013, Maisel et al. 2015). The hypotonic aqueous formulation promotes mucus swelling, thus facilitating an increase in pore sizes and reduction of viscosity in the solvent phase, resulting in increased mucus permeability (Nordgård and Draget 2018).

These exogenous ion strategies have, however, mainly been proven successful in simple mucin dispersion models and their application remains to be confirmed *in vivo*.

12.3.4 pH Shift Strategies

The degree of mucin charge and conformation of mucin strands are strongly pH dependent. *Helicobacter pylori* is known to increase pH in gastric mucus by enshrouding itself in an ammonium cloud shifting pH from 2 to 6. This shift enables the otherwise trapped bacteria to diffuse through the stomach mucus (Abadi 2017, Celli et al. 2009). A similar pH-changing strategy is also observed in the female cervical tract upon sperm arrival, where the vaginal mucus pH is rapidly increased from 4.3 to 7.2. This enables sperm mobility and aids penetration into mucus (Suarez and Pacey 2005, Fox et al. 1973). Such changes in pH evidently alter mucin conformation. For instance, at low pH the mucin charge is decreased, changing the mucin structure from random coil to extended strands, which promotes the exposure of the hydrophobic mucin domains, facilitating aggregation that results in increased viscoelasticity of mucus (Leal et al. 2017, Bhaskar et al. 1991, Lieleg and Ribbeck 2011).

The permeation enhancer salcaprozate sodium (SNAC), approved for oral delivery of the glucagon-like peptide-1 analogue semaglutide, has been shown to buffer local gastric pH, thereby stabilizing and enhancing the gastric absorption of semaglutide. Apart from stabilization of and facilitating absorption of therapeutic peptide, the buffer capacity of SNAC might indeed also affect the gastric mucus barrier by reducing its viscoelastic properties, hence increasing the permeation of semaglutide to reach the absorption site (Buckley et al. 2018, Twarog et al. 2019).

Especially for acidic mucus environments such as the nasal, gastric, and vaginal mucus, the pH shift drug delivery approach could be applied to ideally reduce the viscoelasticity of the mucus and thereby increase penetration into mucus. In contrast, this approach will likely not lead to more favorable viscoelastic properties in the mucus barriers with a pH close to neutral or slightly alkaline.

12.3.5 Mucus Disruption Strategies

Overcoming the mucus barrier can also be achieved by disrupting the mucus mesh network. Mucolytic compounds, e.g., N-acetylcysteine, trypsin, papain, protease, and bromelain, can cleave the disulfide bonds between cross-linked mucin strands thereby reducing mucus viscosity and promoting drug penetration into and through mucus (Ferrari et al. 2001, Suk et al. 2011, Macierzanka et al. 2014, Sanders et al. 2000, Müller et al. 2012). Among the different proteolytic enzymes, papain and proteinase have been reported to disrupt the mucus network more efficiently (Müller et al. 2012). Modification of nanoparticles with papain was shown to induce a three-fold increase in diffusion in mucus as compared to that of unmodified nanoparticles (Müller et al. 2014). Disruption of the mucus barrier can also be achieved by DNase, which hydrolyses DNA, thus hindering its dense entanglement with mucin, reducing the mechanical properties and increasing the pore size within the mucus barrier (Nordgård and Draget 2018, Lai et al. 2009a). However, the effect of DNase alone as a mucolytic is questionable, whereas DNase in combination with N-acetylcysteine seems to induce a synergistic mucolytic effect (Suk et al. 2011, Macierzanka et al. 2014, Dawson et al. 2003, Sanders et al. 2000).

Mucus disruption strategies are highly relevant when targeting conditions with a dysfunctional viscous mucus barrier. However, such strategies are largely avoided in mucus with normal barrier properties due to the likelihood of subsequent mucosal damage and hence increased risk of, e.g., infections. Importantly, immobilization of mucolytic agents on a DDS surface might only induce local mucus disruption sufficient to ease diffusion of the DDS yet without risk of mucosal damage (Nordgård and Draget 2018, Dünnhaupt et al. 2015a).

12.3.6 Mucoadhesion Strategies

The most common mechanism of drug absorption is passive diffusion, which is driven by the concentration gradient of drug across the mucosal barrier (Brodin et al. 2010). Mucus shedding and clearance impair drug absorption by dilution and removal of the drug from the site of absorption. Accordingly, to improve drug bioavailability, mucoadhesive DDSs such as nanoparticles, nanofibers, gels, and microcontainers have been rationally designed to facilitate adhesion to the mucosa for a prolonged period to enhance the concentration gradient of released drug across the barrier (Bernkop-Schnürch et al. 2004, Dünnhaupt et al. 2015b, Boddupalli et al. 2010). Well-characterized polymers with mucoadhesive properties include chitosan, alginate, hydroxypropylmethylcellulose, pectin, etc. (Sandri et al. 2015). Depending on the excipient, mucoadhesion can be driven by several mechanisms, e.g., dehydration of the mucosal surface by hygroscopic polymers, non-covalent interactions with mucins through, e.g., hydrogen bonds, van der Waals forces, and electrostatic interactions due to the anionic nature of mucin, and finally covalent disulfide bonds can be made between thiolated polymers and the cysteine-rich domains of mucins (Dünnhaupt et al. 2015b, Barthelmes et al. 2011, Bernkop-Schnürch et al. 2004, Boddupalli et al. 2010).

12.4 MODELS AND METHODS FOR EVALUATING EFFECTS ON MUCUS BARRIER PROPERTIES

Several considerations must be taken into account when selecting mucus model and experimental methodologies to study mucus interactions. As stated previously, mucus properties and composition vary depending on species and anatomic location. As an example, the dominant mucin in gastric mucus is MUC5AC, whereas it is MUC2 for intestinal mucus (Rodríguez-Piñeiro et al. 2013, Larsson et al. 2013). An ideal mucus model should, to the extent possible, mimic the composition and structure of the native human mucus in question. However, the availability of native human mucus is limited. Despite eventual collection of animal mucus, the use might be limited by the sensitivity of the experimental method and lack of reproducibility, which is why numerous studies use dispersions of commercially available mucin (Groo and Lagarce 2014). In the following section, mucus models and experimental methods for mucus interactions will be reviewed.

12.4.1 Mucus Barrier Models

A variety of mucus models, including isolated native mucus, purified mucin preparations, biosimilar mucus, *in vitro* cell culture models, and mucosal tissue, have been used to study interactions with and within mucus.

Fresh native mucus collected directly from the mucosal tissue represents the most ideal mucus model. However, issues such as inaccessibility, yield, reproducibility, and inter- and intra-specie variation in composition and physical properties complicate its use. For instance, our observations show that porcine intestinal mucus yields vary from 1 to 10 mL per meter intestine in healthy animals. Also, it was reported that for patients suffering from CF, the mucin concentration varied from 10 ± 2 to 47 ± 3 mg/mL (Sanders et al. 2000). Native mucus has been isolated from several species including humans, pigs, horses, and rats (Groo and Lagarce 2014). When studying gastrointestinal mucosa or mucus, pigs are generally the preferred species due to their high similarity to humans as well as reasonable availability from the food industry compared to more ethically problematic use of mucus from, e.g., dogs or monkeys (Kararli 1995).

The crudeness and heterogeneity of native mucus challenge its use in numerous experimental methods. To overcome this obstacle and improve the reproducibility of experiments, mucin may be purified and applied for investigation (Ambort et al. 2012, Georgiades et al. 2014a, Zhao et al. 2012). Only a few commercial mucins are available, i.e., recombinant MUC1, mucin from bovine submaxillary gland, and PGM (Lock et al. 2018). The advantages of using such mucin dispersions include the possibility to easily alter the properties of the reconstituted mucin dispersion, e.g., mucin concentration, ionic strength, pH, and to include other components. However, mucins and especially commercially PGM have been reported to partially lose native mucin properties such as the gel-forming capability probably due to the purification process, and thus might not serve as ideal mucus models (Groo and Lagarce 2014, Lock et al. 2018, Griffiths et al. 2010).

In addition to mucin, mucus also contains lipids, minerals, and non-mucin proteins, which are all important for the integrity of the mucus barrier. It has been shown that the removal of associated lipids reduces the viscosity of canine gastric mucin by 80–85%, and the removal of covalently bound fatty acids led to a further 39% decrease in viscosity (Murty et al. 1984). Lipids and especially phospholipids are known to interact with the non-glycosylated domains of mucins, stabilizing the extended mucin structure in an aqueous environment (Boegh et al. 2013b, 2014, Murty et al. 1984). Thus, to capture a more precise picture of the mucus barrier, all constituents of mucus must be employed in mucus models to fully understand interactions of drugs or DDSs with mucus (Boegh et al. 2013b, 2014, Dawson et al. 2004, Larhed et al. 1998). One of these biosimilar mucus models is reported to be biocompatible with the frequently used intestinal epithelial Caco-2 cell culture model. When applied onto the Caco-2 epithelium it provides protection against effects induced by permeation enhancers and simulated fed-state gastric media (Boegh et al. 2014, Birch et al. 2018). Thus, this biosimilar intestinal mucus model provides a unique opportunity to study the impact of the mucus barrier *in vitro* when assessing the transmucosal permeation and toxicity of drugs, excipients, and DDSs.

Alternative *in vitro* models applied to study the effect of mucus interaction comprise mucus-producing cell lines and co-cultures. Commonly used mucus-producing cell lines include the human bronchial carcinoma cell line Calu-3, the human colon adenocarcinoma-derived cell line HT29 and subpopulations thereof: HT29-MTX and HT29-FU. Calu-3, HT29, and HT29-MTX cells secrete the gastric and respiratory tract mucin MUC5AC, whereas HT29-FU cells primarily secrete the intestinal mucin MUC2 (Lock et al. 2018, Kreda et al. 2007, Lesuffleur et al. 1993). Co-cultures of HT29 and Caco-2 cells are often used for intestinal drug delivery studies as they mimic both mucus-secreting goblet cells (HT29) and intestinal absorptive enterocytes (Caco-2) (Lock et al. 2018, Lea 2015). However mucus thickness, distribution of mucus, and transepithelial electrical resistance (TEER) of the mucosae highly depend on the Caco-2 and HT29 ratio, due to the different properties of the two cell lines, and may thus differ from the *in vivo* situation (Chen et al. 2015, Gustafsson et al. 2012, Lock et al. 2018).

12.4.2 Interactions with the Mucus and the Mucosal Barrier

12.4.2.1 Diffusion Studies in Mucus

A variety of methodologies can be employed to study diffusion within and through mucus. The overall strategy is to study either bulk diffusion of numerous molecules/particles or multiple or single particle/molecule diffusion. Bulk diffusion studies, also known as permeation studies, are frequently reported and used to provide quantitative measurements on the lateral mobility of compounds (Boegh et al. 2015, Kalouta et al. 2020, Marxen et al. 2017, Müller et al. 2012, Griessinger et al. 2015). Bulk diffusion studies can be conducted in setups such as the commonly used permeable filter inserts (e.g., Transwell®), Franz cells, and Ussing chambers (Figure 12.3) (Griessinger et al. 2015, Groo and Lagarce 2014, Lock et al. 2018). In such studies, the donor and acceptor compartments are separated by a barrier such as tissue

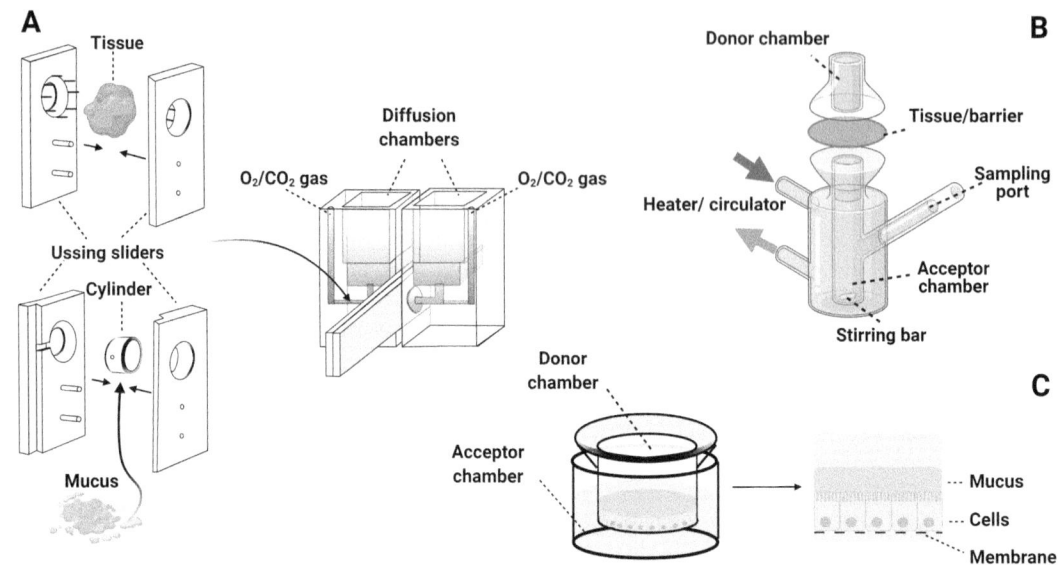

FIGURE 12.3 Illustrations of bulk diffusion methods. (A) Modified Ussing chambers, (B) Franz diffusion cells, and (C) filter inserts. Created with Biorender.com.

or mucus. After applying an amount of drug/particle in the donor compartment, the flux through the mucus barrier to the acceptor compartment can be determined by sample collection at defined time points (Brodin et al. 2010).

Also, single or multiple particle tracking (SPT/MPT) (Figure 12.4) and fluorescent recovery after photobleaching (FRAP) can be utilized to evaluate the mobility of the dynamics of particle or molecule diffusion. Thus, SPT/MPT and FRAP are able to provide behavioral information relating to different modes of particle or molecule interactions within the mucus network (Griessinger et al. 2015, McGlynn et al. 2020, Crater and Carrier 2010, Lai et al. 2007, Yildiz et al. 2015, Olmsted et al. 2001, Gonzales et al. 2015, Raynal et al. 2003, Nordgård et al. 2014). In MPT, the Brownian motion of several fluorescently labeled nano- or micron-sized particles is simultaneously detected in a given medium, such as mucus, using fluorescence video microscopy. By determining particle locations as a function of time, image analysis algorithms can be used to determine trajectories of the particles, and thus calculate time-average mean squared displacement (MSD) and effective diffusivity for the particles (Figure 12.4) (McGlynn et al. 2020, Griessinger et al. 2015). FRAP is also one of the primary techniques used to study the dynamics of single molecule (e.g., proteins) diffusion in mucus. With FRAP, a specific area in the sample is photobleached with a high-intensity laser and as the Brownian motion of the molecules continues, non-fluorescent molecules move into a fluorescent area and fluorescent molecules move into the photobleached area. It is thus possible to measure time and intensity of the fluorescence recovery even for very small entities, which can be used to calculate the diffusion constant for the molecule in a given medium (Meyvis et al. 1999).

12.4.2.2 Biophysical Characterization of Interactions with Mucus

Many biophysical methods can be employed to assess the interactions of drugs, excipients, and DDSs with mucin and mucus. The used methods comprise rheology, quartz crystal microbalance with dissipation monitoring (QCM-D), atomic force microscopy (AFM), and various scattering techniques including, but not limited to, dynamic light scattering (DLS), small-angle X-ray scattering (SAXS), and small-angle neutron scattering (SANS). These techniques are indeed complementary; some provide information about intermolecular interactions with mucin, whereas others elucidate the mechanism of interaction of drug, excipient, or DDS with mucin and whole mucus on a macroscopic level. Some of these methods are illustrated in Figure 12.4.

Advanced microscopic techniques such as AFM, transmission electron microscopy (TEM), cryo-TEM, and scanning electron microscopy (SEM) are reported in the literature to explore interactions with and within mucus and models thereof (Eshel-Green and Bianco-Peled 2016, Genta et al. 1998, Wan et al. 2020). AFM is based on scanning probe microscopy where a cantilever is used to monitor surface topography in length scales from nm to μm (Figure 12.4). By using either a covalently grafted or physically adsorbed mucin layer, topographic images of mucin structure can be obtained (Hong et al. 2005, Wan et al. 2020). Moreover, interactions between particulate systems and mucin can be visualized in both 2D and 3D by applying the test samples to a mica surface (Ferreira et al. 2018), and material properties can be quantified to some extent. In TEM, an electron microscope is applied to provide 2D projections of structures inside a specimen such as a mucin dispersion or mucus with a resolution suitable for size ranges down to approximately 1 to 20 nm, whereas SEM may be applied to generate 2D and 3D images of sample surfaces with a resolution around 10 nm. Upon mixing a mucin dispersion with, e.g., a drug or a particulate DDS, morphological changes due to mucus interaction can be visualized (Genta et al. 1998).

Rheological techniques are relevant when quantifying macroscopic properties of the interaction between mucus and components thereof with drugs, excipients, or DDSs of interest in relation to adhesion,

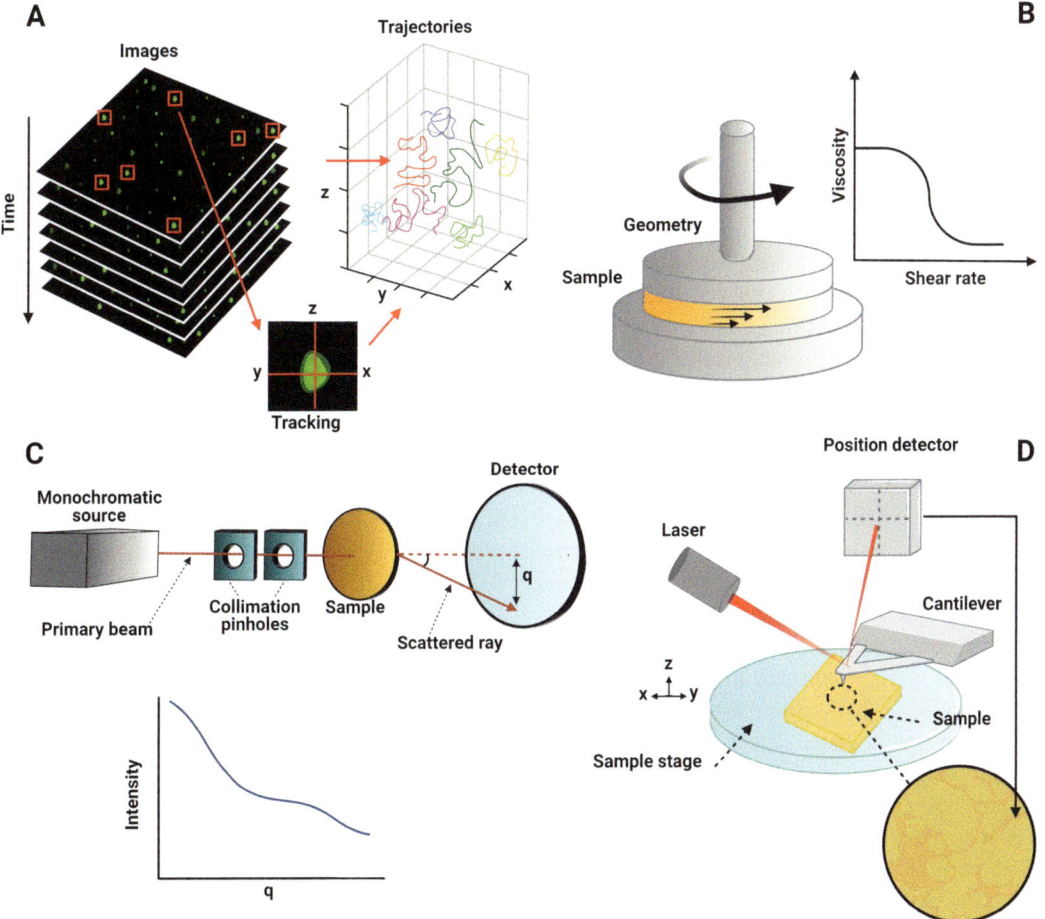

FIGURE 12.4 Illustrations of different methods for mucus/mucin drug or drug delivery system interaction studies. (A) Multiple particle tracking, (B) rheology, (C) small angle X-ray scattering, and (D) atomic force microscopy. Created with Biorender.com.

tensile strength, and viscosity (Figure 12.4) (Boegh and Nielsen 2015, Sotres et al. 2017, Harloff-Helleberg et al. 2017). From viscosity measurements using small deformation rheology, the apparent viscosity (η_a), a parameter related to mucoadhesion, can be calculated (Harloff-Helleberg et al. 2017). Besides mucoadhesion measurements, the material properties directly linked to the mucin network and mucus structure in general can be characterized using small deformation rheology (Boegh et al. 2014). Thus, if an excipient or DDS destabilizes the mucosal matrix, this will be reflected in a decreased elastic modulus, G'.

Another approach is passive microrheology using MPT or diffusion wave spectroscopy (DWS). Here, particles are used to determine mucus microviscosity, elasticity, and heterogeneity of the local microenvironment within a specimen. MPT microrheology is particularly well suited for small samples of complex materials such as mucus, and whereas DWS typically requires up to 1 mL of sample, MPT requires only very low sample volumes (1–50 μL) (Oelschlaeger et al. 2013, McGlynn et al. 2020). Measuring at high frequency and at low moduli range enables quantification of weak mechanical properties that in general cannot be detected using small deformation rheology (Boegh et al. 2015).

Recently, the QCM-D technique has been adapted to study the interaction of polymers, micro- and nanoparticles with immobilized commercial mucins and native gastric mucin (Oh et al. 2015, Wan et al. 2020). QCM-D has proven to be a versatile technique to study both mucoadhesion and penetration into mucus. A layer of mucin or mucus is immobilized on a crystal sensor either by chemical cross-linking or physical absorption (Oh et al. 2015, Wan et al. 2020). Adhesion to and penetration of drugs, excipients, or DDSs into the mucin or mucus layer can be recorded as a microscopic weight gain by changes in the frequency (Δf) in real time. Loss of sample weight can be due to mucin or mucus removal or loss of bound water in the immobilized and hydrated layer due to, e.g., conformational changes of the mucins. The method also provides information about the height of the established layer on the sensor and its viscoelastic properties by dissipation recordings (ΔD) providing, information about structural changes within the sample (Oh et al. 2015).

Within the range of thermal techniques, isothermal titration calorimetry (ITC) and differential scanning calorimetry (DSC) are the most commonly used to assess mucin or mucus interactions with test samples. Such interactions with test samples containing, e.g., drug or excipient molecules or nanoparticles can be quantified using ITC (Xu et al. 2015, Hsein et al. 2015). With this technique, the thermal activity occurring during chemical and biological processes such as interactions can be recorded (Hsein et al. 2015). From this information, the stoichiometry of mucin molecules bound per unit test sample (per nanoparticle) can be calculated using binding curves generated upon the stepwise injection of test sample into mucin-loaded sample cells (Hsein et al. 2015, Menchicchi et al. 2014, Meng-Lund et al. 2014, Zhao et al. 2012). Another thermal technique is DSC, where thermograms of control samples are compared with the ones obtained from mixtures of mucin or mucus with, e.g., nanoparticles, and the adsorption of mucin/mucus to the test samples can be identified (Sonia and Sharma 2013, Yin et al. 2009). A study also reported the use of DSC to explore potential conformational changes on mucus-lined vaginal tissue upon drug interaction (Wang and Lee 2002). Additionally, micro-DSC has been used to explore the role of hydrogen bonding on mucin structures at the supramolecular scale (Lousinian et al. 2018).

Static and dynamic light scattering (SLS and DLS) provide information on both phase behavior and dynamics as well as the structure of the sample in length scale from around 100 nm up to at least 10 μm (Narayanan et al. 2017). In relation to mucin and mucus interactions with test material, DLS analysis of mixtures of mucin dispersions with nanoparticles or similar DDSs in different concentrations can provide information on whether the colloidal behavior of mucin aggregates is affected in terms of size and zeta-potential (Barbero et al. 2016, Griffiths et al. 2015, Wong et al. 2014, Cao et al. 1999). By comparing particle size distribution and polydispersity index, information on adhesive interactions can be obtained (Wong et al. 2014). Mucin dispersions tend to form large aggregates with high polydispersity, but upon interaction between mucin and particulate systems, the mean diameter value is typically increased significantly (Wong et al. 2014). Zeta-potential represents the surface charge of the molecules or DDSs measured, and is typically measured using the same instrument as for DLS (Wong et al. 2014).

Large-scale facility scattering techniques provide high-resolution structural analysis at a length scale of 1–100 nm, offering detailed structural information (Narayanan et al. 2017) leading to further understanding of mucoadhesion behavior (Di Cola et al. 2019). Recently, SANS was used to study inter-actions of emulsions (Pereira de Sousa et al. 2015), polymers (Griffiths et al. 2010), and a cross-linker (Georgiades et al. 2014b) to mucin dispersions. SAXS has been used to study hydration and temperature-induced changes in porcine mucus (Znamenskaya et al. 2012). Both SAXS and SANS have been used to explore the structure of purified mucin (Georgiades et al. 2014a) and mucin in simulated nasal fluid (Di Cola et al. 2019). Interestingly, a novel method based on SAXS and SANS is established to explore the ability of nanoemulsions to penetrate in distances of mm into a mucin matrix, providing direct evi-dence of changes occurring in the mucin network induced upon such interactions (Di Cola et al. 2019). By complementing SAXS with SANS, a more detailed understanding of the porous structure formation within a mucin matrix can be obtained, as SANS provides more information on the cysteine-rich regions of glycoproteins, i.e., regions related to pore formation (Di Cola et al. 2019). Spin-echo SANS has been used to explore structural changes in 0.5 µm length scale in mucus upon interaction with nanoparticles (Georgiades et al. 2015).

12.4.2.3 Ex vivo *Retention Studies*

Mucus shedding is a significant challenge for mucosal drug delivery as it results in loss of drug and potential exposure to off-target sites. Mucoadhesive strategies intend to prolong the retention of the DDS at or near the mucosa, enhancing the drug concentration gradient across the barrier, thus improving drug absorption. Force measurements and displacement readings by texture profile analysis have been used to assess the mucoadhesiveness of, amongst others, polymers, DDSs such as tablets, films, and patches to discs prepared from mucin or to excised *ex vivo* mucosal tissue, e.g., porcine buccal, sublingual, and intestinal mucosa (Szymańska et al. 2014, Sogias et al. 2012, Nho et al. 2014, Mendes et al. 2018, Samprasit et al. 2015). The resilience of mucoadhesive DDSs such as microparticles and microcontainers to washout by mucus shedding or exposure to fluid flow has been assessed using *ex vivo* retention models. By this method, the retention of drug or DDS at the mucosa is indirectly determined by quantifying the loss of drug or DDS after washout by a flow of liquid across *ex vivo* mucosal tissue (Madsen et al. 2013, Mosgaard et al. 2019).

12.4.2.4 In vivo *Evaluation of Mucus and Mucosal Barrier Effects*

Several approaches exist on how to study the mucosal barrier properties *in vivo*. Upon method selec-tion, it is obviously of utmost importance to consider inter-species variation. As an example, the MUC type expression varies across species, e.g., rabbits having unique corneal mucin expression compared to humans and dogs (Leonard et al. 2016).

In vivo studies focusing on the mucosal barrier include absorption studies, assessment of the integrity of the mucosal barrier post-administration (morphological studies of the mucosal barrier, immunohis-tochemistry to assess both mucus and the cellular barrier) as well as mechanistic studies to understand interactions between the DDS and the mucus matrix. When considering DDSs developed to overcome the mucus barrier, it is highly relevant not only to explore the bioavailability of the drug, but also to evaluate the safety issues in relation to the mucosal surface, as the integrity should remain intact or regenerate within a limited time to prevent the absorption of unwanted substances (Mouez et al. 2014). Evaluation of the effects of orally administered DDSs *in vivo* on the mucus and the mucosal barrier can be assessed in various ways. One strategy is to dose fluorophore-labelled drug or DDS by oral gavage to, e.g., rats and euthanize the animals at the time points of interest post-administration, remove the intestinal tissue, and cut it in the longitudinal direction in sections at 10 µm intervals (Nie et al. 2019). After washing, snap freezing, and staining of cytoskeleton and nuclei, samples of the mucosal barrier can be inspected using confocal microscopy (He et al. 2018, Lian et al. 2013). Note should be taken that the procedure may reduce the amount of residing mucus. Another approach is to evaluate mucoadherence by *in situ* closed-loop rat intestinal perfusion studies (Nielsen et al. 2016). Here, the intestinal segment of interest is isolated and cannulated, and the DDS administered after intestinal washing. Samples are collected via the cannula at defined time points, providing information on adherence of the DDS to the intestinal mucosa. To monitor bioavailability, blood samples can be collected simultaneously. Subsequent to euthanization, intestinal tissue can be collected and mucosal morphology inspected using light microscopy (Nielsen et al. 2016). Likewise, a morphological study of mucosal surfaces is also reported in rabbits after nasal administration in combination with bioavailability assessment (Mouez et al. 2014).

12.5 FUTURE PERSPECTIVES

To enhance efficient and safe drug delivery after mucosal drug administration, further understandings of the mucus not only as a simple steric, but rather a dynamic, chemical, physical, and metabolic barrier are required. The properties of mucus are highly variable depending on anatomical site, health and disease state, and between species. For practical reasons, very simple models of mucin dispersions have most often been applied in studies on drug delivery strategies to exploit and overcome the barrier. However, it is clear that more representative models of both healthy and disease state mucus should be developed, and orthogonal methodologies should be established and employed to achieve a comprehensive understanding of this complex biological matrix. Several individual strategies and technologies to improve mucosal drug delivery are investigated and applied, yet often not fully understood. Explanations of their mode of action tend to be somewhat speculative, and evidence of direct clinical translation of this is sparse. Strategies for non-targeted extensive disruption of the mucus barrier cannot be uncritically implemented without thoroughly considering the impact on safety by disrupting the mucus throughout an entire location, and thereby inducing a risk of exposing and compromising the underlying epithelium. Optimal mucosal drug delivery depends on the combination of, e.g., mucoadhesive or mucus-penetrating compounds with for example mucolytic enzymes either co-administered or co-formulated in a DDS. By directly incorporating or immobilizing functional excipients together with the drug to be delivered and thereby ensuring co-localization, it can be anticipated that only local microenvironment mucus effects are induced. To our knowledge, such head-to-head comparisons between the effect of co-administered and co-formulated excipients and drug have yet not been investigated. To design, apply, and understand the mechanisms for such approaches, more representative models and high-resolution orthogonal methodologies should be further developed.

ACKNOWLEDGMENTS

To the Novo Nordisk Foundation for funding to the Center for Biopharmaceuticals and Biobarriers in Drug Delivery (BioDelivery; Grand Challenge Program; NNF16OC0021948; HMN, JSM & MBS) and to the Lundbeck Foundation (R303-2018-2968; SHH).

REFERENCES

Abadi, A. T. B. "Strategies Used by Helicobacter Pylori to Establish Persistent Infection." *World Journal of Gastroenterology* 23, no. 16 (2017): 2870–82. doi:10.3748/wjg.v23.i16.2870.

Adler, A. F., and K. W. Leong. "Emerging Links Between Surface Nanotechnology and Endocytosis: Impact on Nonviral Gene Delivery." *Nano Today* 5, no. 6 (2010): 553–69. doi:10.1016/j.nantod.2010.10.007.

Ali, M. S., and J. P. Pearson. "Upper Airway Mucin Gene Expression: A Review." *Laryngoscope* 117, no. 5 (2007): 932–8. doi:10.1097/MLG.0b013e3180383651.

Ambort, D., M. E. V. Johansson, J. K. Gustafsson, H. E. Nilsson, A. Ermund, B. R. Johansson, P. J. B. Koeck, H. Hebert, and G. C. Hansson. "Calcium and PH-Dependent Packing and Release of the Gel-Forming MUC2 Mucin." *PNAS* 109, no. 15 (2012): 5645. doi:10.1073/pnas.1120269109.

An, G., B. Wei, Baoyun Xia, J. M. McDaniel, T. Ju, R. D. Cummings, J. Braun, and L. Xia. "Increased Susceptibility to Colitis and Colorectal Tumors in Mice Lacking core 3–Derived O-Glycans." *Journal of Experimental Medicine* 204, no. 6 (2007): 1417–29. doi:10.1084/jem.20061929.

Atuma, C., V. Strugala, A. Allen, and L. Holm. "The Adherent Gastrointestinal Mucus Gel Layer: Thickness and Physical State In Vivo." *American Journal of Physiology. Gastrointestinal & Liver Physiology* 280, no. 5 (2001): G922–G9.

Bansil, R., and B. S. Turner. "Mucin Structure, Aggregation, Physiological Functions and Biomedical Applications." *Current Opinion in Colloid & Interface Science* 11, no. 2 (2006): 164–70. doi:10.1016/j.cocis.2005.11.001.

Bansil, R., and B. S. Turner. "The Biology of Mucus: Composition, Synthesis and Organization." *Advanced Drug Delivery Reviews* (2017). doi:10.1016/j.addr.2017.09.023.

Barbero, N., M. Marenchino, R. Campos-Olivas, S. Oliaro-Bosso, L. Bonandini, J. Boskovic, G. Viscardi, and S. Visentin. "Nanomaterial–Protein Interactions: The Case of Pristine and Functionalized Carbon Nanotubes and Porcine Gastric Mucin." *Journal of Nanoparticle Research* 18, no. 4 (2016): 84. doi:10.1007/s11051-016-3388-z.

Barthelmes, J., S. Dünnhaupt, J. Hombach, and A. Bernkop-Schnürch. "Thiomer Nanoparticles: Stabilization via Covalent Cross-Linking." *Drug Delivery* 18, no. 8 (2011): 613–9. doi:10.3109/10717544.2011.621986.

Bernkop-Schnürch, A., A. H. Krauland, V. M. Leitner, and T. Palmberger. "Thiomers: Potential Excipients for Non-Invasive Peptide Delivery Systems." *European Journal of Pharmaceutics & Biopharmaceutics* 58, no. 2 (2004): 253–63. doi:10.1016/j.ejpb.2004.03.032.

Bhaskar, K. R., D. H. Gong, R. Bansil, S. Pajevic, J. A. Hamilton, B. S. Turner, and J. T. LaMont. "Profound Increase in Viscosity and Aggregation of Pig Gastric Mucin at Low pH." *American Journal of Physiology. Gastrointestinal & Liver Physiology* 261, no. 5 (1991): G827–G32. doi:10.1152/ajpgi.1991.261.5.G827.

Birch, D., R. G. Diedrichsen, P. C. Christophersen, H. Mu, and H. M. Nielsen. "Evaluation of Drug Permeation Under Fed State Conditions Using Mucus-Covered Caco-2 Cell Epithelium." *European Journal of Pharmaceutical Sciences* 118 (2018): 144–53. doi:10.1016/j.ejps.2018.02.032.

Boddupalli, B. M., Z. N. K. Mohammed, R. A. Nath, and D. Banji. "Mucoadhesive Drug Delivery System: An Overview." *Journal of Advanced Pharmaceutical Technology & Research* 1, no. 4 (2010): 381–7. doi:10.4103/0110-5558.76436.

Boegh, M., and H. M. Nielsen. "Mucus as a Barrier to Drug Delivery - Understanding and Mimicking the Barrier Properties." *Basic & Clinical Pharmacology & Toxicology* 116, no. 3 (2015): 179–86. doi:10.1111/bcpt.12342.

Boegh, M., C. Foged, A. Müllertz, and H. Mørck Nielsen. "Mucosal Drug Delivery: Barriers, In Vitro Models and Formulation Strategies." *Journal of Drug Delivery Science & Technology* 23, no. 4 (2013a): 383–91. doi:10.1016/S1773-2247(13)50055-4.

Boegh, M., S. G. Baldursdottir, M. H. Nielsen, A. Müllertz, and H. M. Nielsen. "Development and Rheological Profiling of Biosimilar Mucus *Nord Rheol Soc Annu Trans*" 21 (2013b): 233–40.

Boegh, M., S. G. Baldursdottir, A. Mullertz, and H. M. Nielsen. "Property Profiling of Biosimilar Mucus in a Novel Mucus-Containing In Vitro Model for Assessment of Intestinal Drug Absorption." *European Journal of Pharmaceutics & Biopharmaceutics* 87, no. 2 (2014): 227–35. doi:10.1016/j.ejpb.2014.01.001.

Boegh, M., M. Garcia-Diaz, A. Mullertz, and H. M. Nielsen. "Steric and Interactive Barrier Properties of Intestinal Mucus Elucidated by Particle Diffusion and Peptide Permeation." *European Journal of Pharmaceutics & Biopharmaceutics* 95, no. A (2015): 136–43. doi:10.1016/j.ejpb.2015.01.014.

Brockhausen, I. "Sulphotransferases Acting on Mucin-Type Oligosaccharides." *Biochemical Society Transactions* 31, no. 2 (2003): 318–25. doi:10.1042/bst0310318.

Brodin, B., B. Steffansen, and C. Nielsen. "Passive Diffusion of Drug Substances: The Concepts of Flux and Permeability." In *Molecular Biopharmaceutics: Aspects of Drug Characterisation, Drug Delivery and Dosage Form Evaluation*, 135–51. London, Great Britain: Pharmaceutical Press, 2010.

Buckley, S. T., T. A. Baekdal, A. Vegge, S. J. Maarbjerg, C. Pyke, J. Ahnfelt-Ronne, K. G. Madsen, S. G. Scheele, T. Alanentalo, R. K. Kirk, B. L. Pedersen, R. B. Skyggebjerg, A. J. Benie, H. M. Strauss, P. O. Wahlund, S. Bjerregaard, E. Farkas, C. Fekete, F. L. Sondergaard, J. Borregaard, M. L. Hartoft-Nielsen, and L. B. Knudsen. "Transcellular Stomach Absorption of a Derivatized Glucagon-Like peptide-1 Receptor Agonist." *Science Translational Medicine* 10, no. 467 (2018). doi:10.1126/scitranslmed.aar7047.

Cao, X., R. Bansil, K. R. Bhaskar, B. S. Turner, J. T. LaMont, N. Niu, and N. H. Afdhal. "pH-Dependent Conformational Change of Gastric Mucin Leads to Sol-Gel Transition." *Biophysical Journal* 76, no. 3 (1999): 1250–8. doi:10.1016/s0006-3495(99)77288-7.

Carlson, T. L., J. Y. Lock, and R. L. Carrier. "Engineering the Mucus Barrier." *Annual Review of Biomedical Engineering* 20, no. 1 (2018): 197–220. doi:10.1146/annurev-bioeng-062117-121156.

Celli, J. P., B. S. Turner, N. H. Afdhal, S. Keates, I. Ghiran, C. P. Kelly, R. H. Ewoldt, G. H. McKinley, P. So, S. Erramilli, and R. Bansil. "Helicobacter pylori Moves Through Mucus by Reducing Mucin Viscoelasticity." *PNAS* 106, no. 34 (2009): 14321. doi:10.1073/pnas.0903438106.

Chen, E. Y. T., N. Yang, P. M. Quinton, and W. Chin. "A New Role for Bicarbonate in Mucus Formation." *American Journal of Physiology. Lung Cellular & Molecular Physiology* 299, no. 4 (2010): L542–L9. doi:10.1152/ajplung.00180.2010.

Chen, Y., Y. Lin, K. M. Davis, Q. Wang, J. Rnjak-Kovacina, C. Li, R. R. Isberg, C. A. Kumamoto, J. Mecsas, and D. L. Kaplan. "Robust Bioengineered 3D Functional Human Intestinal Epithelium." *Scientific Reports* 5, no. 1 (2015): 13708. doi:10.1038/srep13708.

Crater, J. S., and R. L. Carrier. "Barrier Properties of Gastrointestinal Mucus to Nanoparticle Transport." *Macromolecular Bioscience* 10, no. 12 (2010): 1473–83. doi:10.1002/mabi.201000137.

Creeth, J. M. "Constituents of Mucus and Their Separation." *British Medical Bulletin* 34, no. 1 (1978): 17–24. doi:10.1093/oxfordjournals.bmb.a071454.

Crowther, R. S., C. Marriott, and S. L. James. "Cation Induced Changes in the Rheological Properties of Purified Mucus Glycoprotein Gels." *Biorheology* 21, no. 1–2 (1984): 253–63. doi:10.3233/BIR-1984-211-227.

d'Angelo, I., C. Conte, M. I. La Rotonda, A. Miro, F. Quaglia, and F. Ungaro. "Improving the Efficacy of Inhaled Drugs in Cystic Fibrosis: Challenges and Emerging Drug Delivery Strategies." *Advanced Drug Delivery Reviews* 75 (2014): 92–111. doi:10.1016/j.addr.2014.05.008.

Dawes, C. "Salivary Flow Patterns and the Health of Hard and Soft Oral Tissues." *Journal of the American Dental Association* 139, no. Suppl. (2008): 18s–24s. doi:10.14219/jada.archive.2008.0351.

Dawson, M., D. Wirtz, and J. Hanes. "Enhanced Viscoelasticity of Human Cystic Fibrotic Sputum Correlates with Increasing Microheterogeneity in Particle Transport." *Journal of Biological Chemistry* 278, no. 50 (2003): 50393–401. doi:10.1074/jbc.M309026200.

Dawson, M., E. Krauland, D. Wirtz, and J. Hanes. "Transport of Polymeric Nanoparticle Gene Carriers in Gastric Mucus." *Biotechnology Progress* 20, no. 3 (2004): 851–7. doi:10.1021/bp0342553.

Dekker, J., W. M. O. Van Beurden-Lamers, A. Oprins, and G. J. Strous. "Isolation and Structural Analysis of Rat Gastric Mucus Glycoprotein Suggests a Homogeneous Protein Backbone." *Biochemical Journal* 260, no. 3 (1989): 717–23. doi:10.1042/bj2600717.

des Rieux, A., V. Fievez, M. Garinot, Y. Schneider, and V. Préat. "Nanoparticles as Potential Oral Delivery Systems of Proteins and Vaccines: A Mechanistic Approach." *Journal of Controlled Release* 116, no. 1 (2006): 1–27. doi:10.1016/j.jconrel.2006.08.013.

Di Cola, E., L. Cantu, P. Brocca, V. Rondelli, G. C. Fadda, E. Canelli, P. Martelli, A. Clementino, F. Sonvico, R. Bettini, and E. Del Favero. "Novel O/W Nanoemulsions for Nasal Administration: Structural Hints in the Selection of Performing Vehicles with Enhanced Mucopenetration." *Colloids & Surfaces, Part B: Biointerfaces* 183 (2019): 110439. doi:10.1016/j.colsurfb.2019.110439.

Duncan, G. A., J. Jung, J. Hanes, and J. S. Suk. "The Mucus Barrier to Inhaled Gene Therapy." *Molecular Therapy* 24, no. 12 (2016): 2043–53. doi:10.1038/mt.2016.182.

Dünnhaupt, S., J. Barthelmes, S. Köllner, D. Sakloetsakun, G. Shahnaz, A. Düregger, and A. Bernkop-Schnürch. "Thiolated Nanocarriers for Oral Delivery of Hydrophilic Macromolecular Drugs." *Carbohydrate Polymers* 117 (2015a): 577–84. doi:10.1016/j.carbpol.2014.09.078.

Dünnhaupt, S., O. Kammona, C. Waldner, C. Kiparissides, and A. Bernkop-Schnürch. "Nano-Carrier Systems: Strategies to Overcome the Mucus Gel Barrier." *European Journal of Pharmaceutics & Biopharmaceutics* 96 (2015b): 447–53. doi:10.1016/j.ejpb.2015.01.022.

Elborn, J. S. "Cystic Fibrosis." *Lancet* 388, no. 10059 (2016): 2519–31. doi:10.1016/S0140-6736(16)00576-6.

Ensign, L. M., C. S. Schneider, J. S. Suk, R. Cone, and J. Hanes. "Mucus Penetrating Nanoparticles: Biophysical Tool and Method of Drug and Gene Delivery." *Advanced Materials* 24, no. 28 (2012): 3887–94. doi:10.1002/adma.201201800.

Ensign, L. M., T. E. Hoen, K. Maisel, R. A. Cone, and J. S. Hanes. "Enhanced Vaginal Drug Delivery Through the Use of Hypotonic Formulations That Induce Fluid Uptake." *Biomaterials* 34, no. 28 (2013): 6922–9. doi:10.1016/j.biomaterials.2013.05.039.

Ermund, A., L. N. Meiss, J. K. Gustafsson, and G. C. Hansson. "Hyper-Osmolarity and Calcium Chelation: Effects on Cystic Fibrosis Mucus." *European Journal of Pharmacology* 764 (2015): 109–17. doi:10.1016/j.ejphar.2015.06.051.

Eshel-Green, T., and H. Bianco-Peled. "Mucoadhesive Acrylated Block Copolymers Micelles for the Delivery of Hydrophobic Drugs." *Colloids & Surfaces, Part B: Biointerfaces* 139 (2016): 42–51. doi:10.1016/j.colsurfb.2015.11.044.

Fahy, J. V., and B. F. Dickey. "Airway Mucus Function and Dysfunction." *New England Journal of Medicine* 363, no. 23 (2010): 2233–47. doi:10.1056/NEJMra0910061.

Ferrari, S., C. Kitson, R. Farley, R. Steel, C. Marriott, D. A. Parkins, M. Scarpa, B. Wainwright, M. J. Evans, W. H. Colledge, D. M. Geddes, and Ewfw Alton. "Mucus Altering Agents as Adjuncts for Nonviral Gene Transfer to Airway Epithelium." *Gene Therapy* 8, no. 18 (2001): 1380–6. doi:10.1038/sj.gt.3301525.

Ferreira, L. M. B., J. D. Alonso, C. P. Kiill, N. N. Ferreira, H. H. Buzzá, D. R. Martins de Godoi, D. de Britto, O. B. G. Assis, T. V. Seraphim, J. C. Borges, and M. P. D. Gremião. "Exploiting Supramolecular Interactions to Produce Bevacizumab-Loaded Nanoparticles for Potential Mucosal Delivery." *European Polymer Journal* 103 (2018): 238–50. doi:10.1016/j.eurpolymj.2018.04.013.

Fox, C. A., S. J. Meldrum, and B. W. Watson. "Continuous Measurement by Radio-telemetry of Vaginal pH During Human Coitus." *Journal of Reproduction & Fertility* 33, no. 1 (1973): 69–75. doi:10.1530/jrf.0.0330069.

Freire, A. C., A. W. Basit, R. Choudhary, C. W. Piong, and H. A. Merchant. "Does Sex Matter? The Influence of Gender on Gastrointestinal Physiology and Drug Delivery." *International Journal of Pharmacy* 415, no. 1 (2011): 15–28. doi:10.1016/j.ijpharm.2011.04.069.

Friedl, H., S. Dünnhaupt, F. Hintzen, C. Waldner, S. Parikh, J. P. Pearson, M. D. Wilcox, and A. Bernkop-Schnürch. "Development and Evaluation of a Novel Mucus Diffusion Test System Approved by Self-Nanoemulsifying Drug Delivery Systems." *Journal of Pharmaceutical Sciences* 102, no. 12 (2013): 4406–13. doi:10.1002/jps.23757.

Fu, J., B. Wei, T. Wen, M. E. V. Johansson, X. Liu, E. Bradford, K. A. Thomsson, S. McGee, L. Mansour, M. Tong, J. M. McDaniel, T. J. Sferra, J. R. Turner, H. Chen, G. C. Hansson, J. Braun, and L. Xia. "Loss of Intestinal core 1–Derived O-Glycans Causes Spontaneous Colitis in Mice." *Journal of Clinical Investigation* 121, no. 4 (2011): 1657–66. doi:10.1172/JCI45538.

Garcia-Diaz, M., D. Birch, F. Wan, and H. M. Nielsen. "The Role of Mucus as an Invisible Cloak to Transepithelial Drug Delivery by Nanoparticles." *Advanced Drug Delivery Reviews* 124 (2018): 107–24. doi:10.1016/j.addr.2017.11.002.

Genta, I., M. Costantini, A. Asti, B. Conti, and L. Montanari. "Influence of Glutaraldehyde on Drug Release and Mucoadhesive Properties of Chitosan Microspheres." *Carbohydrate Polymers* 36, no. 2 (1998): 81–8. doi:10.1016/S0144-8617(98)00022-8.

Georgiades, P., E. di Cola, R. K. Heenan, P. D. A. Pudney, D. J. Thornton, and T. A. Waigh. "A Combined Small-Angle X-Ray and Neutron Scattering Study of the Structure of Purified Soluble Gastrointestinal Mucins." *Biopolymers* 101, no. 12 (2014a): 1154–64. doi:10.1002/bip.22523.

Georgiades, P., P. D. A. Pudney, S. Rogers, D. J. Thornton, and T. A. Waigh. "Tea Derived Galloylated Polyphenols Cross-Link Purified Gastrointestinal Mucins." *PLOS ONE* 9, no. 8 (2014b): e105302. doi:10.1371/journal.pone.0105302.

Gerken, T. A. "Biophysical Approaches to Salivary Mucin Structure, Conformation and Dynamics." *Critical Reviews in Oral Biology & Medicine* 4, no. 3 (1993): 261–70. doi:10.1177/10454411930040030201.

Gipson, I. K. 2005. "Human Endocervical Mucins." In *New Mechanisms for Tissue-Selective Estrogen-Free Contraception*. Berlin/Heidelberg, Germany: Springer.

Gonzales, G. B., G. Smagghe, A. Mackie, C. Grootaert, B. Bajka, N. Rigby, K. Raes, and J. Van Camp. "Use of Metabolomics and Fluorescence Recovery After Photobleaching to Study the Bioavailability and Intestinal Mucus Diffusion of Polyphenols from Cauliflower Waste." *Journal of Functional Foods* 16 (2015): 403–13. doi:10.1016/j.jff.2015.04.031.

Greaves, J. L., and C. G. Wilson. "Treatment of Diseases of the Eye with Mucoadhesive Delivery Systems." *Advanced Drug Delivery Reviews* 11, no. 3 (1993): 349–83. doi:10.1016/0169-409X(93)90016-W.

Griesser, J., G. Hetényi, C. Federer, C. Steinbring, H. Ellemunter, K. Niedermayr, and A. Bernkop-Schnürch. "Highly Mucus Permeating and Zeta Potential Changing Self-Emulsifying Drug Delivery Systems: A Potent Gene Delivery Model for Causal Treatment of Cystic Fibrosis." *International Journal of Pharmacy* 557 (2019): 124–34. doi:10.1016/j.ijpharm.2018.12.048.

Griessinger, J., S. Dunnhaupt, B. Cattoz, P. Griffiths, S. Oh, S. Borrós i Gómez, M. Wilcox, J. Pearson, M. Gumbleton, M. Abdulkarim, I. Pereira de Sousa, and A. Bernkop-Schnürch. "Methods to Determine the Interactions of Micro- and Nanoparticles with Mucus." *European Journal of Pharmaceutics & Biopharmaceutics*. Pearson: M. Gumbleton. Abdulkarim, I 96 (2015): 464–76. doi:10.1016/j.ejpb.2015.01.005.

Griffiths, P. C., P. Occhipinti, C. Morris, R. K. Heenan, S. M. King, and M. Gumbleton. "PGSE-NMR and SANS Studies of the Interaction of Model Polymer Therapeutics with Mucin." *Biomacromolecules* 11, no. 1 (2010): 120–5. doi:10.1021/bm9009667.

Griffiths, P. C., B. Cattoz, M. S. Ibrahim, and J. C. Anuonye. "Probing the Interaction of Nanoparticles with Mucin for Drug Delivery Applications Using Dynamic Light Scattering." *European Journal of Pharmaceutics & Biopharmaceutics* 97, no. A (2015): 218–22. doi:10.1016/j.ejpb.2015.05.004.

Groo, A. C., and F. Lagarce. "Mucus Models to Evaluate Nanomedicines for Diffusion." *Drug Discovery Today* 19, no. 8 (2014): 1097–108. doi:10.1016/j.drudis.2014.01.011.

Gustafsson, J. K., A. Ermund, M. E. Johansson, A. Schutte, G. C. Hansson, and H. Sjovall. "An Ex Vivo Method for Studying Mucus Formation, Properties, and Thickness in Human Colonic Biopsies and Mouse Small and Large Intestinal Explants." *American Journal of Physiology. Gastrointestinal & Liver Physiology* 302, no. 4 (2012): G430–G8. doi:10.1152/ajpgi.00405.2011.

Guzman-Aranguez, Ana, and Pablo Argüeso. "Structure and Biological Roles of Mucin-Type O-Glycans at the Ocular Surface." *Ocular Surface* 8, no. 1 (2010): 8–17. doi:10.1016/s1542-0124(12)70213-6.

Harloff-Helleberg, S., K. J. Vissing, and H. M. Nielsen. "Assessment of Mucoadhesion Using Small Deformation Rheology Revisited *Nord Rheol Soc Annu Trans*" 25 (2017): 63–9.

He, Z., Z. Liu, H. Tian, Y. Hu, L. Liu, K. W. Leong, H. Mao, and Y. Chen. "Scalable Production of Core–Shell Nanoparticles by Flash Nanocomplexation to Enhance Mucosal Transport for Oral Delivery of Insulin." *Nanoscale* 10, no. 7 (2018): 3307–19. doi:10.1039/C7NR08047F.

Hong, Z., B. Chasan, R. Bansil, B. S. Turner, K. R. Bhaskar, and N. H. Afdhal. "Atomic Force Microscopy Reveals Aggregation of Gastric Mucin at Low pH." *Biomacromolecules* 6, no. 6 (2005): 3458–66. doi:10.1021/bm0505843.

Hsein, H., G. Garrait, E. Beyssac, and V. Hoffart. "Whey Protein Mucoadhesive Properties for Oral Drug Delivery: Mucin-Whey Protein Interaction and Mucoadhesive Bond Strength." *Colloids & Surfaces, Part B: Biointerfaces* 136 (2015): 799–808. doi:10.1016/j.colsurfb.2015.10.016.

Huckaby, J. T., and S. K. Lai. "Pegylation for Enhancing Nanoparticle Diffusion in Mucus." *Advanced Drug Delivery Reviews* 124 (2018): 125–39. doi:10.1016/j.addr.2017.08.010.

Johansson, M. E. "Mucus Layers in Inflammatory Bowel Disease." *Inflammatory Bowel Diseases* 20, no. 11 (2014): 2124–31. doi:10.1097/mib.0000000000000117.

Johansson, M. E. V., D. Ambort, T. Pelaseyed, A. Schütte, J. K. Gustafsson, A. Ermund, D. B. Subramani, J. M. H. Larsson, K. A. Thomsson, J. H. Bergström, S. van der Post, A. M. Rodriguez-Piñeiro, H. Sjövall, M. Bäckström, and G. C. Hansson. "Composition and Functional Role of the Mucus Layers in the Intestine." *Cellular & Molecular Life Sciences* 68, no. 22 (2011): 3635. doi:10.1007/s00018-011-0822-3.

Johansson, M. E. V., H. Sjövall, and G. C. Hansson. "The Gastrointestinal Mucus System in Health and Disease." *Nature Reviews. Gastroenterology & Hepatology* 10, no. 6 (2013): 352–61. doi:10.1038/nrgastro.2013.35.

Kalouta, K., M. B. Stie, C. Janfelt, I. S. Chronakis, J. Jacobsen, H. M. Nielsen, and V. Foderà. "Electrospun α-Lactalbumin Nanofibers for Site-Specific and Fast-Onset Delivery of Nicotine in the Oral Cavity: An In Vitro, Ex Vivo, and Tissue Spatial Distribution Study." *Molecular Pharmaceutics* 17, no. 11 (2020): 4189–200. doi:10.1021/acs.molpharmaceut.0c00642.

Kararli, T. T. "Comparison of the Gastrointestinal Anatomy, Physiology, and Biochemistry of Humans and Commonly Used Laboratory Animals." *Biopharmaceutics & Drug Disposition* 16, no. 5 (1995): 351–80.

Karlsson, N. G., A. Herrmann, H. Karlsson, M. E. Johansson, I. Carlstedt, and G. C. Hansson. "The Glycosylation of Rat Intestinal Muc2 Mucin Varies Between Rat Strains and the Small and Large Intestine. A Study of O-Linked Oligosaccharides by a Mass Spectrometric Approach." *Journal of Biological Chemistry* 272, no. 43 (1997): 27025–34.

Kreda, S. M., S. F. Okada, C. A. Van Heusden, W. O'Neal, S. Gabriel, L. Abdullah, C. W. Davis, R. C. Boucher, and E. R. Lazarowski. "Coordinated Release of Nucleotides and Mucin from Human Airway Epithelial Calu-3 Cells." *Journal of Physiology* 584, no. 1 (2007): 245–59. doi:10.1113/jphysiol.2007.139840.

Lacroix, G., V. Gouyer, F. Gottrand, and J. L. Desseyn. "The Cervicovaginal Mucus Barrier." *International Journal of Molecular Sciences* 21, no. 21 (2020): 8266. doi:10.3390/ijms21218266.

Laffleur, F., F. Hintzen, G. Shahnaz, D. Rahmat, K. Leithner, and A. Bernkop-Schnürch. "Development and In Vitro Evaluation of Slippery Nanoparticles for Enhanced Diffusion Through Native Mucus." *Nanomedicine* 9, no. 3 (2014): 387–96. doi:10.2217/nnm.13.26.

Lai, S. K., E. D. Hanlon, S. Harrold, S. T. Man, Y. Y. Wang, R. Cone, and J. Hanes. "Rapid Transport of Large Polymeric Nanoparticles in Fresh Undiluted Human Mucus." *PNAS* 104, no. 5 (2007): 1482. doi:10.1073/pnas.0608611104.

Lai, S. K., Y. Y. Wang, and J. Hanes. "Mucus-Penetrating Nanoparticles for Drug and Gene Delivery to Mucosal Tissues." *Advanced Drug Delivery Reviews* 61, no. 2 (2009a): 158–71. doi:10.1016/j.addr.2008.11.002.

Lai, S. K., Y. Y. Wang, D. Wirtz, and J. Hanes. "Micro- and Macrorheology of Mucus." *Advanced Drug Delivery Reviews* 61, no. 2 (2009b): 86–100. doi:10.1016/j.addr.2008.09.012.

Lai, S. K., Y. Y. Wang, R. Cone, D. Wirtz, and J. Hanes. ""Altering mucus rheology to "solidify" Human Mucus at the Nanoscale." *PLOS ONE* 4, no. 1 (2009c): e4294. doi:10.1371/journal.pone.0004294.

Larhed, A. W., P. Artursson, and E. Björk. "The Influence of Intestinal Mucus Components on the Diffusion of Drugs." *Pharmaceutical Research* 15, no. 1 (1998): 66–71. doi:10.1023/a:1011948703571.

Larsson, J. M. H., H. Karlsson, H. Sjövall, and G. C. Hansson. "A Complex, but Uniform O-Glycosylation of the Human MUC2 Mucin from Colonic Biopsies Analyzed by NanoLC/MSn." *Glycobiology* 19, no. 7 (2009): 756–66. doi:10.1093/glycob/cwp048.

Larsson, J. M. H., H. Karlsson, J. G. g. Crespo, M. E. V. Johansson, L. Eklund, H. Sjövall, and G. C. Hansson. "Altered O-Glycosylation Profile of MUC2 Mucin Occurs in Active Ulcerative Colitis and Is Associated with Increased Inflammation." *Inflammatory Bowel Diseases* 17, no. 11 (2011): 2299–307. doi:10.1002/ibd.21625.

Larsson, J. M. H., K. A. Thomsson, A. M. Rodríguez-Piñeiro, H. Karlsson, and G. C. Hansson. "Studies of Mucin in Mouse Stomach, Small Intestine, and Colon. III. Gastrointestinal Muc5ac and Muc2 Mucin O-Glycan Patterns Reveal a Regiospecific Distribution." *American Journal of Physiology. Gastrointestinal & Liver Physiology* 305, no. 5 (2013): G357–G63. doi:10.1152/ajpgi.00048.2013.

Lea, T. "Caco-2 Cell Line." In *The Impact of Food Bioactives on Health: In Vitro and Ex Vivo Models*, edited by K. Verhoeckx, P. Cotter, I. López-Expósito, C. Kleiveland, T. Lea, A. Mackie, T. Requena, D. Swiatecka, and H. Wichers, 103–11. Cham: Springer International Publishing, 2015.

Leal, J., H. D. C. Smyth, and D. Ghosh. "Physicochemical Properties of Mucus and Their Impact on Transmucosal Drug Delivery." *International Journal of Pharmacy* 532, no. 1 (2017): 555–72. doi:10.1016/j.ijpharm.2017.09.018.

Lehr, C. M., F. G. J. Poelma, H. E. Junginger, and J. J. Tukker. "An Estimate of Turnover Time of Intestinal Mucus Gel Layer in the Rat In Situ Loop." *International Journal of Pharmacy* 70, no. 3 (1991): 235–40. doi:10.1016/0378-5173(91)90287-X.

Leonard, B. C., B. Yañez-Soto, V. K. Raghunathan, N. L. Abbott, and C. J. Murphy. "Species Variation and Spatial Differences in Mucin Expression from Corneal Epithelial Cells." *Experimental Eye Research* 152 (2016): 43–8. doi:10.1016/j.exer.2016.09.001.

Lesuffleur, T., N. Porchet, J. P. Aubert, D. Swallow, J. R. Gum, Y. S. Kim, F. X. Real, and A. Zweibaum. "Differential Expression of the Human Mucin Genes MUC1 to MUC5 in Relation to Growth and Differentiation of Different Mucus-Secreting HT-29 Cell Subpopulations." *Journal of Cell Science* 106, no. 3 (1993): 771–83.

Lian, H., T. Zhang, J. Sun, X. Liu, G. Ren, L. Kou, Y. Zhang, X. Han, W. Ding, X. Ai, C. Wu, L. Li, Y. Y. Wang, Y. Sun, S. Wang, and Z. He. "Enhanced Oral Delivery of Paclitaxel Using Acetylcysteine Functionalized Chitosan-Vitamin E Succinate Nanomicelles Based on a Mucus Bioadhesion and Penetration Mechanism." *Molecular Pharmaceutics* 10, no. 9 (2013): 3447–58. doi:10.1021/mp400282r.

Lieleg, O., and K. Ribbeck. "Biological Hydrogels as Selective Diffusion Barriers." *Trends in Cell Biology* 21, no. 9 (2011): 543–51. doi:10.1016/j.tcb.2011.06.002.

Lieleg, O., I. Vladescu, and K. Ribbeck. "Characterization of Particle Translocation Through Mucin Hydrogels." *Biophysical Journal* 98, no. 9 (2010): 1782–9. doi:10.1016/j.bpj.2010.01.012.

Lillehoj, E. P., K. Kato, W. Lu, and K. C. Kim. "Chapter Four: Cellular and Molecular Biology of Airway Mucins." In *International Review of Cell and Molecular Biology*, edited by K. W. Jeon, 139–202. Cambridge, MA: Academic Press, 2013.

Lock, J. Y., T. L. Carlson, and R. L. Carrier. "Mucus Models to Evaluate the Diffusion of Drugs and Particles." *Advanced Drug Delivery Reviews* 124 (2018): 34–49. doi:10.1016/j.addr.2017.11.001.

Lousinian, S., A. R. Mackie, N. M. Rigby, C. Panayiotou, and C. Ritzoulis. "Microcalorimetry of the Intestinal Mucus: Hydrogen Bonding and Self-Assembly of Mucin." *International Journal of Biological Macromolecules* 112 (2018): 555–60. doi:10.1016/j.ijbiomac.2018.01.185.

Macierzanka, A., A. R. Mackie, B. H. Bajka, N. M. Rigby, F. Nau, and D. Dupont. "Transport of Particles in Intestinal Mucus Under Simulated Infant and Adult Physiological Conditions: Impact of Mucus Structure and Extracellular DNA." *PLOS ONE* 9, no. 4 (2014): e95274. doi:10.1371/journal.pone.0095274.

Madsen, K. D., C. Sander, S. G. Baldursdottir, A. M. L. Pedersen, and J. Jacobsen. "Development of an ex vivo Retention Model Simulating Bioadhesion in the Oral Cavity Using Human Saliva and Physiologically Relevant Irrigation Media." *International Journal of Pharmacy* 448, no. 2 (2013): 373–81. doi:10.1016/j.ijpharm.2013.03.031.

Maisel, K., S. Chattopadhyay, T. Moench, C. Hendrix, R. Cone, L. M. Ensign, and J. Hanes. "Enema Ion Compositions for Enhancing Colorectal Drug Delivery." *Journal of Controlled Release* 209 (2015): 280–7. doi:10.1016/j.jconrel.2015.04.040.

Mantelli, F., and P. Argüeso. "Functions of Ocular Surface Mucins in Health and Disease." *Current Opinion in Allergy & Clinical Immunology* 8, no. 5 (2008): 477–83. doi:10.1097/ACI.0b013e32830e6b04.

Marxen, E., M. D. Mosgaard, A. M. L. Pedersen, and J. Jacobsen. "Mucin Dispersions as a Model for the Oromucosal Mucus Layer in In Vitro and Ex Vivo Buccal Permeability Studies of Small Molecules." *European Journal of Pharmaceutics & Biopharmaceutics* 121 (2017): 121–128. doi:10.1016/j.ejpb.2017.09.016.

Mastropasqua, R., L. Agnifili, and L. Mastropasqua. "Structural and Molecular Tear Film Changes in Glaucoma." *Current Medicinal Chemistry* 26, no. 22 (2019): 4225–40. doi:10.2174/0929867325666181009153212.

Matthews, L. W., S. Spector, J. Lemm, and J. L. Potter. "Studies on Pulmonary Secretions. I. The Over-All Chemical Composition of Pulmonary Secretions from Patients with Cystic Fibrosis, Bronchiectasis, and Laryngectomy." *American Review of Respiratory Disease* 88 (1963): 199–204. doi:10.1164/arrd.1963.88.2.199.

McGlynn, J. A., N. Wu, and K. M. Schultz. "Multiple Particle Tracking Microrheological Characterization: Fundamentals, Emerging Techniques and Applications." *Journal of Applied Physics* 127, no. 20 (2020). doi:10.1063/5.0006122, PubMed: 201101.

Menchicchi, B., J. P. Fuenzalida, K. B. Bobbili, A. Hensel, M. J. Swamy, and F. M. Goycoolea. "Structure of Chitosan Determines Its Interactions with Mucin." *Biomacromolecules* 15, no. 10 (2014): 3550–8. doi:10.1021/bm5007954.

Mendes, A. C., J. S. Moreno, M. Hanif, T. E. L. Douglas, M. Chen, and I. S. Chronakis. "Morphological, Mechanical and Mucoadhesive Properties of Electrospun Chitosan/Phospholipid Hybrid Nanofibers." *International Journal of Molecular Sciences* 19, no. 8 (2018): 2266. doi:10.3390/ijms19082266.

Meng-Lund, E., C. Muff-Westergaard, C. Sander, P. Madelung, and J. Jacobsen. "A Mechanistic Based Approach for Enhancing Buccal Mucoadhesion of Chitosan." *International Journal of Pharmacy* 461, no. 1–2 (2014): 280–5. doi:10.1016/j.ijpharm.2013.10.047.

Meyvis, T. K. L., S. C. De Smedt, P. Van Oostveldt, and J. Demeester. "Fluorescence Recovery After Photobleaching: A Versatile Tool for Mobility and Interaction Measurements in Pharmaceutical Research." *Pharmaceutical Research* 16, no. 8 (1999): 1153–62. doi:10.1023/A:1011924909138.

Miquel-Clopés, A., E. G. Bentley, J. P. Stewart, and S. R. Carding. "Mucosal Vaccines and Technology." *Clinical & Experimental Immunology* 196, no. 2 (2019): 205–14. doi:10.1111/cei.13285.

Mosgaard, M. D., S. Strindberg, Z. Abid, R. S. Petersen, L. H. E. Thamdrup, A. J. Andersen, S. S. Keller, A. Müllertz, L. H. Nielsen, and A. Boisen. "Ex Vivo Intestinal Perfusion Model for Investigating Mucoadhesion of Microcontainers." *International Journal of Pharmacy* 570 (2019):118658. doi:10.1016/j.ijpharm.2019.118658.

Mouez, A. M., N. M. Zaki, S. Mansour, and A. S. Geneidi. "Bioavailability Enhancement of Verapamil HCl via Intranasal Chitosan Microspheres." *European Journal of Pharmaceutical Sciences* 51 (2014): 59–66. doi:10.1016/j.ejps.2013.08.029.

Mrsny, R., A. Daugherty, S. Short, R. Widmer, M. Siegel, and G. A. Keller. "Distribution of DNA and Alginate in Purulent Cystic Fibrosis Sputum: Implications to Pulmonary Targeting Strategies." *Journal of Drug Targeting* 4, no. 4 (1996): 233–43. doi:10.3109/10611869608995625.

Müller, C., K. Leithner, S. Hauptstein, F. Hintzen, W. Salvenmoser, and A. Bernkop-Schnürch. "Preparation and Characterization of Mucus-Penetrating Papain/Poly(Acrylic Acid) Nanoparticles for Oral Drug Delivery Applications." *Journal of Nanoparticle Research* 15, no. 1 (2012): 1353. doi:10.1007/s11051-012-1353-z.

Müller, C., G. Perera, V. König, and A. Bernkop-Schnürch. "Development and In Vivo Evaluation of Papain-Functionalized Nanoparticles." *European Journal of Pharmaceutics & Biopharmaceutics* 87, no. 1 (2014): 125–31. doi:10.1016/j.ejpb.2013.12.012.

Murty, V. L. N., J. Sarosiek, A. Slomiany, and B. L. Slomiany. "Effect of Lipids and Proteins on the Viscosity of Gastric Mucus Glycoprotein." *Biochemical & Biophysical Research Communications* 121, no. 2 (1984): 521–9. doi:10.1016/0006-291X(84)90213-4.

Narayanan, T., H. Wacklin, O. Konovalov, and R. Lund. "Recent Applications of Synchrotron Radiation and Neutrons in the Study of Soft Matter." *Crystallography Reviews* 23, no. 3 (2017): 160–226. doi:10.1080/0889311X.2016.1277212.

Nawroth, J. C., A. M. van der Does, A. R. Firth, and E. Kanso. "Multiscale Mechanics of Mucociliary Clearance in the Lung." *Philosophical Transactions of the Royal Society of London Series B* 375, no. 1792 (2020): 20190160. doi:10.1098/rstb.2019.0160.

Nho, Y. C., J. S. Park, and Y. M. Lim. "Preparation of Poly(Acrylic Acid) Hydrogel by Radiation Crosslinking and Its Application for Mucoadhesives." *Polymers* 6, no. 3 (2014): 890–8. doi:10.3390/polym6030890.

Nie, T., Z. He, Y. Zhou, J. Zhu, K. Chen, L. Liu, K. W. Leong, H. Q. Mao, and Y. Chen. "Surface Coating Approach to Overcome Mucosal Entrapment of DNA Nanoparticles for Oral Gene Delivery of Glucagon-Like Peptide 1." *ACS Applied Materials & Interfaces* 11, no. 33 (2019): 29593–603. doi:10.1021/acsami.9b10294.

Nielsen, L. H., A. Melero, S. S. Keller, J. Jacobsen, T. Rades, A. Müllertz, and A. Boisen Garrigues, T. Rades, A. Müllertz, and A. Boisen. "Polymeric Microcontainers Improve oral Bioavailability of Furosemide." *International Journal of Pharmaceutics* 504, no. 1 (2016): 98–109. doi:10.1016/j.ijpharm.2016.03.050.

Nordgård, C. T., and K. I. Draget. "Co Association of Mucus Modulating Agents and Nanoparticles for Mucosal Drug Delivery." *Advanced Drug Delivery Reviews* 124 (2018): 175–83. doi:10.1016/j.addr.2018.01.001.

Nordgård, C. T., U. Nonstad, M. Ø. Olderøy, T. Espevik, and K. I. Draget. "Alterations in Mucus Barrier Function and Matrix Structure Induced by Guluronate Oligomers." *Biomacromolecules* 15, no. 6 (2014): 2294–300. doi:10.1021/bm500464b.

Oelschlaeger, C., M. Cota Pinto Coelho, and N. Willenbacher. "Chain Flexibility and Dynamics of Polysaccharide Hyaluronan in Entangled Solutions: A High Frequency Rheology and Diffusing Wave Spectroscopy Study." *Biomacromolecules* 14, no. 10 (2013): 3689–96. doi:10.1021/bm4010436.

Oh, Sejin, Matthew Wilcox, Jeffrey P. Pearson, and Salvador Borrós. "Optimal Design for Studying Mucoadhesive Polymers Interaction with Gastric Mucin Using a Quartz Crystal Microbalance with Dissipation (QCM-D): Comparison of Two Different Mucin Origins." *European Journal of Pharmaceutics & Biopharmaceutics* 96 (2015): 477–83. doi:10.1016/j.ejpb.2015.08.002.

Okumura, Ryu, and Kiyoshi Takeda. "Roles of Intestinal Epithelial Cells in the Maintenance of Gut Homeostasis." *Experimental & Molecular Medicine* 49, no. 5 (2017): e338–e. doi:10.1038/emm.2017.20.

Olmsted, S. S., J. L. Padgett, A. I. Yudin, K. J. Whaley, T. R. Moench, and R. A. Cone. "Diffusion of Macromolecules and Virus-Like Particles in Human Cervical Mucus." *Biophysical Journal* 81, no. 4 (2001): 1930–7. doi:10.1016/s0006-3495(01)75844-4.

Pedersen, A. M. L., C. E. Sørensen, G. B. Proctor, G. H. Carpenter, and J. Ekström. "Salivary Secretion in Health and Disease." *Journal of Oral Rehabilitation* 45, no. 9 (2018): 730–46. doi:10.1111/joor.12664.

Pelaseyed, T., J. H. Bergström, J. K. Gustafsson, A. Ermund, G. M. H. Birchenough, A. Schütte, S. van der Post, F. Svensson, A. M. Rodríguez-Piñeiro, E. E. L. Nyström, C. Wising, M. E. V. Johansson, and G. C. Hansson. "The Mucus and Mucins of the Goblet Cells and Enterocytes Provide the First Defense Line of the Gastrointestinal Tract and Interact with the Immune System." *Immunologic Research* 260, no. 1 (2014): 8–20. doi:10.1111/imr.12182.

Pereira de Sousa, I., B. Cattoz, M. D. Wilcox, P. C. Griffiths, R. Dalgliesh, S. Rogers, and A. Bernkop-Schnürch. "Nanoparticles Decorated with Proteolytic Enzymes, a Promising Strategy to Overcome the Mucus Barrier." *European Journal of Pharmaceutics & Biopharmaceutics* 97, no. A (2015a): 257–64. doi:10.1016/j.ejpb.2015.01.008.

Pereira de Sousa, I., C. Steiner, M. Schmutzler, M. D. Wilcox, G. J. Veldhuis, J. P. Pearson, C. W. Huck, W. Salvenmoser, and A. Bernkop-Schnürch. "Mucus Permeating Carriers: Formulation and Characterization of Highly Densely Charged Nanoparticles." *European Journal of Pharmaceutics & Biopharmaceutics* 97, no. A (2015b): 273–9. doi:10.1016/j.ejpb.2014.12.024.

Perera, G., M. Zipser, S. Bonengel, W. Salvenmoser, and A. Bernkop-Schnürch. "Development of Phosphorylated Nanoparticles as Zeta Potential Inverting Systems." *European Journal of Pharmaceutics & Biopharmaceutics* 97, no. A (2015): 250–6. doi:10.1016/j.ejpb.2015.01.017.

Prüfert, F., F. Fischer, C. Leichner, S. Zaichik, and A. Bernkop-Schnürch. "Development and In Vitro Evaluation of Stearic Acid Phosphotyrosine Amide as New Excipient for Zeta Potential Changing Self-Emulsifying Drug Delivery Systems." *Pharmaceutical Research* 37, no. 4 (2020): 79. doi:10.1007/s11095-020-02802-2.

Pullan, R. D., G. A. Thomas, M. Rhodes, R. G. Newcombe, G. T. Williams, A. Allen, and J. Rhodes. "Thickness of Adherent Mucus Gel on Colonic Mucosa in Humans and Its Relevance to Colitis." *Gut* 35, no. 3 (1994): 353–9.

Raynal, B. D., T. E. Hardingham, J. K. Sheehan, and D. J. Thornton. "Calcium-Dependent Protein Interactions in MUC5B Provide Reversible Cross-Links in Salivary Mucus." *Journal of Biological Chemistry* 278, no. 31 (2003): 28703–10. doi:10.1074/jbc.M304632200.

Rodríguez-Piñeiro, A. M., J. H. Bergström, A. Ermund, J. K. Gustafsson, A. Schütte, M. E. V. Johansson, and G. C. Hansson. "Studies of Mucus in Mouse Stomach, Small Intestine, and Colon. II. Gastrointestinal Mucus Proteome Reveals Muc2 and Muc5ac Accompanied by a Set of Core Proteins." *American Journal of Physiology. Gastrointestinal & Liver Physiology* 305, no. 5 (2013): G348–G56. doi:10.1152/ajpgi.00047.2013.

Round, A. N., T. J. McMaster, M. J. Miles, A. P. Corfield, and M. Berry. "The Isolated MUC5AC Gene Product from Human Ocular Mucin Displays Intramolecular Conformational Heterogeneity." *Glycobiology* 17, no. 6 (2007): 578–85. doi:10.1093/glycob/cwm027.

Sakata, T., and W. V. Engelhardt. "Luminal Mucin in the Large Intestine of Mice, Rats and Guinea Pigs." *Cell & Tissue Research* 219, no. 3 (1981): 629–35. doi:10.1007/BF00210000.

Samprasit, W., R. Kaomongkolgit, M. Sukma, T. Rojanarata, T. Ngawhirunpat, and P. Opanasopit. "Mucoadhesive Electrospun Chitosan-Based Nanofibre Mats for Dental Caries Prevention." *Carbohydrate Polymers* 117 (2015): 933–40. doi:10.1016/j.carbpol.2014.10.026.

Sanders, N. N., S. C. De Smedt, E. Van Rompaey, P. Simoens, F. De Baets, and J. Demeester. "Cystic Fibrosis Sputum: A Barrier to the Transport of Nanospheres." *American Journal of Respiratory & Critical Care Medicine* 162, no. 5 (2000): 1905–11. doi:10.1164/ajrccm.162.5.9909009.

Sandri, G., S. Rossi, F. Ferrari, M. C. Bonferoni, and C. Caramella. "Mucoadhesive Polymers as Enabling Excipients for Oral Mucosal Drug Delivery." In *Oral Mucosal Drug Delivery and Therapy*, edited by M. Rathbone, S. Senel, and I. Pather, 53–88. Boston, MA: Springer, 2015.

Sigurdsson, H. H., J. Kirch, and C. M. Lehr. "Mucus as a Barrier to Lipophilic Drugs." *International Journal of Pharmacy* 453, no. 1 (2013): 56–64. doi:10.1016/j.ijpharm.2013.05.040.

Sogias, I. A., A. C. Williams, and V. V. Khutoryanskiy. "Chitosan-Based Mucoadhesive Tablets for Oral Delivery of Ibuprofen." *International Journal of Pharmacy* 436, no. 1–2 (2012): 602–10. doi:10.1016/j.ijpharm.2012.07.007.

Sonia, T. A., and Chandra P. Sharma. "N-hydroxypropyltrimethylammonium Polydimethylaminoethylmethacrylate Sub-Microparticles for Oral Delivery of Insulin: An In Vitro Evaluation." *Colloids & Surfaces, Part B: Biointerfaces* 107 (2013): 205–12. doi:10.1016/j.colsurfb.2013.01.057.

Sotres, J., S. Jankovskaja, K. Wannerberger, and T. Arnebrant. "Ex-Vivo Force Spectroscopy of Intestinal Mucosa Reveals the Mechanical Properties of Mucus Blankets." *Scientific Reports* 7, no. 1 (2017): 7270. doi:10.1038/s41598-017-07552-7.

Suarez, S. S., and A. A. Pacey. "Sperm Transport in the Female Reproductive Tract." *Human Reproduction* 12, no. 1 (2005): 23–37. doi:10.1093/humupd/dmi047.

Suk, J. S., N. J. Boylan, K. Trehan, B. C. Tang, C. S. Schneider, J. M. Lin, M. P. Boyle, P. L. Zeitlin, S. K. Lai, M. J. Cooper, and J. Hanes. "N-Acetylcysteine Enhances Cystic Fibrosis Sputum Penetration and Airway Gene Transfer by Highly Compacted DNA Nanoparticles." *Molecular Therapy* 19, no. 11 (2011): 1981–9. doi:10.1038/mt.2011.160.

Szymańska, E., K. Winnicka, A. Amelian, and U. Cwalina. "Vaginal Chitosan Tablets with Clotrimazole-Design and Evaluation of Mucoadhesive Properties Using Porcine Vaginal Mucosa, Mucin and Gelatine." *Chemical & Pharmaceutical Bulletin* 62, no. 2 (2014): 160–7. doi:10.1248/cpb.c13-00689.

Taherali, F., F. J. Varum, and A. W. Basit. "A Slippery Slope: On the Origin, Role and Physiology of Mucus." *Advanced Drug Delivery Reviews* 124 (2018): 16–33. doi:10.1016/j.addr.2017.10.014.

Thim, L., F. Madsen, and S. S. Poulsen. "Effect of Trefoil Factors on the Viscoelastic Properties of Mucus Gels." *European Journal of Clinical Investigation* 32, no. 7 (2002): 519–27. doi:10.1046/j.1365-2362.2002.01014.x.

Twarog, C., S. Fattah, J. Heade, S. Maher, E. Fattal, and D. J. Brayden. "Intestinal Permeation Enhancers for Oral Delivery of Macromolecules: A Comparison Between Salcaprozate Sodium (SNAC) and Sodium Caprate (C10)." *Pharmaceutics* 11, no. 2 (2019): 78. doi:10.3390/pharmaceutics11020078.

Varum, F. J., F. Veiga, J. S. Sousa, and A. W. Basit. "Mucus Thickness in the Gastrointestinal Tract of Laboratory Animals." *Journal of Pharmacy & Pharmacology* 64, no. 2 (2012): 218–27. doi:10.1111/j.2042-7158.2011.01399.x.

Veerman, E. C. I., P. A. M. van den Keijbus, K. Nazmi, W. Vos, J. E. van der Wal, E. Bloemena, J. G. M. Bolscher, and A. V. Nieuw Amerongen. "Distinct Localization of MUC5B Glycoforms in the Human Salivary Glands." *Glycobiology* 13, no. 5 (2003): 363–6. doi:10.1093/glycob/cwg037.

Wan, F., M. Herzberg, Z. Huang, T. Hassenkam, and H. M. Nielsen. "A Free-Floating Mucin Layer to Investigate the Effect of the Local Microenvironment in Lungs on Mucin-Nanoparticle Interactions." *Acta Biomaterialia* 104 (2020): 115–23. doi:10.1016/j.actbio.2020.01.014.

Wang, Y. Y., and C. H. Lee. "Characterization of a Female Controlled Drug Delivery System for Microbicides." *Contraception* 66, no. 4 (2002): 281–7. doi:10.1016/S0010-7824(02)00354-2.

Wang, Y. Y., S. K. Lai, J. S. Suk, A. Pace, R. Cone, and J. Hanes. ""Addressing the PEG mucoadhesivity paradox to engineer nanoparticles that "Slip" Through the Human Mucus Barrier." *Angewandte Chemie International Edition in English* 47, no. 50 (2008): 9726–9. doi:10.1002/anie.200803526.

Wong, P. T., S. H. Wang, S. Ciotti, P. E. Makidon, D. M. Smith, Y. Fan, C. F. Schuler, and J. R. Baker. "Formulation and Characterization of Nanoemulsion Intranasal Adjuvants: Effects of Surfactant Composition on Mucoadhesion and Immunogenicity." *Molecular Pharmaceutics* 11, no. 2 (2014): 531–44. doi:10.1021/mp4005029.

Xu, Q., L. M. Ensign, N. J. Boylan, A. Schön, X. Gong, J. Yang, N. W. Lamb, S. Cai, T. Yu, E. Freire, and J. Hanes. "Impact of Surface Polyethylene Glycol (PEG) Density on Biodegradable Nanoparticle Transport in Mucus Ex Vivo and Distribution In Vivo." *ACS Nano* 9, no. 9 (2015): 9217–27. doi:10.1021/acsnano.5b03876.

Yang, M., S. K. Lai, Y. Y. Wang, W. Zhong, C. Happe, M. Zhang, J. Fu, and J. Hanes. "Biodegradable Nanoparticles Composed Entirely of Safe Materials That Rapidly Penetrate Human Mucus." *Angewandte Chemie International Edition in English* 50, no. 11 (2011): 2597–600. doi:10.1002/anie.201006849.

Yildiz, H. M., C. A. McKelvey, P. J. Marsac, and R. L. Carrier. "Size Selectivity of Intestinal Mucus to Diffusing Particulates Is Dependent on Surface Chemistry and Exposure to Lipids." *Journal of Drug Targeting* 23, no. 7–8 (2015): 768–74. doi:10.3109/1061186X.2015.1086359.

Yin, L., J. Ding, C. He, L. Cui, C. Tang, and C. L. Yin. "Drug Permeability and Mucoadhesion Properties of Thiolated Trimethyl Chitosan Nanoparticles in Oral Insulin Delivery." *Biomaterials* 30, no. 29 (2009): 5691–700. doi:10.1016/j.biomaterials.2009.06.055.

Yu, M., J. Wang, Y. Yang, C. Zhu, Q. Su, S. Guo, J. Sun, Y. Gan, X. Shi, and H. Gao. "Rotation-Facilitated Rapid Transport of Nanorods in Mucosal Tissues." *Nano Letters* 16, no. 11 (2016): 7176–82. doi:10.1021/acs.nanolett.6b03515.

Yu, M., L. Xu, F. Tian, Q. Su, N. Zheng, Y. Yang, J. Wang, A. Wang, C. Zhu, S. Guo, X. Zhang, Y. Gan, X. Shi, and H. Gao. "Rapid Transport of Deformation-Tuned Nanoparticles Across Biological Hydrogels and Cellular Barriers." *Nature Communications* 9, no. 1 (2018): 2607. doi:10.1038/s41467-018-05061-3.

Zhao, Y., L. Chen, G. E. Yakubov, T. Aminiafshar, L. Han, and G. Lian. "Experimental and Theoretical Studies on the Binding of Epigallocatechin Gallate to Purified Porcine Gastric Mucin." *Journal of Physical Chemistry. Part B* 116, no. 43 (2012): 13010–6. doi:10.1021/jp212059x.

Znamenskaya, Y., J. Sotres, J. Engblom, T. Arnebrant, and V. Kocherbitov. "Effect of Hydration on Structural and Thermodynamic Properties of Pig Gastric and Bovine Submaxillary Gland Mucins." *Journal of Physical Chemistry. Part B* 116, no. 16 (2012): 5047–55. doi:10.1021/jp212495t.

Directing Therapies to Lysosomes

13

Satya Siva Kishan Yalamarty, Xiang Li, Nina Filipczak and Vladimir Torchilin

Contents

13.1 INTRODUCTION

13.1.1 Lysosomes Structure and Discovery

Lysosomes were discovered in the 1950s. The Belgian biochemist Christian de Duve was working on purifying proteins found in rat livers when he stumbled upon bag-shaped intracellular structures. He called them the Greek word for "digestive body", because the contents of this bag were highly acidic, and contained enzymes that could break down practically any biomolecule (De Duve et al. 1955). In 1974, De Duve received the Nobel Prize for his discovery (Bowers 1998).

Since their discovery it has been shown that lysosomes exist in cells in many forms, differing in size and internal structure. Lysosomes appear as dense bodies in the cytoplasm, originally defined as

DOI: 10.1201/9781003092773-15

membrane vacuoles containing acid hydrolases with sizes of 0.2–0.3 μm. However, the lysosomal structure is very diverse and may be spherical, ovoid, or irregular in shape, with a matrix of varying degrees of
homogeneity. The morphological heterogeneity of the lysosomal population in the cytoplasm is a reflection of their different activity in a given, relevant functional state. Lysosomes are formed from the Golgi
sacs as primary lysosomes. Lysosomes are formed from the inner Golgi sacs which, in turn, are derived
from rough endoplasmic reticulum. These three components are sometimes referred to as the GERL
(Novikoff and Yam 1978).

Secondary lysosomes arise in two ways, namely by joining the primary lysosomes with a phagosome
containing the material intended for catabolite decomposition collected from the outside (heterophagy),
or by joining with cytosegregosomes, i.e., with those cell regions that have been separated from the rest
of the cytoplasm by the environment of their specific membrane (autophagy). The size and morphology of
secondary lysosomes depend on the type, structure, and chemical composition of the digestible material
and the advancement of lytic processes. Secondary lysosomes can be additionally divided into phagosomes, digestive vacuoles, or autophagosomes based on the digested material.

The activity of lysosomal hydrolases depends primarily on the pH of the environment. Lysosomes are
cellular organelles also characterized by a low pH, ranging from 3.5 to 5.5. The acidic pH facilitates the
activity of lysosomal hydrolases. Pre-hydrolysis of a number of protein substrates later increases the susceptibility of their macromolecules to further enzymatic degradation. An individual feature of lysosomes
is the latency of their enzymatic systems, i.e., the phenomenon of latent enzymatic activity. It consists of
"closing" the enzymes within the structure of the lysosome so that their activity is fully revealed only after
the destruction of these organelles by the action of physical or chemical factors (Figure 13.1).

Lysosomes have long been considered an intracellular digestive system, degrading material phagocytosed or engulfed by pinocytosis (Ericsson 1969). It is now known that lysosomes perform a number of
other functions. They participate in the natural metabolic turnover and ensure that glandular cells break
down their secretions in the presence of limited demand for them. They can also modify and activate
these secretions thanks to controlled proteolysis (Wiederanders et al. 1978).

It has now been observed that the lysosomal space contains about 100 different types of enzyme
proteins, mainly hydrolases, which are involved in the degradation of protein, carbohydrate, and fat cell

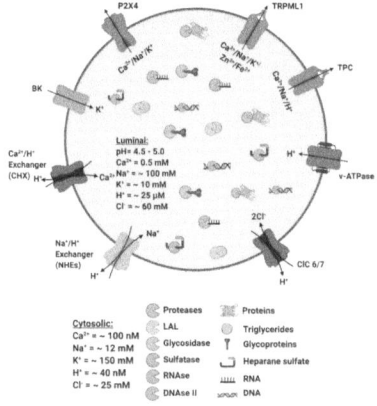

FIGURE 13.1   Ion channels and transporters present in the lysosomal membrane. Lysosomal light contains a
set of soluble substances and hydrolytic enzymes: proteases that break down proteins, acid lipase that breaks
down triglycerides, glycoprotein glycosidases and sulfatases that break down heparan sulfate, and nucleases
that break down nucleic acids. Among the ion channels and transporters present in the lysosomal membrane,
the following are distinguished: vacuolar H + -ATPase (vATPase; proton pump), chloride channel (ClC); ClC
family, which converts cytosolic Cl– to lysosomal H$^+$ (ClC-6 and ClC-7), K$^+$ channels (BK), non-selective ion
channels (TRPML); Ca^{2+}, Na$^+$, K$^+$, Zn^{2+}, and Fe^{2+} permeable, P2X4 channel; Ca^{2+}, Na$^+$, and K$^+$ permeable and
dual-pore (TPC) channels; permeable to H$^+$, Ca^{2+}, and Na$^+$. Ion transporters include Na$^+$/H$^+$ (NHE) exchangers
and Ca^{2+}/H$^+$ (CHX) exchangers (Trivedi, Bartlett, and Pulinilkunnil 2020).

structures, as well as proteoglycans, i.e., all types of cell-building substances. In 1972, Barrett provided the following list of six major groups of lysosomal enzymes, namely: (1) thiol carboxylic hydrolases (lipases, phospholipases, esterases, thioesterases); (2) hydrolases affecting phosphorus-containing linkages (acid phosphatase, phosphoprotein phosphatase, phosphoamidase, phosphatidyl phosphatase, phospholipase C, ribonuclease, deoxyribonuclease II, acid pyrophosphatase, phosphodiodiesterase, and exonuclease); (3) sulfate esterases (arylsulfatase A and B); (4) glucosidases (lysozyme, hyaluronidase, neuraminidase, β-glucuronidase, N-acetyl-pD-glucosaminidase, β-glucosidase); (5) peptidases and amidases (cathepsins A, B, D, E, acid carboxypeptidase, collagenase); (6) other. These enzymes appear in the early stages of fetal life, and their activity changes with the aging of the organism (Barrett 1984; Xu and Ren 2015). It is now known that the lysosomal system is an important element involved in the morphogenesis of tissues and organs, and its action has been described as physiological destruction (Dice et al. 1978).

13.1.2 The Lysosome as a Signaling Hub

It is also known that the lysosomal apparatus is a natural, highly dynamic system that takes part in the early adaptive responses of the organism (Figure 13.2), and is involved in maintaining internal homeostasis (Desjardins 1995). Damage to the lysosomes can cause cell death, although controlled destabilization can take place under physiological conditions. The lysosomal system provides specific protection of the cell against stress factors.

Lysosomes also contribute to the extremely important processes of autophagy, allowing the cell to use its own organelle as a source of various resources and to fight against diseases and aging processes. Their discoverer himself – De Duve – called lysosomes "suicide bags". In the case of improper metabolite management, e.g., during fasting, the lysosomal compartment is one of the first to react with the activation of specific defense mechanisms (Perera and Zoncu 2016). Recent studies show that the processes

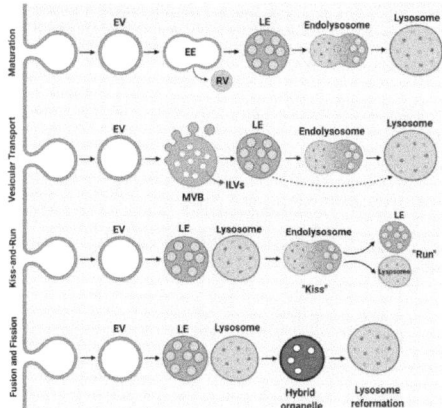

FIGURE 13.2 Phagosome biogenesis: schematic representation of the steps leading to phagosome biogenesis. Maturation: the biogenesis of lysosomes begins with the formation of endocytic vesicles (EV) from the cell membrane and their maturation into late endosomes, and then into the lysosome. The degradation load is provided by recycling vesicles (RVs) while the material to be lysosomally degraded is transported through the late endosomes. Vesicular transport: endosomal carrier vesicles (ECV) and multivesicular bodies (MVB) carrying intraluminal vesicles (ILV) are involved in this phenomenon, which mobilizes the load from early to late endosomes and then to lysosomes. They can also mobilize charge directly from the mature late endosome to the lysosomes. Kiss and Run phenomenon: Transiently the late endosome membrane (kiss) binds to the lysosome by forming fusion pores that allow the contents of the granules to be released by charge transfer and the resulting dissociation ("run") of the late endosomes from the lysosomes. Fusion and Fission: the phagosomes combine with the lysosomes to form hybrid organelles, or phagolysosomes, in which the digestion of the charge occurs (Trivedi, Bartlett, and Pulinilkunnil 2020).

inside lysosomes are mainly related to their ability to fuse and split (Saffi and Botelho 2019), exocytosis (Corrotte and Castro-Gomes 2019), positioning (de Araujo et al. 2020), and the formation of a membrane interface (Wong et al. 2019). Lysosomes are also able to reorganize inside cells toward the periphery of the cell, or to the perinuclear region (de Araujo et al. 2020). The membrane of the lysosome is also a place of contact with other organelles, which ensures the exchange of information between signaling pathways and restoration of ionic balance.

The multitude of functions performed by lysosomes makes them a molecular target for many therapies. However, for such therapies to be effective, it is necessary not only to deliver the drug but also to release it, which is associated with the participation of such processes as phagocytosis (Champion, Walker, and Mitragotri 2008), clathrin-dependent endocytosis, caveolae-mediated endocytosis (Doherty and McMahon 2009; Canton and Battaglia 2012), clathrin- and caveolae-independent endocytosis (Damm et al. 2005), and transcytosis (Tuma and Hubbard 2003).

13.1.3 Lysosome Dysfunction and Its Importance

Genetically determined disturbances in the activity of lysosomal enzymes lead to the deposition of products of incomplete catabolic transformations inside the cell organelles (mainly in lysosomes) and damage to the functions of the affected cell systems. This is known as lysosomal storage disease. This causes the growth of typical histochemical and ultrastructural changes, which are characterized by the enlargement of the affected cells, and thus of entire organs (Ballabio and Gieselmann 2009). On the other hand, an increase in the activity of some lysosomal enzymes can also be a pathogenic factor. The destabilization of lysosomal membranes is a pathogenic factor in rheumatic diseases, and in neoplastic diseases due to increased activity of lysosomal enzymes. In cancer that activity is particularly high during the period of metastasis formation. Another feature associated with the cancers involves enhancement of the autophagy–lysosome system, which enables efficient nutrient scavenging and growth in nutrient-poor microenvironments (White 2015).

Nowadays it is known that lysosomal dysfunction is connected with neurodegenerative diseases like Parkinson's disease, Alzheimer's disease, and Huntington's disease. The impaired ability of the autophagy–lysosome system to remove degraded materials leads to a domino effect that eventually compromises the viability of neuronal cells (Nixon 2013).

The ability to modulate lysosome activity is a key element in the treatment of lysosomal storage disorders (LSD), neuronal degeneration, cardiovascular diseases, infectious diseases, and autoimmune diseases. Advances in the field of targeted drug delivery allow for a more effective fight against diseases associated with lysosome dysfunction.

13.2 TARGETING THERAPIES FOR LYSOSOMES

Therapies targeted to endolysosomal pathways offer several advantages. First, to be able to utilize the specific upregulated membrane proteins in certain indications and second, to benefit from targeting the cargo to the specific organelles such as lysosomes and endosomes and treat the diseases associated with these organelles. Active targeting of the drug cargo can be achieved by either macromolecule-containing targeting moieties or complexing to a ligand. This targeting causes more buildup of the cargo inside the target than accumulation in unnecessary sites, essentially decreasing the toxicity. Ligand-targeted internalization is achieved by receptor-meditated endocytosis. Furthermore, it is necessary to pick the right ligand because the intracellular trafficking can thus be readily controlled by ligand choice. Clathrin-dependent receptor-mediated endocytosis typically ends up in lysosomes whereas clathrin-independent receptor mediated endocytosis ends up in endosomes (Bareford and Swaan 2007). Effective therapies can be developed by selecting the appropriate ligands that target either endosomes or lysosomes to treat indications such as cancer (Castino, Démoz, and Isidoro 2003), Alzheimer's disease (Tate and Mathews 2006), lysosomal storage diseases, cardiovascular diseases (Schiattarella and Hill 2016), and even infectious diseases (Sharma et al. 2018). Physicochemical properties such as size, shape, and particle charge play a key role in selective internalization and entrapment of the particles (Canton and Battaglia 2012). The particle size plays a key role in determining the endocytic pathway it is going to enter after internalization (Shang, Nienhaus, and Nienhaus 2014). For example, if the particle size is in the range of 100–300 nm the internalization happens via clathrin-mediated endocytosis, but if the particle size is 50–80 nm, the endocytosis is caveole-mediated (Rothberg et al. 1992; Anderson 1998; Kurzchalia and Partan 1999). Furthermore, properties such as surface properties and hydrophobicity also play an important role in internalization and organelle targeting. Cationic nanoparticles escape from the endosome due to a "proton sponge effect" which could help the nanoparticles evade the acidic lysosomes. Moreover, positively charged nanoparticles also show high internalization due to surface interaction between negatively charged cell surfaces (Canton and Battaglia 2012).

An accumulation of crude large molecule substrates can be caused due to malfunction of the lysosomal machinery and could have an impact on the cell homeostasis. This disruption of the homeostasis can cause pathological conditions such as cancer, neurodegenerative diseases, lysosomal storage diseases, and autoimmune diseases. Ebrahimi-Fakhari et al. suggested that any disruption of lysosome-mediated autophagy and inhibition of phagosome maturation can cause several lysosomal diseases (Ebrahimi-Fakhari et al. 2014). Targeting of the lysosomal pathways and delivering the bioactive molecules to the endolysosomal pathway can be highly beneficial and adds another facet in treating the above-mentioned diseases. Using certain targeting ligands such as antibodies, proteins, aptamers, and lectins to target certain specific markers in the disease indications can be a way to achieve the desired effect. Targeting the cell surface receptors such as transferrin and folate can be another way to target the endolysosomal pathway (Sakhrani and Padh 2013). The delivery of large molecules such as proteins/peptides poses a challenge to the delivery of the biomolecules intracellularly. However, with advanced drug delivery systems, we can overcome this problem and improve the accumulation of those molecules in lysosome.

13.2.1 Therapeutic Indications to Target Lysosomes

13.2.1.1 Cancer

Lysosomes play an important role in cancer development, and alterations in the lysosomal content, composition, and distribution can lead to cancer. As mentioned earlier lysosomes play an important role in autophagy, and any disruption of the lysosomal machinery such as their trafficking, augmented expression of cathepsins, and their instability can all cause high metastasizing and rapidly developing cancer (Fehrenbacher and Jäättelä 2005). Angiogenesis an important characteristic of highly invasive cancer, and upregulation and trafficking of the lysosomal enzymes could cause this. Cathepsin proteases are the lysosomal hydrolases that can either suppress or promote tumor growth. Their ability to suppress or promote depends on their location. For example cytosolic cathepsins can initiate the apoptotic pathway by lysosomal membrane permeabilization and thus suppress tumor growth (Kirkegaard and Jäättelä 2009). However, the extracellular cathepsins can initiate tumor-promoting proteins due to their ability to break the basement membrane (Repnik et al. 2012). Moreover, cancer progression and metastasis have been associated with hydrolases such as cathepsins B, E, and S (Withana et al. 2012; Small et al. 2013; Keliher et al. 2013).

Lysosomal membrane proteins can be potential targets with essential functions with certain cancer therapeutics. Much research has been done on luminal lysosomal hydrolases. Lysosome-associated membrane protein 1 (LAMP-1) and LAMP-2 are the two major membrane proteins and can be considered the most abundant of the outer membrane proteins (Saftig and Klumperman 2009; Saftig, Schröder, and Blanz 2010). These proteins carry out essential functions such as lysosome acidification, chaperone-mediated autophagy (CMA), and metabolite transportation (Saftig and Klumperman 2009). Evidence of cell-cell adhesion and migration is seen in the metastatic colon cancer where LAMP-1 is overexpressed on the cell surface (Furuta et al. 2001). Furthermore, the H^+-ATPase (V-ATPase) is a lysosomal membrane protein that pumps hydrogen ions into the lumen of the lysosome, increasing the proton concentration inside the lumen and thus decreasing the pH of the lysosome. Lower pH in the tumor microenvironment promotes invasive metastatic tumors, and V-ATPase plays an important role in endosomal trafficking by decreasing the pH of extracellular matrix by proton extrusion causing an acidic tumor microenvironment (Dettmer et al. 2006). Targeting this membrane protein could act as a cancer therapeutic by decreasing the proton extrusion which in turn increases the pH to decrease tumor metastasis and progression (Fais et al. 2007). The master effector in E2F1 (a transcription factor that regulates important biological functions such as growth and malignancy)-mediated lysosomal trafficking, mTOR1 activation, and autophagy in tumors is V-ATPase. Metastatic tumors overexpressing E2F1 can be inhibited by targeting V-ATPase lysosomal membrane protein (Meo-Evoli et al. 2015). Recent studies show that any malfunctions in sphingolipid metabolism also cause cancer either by decreased levels of ceramide (a proapoptotic lipid) or increased levels of sphingosine 1-phosphate (a proliferative lipid) which gives us a target to fix. The enzyme responsible could be acid sphingomyelinase (ASM) (Petersen et al. 2013; Savić and Schuchman 2013).

Lysosome membrane permeabilization (LMP) causes necrosis, autophagy, and apoptosis by liberating the enzymes into the cytosol, especially cathepsins (Patricia Boya and Kroemer 2008). LMP is a complex process with varying levels of permeabilization. Limited release of the lysosomal enzymes causes apoptosis whereas extensive release of these enzymes would cause necrosis which is of major interest in cancer therapy. Cancer cells usually mutate and cause disruptions in the apoptotic pathways which protects them from cell death (Aits, Jäättelä, and Nylandsted 2015). Reactive oxygen species (ROS) are among the many stimuli that can induce LMP and cause cathepsins to be released into the cytosol from the lysosomal lumen. Phospholipases A2 are activated due to the ROS which could degrade membrane phospholipids which in turn can breakdown the membrane and release the enzymes into the cytosol (Kurz et al. 2008). Most tumor microenvironments have higher levels of ROS which can be used as a target for cancer therapy. Furthermore, sphingosine and ceramide accumulation can also induce LMP (LeGendre, Breslin, and Foster 2015). In recent studies, it was found that RNA-dependent protein kinase R (PKR) plays a significant role in regulating misfolded protein clearance and inhibits their clearance via the exosomes and lysosomes which plays a key role in cancer cells. Apar et al. verified this claim using two PKR-associated compounds (Pac1 and 2) where Pac1 binds to the PI4K2A and disrupts the PKR/PI4K2A complex thereby destabilizing the lysosome membrane and causing cell death. This was further verified in lung and breast xenograft mouse models (Pataer et al. 2020).

Since LMP is a dynamic process, quantifying and visualization is a challenging process. Some of the methods are about detecting enzymatic activity and tracking lysosomes where we can visualize LMP using a fluorescent antibody against galectins to monitor LMP. Each of the assays and techniques have their own intrinsic technical hurdles to accurately measure the LMP. The complexity of the LMP process makes it biologically challenging as well. A careful selection of the methods and their complementary methods is necessary to measure LMP with accuracy and precision (Patricia Boya and Kroemer 2008; Aits, Jäättelä, and Nylandsted 2015; Repnik, Česen, and Turk 2014).

Alternatively, there are proteins that can protect the lysosomal membrane and inhibit LMP: heat shock protein (HSP70), LAMP-1, and LAMP-2 (Česen et al. 2012). Of the above-mentioned HSP70 investigated, it has heat-inducible and constitutively active protein components (Cuervo and Wong 2014). HSP70 is considered a very conservative chaperone protein. Many lysosomal proteins can be modulated using HSP70 specifically binding to bis- monoglycerophosphate, which activates ASM, in turn breaking down the lipid sphingomyelin. Inhibition of HSP70 can reduce ASM and should increase LMP in cancer cells (Saftig and Sandhoff 2013).

The alteration of lysosomal acidification in cancer cells can be exploited in targeting therapies. Typically, lysosomes are highly acidic and when a basic drug when enters the lysosome it causes protonation and thus their movement outside of the membrane is hindered. This defective acidification of lysosomes may prevent the basic drugs being accumulated inside the lysosome and hence leave more in the cytosol. This strategy can be exploited in cancer cells by targeting therapies to lysosomes. Strategies specifically targeting the lysosomes that enhance the concentration of the drug in the cytosol and activation of LMP can be used in more resistant cancers (Česen et al. 2012; Fehrenbacher and Jäättelä 2005; Piao and Amaravadi 2016). Some strategies for targeting lysosomes could use lysosmotropic agents, nanocarriers, metal chelators, and micelles.

The usage of lysosmotropic agents to treat cancer could utilize the lysosomal death pathways to treat cancer in addition to the conventional therapies. Contrary to hydrophobically weak bases that accumulate in lysosomes and get trapped, lysosmotropic agents are moderately basic with amino groups, that would assist in penetrating the cell membrane and activating lysosome membrane permeabilization. This process of membrane permeabilization would release the hydrolytic enzymes in the cytosol and trigger the apoptotic pathways in the cell leading to the death of the cell (Ndolo et al. 2012). Drugs such as chloroquine, chlorpromazine, thioridazine, aripiprazole, imipramine, and desipramine all have lysosmotropic properties (Firestone, Pisano, and Bonney 1979; Bhat and Hickey 2000). Many lysosmotropic detergents have been used successfully in *in vitro* models and *in vivo* xenograft models to show anticancer efficacy (Ostenfeld et al. 2008). Recently, Koshkaryev et al. have tracked the localization of liposomes modified with octadecyl-rhodamine B, a lysosmotropic detergent, into the lysosomes. This was confirmed by comparing these liposome localizations along with lysosomal markers unlike the plain liposomes (Koshkaryev et al. 2011).

Biodegradable polymers such as poly (DL-lactide-co-glycolide) (PLGA) and poly (DL-lactide) (PLA) showed increased accumulation in the lysosomes and subsequently showed enhanced lysosomal membrane destabilization (Baltazar et al. 2012). Research groups such as Gao's have shown the use of multifunctional Au–ZnO hybrid nanoparticles distorts the LMP process thereby enhancing LMP-induced apoptosis (Gao et al. 2014). Domenech et al. have shown the benefits of targeting epidermal growth factor (EGF) using magnetic iron oxide nanoparticles (MNPs) that induce LMP. They were able to achieve this by the surface modification of the MNPs with EGF, treating them in the presence of alternating magnetic fields (AMF) which assists in increased lysosomal membrane permeability and thus release of the lysosomal contents (Domenech et al. 2013). Increased LMP is directly proportional to the ROS levels in the cells causing cell death in cancer cells. They also claimed that targeting the MNPs to EGFR can enhance selectivity of the nanoparticles towards the tumor and decrease cell proliferation and that increased cell death of cancer cells alone could reduce off-target effects since EGFR is significantly overexpressed in certain cancers. Targeting the lysosomal hydrolase cathepsin B (Cat B) has been done by several research groups. This was done with the help of its substrate, a tetra peptide Gly-Leu-Phe-Gly (GLPG). A sorbitol scaffold linked to octa-guanidine and GLPG was effective in delivering doxorubicin to the cancer site (Maniganda et al. 2014). Figure 13.3 shows the schematic of the sorbitol scaffold along with the tetrapeptide used to target the lysosomes in cancer cells. Liu et al. used a natural protein, sericin, to functionalize mesoporous silica nanoparticles to target lysosomes. The low pH in the lysosomes cleaved sericin and mesoporous silica nanoparticles. The burst release of the drug and the hydrolytic enzymes of lysosomes were used in the reversal of multidrug resistance in cancer (Liu et al. 2017).

There has been a recent trend toward theranostic (both therapeutic and diagnostic) approaches in cancer where multifunctional nanomicelles were used to deliver fluorescent probes and the NIR photosensitizer, R16FP. Upon NIR irradiation the fluorescent probes lit up the lysosomes and the R16FP disrupted the lysosomes by increasing reactive oxygen species in the cells (Tian et al. 2014).

Micronutrients such as iron and copper are overconsumed by the cancer cells compared to normal cells due to their higher metabolic demands. This property can be exploited using metal chelators targeted to lysosomes (Goodman, Brewer, and Merajver 2004). Approaches to deprive the cancer cells of available metal ions using metal chelators open a door to a new chemotherapeutic tool. Chelators such as dipyridyl-thio-semi-carbazones chelate iron and copper ions to form redox-active complexes subsequently resulting in LMP. These chelators also accumulate in the lysosomes due to their ionization properties. Albumin nanoparticles containing 4,4,-di-methyl-3-thiosemicarbazone (Dp44mT) were used to target lysosomes and thus increased the selectivity and efficacy of the chelator (Merlot et al. 2015).

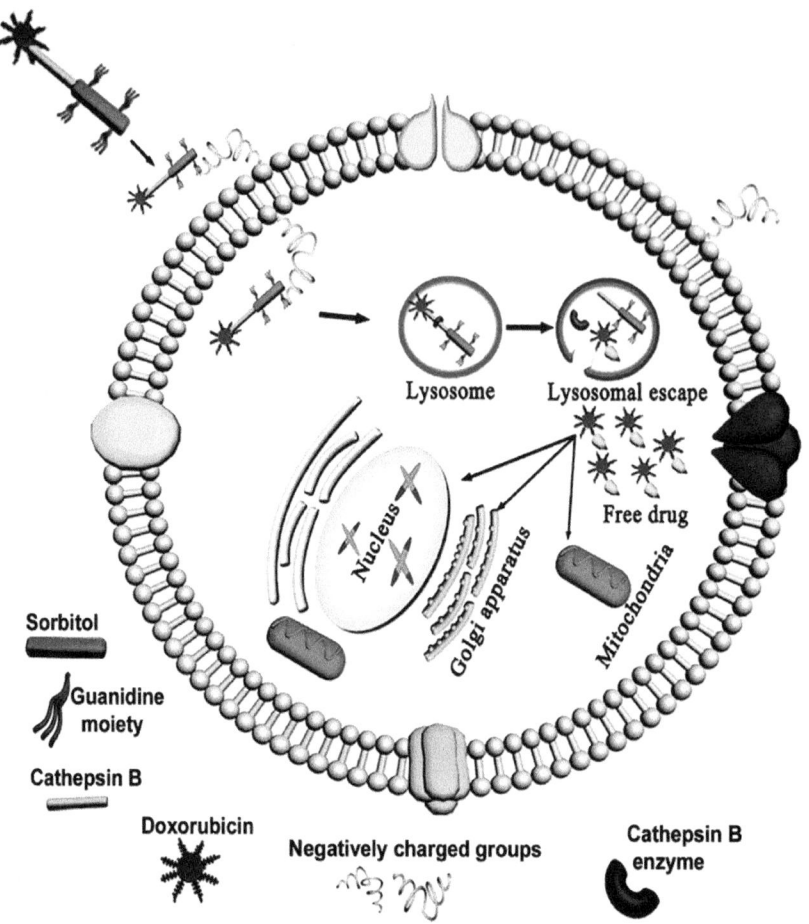

FIGURE 13.3 Mechanism of the internalization of sorbital backbone of the tetrapeptide and their electrostatic interaction of guanidine groups and the negatively charged molecules in the lipid bilayer. The doxorubicin is released intracellularly due to cathepsin B enzyme activity in the lysosome (Maniganda et al. 2014).

13.2.1.2 Neurodegenerative Diseases

There is a lot of evidence of defective endolysosomal pathways showing that the accumulation of undigested defective protein can cause several neurodegenerative diseases such as Alzheimer's disease (AD), Parkinson's disease (PD), amylotropic lateral sclerosis, and Huntington's disease. Amyloid precursor protein (APP) is a transmembrane protein present in both the cell surface and intracellular organelles including the trans-Golgi network (TGN) and endosomes (Vetrivel and Thinakaran 2006; De Strooper and Annaert 2000). β-amyloid (Aβ) peptide is generated from endosomes because a portion of the APP protein is internalized from the cell surface (Vetrivel and Thinakaran 2006; Selkoe et al. 1996; Perez et al. 1999). This Aβ peptide is an important factor in the AD pathophysiology (Hardy and Selkoe 2002). There are two predominant pathways that APP follows; one of the pathways generates Aβ peptide while the other does not. Besides ending in lysosomes, the α-secretory pathway inhibits the production of Aβ peptide because this enzyme cleaves the Aβ peptide region in APP and hence this pathway has no role in AD pathogenesis (Buxbaum et al. 1998; Lopez-Perez et al. 2001; Lammich et al. 1999; Parvathy et al. 1999). However, the second pathway, the β-secretase pathway, cleaves APP at particular areas where Aβ peptide is generated. This Aβ-peptide generated intracellularly is released into the extracellular space and forms β-amyloid plaque, a hallmark of AD and other neurogenerative diseases (Vetrivel and Thinakaran 2006; De Strooper and Annaert 2000).

Research within the past decade has shown enough evidence that along with the understanding of the proteases causing the β-amylogenic APP processing, there are also endocytic alterations in the neuronal cells of AD and AD-like diseases. Brian tissue samples from AD patients show enlarged endosomes where Aβ overproduction is seen. This shows evidence of altered endocytic mechanisms with the pathophysiological events of AD (Nixon 2005; Nixon, Mathews, and Cataldo 2001). Moreover, this brain tissue was from individuals who had the earliest stages of the disease telling us that endocytic alterations could be the reason for the early onset of the disease and serve as a marker for disease progression (Cataldo et al. 1997, 2000). Furthermore, there is evidence that enlarged endosomes are not a consequence of Aβ accumulation. This was corroborated in patients having familial AD history who showed β-amyloid plaques but no enlarged neuronal endosomes (Cataldo et al. 2001). Therefore, in sporadic AD, the cause could be altered endocytic machinery that drives the overproduction of Aβ peptide. Models have been built to predict the early onset of AD based on the alterations in endocytic functions. Several research groups have studied the Aβ level in neuronal endocytic compartments since the detection sensitivity for Aβ is very low. This was achieved by immunolabeling the brain samples (Gouras et al. 2000; Takahashi et al. 2002, 2004; Cataldo et al. 2004). There is also evidence that the abnormal endocytic system in the neuronal cells caused the increase in the soluble Aβ (not deposited as extracellular plaques) (Cataldo et al. 2004).

Accumulation of Aβ peptide in the brain is a hallmark pathophysiological feature of AD. There are several reasons this could happen, for example, the imbalance between Aβ production and clearance, neuroinflammation, nucleation of Aβ oligomers, interaction of Aβ with cofactors, and so on. But if endocytic alterations subsequently result in increased accumulation of Aβ peptide, we can use this information to develop therapies to target these endocytic compartments and maybe even use it as a preventative treatment. Several research groups have developed nanocarriers to enhance the clearance of Aβ. Acetylcholine was delivered to the lysosomes of neuronal brain cells using single-wall carbon nanotubes (SWCN) and tested in an *in vivo* mouse model for efficacy. However, there were safety and toxicity concerns that arose due to the non-biodegradable nature of SWCN (Yang et al. 2010; Xue et al. 2014). Biologically friendly apolipoprotein-E3 was used in a reconstituted model of high-density lipoprotein (ApoE3-rHDL) to act as a nanomedicine for AD to target the neuronal lysosomes since it has high affinity for Aβ (Song et al. 2014). Normal mTOR signaling and lysosomal enzyme insufficiency were reversed by restoring normal autophagy using functionalized SWNT to increase the clearance of amyloid products (Xue et al. 2014).

13.2.1.3 Autoimmune Diseases

Changes in the lysosomal membrane and enzymes are a distinguishing factor in autoimmune diseases. Many signal transduction pathways such as MHC class-II maturation, antigen processing and presenting, and antigen trafficking are regulated by lysosomes and any change, alteration, or dysfunction in lysosomal function causes abnormal immune responses (Bohgaki and Atsumi 2014; Wang and Muller 2015; Yang, Goronzy, and Weyand 2015). Lysosomal malfunction also causes increased T cell activity due to atypical presentation and maturation by antigen-presenting cells (APCs) in autoimmune diseases such as systemic lupus erythematosus (SLE) (Wang and Law 2015). Autoimmune diseases such as SLE, rheumatoid arthritis (RA), and Sjögren's syndrome (SS) develop due to abnormalities in lysosomes and their pathways that are responsible for normal autophagy processes (Wang and Law 2015; Bohgaki and Atsumi 2014). Lysosmotropic reagents can be used to alter the lysosomal function in autoimmune diseases which could increase the pH of the lysosome. Hydroxychloroquine is a compound that accumulates in the lysosome and increases its pH and has been used in encephalomyelitis animal models. Gold nanoparticles (AuNP) also accumulate in the lysosome more than the typical sodium aurothiomalate treatment. AuNP treatment also has lower toxicity and can also neutralize superoxide radicals and thereby elicit an antioxidant effect (Ghadially 1979).

13.2.1.4 Other Indications

Other common indications where lysosomes are targeted could include lysosomal storage diseases (LSDs), infectious diseases, and cardiovascular diseases. LSDs are due to undigested substrate accumulation in the lysosomes due to abnormal functioning of the lysosomal enzymes, a cofactor, or transport protein (Parenti, Andria, and Ballabio 2015). Some of the clinical manifestations for LSDs include disruption of calcium homeostasis, abnormal autophagy, and high reactive oxygen species, usually seen in children (Lara-Aguilar, Juárez-Vázquez, and Medina-Lozano 2011). Conventional approaches for LSDs include enzyme replacement therapy, gene therapy (use of adeno-associated virus), liver transplant, stem cell transplant, bone marrow transplant, and substrate reduction therapies (Ortolano et al. 2014; Watson et al. 2006). Gregoriadis et al. and Thekkedath et al. used liposomes to target hydrolytic enzymes such as β-glucosidase, α-mannosidase, and neuraminidase to digest their substrates and also used polyethyleneglycol (PEG)-coated liposomes for passive targeting (Gregoriadis and Ryman 1972; Thekkedath, Koshkaryev, and Torchilin 2013). Cell-penetrating peptides such as RGD have been used to functionalize the cell surface in order to better target the cells in recent years (Cabrera et al. 2016). The use of polymeric nanoparticles to deliver the enzymes to lysosomes is also getting popular. Gold nanoparticles have shown great efficacy in delivering the enzymes to lysosomes when conjugated with cell-penetrating peptides or lysosomal sorting peptides that target the lysosome with minimal toxicity (Dekiwadia, Lawrie, and Fecondo 2012). Transmembrane proteins such as intercellular adhesion molecule (ICAM-1) can act as a target in LSDs as they are overexpressed. Certain research groups have exploited this target by functionalizing nanoparticles with anti-ICAM-1 antibodies to efficiently target the enzymes to the target site and increase enzyme function in the body overall since LSDs are a multiorgan indication (Muro, Schuchman, and Muzykantov 2006; Hsu, Hoenicka, and Muro 2015; Rappaport, Garnacho, and Muro 2014).

Microbial infections caused by *Salmonella*, *Mycobacterium tuberculosis*, *Chlamydia*, *Brucella abortus*, *Brucella leishmania*, and *Yersinia*, etc., enter the host macrophages and halt the phagosome maturation by altering the acidic environment and use several strategies to bypass the fusion of phagosome with lysosome. Drugs that could enhance the phagosome maturation and cause the fusion of phagosome with lysosome could help overcome the microbial infections. To aid in the phagolysosome maturation, researchers have explored the physicochemical properties of drugs such as hydrophobicity and micron-sized particles to achieve the desired outcome. Another avenue researchers have explored is to activate autophagy and kill the bacterial cells inside the host and further activate programmed cell death (Underhill 2005; Zabirnyk, Yezhelyev, and Seleverstov 2007).

Autophagy plays an important role in cardiovascular diseases such as ischemic heart disease, cardiac hypertrophy and failure, cardiac arrhythmia, cardiac lysosomal storage diseases, and chemotherapy-induced cardiotoxicity (Schiattarella and Hill 2016). Autophagy done in the right dosage can be cardioprotective. However, too low or too high autophagy can be fatal. Therapies for diseases such as ischemic heart disease and cardiac hypertrophy have been characterized by increased cardiomyocyte autophagy and by a search for targets to achieve that result (Gurusamy et al. 2009; Huang et al. 2010; Nakai et al. 2007). Chemotherapy- induced cardiotoxicity is common for anticancer drugs. Increased autophagy was shown in animal models suggesting restoration of normal autophagy may be ideal in treating chemotherapy-induced cardiotoxicity (Lu et al. 2009). Targets such as mTOR1 are essential for therapies to restore normal autophagy and hence address the cardiovascular diseases caused by abnormal autophagy (Thoreen et al. 2009).

13.3 LYSOSOMES AS A DIAGNOSTIC TARGET

Lysosomes are involved in a wide variety of cellular biological activities. Visualizing lysosomes and detecting their active species, specific microenvironment, and key physiological processes not only help improve our understanding at the molecular level of how lysosomes participate in biological activities, but they also provide important guidance for treating various diseases.

As an important acidic organelle in eukaryotic cells, lysosomes contain more than 60 kinds of acid hydrolases, cathepsins, and various specific membrane proteins. Several reactive small molecules in the lysosome participate in lysosomal biochemical reactions that influence cellular physiological activities. These reactive small molecules include the hydrogen ion (H^+), reactive oxygen species (ROSs, including hydrogen peroxide and hypochlorous acid), reactive nitrogen species (NO and nitrosyl hydrogen), reducing species (the thiol compounds cysteine, hydrogen sulfide, homocysteine, and glutathione), and ions (metal cations and anions) (Yu, Xiao, and Jin 2012; Li et al. 2015; Kim et al. 2015). Thus, research on these lysosomal molecules is of great importance for the diagnosis and treatment of lysosome-related diseases.

Fluorescent probes are powerful tools that have garnered much interest in applications involving the study of cells at the subcellular level. Several lysosome-targeting fluorescent probes have been designed and synthesized to quantitatively and effectively detect temporal and spatial changes in the distribution of reactive small molecules. These fluorescent probes have been specifically designed with highly reactive groups such as primary amino and hydroxyl groups and can be easily conjugated or incorporated into nanoscale preparations to achieve molecular imaging of lysosomes at cellular, tissue, and organismic levels.

The methods used to target lysosomes have been based on mechanisms that take advantage of the physicochemical characteristics of the lysosome itself (Wu et al. 2011; Fan et al. 2012; Boya et al. 2003; Yu et al. 2014). (1) First, some amines with low molecular weights have been used as lysosome-targeting probes. The weak alkalinity levels of amines help such probes to selectively accumulate in the acidic (pH = 4.5–5.5) environment of the lysosome. (2) Some molecules with high molecular weights have also been used as lysosome-targeting probes. These probes enter the cells by being endocytosed and reach the lysosomes through a metabolic pathway. (3) Finally, substrates of the characteristic hydrolases or membrane proteins of the lysosomes have been used as specifically lysosome- recognizing probes as well.

13.3.1 Lysosomal Fluorescent Probes Based on pH Values

The acidic (pH = 4.5–5.0) environment in lysosomes is important for the activity of various biochemical processes of the lysosome. Because the pH of the lysosome is more acidic than the cytoplasm (pH = 7.0–7.3), the functional probes detecting H^+ can be used to locate the lysosome in cells and monitor the pH value of the lysosome and the related intracellular diseases. A series of lysosome-targeting pH-monitoring fluorescent probes (Superior LysoProbes) have been synthesized using the click reaction and have shown the ability to label acidic organelles and monitor lysosomal pH (Figure 13.4) (Chen et al. 2015). Superior LysoProbes combined with confocal laser scanning microscopy have been used to realize a detection of changes of lysosome morphology during the apoptosis response to lobaplatin elicited in human chloangiocarcinoma (CCA) RBE cells. By taking advantage of lysosomal membrane proteins being heavily glycosylated with numerous N-linked glycans, researchers have effected a binding between the parent spirocyclic fluorophore rhodamine and the polysaccharides to convert the rhodamine structures from a cyclic amide form to a linear amide form; this product has been shown to display measurable absorbance and fluorescence in the visible light region and to preferentially localize in the lysosome.

13.3.2 Lysosomal Fluorescent Probes Based on Their Reactions with Specific Molecules in Lysosomes

Cysteine (Cys), homocysteine (Hcy), and glutathione (GSH) are three important and universal thiols with important physiological functions. The relative amounts of sulfhydryl compounds in an organism are closely related to many diseases. For example, an abnormal cysteine content can cause yellowing of the hair, edema, lung dysfunction, and slow growth of children (Kand et al. 2015). Determining the amounts

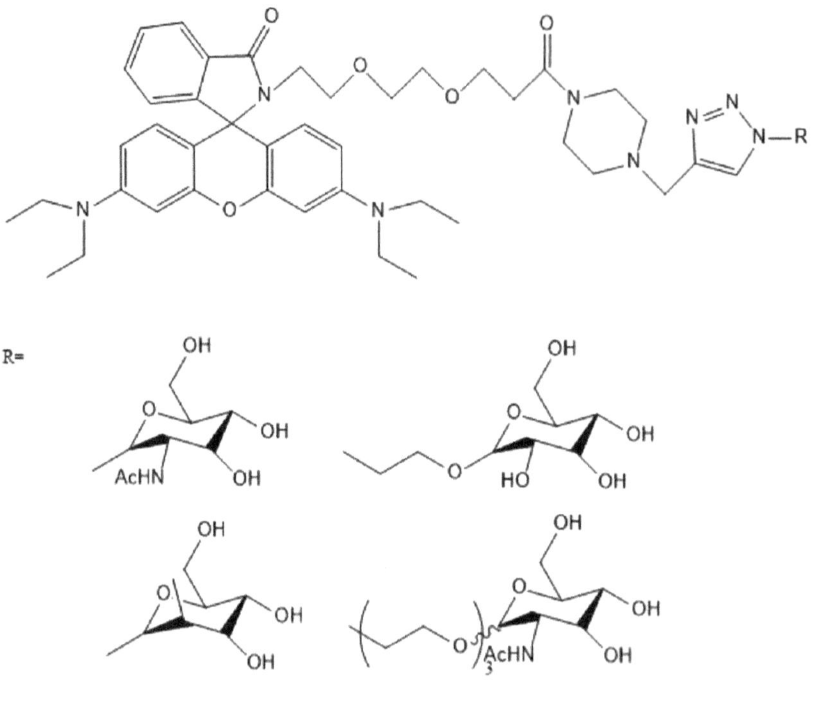

FIGURE 13.4 Rhodamine-based fluorescent probe designed to take advantage of the low pH in lysosomes.

of sulfhydryl compounds in organelles can help improve our understanding of certain important biological processes. Lysosome-specific fluorescent probes have been used to help elucidate the functions of lysosomal thiols. Nucleophilic substitution is a basic mechanism for reactions involving fluorescent thiol probes containing the 2,4-dinitrobenzenesulfonyl group. An efficient 1,8-naphthalimide-based two-photon fluorophore probe involving conjugation of a 2,4-dinitrobenzenesulfonyl chloride and morpholine has been designed. This probe exhibited high selectivity and quantitative sensitivity towards lysosomal thiols by way of turned-on fluorescence, and was shown to allow an effective monitoring of the total level of thiols in lysosomes (Fan et al. 2016).

ROS play an important role not only in many physiological processes, but also in the treatments of some diseases including cancers, neurological disorders, and cardiovascular diseases. Of the various ROS, hydrogen peroxide has become an especially important biomarker. While it is responsible for host defense, immune response, and cell signal transduction, at abnormally high levels it also causes oxidative damage to intracellular proteins, leading to accelerated aging or disease. Therefore, determining the amount of hydrogen peroxide in living cells is very important (Zhou et al. 2015; Abo et al. 2014; Bortolozzi et al. 2014). Hydrogen peroxide probes are often designed based on chemical reactions related to hydrogen peroxide, such as the oxidations of phosphine, dihydrorhodamine, and dihydrophenoxazine. In addition, probes have also been developed based on hydrogen peroxide that effect cleavage of compounds such as m-aminophenol and hydroquinone and compounds containing borate, aromatic sulfonyl, and benzyl groups (Schaferling, Grogel, and Schreml 2011). The fluorescence detection can also be achieved through the reaction of hydrogen peroxide and metalloenzymes, imitating the redox reaction occurring in the organism. A two-photon probe (Figure 13.5) with naphthimide as the parent structure, morpholine as the lysosomal-positioning group, and a borate substituent as the site of reaction with hydrogen peroxide has been synthesized (Ren et al. 2016). This probe has been used to image endogenous and exogenous hydrogen peroxide in living cells and monitor the changes in hydrogen peroxide levels in lysosomes (Figure 13.6).

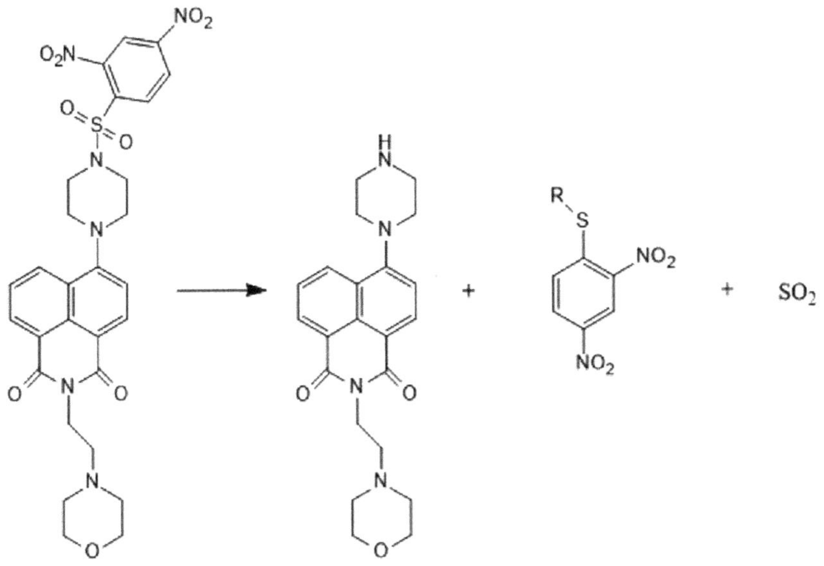

FIGURE 13.5 Fluorescent probe based on its reaction with sulfhydryl compounds.

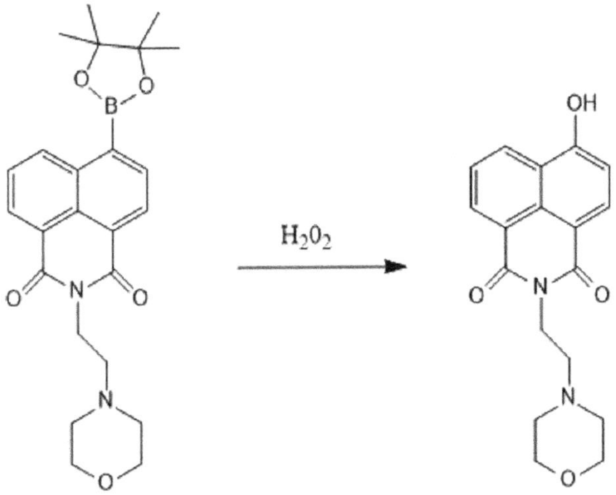

FIGURE 13.6 A fluorescent probe based on its reaction with ROSs.

ATP plays a major role in cell energy metabolism, and it is also used as an indicator of cell viability and injury. The lysosomes of astrocytes and microglia contain large amounts of ATP, which can be released as an important signaling molecule depending on Ca^{2+} exocytosis. Conjugated polymers can greatly enhance the fluorescence signal and then serve as a good optical platform for sensitive detection. Water-soluble polythiophene derivatives can be used for highly sensitive fluorescence detection of DNA, proteins, and small biological molecules, with high sensitivity, at a low detection limit (especially for ATP), and good biocompatibility (Huang et al. 2016) (Figure 13.7). These derivatives have been designed with various side chains containing different imidazolium salt groups acting as binding sites for electrostatic interaction with anions. These polymers apparently undergo random coil isomerization in liquids and combine with ATP through electrostatic interactions to form aggregates and have allowed successful real-time monitoring of ATP in lysosomes.

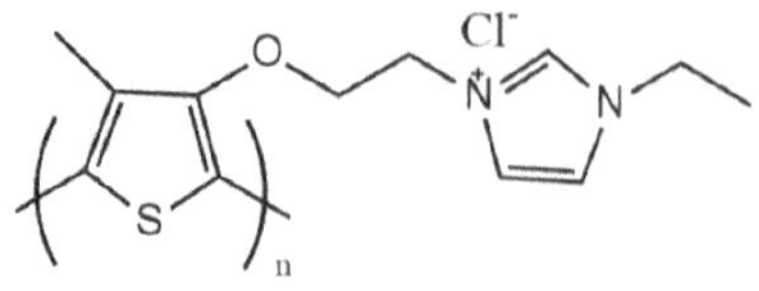

FIGURE 13.7   Fluorescent probe based on its reaction with ATP.

13.3.3 Lysosomal Fluorescent Probes Based on Their Reactions with Enzymes in Lysosomes

Enzymes in lysosomes are important to provide the ability of cells to digest themselves, and are closely involved in the decomposition of proteins, lipids, and carbohydrates. Insufficient quantities of enzymes in the lysosome can lead to a series of inherited lysosomal storage disorders (LSDs). For example, insufficient secretion of lysosomal esterase can cause Wolman's disease includes symptoms such as diarrhea, bloating, hepatomegaly and weight loss. A probe for targeting lysosomal enzyme activity (Figure 13.8) was designed to consist of three parts: the epoxysuccinyl structural unit that reacts with the active center of cysteine protease, the fluorescent signal unit (biotin), and the lysosome-penetrating peptide containing arginine residues. This probe has been confirmed as recognizing the cathepsin family members in lysosomes (Greenbaum et al. 2002).

Another probe was also developed to detect nitroreductase in lysosomes. This probe was designed to use morpholine as the lysosome-targeting group, and 4-nitro-1,8-naphthimide as both the fluorescent chromophore and the unit that reacts with nitroreductase (Figure 13.9) (Zhou et al. 2016). The mechanism of this probe has been shown to be derived from the reduction reaction catalyzed by nitroreductase, and the fluorescence of the probe was observed to be significantly enhanced after the probe was reduced to 4-amino-1,8-naphthimide. The detection limit of this probe for nitroreductase was measured to be 2.2 ng/mL, hence this probe can be used for fluorescence imaging of nitroreductase in hypoxic conditions. The results of the study showed that in hypoxic conditions, the level of nitroreductase in the lysosomes was higher than that in the cytoplasm.

Lysosomal probes have been applied to the fluorescence imaging of various cancer cells and can be used to demonstrate the dynamic monitoring of various substances in lysosomes in biological systems. By determining the amounts of various lysosome enzymes, many cells at different stages have been

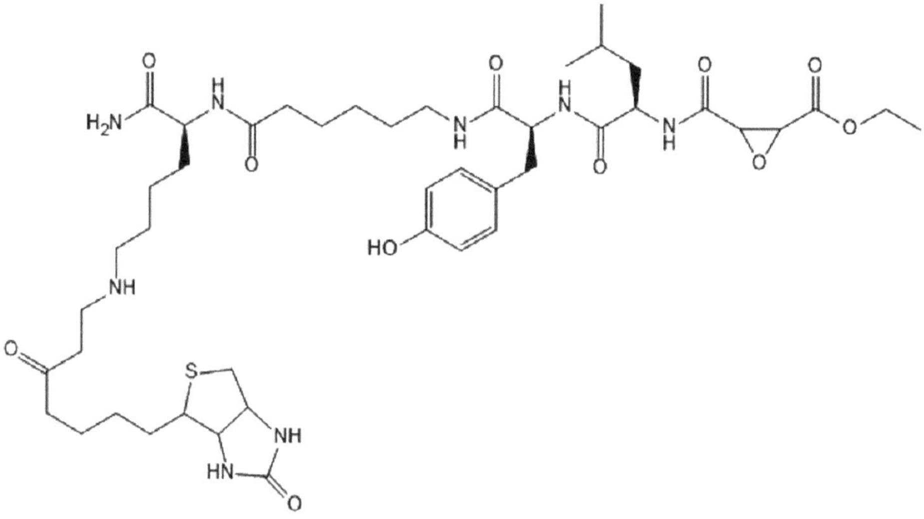

FIGURE 13.8   Fluorescent probe based on its reaction with cathepsins.

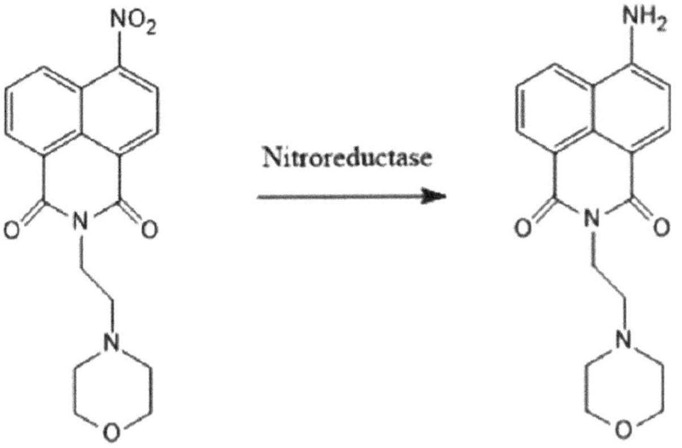

FIGURE 13.9 Fluorescent probe based on its reaction with nitroreductase.

quantitatively analyzed. In-depth research using lysosomal probes is expected to help further understanding of the molecular mechanisms of biological activities involved in lysosomes, as well as the causes and factors controlling lysosome-related diseases. The use of lysosomal probes for early diagnosis and even late treatment of diseases is expected to become one of the important directions of development in this field.

13.4 SUMMARY

The ability to target lysosomes unlocks a great potential in developing new therapies and also diagnostic tools to address a myriad of indications. Lysosomes have been traditionally viewed as the suicidal bags of the cells. However, with the recent developments outlined in this chapter it is clear that there are additional, important cellular pathways that lysosomes interact within a cell, which can be exploited to target certain indications. The therapeutic potential in targeting endolysosomal pathways is enormous. Lysosomes also participate in autophagy, an important cellular process that controls various functions inside the cell. Furthermore, the diagnostic applications in lysosomes are also likely to be very useful in the early detection of diseases which may result in a paradigm shift in the treatment of diseases. More research has to be done to explore and understand the processes lysosomes are involved in inside the cell to develop more smart therapies and diagnostics.

REFERENCES

Abo, M., R. Minakami, K. Miyano, M. Kamiya, T. Nagano, Y. Urano, and H. Sumimoto. "Visualization of Phagosomal Hydrogen Peroxide Production by a Novel Fluorescent Probe That Is Localized via SNAP-Tag Labeling." *Analytical Chemistry* 86, no. 12 (2014): 5983–90. doi:10.1021/ac501041w.

Aits, Sonja, Marja Jäättelä, and Jesper Nylandsted. "Methods for the Quantification of Lysosomal Membrane Permeabilization: A Hallmark of Lysosomal Cell Death." *Methods in Cell Biology* 126 (2015): 261–85.

Anderson, Richard G. W. "The Caveolae Membrane System." *Annual Review of Biochemistry* 67, no. 1 (1998): 199–225.

Ballabio, A., and V. Gieselmann. "Lysosomal Disorders: From Storage to Cellular Damage." *Biochimica & Biophysica Acta* 4, no. 4 (2009) 1793: 684–96. doi:10.1016/j.bbamcr.2008.12.001.

Baltazar, Gabriel C., Sonia Guha, Wennan Lu, Jason Lim, Kathleen Boesze-Battaglia, Alan M. Laties, Puneet Tyagi, Uday B. Kompella, and Claire H. Mitchell. "Acidic Nanoparticles Are Trafficked to Lysosomes and Restore an Acidic Lysosomal pH and Degradative Function to Compromised ARPE-19 Cells." *PLOS ONE* 7, no. 12 (2012): e49635.

Bareford, Lisa M., and Peter W. Swaan. "Endocytic Mechanisms for Targeted Drug Delivery." *Advanced Drug Delivery Reviews* 59, no. 8 (2007): 748–58.

Barrett, A. J. "Proteolytic and Other Metabolic Pathways in Lysosomes." *Biochemical Society Transactions* 12, no. 6 (1984): 899–902. doi:10.1042/bst0120899.

Bhat, Meenakshi, and Anthony J. Hickey. "Effect of Chloroquine on Phagolysosomal Fusion in Cultured Guinea Pig Alveolar Macrophages: Implications in Drug Delivery." *AAPS PharmSci* 2, no. 4 (2000): 12–8.

Bohgaki, Toshiyuki, and Tatsuya Atsumi. "Autophagy in Autoimmune Disease." *Japanese Journal of Clinical Immunology* 37, no. 3 (2014): 125–32. doi:10.2177/jsci.37.125. https://europepmc.org/abstract/MED/24974923.

Bortolozzi, R., S. von Gradowski, H. Ihmels, K. Schäfer, and G. Viola. "Selective Ratiometric Detection of H2O2 in Water and in Living Cells with Boronobenzo[b]Quinolizinium Derivatives." *Chemical Communications* 50, no. 60 (2014): 8242–5. doi:10.1039/c4cc02283a.

Bowers, William E. "Christian de Duve and the Discovery of Lysosomes and Peroxisomes." *Trends in Cell Biology* 8, no. 8 (1998): 330–3. doi:10.1016/S0962-8924(98)01314-2. https://www.sciencedirect.com/science/article/pii/S0962892498013142.

Boya, P., K. Andreau, D. Poncet, N. Zamzami, J. L. Perfettini, D. Metivier, D. M. Ojcius, M. Jäättelä, and G. Kroemer. "Lysosomal Membrane Permeabilization Induces Cell Death in a Mitochondrion-Dependent Fashion." *Journal of Experimental Medicine* 197, no. 10 (2003): 1323–34. doi:10.1084/jem.20021952.

Boya, Patricia, and Guido Kroemer. "Lysosomal Membrane Permeabilization in Cell Death." *Oncogene* 27, no. 50 (2008): 6434–51.

Buxbaum, Joseph D., Kang-Nian Liu, Yuxia Luo, Jennifer L. Slack, Kim L. Stocking, Jacques J. Peschon, Richard S. Johnson, Beverly J. Castner, Douglas Pat Cerretti, and Roy A. Black. "Evidence That Tumor Necrosis Factor α Converting Enzyme Is Involved in Regulated α-Secretase Cleavage of the Alzheimer Amyloid Protein Precursor." *Journal of Biological Chemistry* 273, no. 43 (1998): 27765–7.

Cabrera, Ingrid, Ibane Abasolo, José L. Corchero, Elisa Elizondo, Gil Pilar Rivera, Evelyn Moreno, Jordi Faraudo, Santi Sala, Dolores Bueno, Elisabet González-Mira, M. Rivas, M. Melgarejo, D. Pulido, F. Albericio, M. Royo, A. Villaverde, M. F. García-Parajo, S. Schwartz, N. Ventosa, and J. Veciana. "α-Galactosidase-A Loaded-Nanoliposomes with Enhanced Enzymatic Activity and Intracellular Penetration." *Advanced Healthcare Materials* 5, no. 7 (2016): 829–40.

Canton, Irene, and Giuseppe Battaglia. "Endocytosis at the Nanoscale." *Chemical Society Reviews* 41, no. 7 (2012): 2718–39.

Castino, Roberta, Marina Démoz, and Ciro Isidoro. "Destination 'Lysosome': A Target Organelle for Tumour Cell Killing?. " *Journal of Molecular Recognition* 16, no. 5 (2003): 337–48.

Cataldo, Anne M., Jody L. Barnett, Cristiana Pieroni, and Ralph A. Nixon. "Increased Neuronal Endocytosis and Protease Delivery to Early Endosomes in Sporadic Alzheimer's Disease: Neuropathologic Evidence for a Mechanism of Increased β-Amyloidogenesis." *Journal of Neuroscience* 17, no. 16 (1997): 6142–51.

Cataldo, Anne M., Suzana Petanceska, Nicole B. Terio, Corrinne M. Peterhoff, Robert Durham, Marc Mercken, Pankaj D. Mehta, Joseph Buxbaum, Vahram Haroutunian, and Ralph A. Nixon. "Aβ Localization in Abnormal Endosomes: Association with Earliest Aβ Elevations in AD and Down Syndrome." *Neurobiology of Aging* 25, no. 10 (2004): 1263–72.

Cataldo, Anne M., Corrinne M. Peterhoff, Juan C. Troncoso, Teresa Gomez-Isla, Bradley T. Hyman, and Ralph A. Nixon. "Endocytic Pathway Abnormalities Precede Amyloid β Deposition in Sporadic Alzheimer's Disease and Down Syndrome: Differential Effects of APOE Genotype and Presenilin Mutations." *American Journal of Pathology* 157, no. 1 (2000): 277–86.

Cataldo, Anne, G. William Rebeck, Bernadino Ghetti, Christine Hulette, Carol Lippa, Christine Van Broeckhoven, Cornelia Van Duijn, Patrick Cras, Nenad Bogdanovic, Thomas Bird, C. Peterhoff, and R. Nixon. "Endocytic Disturbances Distinguish Among Subtypes of Alzheimer's Disease and Related Disorders." *Annals of Neurology* 50, no. 5 (2001): 661–5.

Česen, Maruša Hafner, Katarina Pegan, Aleš Špes, and Boris Turk. "Lysosomal Pathways to Cell Death and Their Therapeutic Applications." *Experimental Cell Research* 318, no. 11 (2012): 1245–51.

Champion, J. A., A. Walker, and S. Mitragotri. "Role of Particle Size in Phagocytosis of Polymeric Microspheres." *Pharmaceutical Research* 25, no. 8 (2008): 1815–21. doi:10.1007/s11095-008-9562-y.

Chen, X., Y. Bi, T. Wang, P. Li, X. Yan, S. Hou, C. E. Bammert, J. Ju, K. M. Gibson, W. J. Pavan, and L. Bi. "Lysosomal Targeting with Stable and Sensitive Fluorescent Probes (Superior LysoProbes): Applications for Lysosome Labeling and Tracking During Apoptosis." *Scientific Reports* 5 (2015): 9004. doi:10.1038/srep09004.

Corrotte, M., and T. Castro-Gomes. "Lysosomes and Plasma Membrane Repair." *Current Topics in Membranes* 84 (2019): 1–16. doi:10.1016/bs.ctm.2019.08.001.

Cuervo, Ana Maria, and Esther Wong. "Chaperone-Mediated Autophagy: Roles in Disease and Aging." *Cell Research* 24, no. 1 (2014): 92–104.

Damm, E. M., L. Pelkmans, J. Kartenbeck, A. Mezzacasa, T. Kurzchalia, and A. Helenius. "Clathrin- and caveolin-1-independent Endocytosis: Entry of Simian Virus 40 into Cells Devoid of Caveolae." *Journal of Cell Biology* 168, no. 3 (2005): 477–88. doi:10.1083/jcb.200407113.

de Araujo, M. E. G., G. Liebscher, M. W. Hess, and L. A. Huber. "Lysosomal Size Matters." *Traffic* 21, no. 1 (2020): 60–75. doi:10.1111/tra.12714.

De Duve, C., B. C. Pressman, R. Gianetto, R. Wattiaux, and F. Appelmans. "Tissue Fractionation Studies. 6. Intracellular Distribution Patterns of Enzymes in Rat-Liver Tissue." *Biochemical Journal* 60, no. 4 (1955): 604–17. doi:10.1042/bj0600604.

De Strooper, Bart, and Wim Annaert. "Proteolytic Processing and Cell Biological Functions of the Amyloid Precursor Protein." *Journal of Cell Science* 113, no. 11 (2000): 1857–70.

Dekiwadia, Chaitali D., Ann C. Lawrie, and John V. Fecondo. "Peptide-Mediated Cell Penetration and Targeted Delivery of Gold Nanoparticles into Lysosomes." *Journal of Peptide Science* 18, no. 8 (2012): 527–34.

Desjardins, M. "Biogenesis of Phagolysosomes: The 'Kiss and Run' Hypothesis." *Trends in Cell Biology* 5, no. 5 (1995): 183–6. doi:10.1016/s0962-8924(00)88989-8.

Dettmer, Jan, Anne Hong-Hermesdorf, York-Dieter Stierhof, and Karin Schumacher. "Vacuolar H+-ATPase Activity Is Required for Endocytic and Secretory Trafficking in Arabidopsis." *Plant Cell* 18, no. 3 (2006): 715–30.

Dice, J. F., C. D. Walker, B. Byrne, and A. Cardiel. "General Characteristics of Protein Degradation in Diabetes and Starvation." *Proceedings of the National Academy of Sciences of the United States of America* 75, no. 5 (1978): 2093–7. doi:10.1073/pnas.75.5.2093.

Doherty, G. J., and H. T. McMahon. "Mechanisms of Endocytosis." *Annual Review of Biochemistry* 78 (2009): 857–902. doi:10.1146/annurev.biochem.78.081307.110540.

Domenech, Maribella, Ileana Marrero-Berrios, Madeline Torres-Lugo, and Carlos Rinaldi. "Lysosomal Membrane Permeabilization by Targeted Magnetic Nanoparticles in Alternating Magnetic Fields." *ACS Nano* 7, no. 6 (2013): 5091–101.

Ebrahimi-Fakhari, Darius, Lara Wahlster, Georg F. Hoffmann, and Stefan Kölker. "Emerging Role of Autophagy in Pediatric Neurodegenerative and Neurometabolic Diseases." *Pediatric Research* 75, no. 1 (2014): 217–26.

Ericsson, J. L. "Studies on Induced Cellular Autophagy. I. Electron Microscopy of Cells with In Vivo Labelled Lysosomes." *Experimental Cell Research* 55, no. 1 (1969): 95–106. doi:10.1016/0014-4827(69)90462-5.

Fais, Stefano, Angelo De Milito, Haiyan You, and Wenxin Qin. "Targeting Vacuolar H+-ATPases as a New Strategy Against Cancer." *Cancer Research* 67, no. 22 (2007): 10627–30.

Fan, F., S. Nie, D. Yang, M. Luo, H. Shi, and Y. H. Zhang. "Labeling Lysosomes and Tracking Lysosome-Dependent Apoptosis with a Cell-Permeable Activity-Based Probe." *Bioconjugate Chemistry* 23, no. 6 (2012): 1309–17. doi:10.1021/bc300143p.

Fan, J., Z. Han, Y. Kang, and X. Peng. "A Two-Photon Fluorescent Probe for Lysosomal Thiols in Live Cells and Tissues." *Scientific Reports* 6 (2016): 19562. doi:10.1038/srep19562.

Fehrenbacher, Nicole, and Marja Jäättelä. "Lysosomes as Targets for Cancer Therapy." *Cancer Research* 65, no. 8 (2005): 2993–5.

Firestone, Raymond A., Judith M. Pisano, and Robert J. Bonney. "Lysosomotropic Agents. 1. Synthesis and Cytotoxic Action of Lysosomotropic Detergents." *Journal of Medicinal Chemistry* 22, no. 9 (1979): 1130–3.

Furuta, Koh, Masato Ikeda, Yoshifuku Nakayama, Kenjiro Nakamura, Masao Tanaka, Naotaka Hamasaki, Masaru Himeno, Stanley R. Hamilton, and J. Thomas August. "Expression of Lysosome-Associated Membrane Proteins in Human Colorectal Neoplasms and Inflammatory Diseases." *American Journal of Pathology* 159, no. 2 (2001): 449–55.

Gao, Wen, Wenhua Cao, Huaibin Zhang, Ping Li, Kehua Xu, and Bo Tang. "Targeting Lysosomal Membrane Permeabilization to Induce and Image Apoptosis in Cancer Cells by Multifunctional Au–ZnO Hybrid Nanoparticles." *Chemical Communications* 50, no. 60 (2014): 8117–20.

Ghadially, F. N. "The Aurosome." *Journal of Rheumatology* 5 (1979): 45–50.

Goodman, V. L., G. J. Brewer, and S. D. Merajver. "Copper Deficiency as an Anti-Cancer Strategy." *Endocrine-Related Cancer* 11, no. 2 (2004): 255–63.

Gouras, Gunnar K., Julia Tsai, Jan Naslund, Bruno Vincent, Mark Edgar, Frederic Checler, Jeffrey P. Greenfield, Vahram Haroutunian, Joseph D. Buxbaum, Huaxi Xu, P. Greengard, and N. R. Relkin. "Intraneuronal Aβ42 Accumulation in Human Brain." *American Journal of Pathology* 156, no. 1 (2000): 15–20.

Greenbaum, D., A. Baruch, L. Hayrapetian, Z. Darula, A. Burlingame, K. F. Medzihradszky, and M. Bogyo. "Chemical Approaches for Functionally Probing the Proteome." *Molecular & Cellular Proteomics* 1, no. 1 (2002): 60–8. doi:10.1074/mcp.t100003-mcp200.

Gregoriadis, Gregory, and Brenda E. Ryman. "Lysosomal Localization of β-Fructofuranosidase-Containing Liposomes Injected into Rats. Some Implications in the Treatment of Genetic Disorders." *Biochemical Journal* 129, no. 1 (1972): 123–33.

Gurusamy, Narasimman, Istvan Lekli, Nikolai V. Gorbunov, Mihaela Gherghiceanu, Lawrence M. Popescu, and Dipak K. Das. "Cardioprotection by Adaptation to Ischaemia Augments Autophagy in Association with BAG-1 Protein." *Journal of Cellular & Molecular Medicine* 13, no. 2 (2009): 373–87.

Hardy, John, and Dennis J. Selkoe. "The Amyloid Hypothesis of Alzheimer's Disease: Progress and Problems on the Road to Therapeutics. " *Science* 297, no. 5580 (2002): 353–6.

Hsu, Janet, Janet Hoenicka, and Silvia Muro. "Targeting, Endocytosis, and Lysosomal Delivery of Active Enzymes to Model Human Neurons by ICAM-1-Targeted Nanocarriers." *Pharmaceutical Research* 32, no. 4 (2015): 1264–78.

Huang, B. H., Z. R. Geng, X. Y. Ma, C. Zhang, Z. Y. Zhang, and Z. L. Wang. "Lysosomal ATP Imaging in Living Cells by a Water-Soluble Cationic Polythiophene Derivative." *Biosensors & Bioelectronics* 83 (2016): 213–20. doi:10.1016/j.bios.2016.04.064.

Huang, Chengqun, Smadar Yitzhaki, Cynthia N. Perry, Wayne Liu, Zoltan Giricz, Robert M. Mentzer, and Roberta A. Gottlieb. "Autophagy Induced by Ischemic Preconditioning Is Essential for Cardioprotection." *Journal of Cardiovascular Translational Research* 3, no. 4 (2010): 365–73.

Kand, D., T. Saha, M. Lahiri, and P. Talukdar. "Lysosome Targeting Fluorescence Probe for Imaging Intracellular Thiols." *Organic & Biomolecular Chemistry* 13, no. 30 (2015): 8163–8. doi:10.1039/c5ob00889a.

Keliher, Edmund J., Thomas Reiner, Sarah Earley, Jenna Klubnick, Carlos Tassa, Andrew J. Lee, Sridhar Ramaswamy, Nabeel Bardeesy, Douglas Hanahan, and Ronald A. DePinho, C. M. Castro, and R. Weissleder. "Targeting Cathepsin E in Pancreatic Cancer by a Small Molecule Allows In Vivo Detection." *Neoplasia* 15, no. 7 (2013): 684-IN3.

Kim, D., G. Kim, S. J. Nam, J. Yin, and J. Yoon. "Visualization of Endogenous and Exogenous Hydrogen Peroxide Using a Lysosome-Targetable Fluorescent Probe." *Scientific Reports* 5 (2015): 8488. doi:10.1038/srep08488.

Kirkegaard, Thomas, and Marja Jäättelä. "Lysosomal Involvement in Cell Death and Cancer." *Biochimica & Biophysica Acta (BBA)-Molecular Cell Research* 1793, no. 4 (2009): 746–54.

Koshkaryev, Alexander, Ritesh Thekkedath, Cinzia Pagano, Igor Meerovich, and Vladimir P. Torchilin. "Targeting of Lysosomes by Liposomes Modified with Octadecyl-Rhodamine B." *Journal of Drug Targeting* 19, no. 8 (2011): 606–14.

Kurz, Tino, Alexei Terman, Bertil Gustafsson, and Ulf T. Brunk. "Lysosomes in Iron Metabolism, Ageing and Apoptosis." *Histochemistry & Cell Biology* 129, no. 4 (2008): 389–406.

Kurzchalia, Teymuras V., and Robert G. Partan. "Membrane Microdomains and Caveolae." *Current Opinion in Cell Biology* 11, no. 4 (1999): 424–31.

Lammich, Sven, Elzbieta Kojro, Rolf Postina, Sandra Gilbert, Roland Pfeiffer, Marek Jasionowski, Christian Haass, and Falk Fahrenholz. "Constitutive and Regulated α-Secretase Cleavage of Alzheimer's Amyloid Precursor Protein by a Disintegrin Metalloprotease." *Proceedings of the National Academy of Sciences* 96, no. 7 (1999): 3922–7.

Lara-Aguilar, Ricardo Alejandro, Clara Ibet Juárez-Vázquez, and Claudina Medina-Lozano. "Therapy of Lysosomal Storage Diseases: Update and Perspectives." *Revista de Investigación Clínica* 63, no. 6 (2011): 651–8.

LeGendre, Onica, Paul A. S. Breslin, and David A. Foster. "(-)-Oleocanthal Rapidly and Selectively Induces Cancer Cell Death via Lysosomal Membrane Permeabilization." *Molecular & Cellular Oncology* 2, no. 4 (2015): e1006077.

Li, H., C. Wang, M. She, Y. Zhu, J. Zhang, Z. Yang, P. Liu, Y. Wang, and J. Li. "Two Rhodamine Lactam Modulated Lysosome-Targetable Fluorescence Probes for Sensitively and Selectively Monitoring Subcellular Organelle pH Change." *Analytica Chimica Acta* 900 (2015): 97–102. doi:10.1016/j.aca.2015.10.021.

Liu, Jia, Qilin Li, Jinxiang Zhang, Lei Huang, Chao Qi, Luming Xu, Xingxin Liu, Guobin Wang, Lin Wang, and Zheng Wang. "Safe and Effective Reversal of Cancer Multidrug Resistance Using Sericin-Coated Mesoporous Silica Nanoparticles for Lysosome-Targeting Delivery in Mice." *Small* 13, no. 9 (2017). PubMed: 1602567.

Lopez-Perez, Elvira, Yue Zhang, Stuart J. Frank, John Creemers, Nabil Seidah, and Frédéric Checler. "Constitutive α-Secretase Cleavage of the β-Amyloid Precursor Protein in the Furin-Deficient LoVo Cell Line: Involvement of the Pro-Hormone Convertase 7 and the Disintegrin Metalloprotease ADAM10." *Journal of Neurochemistry* 76, no. 5 (2001): 1532–9.

Lu, Lihe, Weikang Wu, Jianyun Yan, Xiaohong Li, Yu Huimin, and Yu Xiyong. "Adriamycin-Induced Autophagic Cardiomyocyte Death Plays a Pathogenic Role in a Rat Model of Heart Failure." *International Journal of Cardiology* 134, no. 1 (2009): 82–90.

Maniganda, Santhi, Vandana Sankar, Jyothi B. Nair, K. G. Raghu, and Kaustabh K. Maiti. "A Lysosome-Targeted Drug Delivery System Based on Sorbitol Backbone Towards Efficient Cancer Therapy." *Organic & Biomolecular Chemistry* 12, no. 34 (2014): 6564–9.

Meo-Evoli, Nathalie, Eugènia Almacellas, Francesco Alessandro Massucci, Antonio Gentilella, Santiago Ambrosio, Sara C. Kozma, George Thomas, and Albert Tauler. "V-ATPase: A Master Effector of E2F1-Mediated Lysosomal Trafficking, mTORC1 Activation and Autophagy." *Oncotarget* 6, no. 29 (2015): 28057.

Merlot, Angelica M., Sumit Sahni, Darius J. R. Lane, Ashleigh M. Fordham, Namfon Pantarat, David E. Hibbs, Vera Richardson, Munikumar R. Doddareddy, Jennifer A. Ong, Michael L. H. Huang, D. R. Richardson, and D. S. Kalinowski. "Potentiating the Cellular Targeting and Anti-Tumor Activity of Dp44mT via Binding to Human Serum Albumin: Two Saturable Mechanisms of Dp44mT Uptake by Cells." *Oncotarget* 6, no. 12 (2015): 10374.

Muro, Silvia, Edward H. Schuchman, and Vladimir R. Muzykantov. "Lysosomal Enzyme Delivery by ICAM-1-Targeted Nanocarriers Bypassing Glycosylation-And Clathrin-Dependent Endocytosis." *Molecular Therapy* 13, no. 1 (2006): 135–41.

Nakai, Atsuko, Osamu Yamaguchi, Toshihiro Takeda, Yoshiharu Higuchi, Shungo Hikoso, Masayuki Taniike, Shigemiki Omiya, Isamu Mizote, Yasushi Matsumura, Michio Asahi, K. Nishida, M. Hori, N. Mizushima, and K. Otsu. "The Role of Autophagy in Cardiomyocytes in the Basal State and in Response to Hemodynamic Stress." *Nature Medicine* 13, no. 5 (2007): 619–24.

Ndolo, Rosemary A., Yepeng Luan, Shaofeng Duan, M. Laird Forrest, and Jeffrey P. Krise. "Lysosomotropic Properties of Weakly Basic Anticancer Agents Promote Cancer Cell Selectivity In Vitro." *PLOS ONE* 7, no. 11 (2012): e49366.

Nixon, Ralph A. "Endosome Function and Dysfunction in Alzheimer's Disease and Other Neurodegenerative Diseases." *Neurobiology of Aging* 26, no. 3 (2005): 373–82.

Nixon, Ralph A. "The Role of Autophagy in Neurodegenerative Disease." *Nature Medicine* 19, no. 8 (2013): 983–97. doi:10.1038/nm.3232.

Nixon, Ralph A., Paul M. Mathews, and Anne M. Cataldo. "The Neuronal Endosomal-Lysosomal System in Alzheimer's Disease." *Journal of Alzheimer's Disease* 3, no. 1 (2001): 97–107.

Novikoff, P. M., and A. Yam. "Sites of Lipoprotein Particles in Normal Rat Hepatocytes." *Journal of Cell Biology* 76, no. 1 (1978): 1–11. doi:10.1083/jcb.76.1.1.

Ortolano, Saida, Irene Vieitez, Carmen Navarro, and Carlos Spuch. "Treatment of Lysosomal Storage Diseases: Recent Patents and Future Strategies." *Recent Patents on Endocrine, Metabolic & Immune Drug Discovery* 8, no. 1 (2014): 9–25.

Ostenfeld, Marie Stampe, Maria Høyer-Hansen, Lone Bastholm, Nicole Fehrenbacher, Ole Dines Olsen, Line Groth-Pedersen, Pietri Puustinen, Thomas Kirkegaard-Sørensen, Jesper Nylandsted, and Thomas Farkas. "Anti-Cancer Agent Siramesine Is a Lysosomotropic Detergent That Induces Cytoprotective Autophagosome Accumulation." *Autophagy* 4, no. 4 (2008): 487–99.

Parenti, Giancarlo, Generoso Andria, and Andrea Ballabio. "Lysosomal Storage Diseases: From Pathophysiology to Therapy." *Annual Review of Medicine* 66 (2015): 471–86.

Parvathy, S., Ishrut Hussain, Eric H. Karran, Anthony J. Turner, and Nigel M. Hooper. "Cleavage of Alzheimer's Amyloid Precursor Protein by α-Secretase Occurs at the Surface of Neuronal Cells." *Biochemistry* 38, no. 30 (1999): 9728–34.

Pataer, Apar, Bulent Ozpolat, RuPing Shao, Neil R. Cashman, Steven S. Plotkin, Charles E. Samuel, Steven H. Lin, Nashwa N. Kabil, Jing Wang, Mourad Majidi, B. Fang, J. A. Roth, A. A. Vaporciyan, I. I. Wistuba, M. C. Hung, and S. G. Swisher. "Therapeutic Targeting of the PI4K2A/PKR Lysosome Network Is Critical for Misfolded Protein Clearance and Survival in Cancer Cells." *Oncogene* 39, no. 4 (2020): 801–13.

Perera, R. M., and R. Zoncu. "The Lysosome as a Regulatory Hub." *Annual Review of Cell & Developmental Biology* 32 (2016): 223–53. doi:10.1146/annurev-cellbio-111315-125125.

Perez, Ruth G., Salvador Soriano, Jay D. Hayes, Beth Ostaszewski, Weiming Xia, Dennis J. Selkoe, Xiaohua Chen, Gorazd B. Stokin, and Edward H. Koo. "Mutagenesis Identifies New Signals for β-Amyloid Precursor Protein Endocytosis, Turnover, and the Generation of Secreted Fragments, Including Aβ42." *Journal of Biological Chemistry* 274, no. 27 (1999): 18851–6.

Petersen, Nikolaj H. T., Ole D. Olsen, Line Groth-Pedersen, Anne-Marie Ellegaard, Mesut Bilgin, Susanne Redmer, Marie S. Ostenfeld, Danielle Ulanet, Tobias H. Dovmark, Andreas Lønborg, S. D. Vindeløv, D. Hanahan, C. Arenz, C. S. Ejsing, T. Kirkegaard, M. Rohde, J. Nylandsted, and M. Jäättelä. "Transformation-Associated Changes in Sphingolipid Metabolism Sensitize Cells to Lysosomal Cell Death Induced by Inhibitors of Acid Sphingomyelinase." *Cancer Cell* 24, no. 3 (2013): 379–93.

Piao, Shengfu, and Ravi K. Amaravadi. "Targeting the Lysosome in Cancer." *Annals of the New York Academy of Sciences* 1371, no. 1 (2016): 45.

Rappaport, Jeff, Carmen Garnacho, and Silvia Muro. "Clathrin-Mediated Endocytosis Is Impaired in Type A–B Niemann–Pick Disease Model Cells and Can Be Restored by ICAM-1-Mediated Enzyme Replacement." *Molecular Pharmaceutics* 11, no. 8 (2014): 2887–95.

Ren, M., B. Deng, J. Y. Wang, X. Kong, Z. R. Liu, K. Zhou, L. He, and W. Lin. "A Fast Responsive Two-Photon Fluorescent Probe for Imaging H_2O_2 in Lysosomes with a Large Turn-On Fluorescence Signal." *Biosensors & Bioelectronics* 79 (2016): 237–43. doi:10.1016/j.bios.2015.12.046.

Repnik, Urška, Maruša Hafner Česen, and Boris Turk. "Lysosomal Membrane Permeabilization in Cell Death: Concepts and Challenges." *Mitochondrion* 19, no. A (2014): 49–57.

Repnik, Urška, Veronika Stoka, Vito Turk, and Boris Turk. "Lysosomes and Lysosomal Cathepsins in Cell Death." *Biochimica & Biophysica Acta (BBA): Proteins & Proteomics* 1824, no. 1 (2012): 22–33.

Rothberg, Karen G., John E. Heuser, William C. Donzell, Yun-Shu Ying, John R. Glenney, and Richard G. W. Anderson. "Caveolin, a Protein Component of Caveolae Membrane Coats." *Cell* 68, no. 4 (1992): 673–82.

Saffi, G. T., and R. J. Botelho. "Lysosome Fission: Planning for an Exit." *Trends in Cell Biology* 29, no. 8 (2019): 635–46. doi:10.1016/j.tcb.2019.05.003.

Saftig, Paul, and Judith Klumperman. "Lysosome Biogenesis and Lysosomal Membrane Proteins: Trafficking Meets Function." *Nature Reviews. Molecular Cell Biology* 10, no. 9 (2009): 623–35.

Saftig, Paul, and Konrad Sandhoff. "Killing from the Inside." *Nature* 502, no. 7471 (2013): 312–3.

Saftig, Paul, Bernd Schröder, and Judith Blanz. "Lysosomal Membrane Proteins: Life Between Acid and Neutral Conditions." *Biochemical Society Transactions* 38, no. 6 (2010): 1420–3.

Sakhrani, Niraj M., and Harish Padh. "Organelle Targeting: Third Level of Drug Targeting." *Drug Design, Development & Therapy* 7 (2013): 585.

Savić, Radoslav, and Edward H. Schuchman. "Use of Acid Sphingomyelinase for Cancer Therapy." *Advances in Cancer Research* 117 (2013): 91–115.

Schaferling, M., D. B. M. Grogel, and S. Schreml. "Luminescent Probes for Detection and Imaging of Hydrogen Peroxide." *Microchimica Acta* 174, no. 1–2 (2011): 1–18. doi:101007/s00604-011-0606-3. http://inis.iaea.org/search/search.aspx?orig_q=RN:43005558.

Schiattarella, Gabriele G., and Joseph A. Hill. "Therapeutic Targeting of Autophagy in Cardiovascular Disease." *Journal of Molecular & Cellular Cardiology* 95 (2016): 86–93.

Selkoe, D. J., T. Yamazaki, M. Citron, M. B. Podlisny, E. H. Koo, D. B. Teplow, and C. Haass. "The Role of APP Processing and Trafficking Pathways in the Formation of Amyloid β-Protein a." *Annals of the New York Academy of Sciences* 777, no. 1 (1996): 57–64.

Shang, Li, Karin Nienhaus, and Gerd Ulrich Nienhaus. "Engineered Nanoparticles Interacting with Cells: Size Matters." *Journal of Nanobiotechnology* 12, no. 1 (2014): 1–11.

Sharma, Ankur, Kalpesh Vaghasiya, E. Ray, R. K. Verma, Eupa Ray, and Rahul Kumar Verma "Lysosomal Targeting Strategies for Design and Delivery of Bioactive for Therapeutic Interventions." *Journal of Drug Targeting* 26, no. 3 (2018): 208–21.

Small, Donna M., Roberta E. Burden, Jakub Jaworski, Shauna M. Hegarty, Shaun Spence, James F. Burrows, Cheryl McFarlane, Adrien Kissenpfennig, Helen O. McCarthy, James A. Johnston, B. Walker, and C. J. Scott. "Cathepsin S from Both Tumor and Tumor-Associated Cells Promote Cancer Growth and Neovascularization." *International Journal of Cancer* 133, no. 9 (2013): 2102–12.

Song, Qingxiang, Meng Huang, Lei Yao, Xiaolin Wang, Xiao Gu, Juan Chen, Jun Chen, Jialin Huang, Quanyin Hu, Ting Kang, Rong Zhengxing, Hong Qi, Gang Zheng, Hongzhuan Chen, and Xiaoling Gao. "Lipoprotein-Based Nanoparticles Rescue the Memory Loss of Mice with Alzheimer's Disease by Accelerating the Clearance of Amyloid-Beta." *ACS Nano* 8, no. 3 (2014): 2345–59. doi:10.1021/nn4058215.

Takahashi, Reisuke H., Claudia G. Almeida, Patrick F. Kearney, Yu Fangmin, Michael T. Lin, Teresa A. Milner, and Gunnar K. Gouras. "Oligomerization of Alzheimer's β-Amyloid Within Processes and Synapses of Cultured Neurons and Brain." *Journal of Neuroscience* 24, no. 14 (2004): 3592–9.

Takahashi, Reisuke H., Teresa A. Milner, Feng Li, Ellen E. Nam, Mark A. Edgar, Haruyasu Yamaguchi, M. Flint Beal, Huaxi Xu, Paul Greengard, and Gunnar K. Gouras. "Intraneuronal Alzheimer Aβ42 Accumulates in Multivesicular Bodies and Is Associated with Synaptic Pathology." *American Journal of Pathology* 161, no. 5 (2002): 1869–79.

Tate, Barbara A., and Paul M. Mathews. "Targeting the Role of the Endosome in the Pathophysiology of Alzheimer's Disease: A Strategy for Treatment." *Science of Aging Knowledge Environment* 10, no. 10 (2006): re2.

Thekkedath, Ritesh, Alexander Koshkaryev, and Vladimir P. Torchilin. "Lysosome-Targeted Octadecyl-Rhodamine B-Liposomes Enhance Lysosomal Accumulation of Glucocerebrosidase in Gaucher's Cells In Vitro." *Nanomedicine* 8, no. 7 (2013): 1055–65.

Thoreen, Carson C., Seong A. Kang, Jae Won Chang, Qingsong Liu, Jianming Zhang, Yi Gao, Laurie J. Reichling, Taebo Sim, David M. Sabatini, and Nathanael S. Gray. "An ATP-Competitive Mammalian Target Of Rapamycin Inhibitor Reveals Rapamycin-Resistant Functions of mTORC1." *Journal of Biological Chemistry* 284, no. 12 (2009): 8023–32.

Tian, Jiangwei, Lin Ding, Huangxian Ju, Yongchao Yang, Xilan Li, Zhen Shen, Zhi Zhu, Yu Jun-Sheng, and Chaoyong James Yang. "A Multifunctional Nanomicelle for Real-Time Targeted Imaging and Precise Near-Infrared Cancer Therapy." *Angewandte Chemie* 126, no. 36 (2014): 9698–703.

Trivedi, P. C., J. J. Bartlett, and T. Pulinilkunnil. "Lysosomal Biology and Function: Modern View of Cellular Debris Bin." *Cells* 9, no. 5 (2020). doi:10.3390/cells9051131.

Tuma, P., and A. L. Hubbard. "Transcytosis: Crossing Cellular Barriers." *Physiological Reviews* 83, no. 3 (2003): 871–932. doi:10.1152/physrev.00001.2003.

Underhill, David M. "Phagosome Maturation: Steady as She Goes." *Immunity* 23, no. 4 (2005): 343–4.

Vetrivel, Kulandaivelu S., and Gopal Thinakaran. "Amyloidogenic Processing of β-Amyloid Precursor Protein in Intracellular Compartments." *Neurology* 66, no. 2 (Suppl. 1) (2006): S69–S73.

Wang, F., and S. Muller. "Manipulating Autophagic Processes in Autoimmune Diseases: A Special Focus on Modulating Chaperone-Mediated Autophagy, an Emerging Therapeutic Target." *Frontiers in Immunology* 6 (2015): 252. doi:10.3389/fimmu.2015.00252.

Wang, Linlin, and Helen Ka Wai Law. "The Role of Autophagy in Lupus Nephritis." *International Journal of Molecular Sciences* 16, no. 10 (2015): 25154–67. doi:10.3390/ijms161025154. https://pubmed.ncbi.nlm.nih.gov/26506346. https://www.ncbi.nlm.nih.gov/pmc/articles/PMC4632796/.

Watson, G., J. Bastacky, P. Belichenko, M. Buddhikot, S. Jungles, M. Vellard, W. C. Mobley, and E. Kakkis. "Intrathecal Administration of AAV Vectors for the Treatment of Lysosomal Storage in the Brains of MPS I Mice." *Gene Therapy* 13, no. 11 (2006): 917–25. doi:10.1038/sj.gt.3302735.

White, E. "The Role for Autophagy in Cancer." *Journal of Clinical Investigation* 125, no. 1 (2015): 42–6. doi:10.1172/jci73941.

Wiederanders, B., S. Ansorge, P. Bohley, H. Kirschke, J. Langner, and H. Hanson. "The Age Dependence of Intracellular Proteolysis: Changes of the Substrate Proteins." *Mechanisms of Ageing & Development* 8, no. 5 (1978): 355–62. doi:10.1016/0047-6374(78)90034-9.

Withana, Nimali P., Galia Blum, Mansoureh Sameni, Clare Slaney, Arulselvi Anbalagan, Mary B. Olive, Bradley N. Bidwell, Laura Edgington, Ling Wang, Kamiar Moin, B. F. Sloane, R. L. Anderson, M. S. Bogyo, and B. S. Parker. "Cathepsin B Inhibition Limits Bone Metastasis in Breast Cancer." *Cancer Research* 72, no. 5 (2012): 1199–209.

Wong, Y. C., S. Kim, W. Peng, and D. Krainc. "Regulation and Function of Mitochondria-Lysosome Membrane Contact Sites in Cellular Homeostasis." *Trends in Cell Biology* 29, no. 6 (2019): 500–13. doi:10.1016/j.tcb.2019.02.004.

Wu, Z., M. Tang, T. Tian, J. Wu, Y. Deng, X. Dong, Z. Tan, X. Weng, Z. Liu, C. Wang, and X. Zhou. "A Specific Probe for Two-Photon Fluorescence Lysosomal Imaging." *Talanta* 87 (2011): 216–21. doi:10.1016/j.talanta.2011.09.065.

Xu, H., and D. Ren. "Lysosomal Physiology." *Annual Review of Physiology* 77 (2015): 57–80. doi:10.1146/annurev-physiol-021014-071649.

Xue, Xue, Li-Rong Wang, Yutaka Sato, Ying Jiang, Martin Berg, Dun-Sheng Yang, Ralph A. Nixon, and Xing-Jie Liang. "Single-Walled Carbon Nanotubes Alleviate Autophagic/Lysosomal Defects in Primary Glia from a Mouse Model of Alzheimer's Disease." *Nano Letters* 14, no. 9 (2014): 5110–7. doi:10.1021/nl501839q.

Yang, Z., J. J. Goronzy, and C. M. Weyand. "Autophagy in Autoimmune Disease." *Journal of Molecular Medicine* 93, no. 7 (2015): 707–17. doi:10.1007/s00109-015-1297-8.

Yang, Zhong, Yingge Zhang, Yanlian Yang, Lan Sun, Dong Han, Hong Li, and Chen Wang. "Pharmacological and Toxicological Target Organelles and Safe Use of Single-Walled Carbon Nanotubes as Drug Carriers in Treating Alzheimer Disease." *Nanomedicine: Nanotechnology, Biology & Medicine* 6, no. 3 (2010): 427–41. doi:10.1016/j.nano.2009.11.007. https://www.sciencedirect.com/science/article/pii/S1549963409003396.

Yu, H., Y. Xiao, and L. Jin. "A Lysosome-Targetable and Two-Photon Fluorescent Probe for Monitoring Endogenous and Exogenous Nitric Oxide in Living Cells." *Journal of the American Chemical Society* 134, no. 42 (2012): 17486–9. doi:10.1021/ja308967u.

Yu, K. K., K. Li, J. T. Hou, H. H. Qin, Y. M. Xie, C. H. Qian, and X. Q. Yu. "Rhodamine-Based Lysosome-Targeted Fluorescence Probes: High pH Sensitivity and Their Imaging Application in Living Cells." *RSC Advances* 4, no. 64 (2014): 33975–80. doi:10.1039/c4ra05215c. <Go to ISI>://WOS:000341287300040.

Zabirnyk, Olga, Maksym Yezhelyev, and Oleksandr Seleverstov. "Nanoparticles as a Novel Class of Autophagy Activators." *Autophagy* 3, no. 3 (2007): 278–81.

Zhou, J., W. Shi, L. H. Li, Q. Y. Gong, X. F. Wu, X. H. Li, and H. M. Ma. "A Lysosome-Targeting Fluorescence Off-On Probe for Imaging of Nitroreductase and Hypoxia in Live Cells." *Chemistry: an Asian Journal* 11, no. 19 (2016): 2719–24. doi:10.1002/asia.201600012.

Zhou, X., Y. Kwon, G. Kim, J. H. Ryu, and J. Yoon. "A Ratiometric Fluorescent Probe Based on a Coumarin-Hemicyanine Scaffold for Sensitive and Selective Detection of Endogenous Peroxynitrite." *Biosensors & Bioelectronics* 64 (2015): 285–91. doi:10.1016/j.bios.2014.08.089.

Microtubule Targeting in Cancer Treatment

14

Abdulaziz Alhussan, Sarah Eaton,
Nicholas Palmerley and Devika B. Chithrani

Contents

DOI: 10.1201/9781003092773-16

14.1 MICROTUBULES

14.1.1 What Are Microtubules?

Microtubules are one of the major components of a cell's cytoskeleton that stretches throughout the cell. They are hollow tubes of nearly 25 nm in diameter, making them the largest organelles in the cytoskeleton [1]. Microtubules are composed of tubulin dimer (two alternating protein structures α-tubulin and β-tubulin subunits) constructed into a linear chain of protofilaments. Each microtubule is made up of 13 protofilaments. Microtubules are polar structures which have a fast growing "plus" end, where polymerization occurs, that is ringed by β-tubulin, and a slow growing "minus" end at the nucleation site that is ringed by α-tubulin (Figure 14.1) [2]. Figure 14.1 also shows a schematic of how microtubules constantly change size by going through assembly/elongation (via polymerization) and disassembly/contraction (via depolymerization) [3]. These processes depend on numerous factors, mainly the number of free tubulins and several essential chemical elements and facilitators [1]. Microtubules expand via the addition of new α- and β-tubulins to the microtubule plus end [1]. The free pool of intracellular α- and β-tubulin molecules is in constant dynamic equilibrium with the microtubule's tubulins [4]. The polymerization process is reversible in which the majority of microtubules exist in dynamic instability [5]. In eukaryotic cells, microtubules emerge from an organelle in the center of the cell known as the centrosome or microtubule organizing center (MTOC) with the plus ends always directed outwards in the process of nucleation [1].

14.1.2 Microtubules' Functions

Microtubules have major cellular roles in cell shape, cell movements, endothelial cell biology, and organelles intracellular transportation [1, 3, 6]. However, their role in cell division is most notable. In mitosis, microtubules perform a vital function of creating the mitotic spindle or the spindle apparatus [7]. During mitosis, the spindle apparatus arranges and divides chromosomes to allow the proper distribution of the chromosomes into two daughter cells. The spindle apparatus consists of microtubules, MTOC, and microtubule-associated proteins [1, 8]. Highly dynamic microtubules in the spindle are essential for the success of mitosis. Microtubules can be divided into three subgroups of microtubules that facilitate mitosis: astral, polar, and kinetochore [1]. Astral microtubules extend from the MTOCs and are anchored to the membrane of the cell, preventing the spindle apparatus from being displaced [1]. Polar microtubules

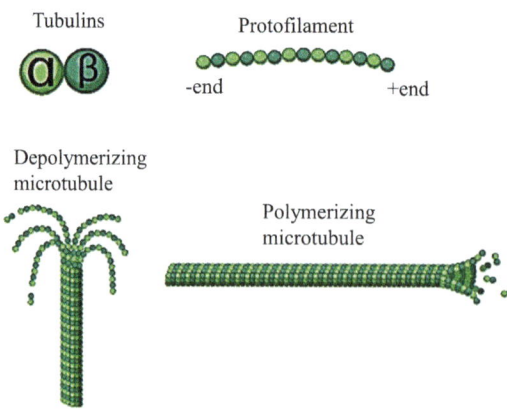

FIGURE 14.1   A schematic shows the components of a microtubule and the processes of polymerization and depolymerization.

connect between two MTOCs, moving them apart, and assist in chromosome separation [1]. Kinetochore microtubules support chromosome separation by invading nuclear space and attaching to chromosomes by a protein complex known as the kinetochore [5, 7, 9]. This important role microtubules play in the cell cycle, via the formation of mitotic spindles which splits chromosomes during cell division, highlights them as a major targeted organelle in cancer treatment.

14.1.3 Microtubule Targeting

Two major polymerization dynamics, treadmilling and dynamic instability, regulate microtubules' biological functions in the cell [1, 5, 6]. Treadmilling describes the phenomenon when the net growth at one end of the microtubule is equal to the net shrinkage at the other end creating a section of filament apparently moving [6]. This process plays an important part in multiple microtubule roles, particularly chromosome polar movement during mitosis anaphase [6]. On the other hand, dynamic instability arises when the plus ends of individual microtubules transition randomly between slow assembling and rapid disassembling states [1]. As a result of the accelerated dynamic instability during mitosis, spindle apparatuses are created and are connected to chromosomes [1]. Regulatory and microtubule-associated proteins can adjust the rate of both treadmilling and dynamic instability. The essence of targeting microtubules is centered around the inhibition of these two key dynamic activities which can disturb the microtubule function involving mitotic spindles causing cell death [1, 5, 6].

In addition to mitosis, microtubules have an essential role in cell interphase such as in vesicular trafficking [10–13]. Figure 14.2a is an illustration of the function of microtubules in intracellular transportation, while Figure 14.2b shows an actual image of microtubules throughout the cell. Microtubules operate like highways within the cell, for molecular motors, i.e., kinesins and dyneins, that move along the microtubules (Figure 14.2a) [9, 12, 14]. These motor proteins act like taxis by transporting cargos, i.e., vesicles or organelles, through the cell to the plus or minus end of the microtubule, as shown in Figure 14.2a. Kinesins and dyneins have similar functions in general, but mainly differ in their direction of movement. Kinesins bring cargoes to the plus end of the microtubule away from the cell center, while dyneins bring cargoes to the minus end of the microtubule towards the cell center (Figure 14.2) [1, 15]. On the other hand, myosin motor protein transport cargo along actin filaments near the cell periphery [3, 4, 10]. These functions of microtubules can be targeted as well.

14.2 MICROTUBULE-TARGETING AGENTS (MTAS)

14.2.1 MTAs Overview

Microtubule-binding agents (MBAs) or microtubule-targeting agents (MTAs) are cancer therapeutic drugs that attach to microtubules and interfere with their dynamic functions. They disturb tubulin's assembly and disassembly which in return, disturbs cell division, usually during mitosis, thus preventing the cell from dividing properly [1, 6]. These drugs are successful in cancer therapy due to the uncontrollable rapid growth of cancer which goes through continuous mitotic divisions making cancer cells more susceptible to mitosis inhibition than noncancerous cells [10, 16]. Colchicine, paclitaxel (PTX), and vinca alkaloids are the first plant-derived MTAs to be discovered and used in cancer treatment [6]. MTAs are one of the most utilized cancer chemotherapeutic drugs and have been used in the treatment of cancer for many years [1, 5, 7, 10, 11, 13, 16]. MTAs could also be used as a supporting treatment for cancers that do not have established specific molecular targets such as the use of docetaxel (DTX) to treat certain types of breast and prostate cancers [9, 10]. The success of different MTAs when used alone or in combination

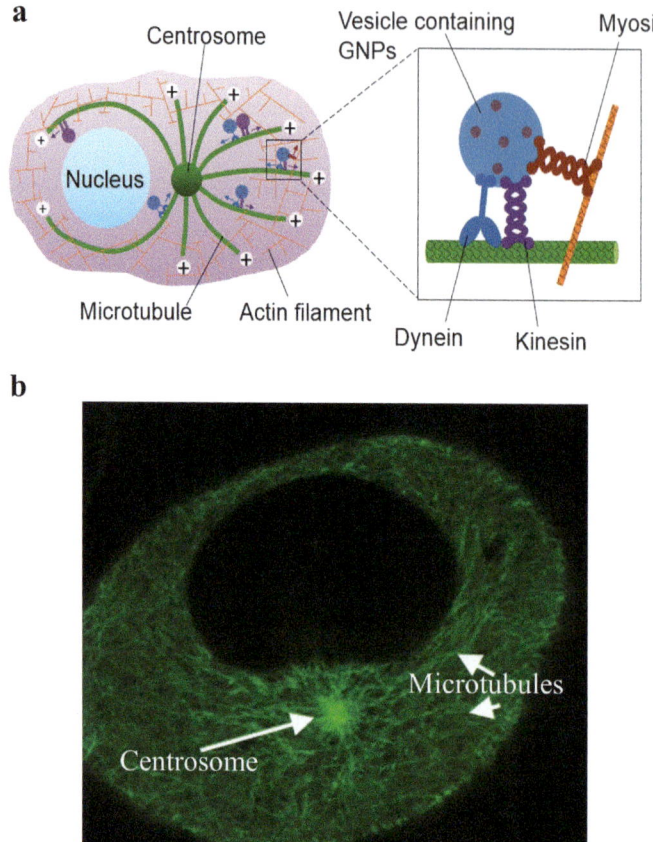

FIGURE 14.2   (a) A diagram showing the transport of vesicles containing gold nanoparticles (GNP) within the microtubule network. (b) A snapshot of a live cell showing a high number of microtubules throughout the cell. Reproduced with permission from open access Creative Common license [14].

with other drugs, in the treatment of a wide variety of both hematopoietic and solid cancers, makes microtubules the most vulnerable cancer target found so far.

MTAs have various mechanisms of action, and they naturally bind to different binding sites on the α-tubulin and β-tubulin making some of them more suitable to certain types of cancer than others [1]. MTAs' ability to attach to a microtubule or to soluble tubulins depends on the tubulin and the microtubule specific binding site location [1]. Three key binding sites have been discovered on the β-tubulin subunits namely the taxane, the vinca, and the colchicine sites, Figure 14.3 [8]. Other binding sites on β-tubulin are also available such as the maytansine and laulimalide sites, as seen in Figure 14.3, but they could interfere with the three major binding sites [4, 10]. Binding sites are also being discovered on the α-tubulin such as the pironetin binding site (Figure 14.3), but they are less used compared to binding sites on β-tubulin [8]. Epothilone and taxane drugs (e.g., DTX and PTX) share the taxane binding site of the β-tubulin subunit, and they both act by stabilizing the microtubule and inhibiting its disassembly [8]. Interestingly, PTX can temporarily attach to the microtubule wall as it uses the wall's molecular pores to reach its binding site [8]. On the other hand, vinca alkaloids, which bind to the vinca site near the GTP-binding site on β-tubulin, and include vinblastine, vinorelbine, vincristine, and vindesine (VDS), operate by obstructing the microtubule polymerization dynamics of spindles [7, 16]. While the colchicine group mainly bind to the colchicine site (Figure 14.3) within the dimer at the interface between α- tubulin and β-tubulin [8]. Some compounds bind to the area at the end of a polymerizing microtubule known as the "GTP cap" where GTP hydrolysis is yet to happen. Others, such as taxanes and epothilones, target the whole microtubule [9].

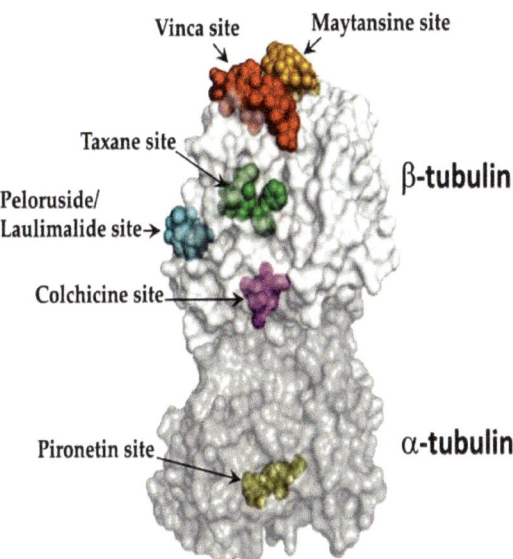

FIGURE 14.3 MTAs' known binding sites on α- and β-tubulins. Reproduced with permission from open access Creative Common license [8].

14.2.2 MTAs' Mechanisms of Action

When used in high concentrations, MTAs either decrease microtubule polymerization by weakening microtubules and reducing their polymer mass, or stimulate microtubule polymerization by strengthening microtubules and growing their polymer mass [1]. Therefore, based on their mechanism of action, MTAs could be divided into two main groups: microtubule destabilizing agents (MDAs) and microtubule-stabilizing agents (MSAs). The first group, which includes vinca alkaloids, colchicine, estramustine, and combretastatins, promotes microtubule depolymerization [1]. The second group promotes and stabilizes microtubule polymerization and includes the taxanes, epothilones, discodermolide, and laulimalide [1]. Lower concentrations of MSAs in the range of nM is usually sufficient for tubulin polymerization induction *in vitro*, whereas higher concentrations in the range of μM are necessary for cancer cell growth inhibition [1, 10].

MTAs interrupt several vital cellular microtubule activities in interphase and in mitosis. Recent studies have shown that MTAs can be lethal to cells that are not undergoing mitosis by affecting cell signaling and the transportation of proteins and other molecules in the microtubule [9, 16]. For instance, MTAs can affect the signaling pathway of mammalian target of rapamycin (mTOR) which is dependent on the affected microtubules dynein, thus inhibiting cancer cell proliferation [2, 17]. MTAs could also delay the repair of radiation-induced DNA damage by interfering with the transportation of DNA repair proteins into the cell's nucleus [11].

However, their most critical action is in disturbing cell proliferation in mitosis. Both MDAs and MSAs intervene with the mitotic spindle formation, thus activating the spindle assembly checkpoint (SAC) [6]. This causes the cell to be suspended in mitosis at the metaphase–anaphase transition and induces self-programmed cell death through apoptosis [6]. Several studies have noticed a weak link between apoptosis and mitotic arrest as there seems to be further mechanisms promoting cell death after MTA treatment [1, 6, 9]. At low concentrations (below those that change microtubule mass), MTAs not only effectively control microtubule dynamics without influencing its polymer mass but could also cause cell death due to their inhibitory effects on spindle dynamics in mitosis [1, 6]. Thus, it is speculated that the mitotic-blocking action of low-concentration MTAs is due to the inhibition of microtubule dynamics rather than the change of microtubule polymer mass. It is important to note that both *in vivo* and *in vitro* studies have demonstrated that this induced cell death by low concentrations of MTAs could be countered by a process known as "mitotic slippage" [2, 6, 7, 12]. This arises when SAC-arrested cells leave mitosis before dividing, thus becoming tetraploid G1 cells which could undergo apoptosis on one pathway or could lead to chromosomal translocations and cancer promotion on another pathway.

14.3 MTAS' CLASSIFICATIONS

14.3.1 Microtubule Destabilizing Agents (MDAs)

14.3.1.1 Vinca Alkaloids

Vinca alkaloids are natural or partially synthetic organic compounds made up of hydrogen, nitrogen, oxygen, and carbon, that are derived from vinca plant alkaloids especially the Madagascar pink periwinkle plant [1]. They were first discovered in the 1950s by Canadian scientists [1]. Vinca alkaloids are famous for their anticancer application due to their cytotoxic effects [8]. They were one of the earliest antimitotic chemotherapeutic drugs to be discovered and used in clinics [1]. They were initially used for treating blood cancer in children, then were upgraded to treat solid and blood cancer in adults [1]. The better understanding of these compounds' mechanism of action has led to the development of several vinca alkaloids including vinblastine (VBL), vinflunine (VFN), vinorelbine (VRL), vincristine (VCR), vindesine (VDS), vincamine (VCA), and vintafolide (VTF) [8, 10, 18, 19].

Only VBL, VCR, and VRL are approved for clinical use in the US [10]. For example, even though VRL is approved to treat advanced breast cancer in other countries, in the US it is only used to treat non-small-cell lung cancer alone or in combined with cisplatin [5, 10]. Similarly, VBL and VCA could be used alone or in combination with other treatment regimens to treat breast cancer, lymphomas, testicular carcinoma, and sarcomas [1, 10, 11]. On the other hand, VTF was approved in 2010 in Europe to treat urothelial cancer [10]. VCR is registered to treat acute leukemia, neuroblastoma, lymphomas, and other diseases [5, 6, 10]. VDS effectiveness has been tested in multiple types of leukemia, malignant melanoma, solid cancers, and some metastatic carcinomas including renal, breast, esophageal, and colorectal [9, 10].

In addition to their mitotic and non-mitotic effects on microtubules in malignant cells discussed in previous sections, vinca alkaloids could affect normal cells, because of microtubules' activities in these cells. This causes plenty of side effects associated with vinca alkaloids including gastrointestinal issues, white blood cell toxicity, nausea, vomiting, dyspnea, chest pain, fever, nervous system toxicity, bone marrow suppression, weakness of immune system, cardiac ischemia, pulmonary effects, hepatic toxicity, and many more [1, 6]. The effect of vinca alkaloids on microtubules could cause obstruction of mitosis and fewer blood cells to be made in the marrow leading to bone marrow suppression, while modification of microtubule dynamics affects neurons and axonal processes and could result in neurotoxicity [1]. The development of some of these semisynthetic analogue drugs could help overcome some of the side effects associated with vinca alkaloids chemotherapy.

14.3.1.2 Colchicine

Colchicine is an alkaloid plant derived from autumn crocus that was first discovered in 1820 and binds to the colchicine site [1]. Colchicine targets microtubules in a similar fashion to vinca alkaloids; at high concentrations it inhibits microtubule polymerization and at low concentrations it stabilizes microtubule dynamics [8, 17]. It is believed that its antitumoral effects, on breast, cervical, esophageal, and lung cancers, could be because of the activation of apoptosis [1, 17]. Even though colchicine agents have some medical uses to prevent and relieve the pain of gout, severe hepatitis, and alcoholic cirrhosis, they have limited uses in cancer treatment due to their potential toxicity to normal tissues [1, 6, 8].

14.3.1.3 Combretastatin

Combretastatins are isolated from members of the *Combretum* genus such as the South African bush willow or *Combretum caffrum* [1]. They are natural phenols (dihydrostilbenes) that display substantial antimitotic and antiproliferative properties by inhibiting tubulin polymerization in cancer cells [1]. Among combretastatins, combretastatin A-4 shows the most successful antineoplastic effects on human solid cancer cell lines [1, 6, 8, 10, 16]. Similar to colchicine, combretastatin binds to the colchicine site on β-tubulin subunit and has anti-mitotic effects. Unlike colchicine, however, they possess angiogenesis properties causing vascular disruption and necrosis to tumors [1, 8, 10]. These effects are more dominant at the tumor core than its boundaries as a result of alteration in the shape of vasculature endothelial cells. Therefore, this class of drugs is best used in combination with other cancer therapeutic drugs for maximum efficacy.

14.3.1.4 Noscapinoids

Noscapine is a phthalide isoquinoline alkaloid, derived from various species of the opium poppy *Papaver somniferum* family that demonstrated antimitotic and antitumoral effects on numerous cancer cell lines [1]. Noscapinoids, a synthetic derivative of noscapine, show improved potential compared to their parent compound by causing microtubule dynamic instability leading to mitotic arrest, cell apoptosis, and boosting tumor regression, with minor toxicity to normal tissues [6, 8, 9]. Increasing noscapinoids' tumor specificity through the use of nanoparticle carriers could enable using them as an effective anticancer drug.

14.3.1.5 Rhizoxin

Rhizoxin is an anticancer agent derived from the fungus *Rhizopus chinensis*. It binds to the maytansine binding site on the β-tubulin that causes obstruction of microtubule assembly and polymerization of tubulin [1]. This leads to cell-cycle arrest, eventually leading to cell death [6]. In addition to these effects, rhizoxin has similar dose-dependent effects to combretastatin of angiogenesis inhibition and suppression of neovascularization [8, 10]. Rhizoxin has been considered as a potential antitumor therapeutic in phase II clinical trials for multiple solid cancers such as melanoma, breast, and head [1]. During clinical trials, rhizoxin showed noticeable toxicity with little efficacy and slow clinical response due to its rapid clearance [1].

14.3.1.6 Maytansine

Maytansine is a cytotoxic agent that is isolated from the *Maytenus* plants [1]. It triggers disassembly of the microtubule and suppresses microtubule dynamic instability by binding to the same maytanisine binding site as the rhizoxins [1]. Its derivative maytansinoids are investigated *in vivo* for their anticancer properties against various cancer cell lines [6]. It has been suggested that maytansinoids may interfere competitively with the binding sites of VBL and VCR on the β-tubulin possibly due to the close proximity of the two binding sites to each other and due to their higher affinity to microtubules [8]. Despite its failure in clinical trials, because of the absence of tumor specificity and undesirable toxicity when used alone, maytansine has been recently approved by the FDA as part of an antibody-drug conjugate (ADC) for the treatment of advanced breast cancer [9].

14.3.1.7 Spongistatin 1

Spongistatin 1 is a unique natural antitumoral agent derived from marine sponges [20]. *In vitro* and *in vivo* studies show its exceptional growth inhibition effects on a range of cancer cell lines, with relatively low toxicity to normal fibroblasts [1]. Spongistatin 1 affects microtubules causing mitotic arrest in prostate cancer cells and inducing apoptosis in primary acute leukaemia cells *in vitro* [20, 21]. *In vivo*, it showed inhibition of melanoma xenograft growth and antimetastatic effects against invasive pancreatic cancer cells [21]. Spongistatin 1 competitively prevents tubulin binding of maytansine site and non-competitively hinders tubulin binding of dolastatin 10 [1, 21].

14.3.1.8 Podophyllotoxin

Podophyllotoxin (PTOX) is a natural plant-based anticancer agent that is mainly isolated from *podophyllum emodi* [1]. PTOX inhibits cell growth by suppressing the polymerization and assembly of tubulin into microtubules, disrupting microtubules assembly and disassembly dynamic equilibrium, promoting cell cycle mitotic arrest and apoptosis, and interfering with the growth of mitotic spindles [3]. These neoplastic effects have been reported in studies of metastatic lung cancer [3].

14.3.1.9 Halichondrin B and Its Analogues

The naturally occurring extract halichondrin B is isolated from the marine sponge *Halichondria*. The synthetic drug eribulin, derived from halichondrin B, is an FDA-approved medication that possesses antineoplastic properties both *in vitro* and *in vivo* [5, 9, 14]. It is used in the US, Canada, and Europe to treat metastatic breast cancer and liposarcoma [5, 9, 14]. It is also being tested to treat other solid cancers including advanced breast cancer, triple negative breast cancer, lung cancer, bladder cancer, prostate cancer, and salivary gland cancer [1, 5, 9, 14, 16]. Just like with most cancer medications, it comes with plenty of side effects such as fatigue, nausea, alopecia, peripheral neuropathy, constipation, pyrexia, and neutropenia [1]. Eribulin binds at the same β-tubulin site as vinca alkaloids at the plus ends of existing microtubules [9]. Its mechanism of action as tubulin-targeting mitotic inhibitor of microtubule dynamics is similar to many other MTAs. Eribulin exerts cytotoxic effects related to its antimitotic activities, in which it stimulates the induction of apoptosis. Eribulin also exhibits non-cytotoxic effects which include vascular remodeling that leads to a decrease in migration and metastatic capability [5, 9].

14.3.1.10 Dolastatins

Dolastatin 10 and its analogue dolastatin 15 are mainly isolated from the marine hare *Dolabella auricularia* [1]. Dolastatin, similar to spongistatin 1, is a non-competitive antimitotic inhibitor to the vinca alkaloids binding site, which implies that the vinca site may contain at least three separate drug-binding areas [21]. Dolastatin 10, its derivative TZT-1016, and dolastatin 15 analogs ILX651 and cemadotin have been tested in cancer clinical trials with various results [10]. Dolastatin 10 is an effective inhibitor of tubulin polymerization microtubule assembly, and tumor cell growth. It comparatively has a longer cell retention time making it one of the most effectives dolastatins [1]. TZT-1016, on the other hand, is more effective in pancreatic carcinoma, Waldenstrom's macroglobulinemia, and diffuse large B-cell lymphoma due to its cytotoxic and antivascular effects that cause hemorrhaging of the vascular system [10].

14.3.2 Microtubule-Stabilizing Agents (MSA)

14.3.2.1 Taxanes

Taxanes such as paclitaxel (PTX) and its semisynthetic analogue docetaxel (DTX) are a group of anti-microtubule anticancer agents that is extracted from the Pacific yew tree [1]. These FDA-approved drugs are widely used in clinics to treat plenty of solid cancers such as ovarian, breast, prostate, and lung cancers in combination with radiotherapy or other chemotherapeutics such as cisplatin [1, 6, 9]. These FDA-approved microtubule-stabilizing drugs bind to the taxane binding site on the β-tubulin down the length of the microtubule but weakly bind to soluble tubulin [1]. Taxanes stimulate modifications of the β-tubulin M-loop which leads to balanced contact between neighboring proto-filaments, thus encouraging microtubule stabilization

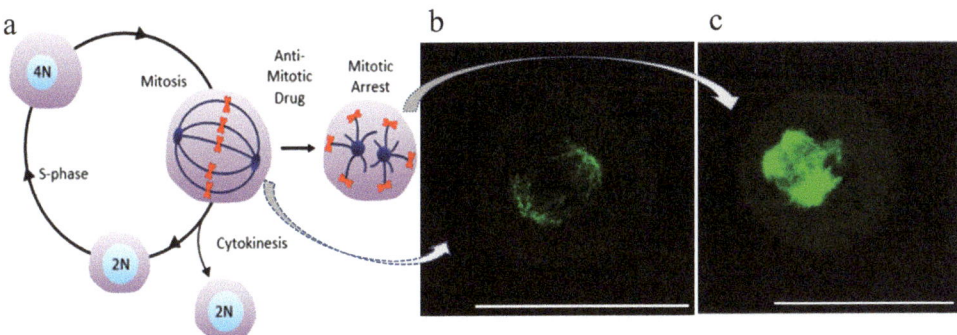

FIGURE 14.4 Role of microtubules in cell division. (a) Schematic diagram illustrating the behavior of microtubules during cell division for a control cell and one treated with an anti-mitotic drug, DTX. (b) Capture of normal mitotic spindles seen for a normal cell division. (c) Capture of asters formation in cells treated with DTX hindering the normal cell division. Reproduced with permission from open access Creative Common license [14].

[6, 8]. It is worth noting that, *in vitro*, small concentrations of paclitaxel stabilize microtubule dynamics without affecting microtubule polymer mass and suppress spindle-microtubule dynamics; this results in mitosis inhibition, blocking cancer cells at metaphase and inhibition of cell division leading to apoptosis [8]. On the other hand, high concentrations of the same compounds lead to an increase in microtubule polymer mass protecting it from disassembly and the breakdown of microtubule dynamics leading to necrosis [6].

Figure 14.4 shows the effects of DTX on cell division (Figure 14.4b) compared to normal cell division conditions (Figure 14.4a). Under regular M phase conditions, normal cells use MTOC and microtubules to form mitotic spindle. Where chromosomes are then segregated equally between two daughter cells. However, when DTX is used, microtubules will be stabilized and the cell will no longer be able to divide properly, thus, it will not be able to continue to anaphase. DTX could lead to several destructive outcomes for the cell including escaping mitosis without division, unequal division, and multinucleation, eventually leading to its death (Figure 14.4b) [15]. The stabilization of microtubules inhibits spindle formation in mitosis thus blocking cell division.

The side effects of taxanes, generally, are similar to those of vinca alkaloids. However, one of the biggest obstacles in treating with taxane drugs is the possible resistance to the drug by cancer cells [6, 8, 10, 14]. This resistance is attributed to many factors, one of which is the overexpression of ATP-binding cassette transporters (ABC transporters) which transport taxanes out of cancer cells, thus decreasing the treatment efficiency [6, 8, 10, 14]. Another factor to consider is β-tubulin mutations which result in undesirable alterations of important parts of the β-tubulin subunit, weakening the ability of taxanes to obstruct microtubules dynamics [1]. Taxane resistance has also been linked to insufficient or defective apoptosis related to either higher activity of anti-apoptotic proteins or lower activity of pro-apoptotic proteins [6].

As a result of cancer cell resistance to taxanes, hypersensitivity, high toxicity, and low solubility, many different synthetic by-products of taxanes have been developed to try to overcome these challenges such as albumin-bound paclitaxel, ortataxel, milataxel, larotaxel, and cabazitaxel [1, 6, 9, 11]. Some of these have been successful in clinical trials such as cabazitaxel which has been approved to treat metastatic prostate cancer, while albumin-bound paclitaxel nanoparticle carriers have been approved for pancreas and breast cancer treatments [5, 12]. The ultimate goal is to design innovative MSAs that will prompt cell death in cancer cells only while sparing normal cells. This could be reached by changing the structures of MSAs in a way that makes them bypass ABC transporters or by binding them to β-tubulins that are only found in resistant cancer cells such as the βIII-tubulin.

14.3.2.2 Epothilones

Epothilones are a novel class of MSAs that compete with taxanes for the taxane binding site on the β-tubulin subunit [1]. They are derived from *Sorangium cellulosum* of the bacterium group myxobacterium.

Epothilones experience fewer side effects and better efficiency compared to taxanes due to their different interaction with the binding site [10]. Like other MSAs they stabilize microtubules, promote microtubule assembly, and inhibit microtubule dynamics, preventing proper cell division and eventually leading to cell death. Epothilones also have the ability to maintain their cytotoxicity in more resistant cancer cells since they are less bound by P-glycoprotein compared to paclitaxel or docetaxel [10]. There are a few epothilone drugs that are being evaluated in clinical trials for different types of cancer including epothilone A, epothilone B, epothilone D, and ixabepilone [1]. The latter is approved to treat metastatic breast cancer and is being tested on breast, cervical, colorectal, renal, and triple negative breast cancer [7].

14.3.2.3 Other MSAs

There are some other MSAs that bind at the same taxane site or at specific sites different from the taxane site. They also stabilize microtubules, enhance microtubule polymerization, and induce cancer cell deaths with varying cytotoxicity and effectiveness. They include estramustine, patupilone, peloruside, discodermolide, sarcodictyins, eleutherobin, and laulimalide [1].

14.4 LIMITATIONS OF MTAS

As discussed in previous sections, MTAs have a plethora of side effects that limit their usability in clinic. These sides effects include peripheral neuropathy, neurotoxicity, hypersensitivity, bone marrow suppression, stomatitis, nausea, vomiting, and diarrhea [1]. Any of these effects could require an interruption of treatment which gives time to the tumor to develop resistance to the treatment. Drug resistance may be attributed to P-glycoprotein which is a multidrug transporter that is often over-expressed in several cancers [3]. P-glycoprotein detects and removes drugs from cancer cells which considerably lowers the drug concentration in them [10]. It has been suggested that cancer may also develop resistance by one or more of the following mechanisms: having mutations that would obstruct endocytosis, or β-tubulin mutations that would affect the proper binding of the drug to its site, or by modification in the apoptosis signaling pathway that could prevent apoptosis, albeit this is still under investigation [1, 3, 10, 16].

Unfortunately, poor absorption of the chemotherapeutic can lead to low concentrations of the drug in the tumor and higher concentrations in normal tissues which limits the administered dose in clinics. This can heavily affect the therapy effectiveness and accordingly increase the drug toxicity. It is also important to note that variations between patients may result in different bioavailability and dissimilar tolerance to the administered drug leading to a wide range of results [1, 14, 22]. This can be seen with many anticancer drugs that show promising activity *in vitro* but fail clinical trials. Problems associated with limited passage through the blood–brain barrier (BBB) and drugs' poor water solubility are also common [9, 22, 23]. Chemotherapeutics with lower solubility could decrease drug absorption which reduces the delivery of the anticancer agents to the tumor [14]. This effect could be amplified for larger molecules that have low penetrability into the tumor [22].

14.5 NEXT GENERATION OF MTAS

According to the National Library of Medicine (NLM) established by the National Institutes of Health (NIH), thousands of clinical trials involving one or more MTAs are taking place as of 2020 [24]. Some of these MTAs are of the so-called "new generation" of MTAs that are synthetic or semisynthetic antimitotic agents developed to address the pharmacokinetic and pharmacodynamic imperfections of the old generation of MTAs [6]. Ideally, a microtubule-targeting compound would only target cancer cells and spare normal cells. However, this is far from feasible in clinics at this time. Nevertheless, novel MTAs should be unique in their approach of targeting microtubules and should have certain features that would make them overcome any limitations of their older natural counterparts.

One method would be to develop drugs with low affinity to P-glycoprotein or incorporate P-glycoprotein inhibitors to the drug [1]. Another technique would be to develop drugs that would target binding sites on the lesser used α-tubulin or drugs that would target multiple binding sites simultaneously or drugs that would have a different mechanism of action. This would decrease the toxicity of the antimitotic drug by allowing the use of lower concentrations [1]. Targeting tumor vasculature via a combination of MTAs and anti-vascular medications could ease delivery of the drug to the tumor which would affect the function of blood vessels leading to cancer cell death via hypoxia [10]. Understanding all possible pathways of drug resistance by cancer could help in developing new drugs that would find their ways around these pathways or drugs that would have new mechanisms of action against drug-resisting cancers.

There have been a few successful cases of MTAs that might be of use in clinics in the near future. One example is Microtubins, novel synthetic microtubule inhibitors that do not bind to the vinca or colchicine β-tubulin binding sites [14]. Microtubins show promising results on patient-derived brain cancer cells and multidrug-resistant small cell lung cancer cells by restraining microtubule polymerization, reducing cancer cell proliferation by arresting them in mitosis, activating the spindle assembly checkpoint, and triggering programmed cell death. Another notable recent example is the use of low concentrations of paclitaxel in combination with Carba1, a carbazole, that promotes synergistic cytotoxic effects on cancer cells *in vitro* and *in vivo*. Unlike paclitaxel, Carba1 is an MDA with an opposite mechanism of action that binds to the colchicine binding site of β-tubulin [2].

Most chemotherapeutic drugs are administered orally or intravenously. Unfortunately, a very small percentage of the drug reaches the tumor site while the rest circulates through the rest of the body [1, 25]. This might necessitate increasing the dose to have higher concentrations of the drug reaching the tumor which in return would induce life-threatening toxicity in healthy tissues in many cases. Thus, liposomes and lipid-based and polymer-based drugs offer a promising solution for tumor-targeted delivery by allowing for the delivery of a significant amount of the drug to the tumor with minimal cytotoxicity to normal tissues which will further reduce side effects [25–30]. The encapsulated medications could be designed to have water-soluble polymers which makes them more soluble [27]. The design could also control the release of the anticancer drug precisely in the tumor by making use of the acidic nature of the tumor microenvironment [31].

In certain cases, nanoparticles could be used as drug carriers to facilitate the drug delivery into the cell. Using nanoparticles as carriers of the drug boosts microtubule inhibition and decreases their high cytotoxicity by favorably targeting cancer cells [26]. It has been demonstrated in recent studies that spherical gold nanoparticles (GNPs) functionalized with an RGD peptide and polyethylene glycol (PEG) have better circulation through the blood vessels and significantly improve the cellular uptake of GNPs [15, 26–28, 31–34]. While GNPs of 50 nm diameter have the optimum uptake in monolayer cell cultures, GNPs of sizes closer to 15 nm diameter are thought to have a higher probability of penetrating through a monoculture three-dimensional (3D) *in vitro* tissue-like structure [23]. Drug-carrier GNPs enter cells mainly through the interactions between their surface proteins and cell membrane receptors until they reach microtubules [32]. The cell membrane allows receptor-bound nanoparticles containing membrane proteins to enter the cell by forming a vesicle (endosome) around them in a process known as endocytosis [32]. Endosome contents go into several handling routes such as into lysosomes for the processing of large proteins, or into the cell membrane to exit the cell through exocytosis [35].

One promising approach for tumor-targeted drug delivery is the use of PTX analogues that bind to a thiolated gold nanoparticle (GNP) delivery system [29]. Preliminary animal *in vivo* studies of the new nanomedicine CYT-21625, which consists of a 27 nm thiolated polyethylene glycol (PEG-thiol) GNP bonded with tumor necrosis factor alpha (TNFα) and PTX analogues, demonstrate an increase in the efficacy of PTX by selectively delivering it into the tumor [29]. This newly developed nanomedicine, CYT-21625, also aids with the slow-release of PTX, effectively reducing solid tumor volumes over time [29]. Figure 14.5 is a comparison between the pharmacokinetics and tumor-accumulation profiles of PTX, CYT-21625, and PTX derivative 5, i.e., compound 5 in B16/F10 tumor burdened C57BL/6 mice. The release of PTX from CYT-21625 was minimal compared to the degradation of compound 5 into PTX (Figure 14.5a). Figures 14.5b and 14.5c, where 50 µg

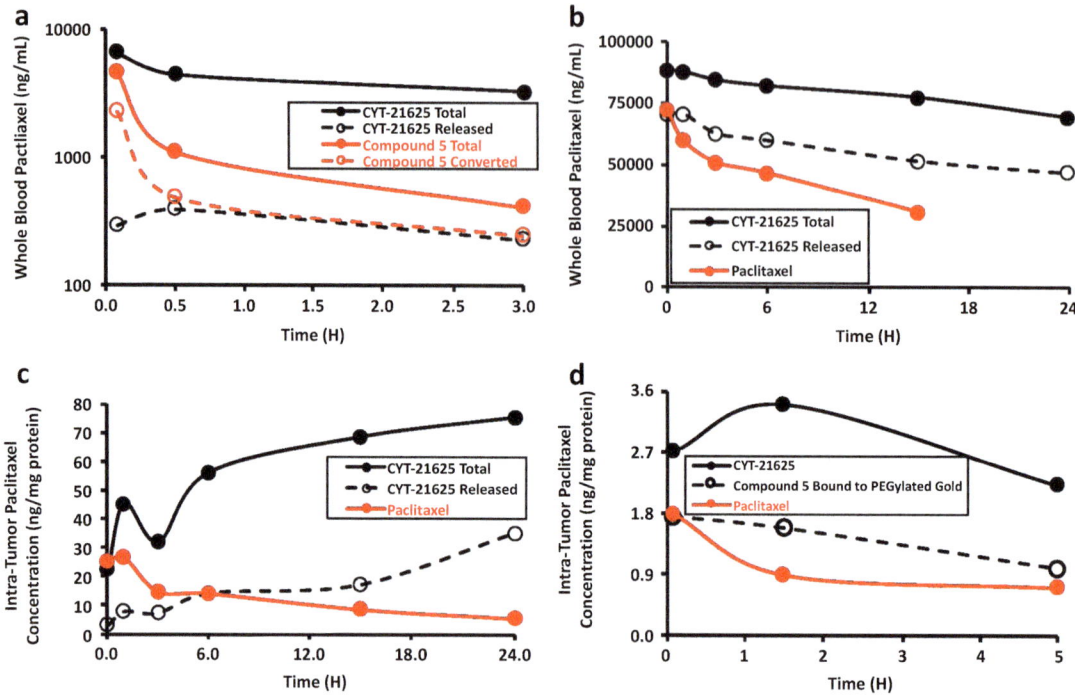

FIGURE 14.5 The pharmacokinetics and tumor-accumulation profiles of PTX, CYT-21625, and compound 5 in B16/F10 tumor burdened C57BL/6 mice. (A) Blood levels of CYT-21625 and compound 5 after injection with 5 µg of compound 5 or the same dose as CYT-21625. (B) Blood levels of CYT-21625, PTX released from CYT-21625, and PTX after injection with 50 µg of either PTX or the equivalent PTX dose on CYT-21625. (C) Tumor levels of CYT-21625, PTX released from CYT21625, and PTX from a similar experiment as described for (B). (D) Tumor levels of CYT-21625, compound 5 bound to PEGylated GNP, and PTX; a total of 5 µg of PTX or its equivalent dose on CYT-21625 was used. Reprinted with permission. Copyright (2016) American Chemical Society [29].

of either PTX or CYT-21625 containing the same amount of PTX was used, show an increase in both the pharmacokinetic exposure and tumor uptake of PTX in the blood (22.5b) and in the tumor (22.5c) using CYT-21625 compared to that of the unaided PTX. Figure 14.5c demonstrates that CYT-21625 has a rapid uptake into tumor cells but with an evident latency between its arrival and its release and conversion into PTX. Figure 14.5d shows that compound 5 bound to PEGylated GNP but without TNF displays a similar uptake into tumor as compared to unaided PTX. This observation confirms the premise that CYT-21625 imitates the entire surgical procedure of isolated limb perfusion (where TNF and chemotherapeutic drug are surgically perfused into neoplasms restricted to the limb resulting in up to 85% response rate) on a single GNP. The advantage of CYT-21625 is that it attacks tumors in two ways, an early attack using TNF and a late attack that involves PTX. The synergic effect of using these two agents causes a series of events starting with vascular leakage, a decrease in tumor interstitial fluid pressure, the release of PTX, and microtubule disturbance, eventually leading to cancer cell death.

14.6 COMBINATION OF MTAS WITH RADIATION THERAPY

MTAs such as docetaxel (DTX) are being used with radiation therapy to treat locally advanced prostate cancer patients. Phase III clinical trials show positive results [36]. A recent study shows that the addition of GNPs into current DTX/radiation would produce a very promising synergistic therapeutic result [37]. This smart combination of cancer therapy is proposed to reduce the required dosages, thus minimizing the damage to healthy tissue surrounding the tumor [37, 38]. GNPs act as a radiosensitizer by boosting local ionizing radiation doses to cancer cells [26, 39]. Gold has a large cross-section for lower energy photons; consequently they absorb the energy of the incident photons and eject electrons in the vicinity of a cancer cell nucleus damaging the DNA and resulting in cell death [35]. On the other hand, DTX has shown remarkable effects when used alone as a cancer therapeutic drug or in combination with ionizing radiation when used as a radiosensitizer [15]. It has been examined as a radiosensitizer *in vitro*, *in vivo*, and in several Phase II clinical trials [15]. It was first introduced in a clinic in 1995, and it is one of the most effective cancer medications in use nowadays [15]. DTX shows radiosensitization effects when in use with ionizing radiation by blocking cells at the most radiosensitive phases of the cell cycle, i.e., the G2/M phases [15]. The synergistic effect of the triple combination of GNPs, DTX, and ionizing radiation has massive prospects to revolutionize cancer treatment.

Figure 14.6 shows a comparison of the triple combination of radiation/GNPs/DTX vs radiation/DTX without GNPs in two cancer cells lines HeLa and MDA-MB-231 [38]. The GNP uptake increases almost 70% in the presence of DTX after 24 h of incubation (Figure 14.6a). The largest level of GNP accumulation is in the G2/M phase due to DTX halting cell division at this phase and allowing more time for GNPs to be accumulated before division. Figure 14.6b demonstrates the effect of the addition of GNPs into the radiation/DTX treatment. It is very evident that the addition of GNPs considerably decreased the survival fraction of cancer cells which indicates the efficacy of the two radiosensitizers', GNPs/DTX, synergic effect. It has also been noted that cells treated with DTX changed their morphology from elongated (Figures 14.6c and 14.6e) to rounded (Figures 14.6d and 14.6f) due to the stabilization effect of DTX on microtubules leading to bundling of microtubules.

The effect of DTX on cells and GNP concentration varies based on the used doses [14, 15, 38]. Most cells dosed with 50 nM DTX are blocked in G2/M phases, while cells dosed with 10 nM DTX are able to divide [15]. When no DTX is used, GNPs are evenly distributed around spindles passing them down to daughter cells. On the other hand, GNPs are unevenly distributed in dividing cells treated with DTX. A 10 nM concentration of DTX allows the cell to go through mitosis but leads to uneven distribution of GNPs in the impaired daughter cells. A 50 nM concentration of DTX results in the assembly of asters with GNPs distributed around the asters, or multinucleation with unsymmetrical distribution of GNPs in the deformed cells with GNPs. DTX also affects the intracellular retention of GNPs typically moving them towards the periphery of the cell. Cells injected with a DTX concentration of 50 nM retain most of their GNP content [15]. It is thought that this is a result of the halt in cell division and the damaged microtubules causing deficiency in the cell's ability to remove GNPs out of the cells [15]. It is also worth mentioning that GNPs did not affect DTX's mechanism of action but DTX did affect the distribution of GNPs in cells [15, 38]. For example, GNPs are closer to the nucleus as shown in Figures 14.6d and 14.6f vs Figures 14.6c and 14.6e, respectively.

14.7 SUMMARY

The crucial role of microtubules as major highways in cells for cargo transportation and their vital function in cell division rendered them a hot target for cancer therapy. Despite the huge success of classical MTAs as anticancer drugs, advances in increasing their effectiveness and safety are still under development. Many taxanes and their derivatives, such PTX and DTX, have been accepted for the treatment of many different types of cancer. Of the epothilones, ixabepilone has already been approved. Of the vinca site binding agents, VBL, VCR, VRL, VFN, VTF, and eribulin are approved for cancer treatment. The mechanism underlying MTAs is based on their suppression of the proper formation of spindle, rather than their impacts on the polymer mass of microtubules. Even though MSAs and MDAs have different effects

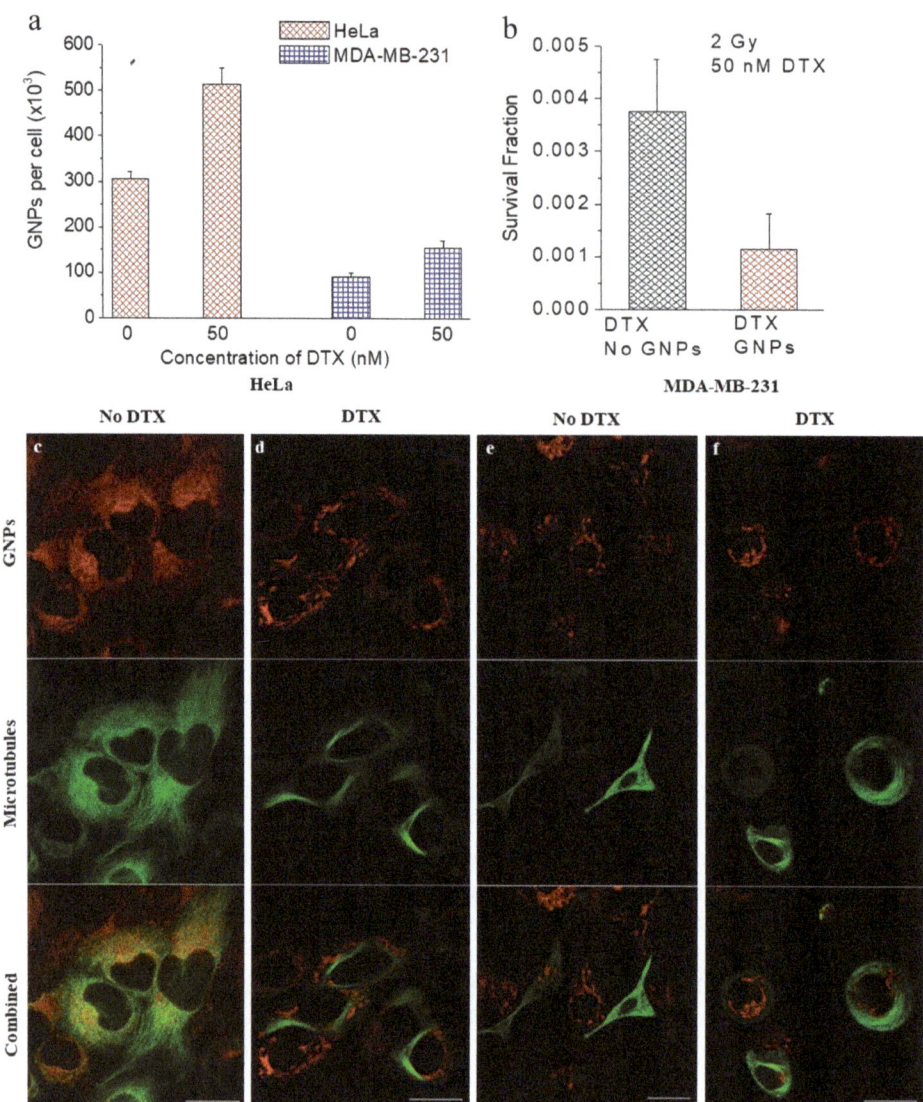

FIGURE 14.6 Cellular uptake of GNPs in MDA-MB-231 and HeLa cells. (a) GNP uptake in the presence of 50 nM DTX (24 h exposure). (b) Survival Fraction in irradiated HeLa cells with DTX and GNP vs DTX with no GNP. (c–f) Confocal images of GNPs (in red) and microtubules (in green) in HeLa and MDA-MB-231, respectively. (c, e) HeLa and MDA-MB-231 not treated with DTX, respectively. (d, f) HeLa and MDA-MB-231 cells treated with 50 nM DTX, respectively. The scale bar is 25 μm. Reproduced with permission from open access Creative Common license [14] and adapted from [38].

at high concentrations, almost all MTAs at low effective concentrations have the same effect of stabilizing microtubules.

Two major challenges of current MTAs are the resistance of cancer cells to the drug and the severe side effects associated with them. To challenge these dilemmas, next-generation antimitotic therapeutics that are structurally modified to prolong their effect and to selectively target cancer cells are being tested. The use of the minimum effective but non-toxic concentrations of MTAs in combination with other drugs or nanoparticles is also being evaluated to overcome MTAs' cytotoxicity. The combined modality of radiation and DTX is already being assessed in clinical trials with the ultimate goal of reducing the side effects by lowering individual dosages [40–47]. The future of MTAs probably lies in isolating new antimitotic agents from the world's biodiverse plant kingdom or synthesizing novel agents that more successfully avoid these adverse difficulties. The contribution of scientists around the world has built a strong foundation of knowledge to introduce new MTAs into the clinic, while other novel MTAs are still under investigation *in vitro* and *in vivo*. This work is opening the door for a bright future to develop effective, personalized, and novel techniques for cancer treatment.

ACKNOWLEDGMENTS

The authors would like to acknowledge the Canada Foundation for Innovation (CFI), the Natural Sciences and Engineering Research Council of Canada (NSERC), NanoMedicines Innovation Network (NMIN), University of Victoria and Kuwait Foundation for the Advancement of Sciences (KFAS) under project code "CB21-63SP-01".

REFERENCES

1. Fojo, T., ed. *The Role of Microtubules in Cell Biology, Neurobiology, and Oncology.* Totowa, NJ: Humana Press, 2008. doi:10.1007/978-1-59745-336-3.
2. Schuemann, J., A. F. Bagley, R. Berbeco, K. Bromma, K. T. Butterworth, H. L. Byrne, B. D. Chithrani, S. H. Cho, J. R. Cook, V. Favaudon, Y. H. Gholami, E. Gargioni, J. F. Hainfeld, F. Hespeels, A.-C. Heuskin, U. M. Ibeh, Z. Kuncic, S. Kunjachan, S. Lacombe, S. Lucas, F. Lux, S. McMahon, D. Nevozhay, W. Ngwa, J. D. Payne, S. Penninckx, E. Porcel, K. M. Prise, H. Rabus, S. M. Ridwan, B. Rudek, L. Sanche, B. Singh, H. M. Smilowitz, K. V. Sokolov, S. Sridhar, Y. Stanishevskiy, W. Sung, O. Tillement, N. Virani, W. Yantasee, and S. Krishnan. "Roadmap for Metal Nanoparticles in Radiation Therapy: Current Status, Translational Challenges, and Future Directions." *Physics in Medicine & Biology* 65, no. 21 (2020): 21RM02. doi:10.1088/1361-6560/ab9159.
3. Mukhtar, E., V. M. Adhami, and H. Mukhtar. "Targeting Microtubules by Natural Agents for Cancer Therapy." *Molecular Cancer Therapeutics* 13, no. 2 (2014): 275–84. doi:10.1158/1535-7163.MCT-13-0791.
4. Loong, H. H., and W. Yeo. "Microtubule-Targeting Agents in Oncology and Therapeutic Potential in Hepatocellular Carcinoma." *OncoTargets & Therapy* 7 (2014): 575–85. doi:10.2147/OTT.S46019.
5. Peronne, L., E. Denarier, A. Rai, R. Prudent, A. Vernet, P. Suzanne, S. Ramirez-Rios, S. Michallet, M. Guidetti, J. Vollaire, D. Lucena-Agell, A.-S. Ribba, V. Josserand, J.-L. Coll, P. Dallemagne, J. F. Díaz, M. Á. Oliva, K. Sadoul, A. Akhmanova, A. Andrieux, and L. Lafanechère. "Two Antagonistic Microtubule Targeting Drugs Act Synergistically to Kill Cancer Cells." bioRxiv.02.06.936849 (2020). doi:10.1101/2020.02.06.936849.
6. Zhang, D., and A. Kanakkanthara. "Beyond the Paclitaxel and Vinca Alkaloids: Next Generation of Plant-Derived Microtubule-Targeting Agents with Potential Anticancer Activity." *Cancers* 12, no. 7 (2020). doi:10.3390/cancers12071721.
7. Čermák, V., V. Dostál, M. Jelínek, L. Libusová, J. Kovář, D. Rösel, and J. Brábek. "Microtubule-Targeting Agents and Their Impact on Cancer Treatment." *European Journal of Cell Biology* 99, no. 4 (2020): 151075. doi:10.1016/j.ejcb.2020.151075.
8. Balachandran, R. S., and E. T. Kipreos. "Addressing a Weakness of Anticancer Therapy with Mitosis Inhibitors: Mitotic Slippage." *Molecular & Cellular Oncology* 4, no. 2 (2017). doi:10.1080/23723556.2016.1277293.
9. Fanale, D., G. Bronte, F. Passiglia, V. Calò, M. Castiglia, F. Di Piazza, N. Barraco, A. Cangemi, M. T. Catarella, L. Insalaco, A. Listì, R. Maragliano, D. Massihnia, A. Perez, F. Toia, G. Cicero, and V. Bazan. "Stabilizing Versus Destabilizing the Microtubules: A Double-Edge Sword for an Effective Cancer Treatment Option?." *Analytical Cellular Pathology* 2015 (2015). doi:10.1155/2015/690916.
10. Poruchynsky, M. S., E. Komlodi-Pasztor, S. Trostel, J. Wilkerson, M. Regairaz, Y. Pommier, X. Zhang, T. K. Maity, R. Robey, M. Burotto, D. Sackett, U. Guha, and A. T. Fojo. "Microtubule-Targeting Agents Augment the Toxicity of DNA-Damaging Agents by Disrupting Intracellular Trafficking of DNA Repair Proteins." *Proceedings of the National Academy of Sciences* 112, no. 5 (2015): 1571–6. doi:10.1073/pnas.1416418112.

11. Serpico, A. F., R. Visconti, and D. Grieco. "Exploiting Immune-Dependent Effects of Microtubule-Targeting Agents to Improve Efficacy and Tolerability of Cancer Treatment." *Cell Death & Disease* 11, no. 5 (2020): 1–7. doi:10.1038/s41419-020-2567-0.

12. Tangutur, A. D., D. Kumar, K. V. Krishna, and S. Kantevari. "Microtubule Targeting Agents as Cancer Chemotherapeutics: An Overview of Molecular Hybrids as Stabilizing and Destabilizing Agents." *Current Topics in Medicinal Chemistry* 17, no. 22 (2017): 2523–37. doi:10.2174/1568026617666170104145640.

13. Senese, S., Y.-C. Lo, A. A. Gholkar, C.-M. Li, Y. Huang, J. Mottahedeh, H. I. Kornblum, R. Damoiseaux, and J. Z. Torres. "Microtubins: A Novel Class of Small Synthetic Microtubule Targeting Drugs That Inhibit Cancer Cell Proliferation." *Oncotarget* 8, no. 61 (2017): 104007–104021. doi:10.18632/oncotarget.21945.

14. Bannister, A., D. Dissanayake, A. Kowalewski, L. Cicon, K. Bromma, and D. B. Chithrani. "Modulation of the Microtubule Network for Optimization of Nanoparticle Dynamics for the Advancement of Cancer Nanomedicine." *Bioengineering* 7, no. 2 (2020). doi:10.3390/bioengineering7020056.

15. Schober, J. M., Y. A. Komarova, O. Y. Chaga, A. Akhmanova, and G. G. Borisy. "Microtubule-Targeting-Dependent Reorganization of Filopodia." *Journal of Cell Science* 120, no. 7 (2007): 1235–44. doi:10.1242/jcs.003913.

16. Schwartz, E. L. "Anti-Vascular Actions of Microtubule-Binding Drugs." *Clinical Cancer Research* 15, no. 8 (2009): 2594–601. doi:10.1158/1078-0432.CCR-08-2710.

17. Sato-Kaneko, F., X. Wang, S. Yao, T. Hosoya, F. S. Lao, K. Messer, M. Pu, N. M. Shukla, H. B. Cottam, M. Chan, D. A. Carson, M. Corr, and T. Hayashi. "Discovery of a Novel Microtubule Targeting Agent as an Adjuvant for Cancer Immunotherapy" [Research article]. *BioMed Research International* (n.d.). Hindawi Publishing. doi:10.1155/2018/8091283.

18. Carlson, K., and A. J. Ocean. "Peripheral Neuropathy with Microtubule-Targeting Agents: Occurrence and Management Approach." *Clinical Breast Cancer* 11, no. 2 (2011): 73–81. doi:10.1016/j.clbc.2011.03.006.

19. Chithrani, B. D., A. A. Ghazani, and W. C. W. Chan. "Determining the Size and Shape Dependence of Gold Nanoparticle Uptake into Mammalian Cells." *Nano Letters* 6, no. 4 (2006): 662–8. doi:10.1021/nl0523960.

20. Moudi, M., R. Go, C. Y. S. Yien, and Mohd Nazre. "Vinca Alkaloids." *International Journal of Preventive Medicine* 4, no. 11 (2013): 1231–5.

21. Rowinsky, E. "The Vinca Alkaloids." *Holland-Frei Cancer Medicine.* 6th ed. 2003. https://www.ncbi.nlm.nih.gov/books/NBK12718/.

22. Zhang, T., W. Chen, X. Jiang, L. Liu, K. Wei, H. Du, H. Wang, and J. Li. "Anticancer Effects and Underlying Mechanism of Colchicine on Human Gastric Cancer Cell Lines In Vitro and In Vivo." *Bioscience Reports* 39, no. 1 (2019). doi:10.1042/BSR20181802.

23. Karahalil, B., S. Yardım-Akaydin, and S. Nacak Baytas. "An Overview of Microtubule Targeting Agents for Cancer Therapy." *Arhiv za Higijenu Rada i Toksikologiju* 70 no. 3 (2019): 160–72. doi:10.2478/aiht-2019-70-3258.

24. Schyschka, L., A. Rudy, I. Jeremias, N. Barth, G. R. Pettit, and A. M. Vollmar. "Spongistatin 1: A New Chemosensitizing Marine Compound That Degrades XIAP." *Leukemia* 22, no. 9 (2008): 1737–45. doi:10.1038/leu.2008.146.

25. Zhigaltsev, I. V., G. Winters, M. Srinivasulu, J. Crawford, M. Wong, L. Amankwa, D. Waterhouse, D. Masin, M. Webb, N. Harasym, L. Heller, M. B. Bally, M. A. Ciufolini, P. R. Cullis, and N. Maurer. "Development of a Weak-Base Docetaxel Derivative That Can Be Loaded into Lipid Nanoparticles." *Journal of Controlled Release* 144, no. 3 (2010): 332–40.

26. Xu, Q., K.-C. Huang, K. TenDyke, J. Marsh, J. Liu, D. Qiu, B. A. Littlefield, K. Nomoto, O. Atasoylu, C. A. Risatti, J. B. Sperry, and A. B. Smith III. "In Vitro and In Vivo Anticancer Activity of (+)-Spongistatin 1." *Anticancer Research* 31, no. 9 (2011): 2773–9.

27. Ardalani, H., A. Avan, and M. Ghayour-Mobarhan. "Podophyllotoxin: A Novel Potential Natural Anticancer Agent." *Avicenna Journal of Phytomedicine* 7, no. 4 (2017): 285–94.

28. US National Library of Medicine (NLM), and *ClinicalTrials.gov.* displayed 1 November 2020. Available at https: clinicaltrials.gov. ct2/.

29. Paciotti, G. F., J. Zhao, S. Cao, P. J. Brodie, L. Tamarkin, M. Huhta, L. D. Myer, J. Friedman, and D. G. I. Kingston. "Synthesis and Evaluation of Paclitaxel-Loaded Gold Nanoparticles for Tumor-Targeted Drug Delivery." *Bioconjugate Chemistry* 27, no. 11 (2016): 2646–57. doi:10.1021/acs.bioconjchem.6b00405.

30. Zhai, J., R. B. Luwor, N. Ahmed, R. Escalona, F. H. Tan, C. Fong, J. Ratcliffe, J. A. Scoble, C. J. Drummond, and N. Tran. "Paclitaxel-Loaded Self-Assembled Lipid Nanoparticles as Targeted Drug Delivery Systems for the Treatment of Aggressive Ovarian Cancer." *ACS Applied Materials & Interfaces* 10, no. 30 (2018): 25174–85. doi:10.1021/acsami.8b08125.

31. Bromma, K., and D. B. Chithrani. "Advances in Gold Nanoparticle-Based Combined Cancer Therapy." *Nanomaterials* 10, no. 9 (2020): 1671. doi:10.3390/nano10091671.

32. Gangjee, A., Y. Zhao, L. Lin, S. Raghavan, E. G. Roberts, A. L. Risinger, E. Hamel, and S. L. Mooberry. "Synthesis and Discovery of Water Soluble Microtubule Targeting Agents That Bind to the Colchicine Site on Tubulin and Circumvent Pgp Mediated Resistance." *Journal of Medicinal Chemistry* 53, no. 22 (2010): 8116–28. doi:10.1021/jm101010n.

33. Steinmetz, M. O., and A. E. Prota. "Microtubule-Targeting Agents: Strategies to Hijack the Cytoskeleton." *Trends in Cell Biology* 28, no. 10 (2018): 776–92. doi:10.1016/j.tcb.2018.05.001.

34. Bromma, K., A. Bannister, A. Kowalewski, L. Cicon, and D. B. Chithrani. "Elucidating the Fate of Nanoparticles Among Key Cell Components of the Tumor Microenvironment for Promoting Cancer Nanotechnology." *Cancer Nanotechnology* 11, no. 1 (2020). doi:10.1186/s12645-020-00064-6.

35. Chithrani, D. B., S. Jelveh, F. Jalali, M. van Prooijen, C. Allen, R. G. Bristow, R. P. Hill, and D. A. Jaffray. "Gold Nanoparticles as Radiation Sensitizers in Cancer Therapy." *Radiation Research* 173, no. 6 (2010): 719–28. doi:10.1667/RR1984.1.

36. Mirjolet, C., J. Boudon, A. Loiseau, S. Chevrier, R. Boidot, A. Oudot, B. Collin, E. Martin, P. A. Joy, N. Millot, and G. Créhange. "Docetaxel-Titanate Nanotubes Enhance Radiosensitivity in an Androgen-Independent Prostate Cancer Model." *International Journal of Nanomedicine* 12 (2017): 6357–64. doi:10.2147/IJN.S139167.

37. Bromma, K., L. Cicon, W. Beckham, and D. B. Chithrani. "Gold Nanoparticle Mediated Radiation Response Among Key Cell Components of the Tumour Microenvironment for the Advancement of Cancer Nanotechnology." *Scientific Reports* 10, no. 1 (2020): 12096. doi:10.1038/s41598-020-68994-0.

38. Bannister, A. H., K. Bromma, W. Sung, M. Monica, L. Cicon, P. Howard, R. L. Chow, J. Schuemann, and D. B. Chithrani. "Modulation of Nanoparticle Uptake, Intracellular Distribution, and Retention with Docetaxel to Enhance Radiotherapy." *British Journal of Radiology* 93, no. 1106 (2020): 20190742. doi:10.1259/bjr.20190742.

39. Schuemann, J., R. Berbeco, B. D. Chithrani, S. Cho, R. Kumar, S. McMahon, S. Sridhar, and S. Krishnan. "Roadmap to Clinical Use of Gold Nanoparticles for Radiosensitization." *International Journal of Radiation Oncology, Biology, Physics* 94, no. 1 (2016): 189–205. doi:10.1016/j.ijrobp.2015.09.032.

40. Alvarez, E. A., A. H. Wolfson, J. M. Pearson, M. P. Crisp, L. E. Mendez, N. C. Lambrou, and J. A. Lucci, 3rd. "A Phase I Study of Docetaxel as a Radio-Sensitizer for Locally Advanced Squamous Cell Cervical Cancer." *Gynecologic Oncology* 113, no. 2 (2009): 195–9.

41. Bridgewater, R. E., J. C. Norman, and P. T. Caswell. "Integrin Trafficking at a Glance." *Journal of Cell Science* 125, no. 16 (2012): 3695.

42. Harari, P. M., J. Harris, M. S. Kies, J. N. Myers, R. C. Jordan, M. L. Gillison, R. L. Foote, M. Machtay, M. Rotman, D. Khuntia, W. Straube, Q. Zhang, and K. Ang. "Postoperative Chemoradiotherapy and Cetuximab for High-Risk Squamous Cell Carcinoma of the Head and Neck: Radiation Therapy Oncology Group RTOG-0234." *Journal of Clinical Oncology* 32, no. 23 (2014): 2486–95.

43. Karasawa, K., K. Ito, T. Takada, F. Matsumoto, T. Haruyama, S. Ito, and K. Ikeda. "2434: Hyperfractionated Radiotherapy with Concurrent Docetaxel for Advanced Head and Neck Cancer." *International Journal of Radiation Oncology Biology Physics* 66, no. 3 (2006): S450–S1.

44. Kiura, K., H. Ueoka, Y. Segawa, M. Tabata, N. Kamei, N. Takigawa, S. Hiraki, Y. Watanabe, A. Bessho, K. Eguchi, N. Okimoto, S. Harita, M. Takemoto, Y. Hiraki, M. Harada, M. Tanimoto, and Okayama Lung Cancer Study Group. "Phase I/II Study of Docetaxel and Cisplatin with Concurrent Thoracic Radiation Therapy for Locally Advanced Non-Small-Cell Lung Cancer." *British Journal of Cancer* 89, no. 5 (2003): 795–802.

45. Kumar, P. "A New Paradigm for the Treatment of High-Risk Prostate Cancer: Radiosensitization with Docetaxel." *Reviews in Urology* 5, no. Suppl. 3 (2003): S71–S7.

46. Kumar, P., and R. Weiss. "Radiosensitization with Docetaxel and 3-D CRT. Results of a Completed Phase I Trial." *Proceeding of American Society of Clinical Oncology* 22, no. 1622 (2003): 404.

47. Varveris, H., M. Mazonakis, M. Vlachaki, S. Kachris, E. Lyraraki, O. Zoras, T. Maris, M. Froudarakis, J. Velegrakis, C. Perysinakis, J. Damilakis, and G. Samonis. "A Phase I Trial of Weekly Docetaxel and Cisplatinum Combined to Concurrent Hyperfractionated Radiotherapy for Non-Small Cell Lung Cancer and Squamous Cell Carcinoma of Head and Neck." *Oncology Reports* 10, no. 1 (2003): 185–95.

Localizing Therapeutics to the Endoplasmic Reticulum

15

Lara Scheherazade Milane

Contents

15.1 ER STRUCTURE AND FUNCTION

The endoplasmic reticulum (ER) is the largest organelle in the eukaryotic cell and the primary roles of the ER are protein synthesis, calcium storage, lipid metabolism, and regulation of the ER stress-autophagy axis.[1] The ER is continuous with the nuclear envelope and form contacts with other organelles and cell structures including mitochondria and microtubules. A portion of the peripheral ER, the cortical ER, connects with the plasma membrane and is important in calcium signaling and muscle contraction. In this way, the ER directly connects the nucleus to the rest of the cell (organelles) as well as the plasma membrane. As illustrated in Figure 15.1, the ER is a dynamic labyrinth of sheets and tubules. As with other organelles, the shape and architecture of the ER alter in response to cellular signals and demand.[1] The nuclear envelope consists of an inner and outer nuclear membrane studded with nuclear pores; the outer nuclear membrane shares luminal space with sheets of the peripheral ER.[1] The ER sheets are studded with ribosomes and are flat with two lipid bilayers and a luminal space of 50 nm in mammals.[1] The ER sheets are most commonly referred to as the rough ER due to the high number of ribosomes. Sheets are the site of protein synthesis, folding, and post-translational modifications.[1] The tubules of the ER also have a 50 nm luminal space, but the tubules have very few ribosomes and are highly plastic.[1] The tubules' function in lipid synthesis, calcium signaling, and organelle contact points.[1] The ratio of sheets to tubules can alter throughout the lifetime of a cell and is different in certain cell types; secretory cells such as beta cells have a higher number of sheets whereas muscle cells, liver cells, and adrenal cells have a higher number

DOI: 10.1201/9781003092773-17

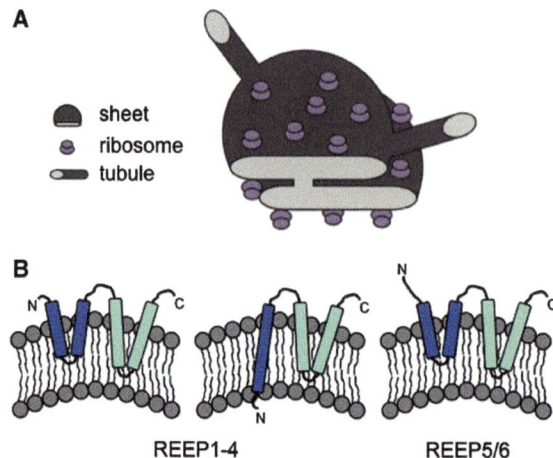

FIGURE 15.1   Endoplasmic reticulum sheets and tubules. (a) ER sheets and tubules have a diameter of 30–50 nm in eukaryotes. Eukaryotic ribosomes are 25–30 nm and localize to the flat regions of ER sheets, giving the sheets a rough appearance (rough ER). Ribosomes are present in much lower numbers on tubules, giving the tubules a more smooth appearance (smooth ER). (b) Models of potential hairpin topologies of REEP family proteins that act as wedges to promote bending of the membrane. Reprinted with permission and under the terms of the Creative Commons Attribution 4.0 International License (http://creativecommons.org /licenses/by/4.0/).[1]

of tubules.[1] The ratio of sheets to tubules is determined by many proteins including reticulons and REEP proteins (1–4 and 5/6), integral membrane proteins that bend ER membranes and enable tubule formation.[1] Atlastins, Rab10, lunapark (Lnp1), and Yop1 also play a role in ER-ER membrane fusion.[1] Climp63, p180, and kinectin are important for ER sheet stabilization.[1]

The ER attaches to microtubules through tip attachment complexes (TACs) and by moving along microtubules with kinesin and dynein motors.[1] The ER forms contacts with microtubules, endosomes, mitochondria, peroxisomes, lipid droplets, the Golgi apparatus, and the plasma membrane.[2] Although the ER is often depicted as being contained to the perinuclear region, the ER can fan out over the entire cell. As the ER functions in protein and lipid synthesis and calcium regulation, forming contacts with these organelles allows the ER to distribute proteins and lipids directly and to manage calcium signaling. The ER lumen has the highest concentration of calcium in the cell (60–500 µM); this compares to 100 µM in the mitochondrial matrix, 100 nM in the nucleus and the cytosol, and 1 nM in the extracellular space.[2] The ER is central in connecting cellular organelles and forming a continuous cell structure with multi-organelle contacts that enable effective maintenance of homeostasis.

15.2 ER DYSFUNCTION AND DISEASE

As illustrated in Figure 15.2, the unfolded protein response (UPR) is one of the main outcomes from ER stress.[3] The UPR is the accumulation of misfolded proteins in the ER lumen.[4] There are three different classes of ER stress sensors: (1) pancreatic ER eIF2α kinase (PERK), double-stranded RNA activated protein kinase-like ER kinase, and PKR-like ER kinase, (2) activating transcription factor 6 (ATF6), and (3) inositol-requiring kinase 1 (IRE1).[4] A simplified depiction of the PERK pathway is illustrated in Figure 15.3. Without oxidative or ER stress, the chaperone GRP78/BiP is bound to each of the ER stress sensors; in conditions of ER stress, the chaperone dissociates and binds unfolded proteins.[4] The UPR either activates cell survival or cell death cascades.[4] The first phase of the UPR is an adaptive phase where

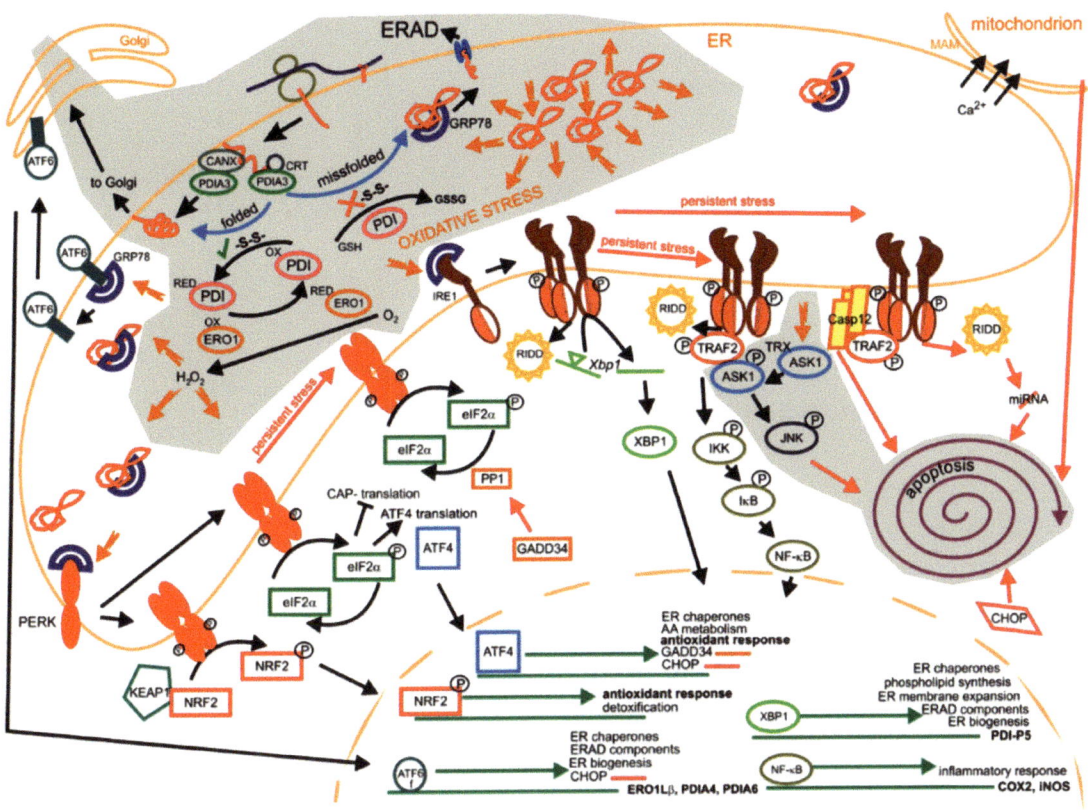

FIGURE 15.2   The unfolded protein response in cell survival and cell death. The three ER sensors include PERK, IRE1, and ATF6. ER stress activates an early adaptive response (black arrows), and if ER stress is unresolved this leads to a late-stage response resulting in survival or death signaling. Correcting ER stress relies on reducing protein burden, load, and misfolding in the ER. Gray areas are associated with oxidative stress. Death can be through mitochondrial apoptosis, CHOP activation, or apoptosis signal-regulating kinase (ASK1) activation. Reprinted with permission and under the terms of the Creative Commons Attribution 4.0 International License (http://creativecommons.org/licenses/by/4.0/).[4]

protein translation is stopped and protein accumulation in the ER is reduced through increased ER chaperones, increased protein disulfate isomerases that catalyze disulfide bonds in proteins, and ER biogenesis.[4] Misfolded proteins are cleared from the ER lumen and degraded in proteasomes in ER-associated degradation (ERAD).[4] If this first phase does not reverse the ER stress then prolonged stress can result in an inflammatory response or cell death via intrinsic apoptosis or through transcription factor C/EBP homologous protein (CHOP) activation.[4]

The N-terminal fragments of ATF6 isoforms are transcription factors that target ER stress response elements (ERSE) on target genes.[4] IRE1 and PERK are kinases. IRE1 activates mitogen protein kinase and the transcription factor XBP-1 that upregulates UPR genes for cell survival or IRE1 signaling can lead to apoptosis through the regulated IRE1 dependent decay (RIDD) process.[4] PERK signaling is mediated by eIF2α which reduced translation and activates the transcription factor ATF4 that increases protein folding genes (in cell survival signaling) or in conjunction with other factors actives pro-apoptotic CHOP.[4]

ER stress and the UPR contribute to cardiovascular disease, neurodegeneration, cancer, and type-2 diabetes mellitus (Figure 15.4). Ischemia from atherosclerosis and mechanical stress results in ER hypoxia which triggers the UPR leading to cardiomyocyte apoptosis.[3] A dysfunctional UPR can directly result in the accumulation of proteins in neurodegenerative disease such as Alzheimer's and Parkinson's disease and sustain neurodegeneration in prion diseases.[4] Calcium excess from the ER can also result

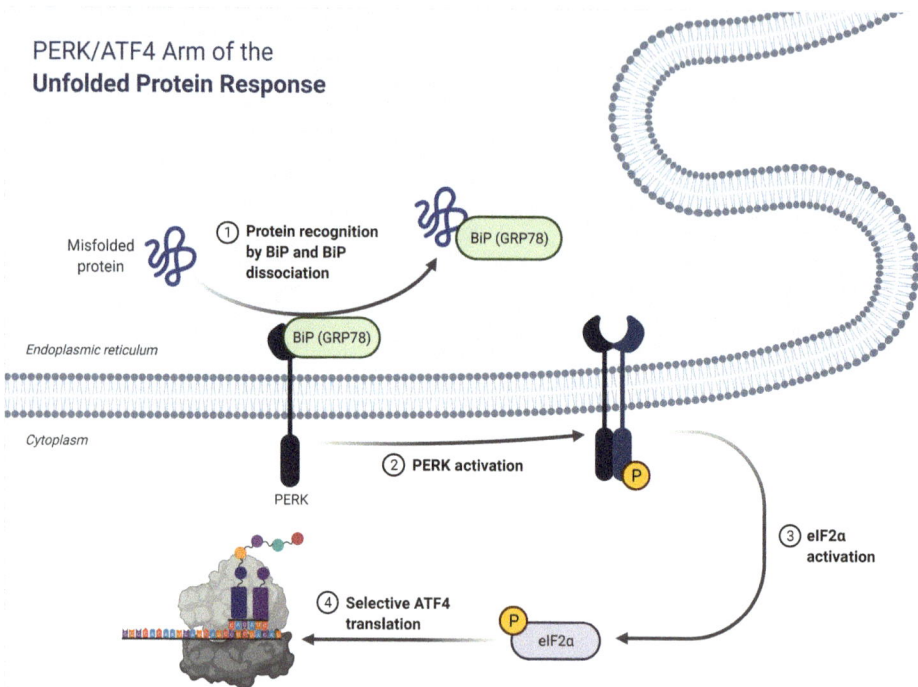

FIGURE 15.3 The PERK/ATF4 arm of the unfolded protein response. Intracellular sensors located at the ER membrane detect misfolded proteins and elicit a cellular response. (1) The dissociation of BiP following the interaction with misfolded proteins leads to (2) the dimerization of PERK (protein kinase R (PKR)-like endo-plasmic reticulum kinase) and its activation by autophosphorylation. (3) PERK subsequently activates eIF2a, driving an imbalance in the translational machinery that (4) leads to the selective translation of ATF4. By Angel Santiago-Lopez, reprinted with permission and credited to Biorender.com.

in neurodengeneration.[3] In cancer, the UPR can trigger autophagy and lead to cellular repair while ER-mitochondrial calcium exchange increases metabolism and cell survival.[3] The UPR in pancreatic beta cells can lead to cell death which contributes to insulin resistance.[3]

The ER stress-autophagy axis is very important for cell survival, and the primary pathway seems to be the IRE1-JNK pathway although there seems to be multiple levels of ER stress-triggered autophagy involving the PERK-ATF-MYC pathway, the IRE1-MAPK8 pathway, ATF6a, IER1-XBP1-LC3 pathway, and calcium signaling to name a few.[5,6] In neurodegenerative disease a lack of autophagy in this feedback loop is detrimental whereas an increase in ER stress-induced autophagy is critical to cancer cell survival.

15.3 ER TARGETING AND NANOMEDICINE

The ER is a very rich organelle for targeting. Protein import and ER targeting are important in the cell, and exploiting the endogenous mechanisms of ER targeting is the ideal strategy for ER-specific drug delivery. For this reason, peptide leader sequences or peptide modified nanoparticles are the ideal approach for targeting ER import pathways. One ER-targeting pathway is the signal recognition particle (SRP) pathway; SRP is a conserved ribonucleoprotein complex.[7] SRP is associated with ribosomes and identifies hydrophobic regions of secretory proteins, and then binds to ER-localized SRP receptors (SR) forming a translocon complex that guides the polypeptide into the ER lumen for continued translation and modification.[7] The SRP dissociates from the ER with GTP hydrolysis.[7]

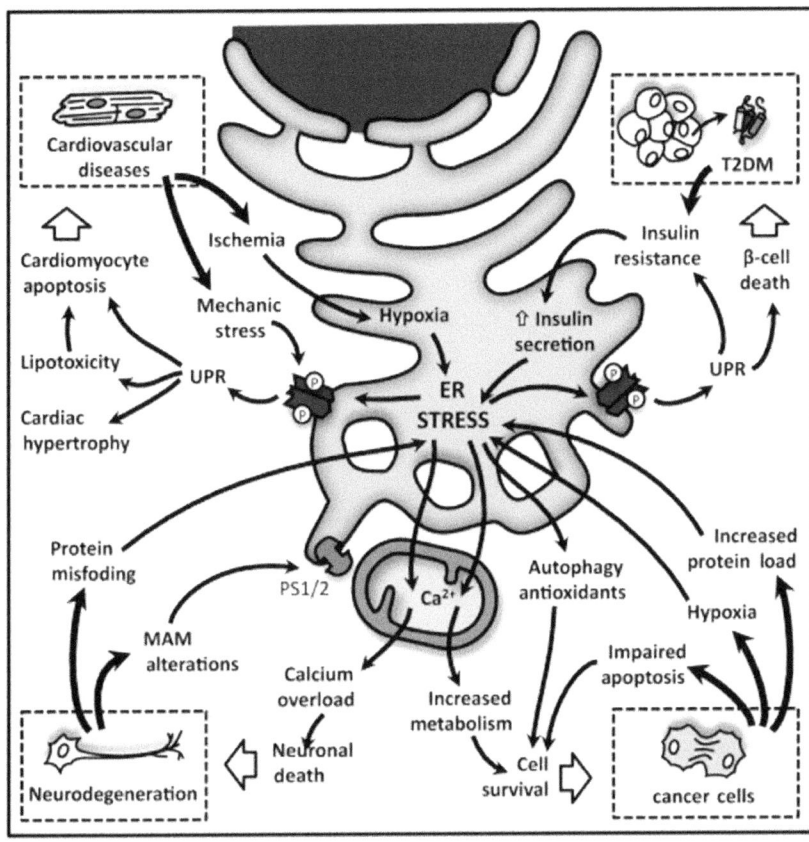

FIGURE 15.4 The ER in pathologies. ER stress contributes to the development of cardiovascular disease, neurodegeneration, Type 2 diabetes mellitus, and cancer. The unfolded protein response (UPR) is central to all of these pathologies. Reprinted with permission from Elsevier.[3]

Some proteins are directed to the ER via a C-terminus transmembrane domain (a tail anchor; TA) that is recognized by the transmembrane recognition complex 40kDa (TRC40, also known as ASNA1).[7] TRC40 recognizes these TA proteins on ribosomes, they are complexed with Bat3-Get4-Ubl4a, and the ATPase chaperone protein Get3 transports the complex to the CAML-WRB receptor in the ER.[7] Additional ER-targeting pathways exist including the ribosome associated SND protein 1 (Snd1) pathway.[7] Once proteins are targeted to the ER they can translocate through a translocon channel such as Sec61 complex.[7] Sec channels can translocate proteins independent of the CAML-WRB and SR receptor engagement.[7]

Effective ER targeting has been achieved with synthetic peptides and recombinant proteins.[8] One such protein was designed as an anti-cancer agent and had three different domains with three different functions: interleukin-24 (IL-24), Tat (GRKKRRQRRRPQ), and Lys-Asp-Glu-Leu (KDEL) domains.[8] The interleukin-24 domain was selected as IL-24 is a pro-apoptotic cytokine in cancer that works at the level of the endoplasmic reticulum.[8] The Tat domain was selected as this is a well-established cell-penetrating peptide derived from human immunodeficiency virus (HIV).[8] The KDEL domain was selected as ER resident proteins contain a C-terminal KDEL sequence.[8] The researchers demonstrated that the peptide enters cells, targets the ER, and induces apoptosis in cancer cells and in nude mice with human lung tumor xenografts.[8] The researchers combined the peptide with YM155, a survivin inhibitor, and demonstrated synergistic efficacy for the combination.[8] Survivin is an inhibitor of apoptosis protein.[8]

An eloquent ER-targeting therapy that was recently developed combines the ideal approach of ER peptide targeting with the benefit of nanomedicine.[9] The investigators developed a dual cell-penetrating peptide-ER targeting peptide construct that they identified as Penetratin (RQIKIWFQNRRMKWKKGG).[9]

Penetratin was conjugated to the surface of polymeric-lipid nanoparticles.[9] Penetratin conjugation increased the cellular uptake and ER localization of the nanoparticles relative to unconjugated nanoparticles and nanoparticles with a Tat peptide.[9] This system is very promising for the future of ER targeting. Optimizing peptides for ER targeting is the most rationale approach for ER localization while the use of a nanoparticle enables the delivery of a range of therapeutics that could be used to treat the ER-associated pathologies identified in Figure 15.4.

Figure 15.5[10] illustrates the considerations and capabilities of ER-targeted nanomedicine. The first consideration is the physical properties of the nanomedicine including shape, size, and charge; these are largely

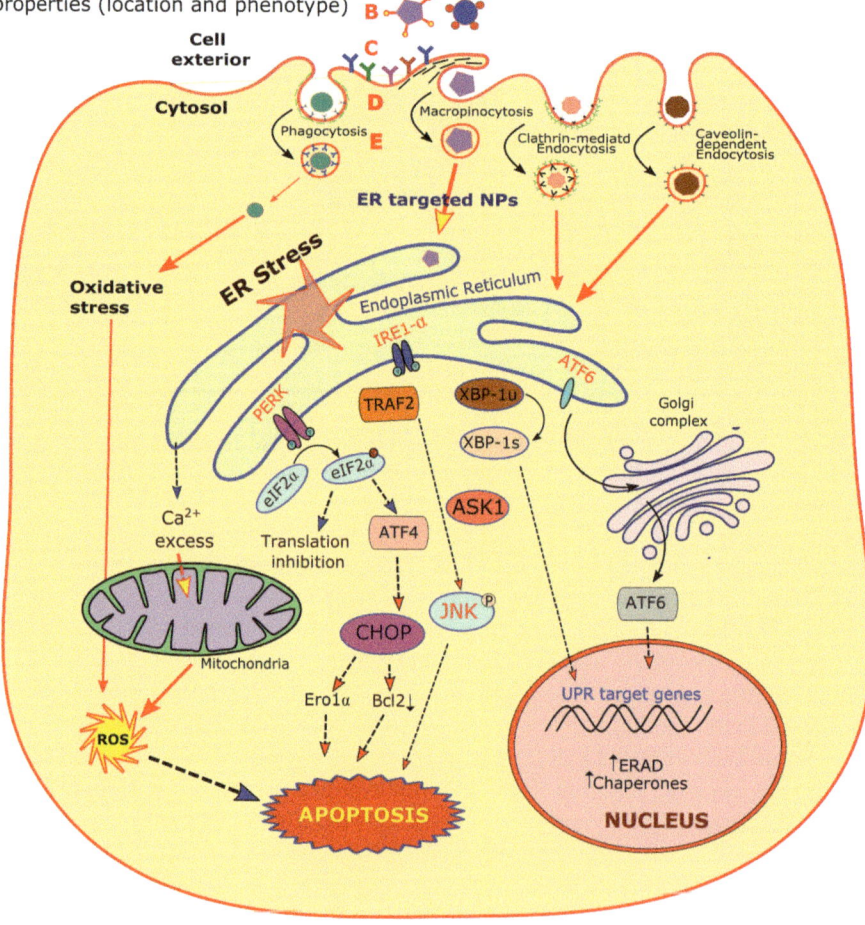

FIGURE 15.5 ER-targeted nanomedicine. Cellular uptake of ER-targeted nanomedicine depends on the physical properties of the nanomedicine including the particle shape, size, and charge. If the nanomedicine is actively targeted to a cell surface receptor, uptake will also depend on the density or targeting ligands on the nanoparticle surface and the expression level of the receptor. The mechanism of internalization (non-specific endocytosis, clathrin-mediated endocytosis, etc.) will determine the rate of cell accumulation and sub-cellular trafficking. ER targeted nanomedicines can contain therapeutics that increase the adaptive phase of the UPR and resolve misfolded proteins, increase ER stress, and sustain the UPR until apoptosis is induced via CHOP or mitochondria, or correct calcium balance. Reprinted with permission and under the terms of the Creative Commons Attribution 4.0 International License (http://creativecommons.org/licenses/by/4.0/).[10]

dictated by the nanoparticle materials and method of synthesis.[10] For actively targeted nanoparticles that are designed to target a specific cell surface receptor, the density of targeting ligands on the nanoparticle as well as the expression level of the receptor will contribute to uptake.[10] An important factor determining the rate of internalization is the mechanism of uptake; if there is active receptor targeting the rate of receptor recycling to the cell membrane will effect uptake as will non-specific endocytosis, clathrin-mediated endocytosis, and caveolin-mediated endocytosis.[10] ER targeting is achieved by conjugating ER-specific peptides to the surface of the nanoparticles. ER-targeted nanomedicine can be designed to either correct ER stress and dysfunction or to induce ER stress and ER stress mediated cell death. For example, increasing the intensity of the adaptive phase of the UPR would be beneficial for treating neurodegenerative disease whereas inducing ER stress/UPR mediated apoptosis would be a treatment strategy for cancer.[10]

15.4 ER THERAPIES AND NANOMEDICINES

Figure 15.6 depicts the role of ER stress in cancer signaling and survival. ER stress in cancer enables cancer survival and proliferation. The most significant axis here is the ER-autophagy axis. ER stress

ER Stress and Cancer Signaling

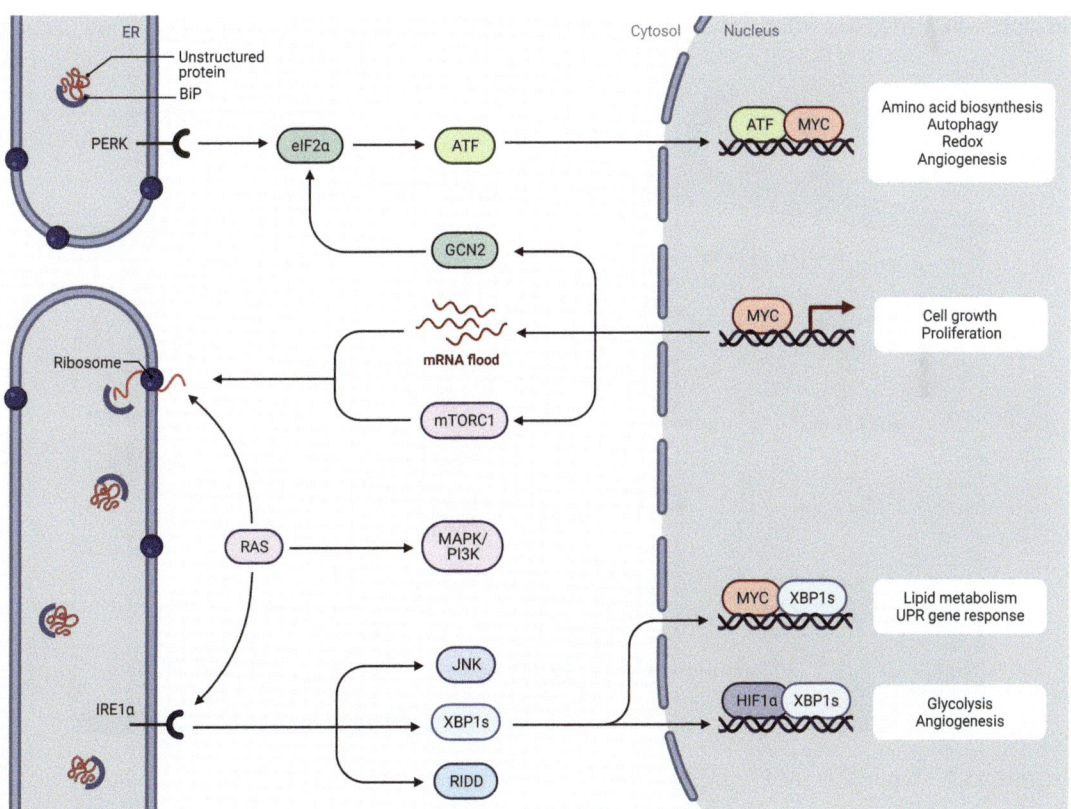

FIGURE 15.6 ER stress and cancer. ER stress in cancer enables cancer survival and proliferation with the most important effect being the ER stress-autophagy feedback loop. ER stress sensors activate transcription factors that induce autophagy, helping a cancer cell to recycle cellular components and survive. Increased mRNA in cancer cells sustains ER stress and this feedback loop. ER stress also leads to transcriptional activation of angiogenesis, glycolysis, proliferation, and amino acid and lipid synthesis. Reprinted with permission and credited to Biorender.com.

promotes autophagy and helps cancer cells to maintain homeostasis through the PERK, eIF2α, ATF, MYC pathway. Increased autophagy contributes to four cancer hallmarks, resisting cell death, sustaining proliferative signaling, enabling replicative immortality, and evading growth suppresion.[11] This same pathway increased amino acid biosynthesis, and angiogenesis. MYC also leads to cell proliferation and an increase in mRNA which results in a feedback loop inducing ER stress that triggers autophagy. The ER stress sensor IRE1α, XBP1s, HIF1α pathway results in aerobic glycolysis and angiogenesis. This is significant as altered bioenergetics and angiogenesis are hallmarks of cancer.[11] The IRE1α, XBP1s, MYC pathway results in lipid metabolism and increased UPR genes which sustain proliferation and survival.

One strategy for treating cancer is to induce the accumulation of misfolded proteins in the ER.[3] Proteosome inhibitors such as bortezomib (approved for multiple myeloma) and ERAD inhibitors such as eeyarestatin I increase the level of misfolded proteins in the ER.[3] Inhibiting chaperones also increases the level of misfolded proteins in the ER; the HSP9 inhibitor 17-allyamino-17-demethoxygeldanamycin (17AAG) and the BiP/GRP78 inhibitor versipelostatin have demonstrated anti-cancer efficacy in pre-clinical models.[3]

A combination nanomedicine for treating cancer has been designed to target the critical ER stress-autophagy feedback loop that propels cancer cell survival.[12] The rationale of this system is illustrated in Figure 15.7. Anodic alumina nanotubes (AANTs) loaded with thapsigargin (TG), an ER stressor, were combined with 3-methyladenine (3-MA) treatment as 3-MA inhibits authophagy.[12] The class III phosphatidylinositol-3 kinase complex PI3K-III is required for autophagy as is microtubule-associated protein 1A/1B-light chain 3 (LC3) association with the phagophore membrane; 3-MA inhibits this process.[12] TG inhibits the sarco/endoplasmic reticulum Ca2+-ATPases (SERCA) channel and induces ER stress.[12] The researchers demonstrated that the AANTs were nontoxic in normal human fibroblasts while combination therapy with 3-MA was effective at treating human triple negative breast cancer cells.[12] This is a very

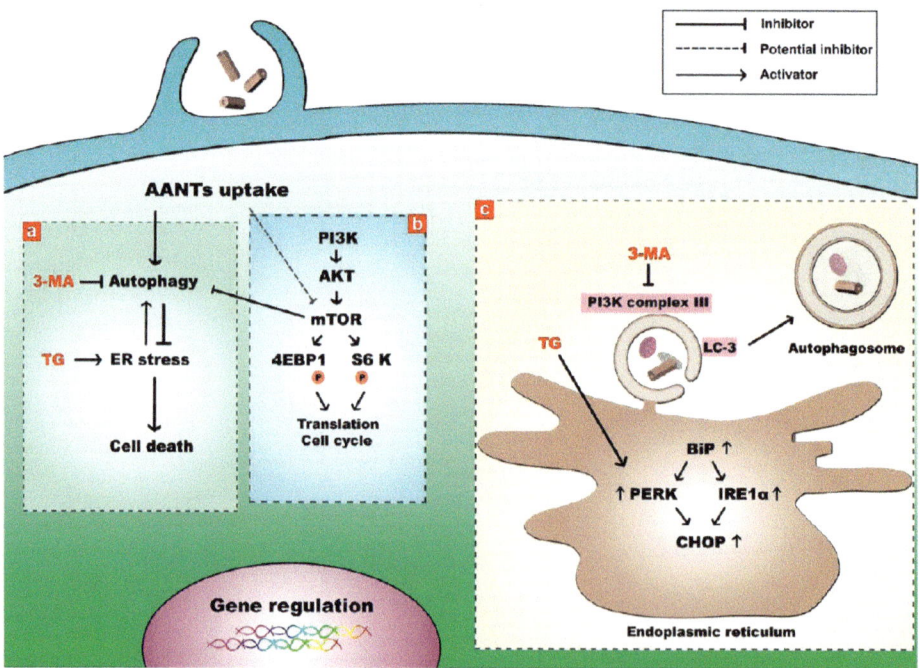

FIGURE 15.7   Nanomedicine for targeting the ER stress-autophagy axis. Anodic alumunia nanotubes (AANTs) loaded with thapsigargin (TG; an ER stressor) were combined with 3-methyladenine (3-MA) treatment as 3-MA inhibits autophagy. Remarkably, AANTs were not toxic in normal human fibroblasts and were very effective at treating human breast cancer. Reprinted with permission from: Wang, Y. et al. Bioinert Anodic Alumina Nanotubes for Targeting of Endoplasmic Reticulum Stress and Autophagic Signaling: A Combinatorial Nanotube-Based Drug Delivery System for Enhancing Cancer Therapy. *ACS Applied Materials & Interfaces* **7**, 27140-27151, doi:10.1021/acsami.5b07557 (2015). Copyright 2015 American Chemical Society.[12]

important strategy to move into *in vivo* models and clinical translation. The lack of toxicity and important ER stress-autophagy targeting could be a transformative cancer treatment.

ER-targeting nanoparticles have been engineered to treat chronic granulomatous disease (CGD), an immunodeficiency disease.[13] CGD is caused by defective NADP oxidase in leukocytes; activated NADP oxidase (NOX2) leads to excessive ROS production which is important for leukocyte signaling and immune activation.[13] Patients with CGD do not mount an efficient immune response to invading pathogens and injury.[13] The investigators who developed this nanomedicine for treating CGD, loaded poly(lactic-coglycolic-acid) (PLGA) nanoparticles with curcumin as curcumin inhibits the sarcoplasmic/endoplasmic reticulum calcium pump (SERCA).[13] The rationale was that the mutant NOX2 in these patients is retained in the ER and drives a UPR which leads to leukocyte apoptosis; inhibiting SERCA could release NOX2 from its chaperon and from ER retention and could restore NADP oxidase function.[13] Active ER targeting was achieved by functionalizing the surface of the nanoparticles with an ER-specific peptide: H-Ala-Ala-Lys-Lys-Ala-Ala-Cys-Cys-Cys-OH.[13] The ER targeted polymeric nanoparticles loaded with curcumin were able to reverse NOX2 accumulation in the ER, decreased leukocyte apoptosis, and increased leukocyte function in C57BL/6 mice.[13] This system is not only an achievement in the treatment of CGD but this system is a flexible platform that could be adapted to target the ER for multiple pathologies by interchanging the cargo (curcumin).

REFERENCES

1. Schwarz, D. S., and M. D. Blower. "The Endoplasmic Reticulum: Structure, Function and Response to Cellular Signaling." *Cellular & Molecular Life Sciences* 73, no. 1 (2016): 79–94. doi:10.1007/s00018-015-2052-6.
2. Phillips, M. J., and G. K. Voeltz. "Structure and Function of ER Membrane Contact Sites with Other Organelles." *Nature Reviews. Molecular Cell Biology* 17, no. 2 (2016): 69–82. doi:10.1038/nrm.2015.8.
3. Bravo, R., V. Parra, D. Gatica, A. E. Rodriguez, N. Torrealba, F. Paredes, Z. V. Wang, A. Zorzano, J. A. Hill, E. Jaimovich, A. F. Quest, and S. Lavandero. *International Review of Cell & Molecular Biology* vol. 301. Edited by Kwang W. Jeon, 215–90. Academic Press, 2013.
4. Milisav, I., D. Šuput, and S. Ribarič. "Unfolded Protein Response and Macroautophagy in Alzheimer's, Parkinson's and Prion Diseases." *Molecules* 20, no. 12 (2015). doi:10.3390/molecules201219865.
5. Ogata, M., S. Hino, A. Saito, K. Morikawa, S. Kondo, S. Kanemoto, T. Murakami, M. Taniguchi, I. Tanii, K. Yoshinaga, S. Shiosaka, J. A. Hammarback, F. Urano, and K. Imaizumi. "Autophagy Is Activated for Cell Survival After Endoplasmic Reticulum Stress." *Molecular & Cellular Biology* 26, no. 24 (2006): 9220–31. doi:10.1128/MCB.01453-06.
6. Lee, W. S., W. H. Yoo, and H. J. Chae. "ER Stress and Autophagy." *Current Molecular Medicine* 15, no. 8 (2015): 735–45. doi:10.2174/1566524015666150921105453.
7. Aviram, N., and M. Schuldiner. "Targeting and Translocation of Proteins to the Endoplasmic Reticulum at a Glance." *Journal of Cell Science* 130, no. 24 (2017): 4079–85. doi:10.1242/jcs.204396.
8. Zhang, J., R. Xu, X. Tao, Y. Dong, X. Lv, A. Sun, and D. Wei. "TAT-IL-24-KDEL-Induced Apoptosis Is Inhibited by Survivin but Restored by the Small Molecular Survivin Inhibitor, YM155, in Cancer Cells." *Oncotarget* 7, no. 24 (2016): 37030–42. doi:10.18632/oncotarget.9458.
9. Kang, J. Y., S. Kim, J. Kim, N. G. Kang, C. S. Yang, S. J. Min, and J. W. Kim. "Cell-Penetrating Peptide-Conjugated Lipid/Polymer Hybrid Nanovesicles for Endoplasmic Reticulum-Targeting Intracellular Delivery." *Journal of Materials Chemistry B* 9, no. 2 (2021): 464–70. doi:10.1039/D0TB01940B.
10. Khan, A. A., K. S. Allemailem, A. Almatroudi, S. A. Almatroodi, A. Mahzari, M. A. Alsahli, and A. H. Rahmani. "Endoplasmic Reticulum Stress Provocation by Different Nanoparticles: An Innovative Approach to Manage the Cancer and Other Common Diseases." *Molecules* 25, no. 22 (2020): 5336.
11. Hanahan, D., and Robert A. Weinberg. "Hallmarks of Cancer: The Next Generation." *Cell* 144, no. 5 (2011): 646–74. doi:10.1016/j.cell.2011.02.013.
12. Wang, Y., G. Kaur, Y. Chen, A. Santos, D. Losic, and A. Evdokiou. "Bioinert Anodic Alumina Nanotubes for Targeting of Endoplasmic Reticulum Stress and Autophagic Signaling: A Combinatorial Nanotube-Based Drug Delivery System for Enhancing Cancer Therapy." *ACS Applied Materials & Interfaces* 7, no. 49 (2015): 27140–51. doi:10.1021/acsami.5b07557.

13. Yen, C.-L., Y. C. Liao, R. F. Chen, Y. F. Huang, W. C. Chung, P. C. Lo, C. F. Chang, P. C. Wu, D. B. Shieh, S. T. Jiang, and C. C. Shieh. "Targeted Delivery of Curcumin Rescues Endoplasmic Reticulum–Retained Mutant NOX2 Protein and Avoids Leukocyte Apoptosis." *Journal of Immunology* 202, no. 12 (2019): 3394–403. doi:10.4049/jimmunol.1801599.

Targeting Mitochondria*

16

Lara Scheherazade Milane

Contents

16.1 MITOCHONDRIAL FUNCTION

Mitochondria are dynamic organelles that undergo perpetual fusion and fission and even fuse with other organelles such as the endoplasmic reticulum.[1,2] The mitochondrial network continually adapts and responds to cellular needs; mitochondria are the ultimate cellular sensors and effectors. Mitochondria are memorized to be the power house of the cell, and are often depicted in illustrations as peanut-shaped organelles in an isolated region of the cell; this notion is drastically inadequate. Mitochondria regulate apoptosis, produce energy (ATP), respond to cell stress such as elevated ROS and the unfolded protein response, and manage mitophagy and autophagy to aid in cell survival.[3,4] If a cell were a city, mitochondria would be the electric company, the grim reaper, the recycling center, and a large portion of the traffic lights.

Mitochondria originated as archaebacteria that were engulfed by the primordial eukaryotic cell in a process referred to as endosymbiosis. This mutually beneficial occurrence provided the mitochondria with a constant supply of nutrients and metabolites while the mitochondria provided the eukaryotic cell with a high number of adenine triphosphate (ATP) molecules for energy. Mitochondria produce ATP through oxidative phosphorylation (OXPHOS) which generates 36 molecules of ATP per molecule of glucose whereas glycolysis (cytoplasmic process and the only energy process before endosymbiosis) produces 2 molecules of ATP per molecule of glucose. The endosymbiosis of mitochondria truly enabled evolution as we know it. Without the increased energy capacity, complex organisms such as humans would not be possible.

---

* Sections of this chapter such as Figure 16.2 and Table 16.1 are reprinted with permission from: Milane, L., Trivedi, M., Singh, A., Talekar, M. & Amiji, M. Mitochondrial biology, targets, and drug delivery. *J Control Release* **207**, 40–58. Copyright © 2015, Elsevier

DOI: 10.1201/9781003092773-18

The inner mitochondrial membrane (IMM) contains the OXPHOS complexes: Complex I (NADH: ubiquinone oxidoreductase), Complex II (succinate: ubiquinone oxidoreductase), Complex III (ubiquinol: cytochrome c oxidoreductase), Complex IV (cytochrome c oxidase), and Complex V (ATP synthase; F1F0-ATPase).[5] ATP is produced by Complex V when the electron transport chain oxidizes NADH which drives the production of ATP from adenosine 5'-diphosphate (ADP).[5] The mitochondrial permeability transition pore (mPTP) complex is a multiprotein channel that spans the IMM and the intermembrane space (IMS) exiting the outer mitochondrial membrane (OMM) for the release of ATP.[6] The mPTP complex also mediates the release of cytochrome c for the induction of apoptosis. The mPTP complex is composed of adenosine nucleotide transporter (ANT) in the IMM, IMS and matrix proteins creatine kinase (CK) and cyclophilin D (CypD), and the voltage-dependent anion channel (VDAC) in the OMM.[6] The capture of ATP for glycolysis occurs through hexokinase 2 (HXK2) association with the mPTP complex.[6]

In addition to energy production, mitochondria mediate cell death through the intrinsic apoptotic pathway.[7] This process is compared to the extrinsic pathway in Figure 16.1. This is a well-characterized pathway regulated by proapoptotic and antiapoptotic B cell lymphoma-2 (Bcl-2) family proteins.[7] Proapoptotic Bcl-2 proteins include Bax and Bak while the anti-apoptotic factors include Bcl-2, Bcl-XL, Bcl-W, Mcl-1, and A1/Bfl-1.[8] The anti-apoptotic factors bind to pro-apoptotic BH3-only proteins (BID,

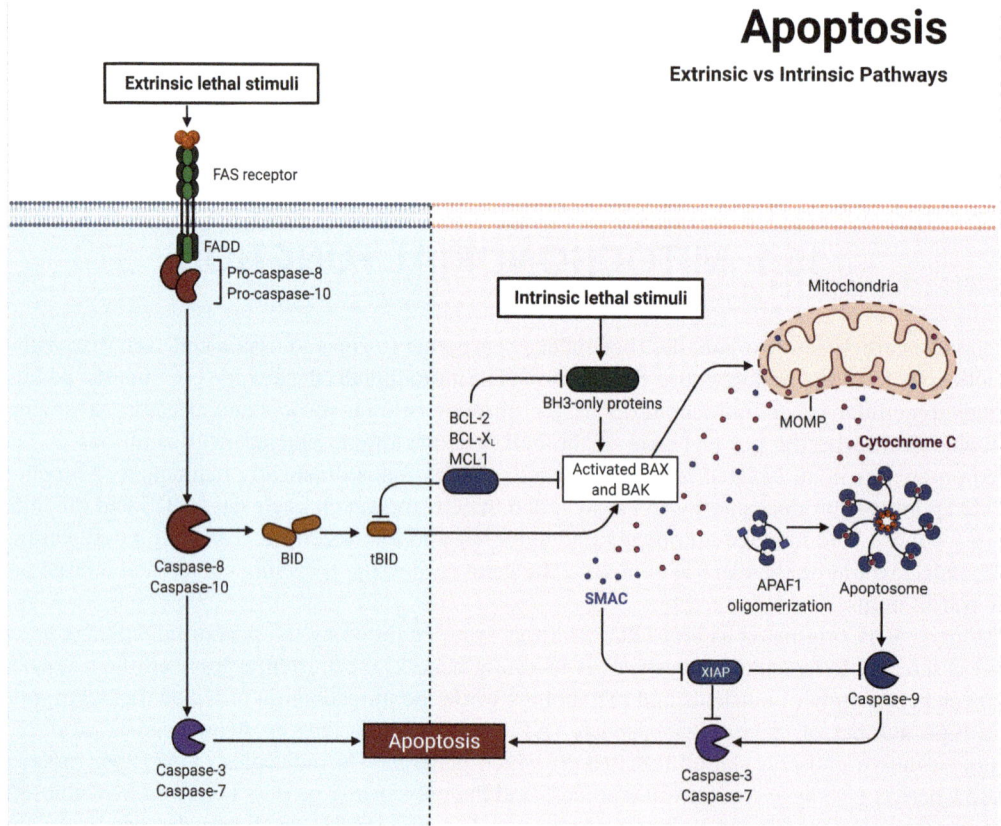

FIGURE 16.1 Extrinsic and intrinsic apoptosis. The external apoptotic pathway involves ligand binding (or auto-stimulation) of a death receptor on the plasma membrane. This leads to pro-caspade 8 and 10 activation, activated caspase 8 and 10, and effector caspase 3 and 7 activation. The intrinsic apoptotic pathway begins with activated Bax or Bak inducing mitochondrial outer membrane permeability (MOMP) which leads to the release of cytochrome c and Smac/Diablo. Smac/Diablo inhibits IAPs while cytochrome c complexes with pro-caspase 9 and apoptosis protease activating factor (APAF-1) to form the apoptosome. The apoptosome then activates caspase 9 which leads to caspase 3 and 7 activity. Reprinted with permission and credited to Biorender.com.

BIM, PUMA/BBC3, BAD, NOXA/PMAIP, BIK/BLK/NBK, BMF, and HRK/DP5) and prevent their activation of Bax and Bak.[8] Activated Bax and Bak bind to the OMM and induce mitochondrial membrane permeabilization and pore formation which leads to the release of cytochrome c, apoptosis inducing factor (AIF), and Smac/Diablo.[9] Pore formation also requires activation by pro-apoptotic BH3-proteins and dimerization of Bax or Bak.[9] AIF fragments, Smac/Diablo binding to the inhibitor of apoptosis (IAP) proteins, and cytochrome c complexes with pro-caspase 9 and apoptosis protease activating factor (APAF-1) to form the apoptosome.[10] The apoptosome activates caspase 9 which leads to effector caspase (3/7) activation.[10]

In addition to energy production and regulation of intrinsic apoptosis, mitochondria regulate reactive oxygen species (ROS) production. Complex I is the primary source of ROS production, and this occurs during OXPHOS.[5] ROS function in cell signaling and can be cell stressors. ROS can trigger autophagy and induce neutrophils to undergo netosis, the formation of DNA-based neutrophil extracellular traps (NETs) to capture pathogenic bacteria.[11] Excessive ROS accumulation can lead to inflammation and cell death and contributes to neurodegenerative disease as well as cancer.[11] ROS-scavenging enzymes help to resolve ROS accumulation but they are not adequate to manage ROS toxicity when a cell is undergoing excessive ROS production.[11]

An important and often overlooked function of mitochondria is in the regulation of mitophagy and autophagy. Mitochondrial stress, excessive ROS, and depleted ATP can induce mitophagy and autophagy to correct mitochondrial and cellular dysfunction.[12,13] Mitophagy is controlled via three pathways. The main mitophagic pathway is the PINK1/Parkin pathway.[14] When there is no mitochondrial stress, PINK1 is trafficked to mitochondria, internalized, and degraded in mitochondria.[14] When there is mitochondrial stress, PINK1 is stabilized on the OMM instead of internalized for degradation.[14] Parkin is then recruited, leading to mitochondrial protein ubiquitinations and mitophagy.[15,16] The Bcl-2 nineteen-kilodalton interacting protein 3 (BNIP3) and Bcl-2 Interacting Protein 3 Like protein (BNIP3L/NIX) pathway involves the recruitment of BNIP3L and NIX to the OMM which then leads to microtubule-associated protein 1A/1B-light chain 3 (LC3-I) binding to the OMM.[12,13] LC3-1 is then conjugated to phosphatidylethanolamine (PE), forming LC3-II.[12,13] The cardiolipin pathway occurs when the IMM protein cardiolipin translocates to the OMM, marking mitochondrial dysfunction.[12,13] As with the BNIP3L/NIX pathway, this then leads to LC3-1 recruitment and eventual mitophagy and autophagy.[13]

16.2 MITOCHONDRIAL DYSFUNCTION AND DISEASE

As illustrated in Figure 16.2 and Table 16.1, there are multiple mitochondrial targets that have applications in treating a range of diseases from cancer to Parkinson's disease.[7] Mitochondrial targets for therapeutic intervention are present in the outer mitochondrial membrane (OMM), inner mitochondrial membrane (IMM), matrix, and intermembrane space (IMS). Targets of the OMM include the fission proteins Drp1 and Fis1, fusion proteins including Mitofusin 1 (Mfn1), the migratory protein Miro, PTEN-induced kinase 1 (Pink1) and associated Parkin, the multi-drug efflux pump P-glycoprotein (Pgp), pro-apoptotic and anti-apoptotic Bcl-2 family member proteins (Bcl2), the voltage-dependent anion channel (VDAC), hexokinase 2 (HXK2), the peripheral benzodiazepine receptor/translocator protein (PBR/TSPO), the translocase of the outer membrane (TOM), the tumor suppressor p53, and the importer for activated fatty acids carnitine palmitotransferase I (CPT1).[7] IMM targets include complexes I–V of the respiratory chain, cytochrome c, uncoupling proteins (UCP2), the adenine nucleotide translocators (ANTs), the translocase of the inner membrane (TIM), and the IMM fusion protein Optic atrophy protein 1 (Opa1).[7] Matrix targets include the silent information regulator proteins (sirtuin), mitochondrial estrogen receptors, components of the TCA cycle, cyclophilin D associated with the mitochondrial permeability transition pore complex (mPTPC; VDAC, ANT, and associated proteins), heat shock proteins (HSP 70), mitochondrial ribosomes, and mitochondrial DNA.[7]

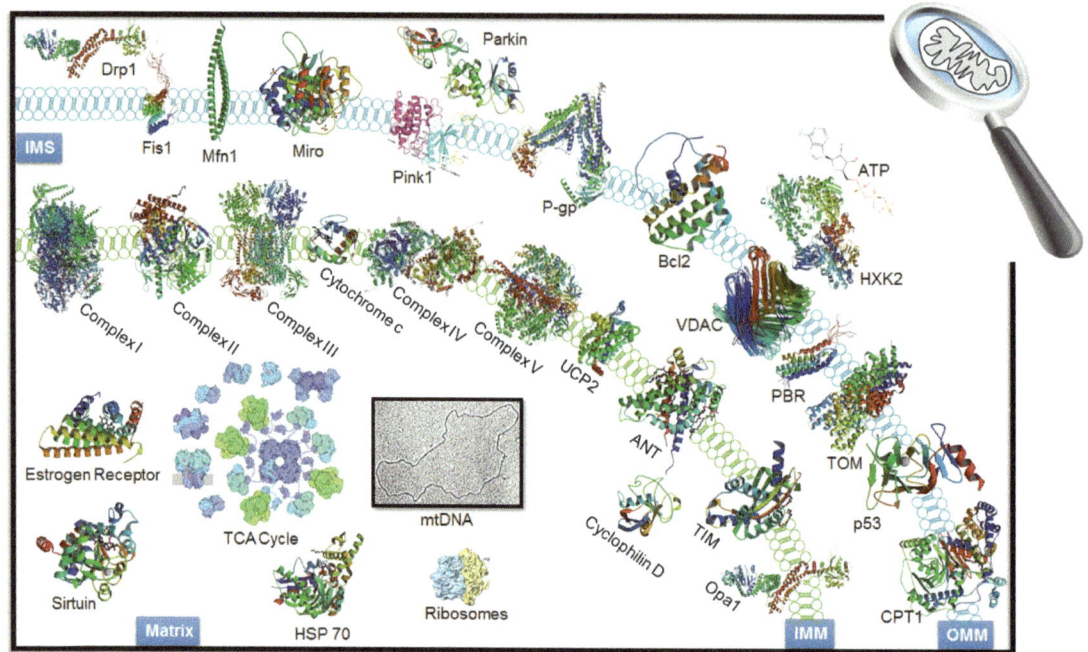

FIGURE 16.2 Mitochondrial targets. Mitochondrial targets exist at the level of the OMM, the IMM, the IMS, and the matrix. These targets are important in many pathologies such as hexokinase 2 (HXK2) inhibition of the Warburg effect in cancer and Parkin induced autophagy in Parkinson's disease. Complex I is a prime target for decreasing ROS. Reprinted with permission from: Milane, L., Trivedi, M., Singh, A., Talekar, M. & Amiji, M. Mitochondrial biology, targets, and drug delivery. *J Control Release* **207**, 40–58. Copyright © 2015, Elsevier.

Specific mitochondrial processes are also therapeutic targets. Senescence is the counterbalance to PINK1/Parkin mediated mitophagy.[17] Cytosolic p53 stabilizes Parkin in the cytosol and prevents mitochondrial association and inhibits mitophagy.[17] Mitophagy and autophagy are lacking in neurogenerative disease, and this is evident from PARK2 mutations that lead to some forms of Parkinson's disease.[16] On the other hand, cancer is associated with loss of or aberrant p53; without p53 to trap Parkin in the cytosol it can readily bind to the OMM to induce mitophagy which aids in cancer cell survival.

There is marked mitochondrial dysfunction in cancer. The most significant dysfunction is that cancer cells are resistant to intrinsic apoptosis as cancer cells are most simply cells that will adapt and change however necessary to confer survival. Resistance to cell death is an important hallmark of cancer.[18] Cancer cells achieve this resistance via multiple mechanisms including overexpression of anti-apoptotic Bcl-2 proteins, apoptosome dysfunction, and mutations.[4,19] One of the hallmarks of cancer is deregulated bioenergetics and increased aerobic glycolysis (the Warburg effect).[18,20–22] Aerobic glycolysis enables cancer cells to reduce ROS accumulation during OXPHOS, generates metabolic intermediates, and enables an energy supply under hypoxic and anoxic conditions.[20–22] Hexokinase 2 (HXK2) enables the Warburg effect by capturing ATP from the mPTP complex for the initiation of glycolysis.[6,20–22] HXK2 binding to the OMM also has anti-apoptotic effects as HXK2 association with the mPTP complex sterically hinders Bax binding to the OMM.[21]

Mitochondrial dysfunction in neurodegenerative disease results from excessive ROS production, decreased OXPHOS, and hyper activation of apoptosis[23,24] For example, β-amyloid accumulation in mitochondria of Alzheimer's disease (AD) patients has been shown to inhibit mitochondrial protein import through the translocase of the outer mitochondrial membrane 40 (TOM40) and induce mPTP opening leading to the release of cytochrome c and the pro-apoptotic cascade.[25] Mitochondrial dysfunction also contributes to rheumatoid arthritis (RA) and type II diabetes mellitus through ROS accumulation in the synovium and beta cells respectively.[26,27] Cardiovascular disease is associated with hypersensitivity to apoptosis and oxidative stress.[28]

TABLE 16.1 Mitochondrial Targets and Substrates[7]

LOCATION	TARGET	DRUG
OMM	Hexokinase	Lonidamine
		3-Bromopyruvate (also a Complex II inhibitor)
		2-Deoxyglucose
	VDAC	Geldanamycin (and its derivatives 17AAG, Ub0, and decyl-ubiquinone)
		Arsenic derivatives (such as AS_2O_3)
		Benzyl isothiocyanate
	Bcl-2 family member proteins	BH3 mimetics such as gossypol, ABT-263 (navitoclax), and ABT-737
		Antimycin A
		α-Tocopheryl succinate
	PBR	PK11195
		Endozepine
		Protoporphyrin IX
		Triakontatetraneuropeptide
		Phospholipase A2
		Ro5-4864
		XK469
		4'-Chlorodiazepam
		BBL22
		FGIN-1-27
		SSR180575
	Forms channels in OMM	Ceramide
	P-gp	P-gp substrates (such as digoxin, fexofenadine, indinavir, vincristine, colchicine, topotecan, paclitaxel)
		P-gp inhibitors (such as ritonavir, cyclosporine, verapamil, erythromycin, ketocoanzole, itraconazole, quinidine)
OMM and IMM	P-gp in OMM; also IMM	Rhodamine 123
IMM	IMM	Triphenylphosphonium
		MitoQ
		MKT-077
		F16
	Complex I inhibitor	Rotenone
		Annonaceous acetogenins
		Metformin
	Complex II	Vitamin E analogs such as α-tocopheryl succinate
	Complex II inhibitor	3-Bromopyruvate
		3-Nitropropionic acid (irreversible inhibitor)
	Complex III inhibitor	Antimycin A
		Myxothiazole
	Complex IV inhibitor	Cyanide
	Complex V	Oligomycin

(Continued)

TABLE 16.1 (Continued) Mitochondrial Targets and Substrates[7]

LOCATION	TARGET	DRUG
		Apoptolidins
		Bz-423
		Resveratrol
		Dindolyl methane
		Aurovertin
		PK11195
	ROS scavengers	Szeto-Schiller peptides
	ANT1 inhibitor	Bongkrekic acid
		Carboxyatractyloside
	MitoK$_{ATP}$ channel blocker	Glibenclamide
		5-Hydroxydecanoic acid
		MCC-134
	MitoK$_{ATP}$ channel opener	Diazoxide
		Nicorandil
		BMS180448
		BMS-191095
	UCP	Carbonyl cyanide M-chlorophenyl hydrazone
		2,4-Dinitrophenol
Matrix	Pyruvate dehydrogenase kinase	Dichloroacetate
	SIRT1	Resveratrol
	Mitochondrial estrogen receptors	Tamoxifen
		Estrogen derivatives
	mtDNA damage	Ciprofloxacin
	Cyclophilin	Cyclosporin A
General intrinsic apoptotic activators/ inducers of mPTPC formation		Paclitaxel
		Anthracyclines
		Arsenic trioxide
		Doxorubicin (ROS generation, Complex I activity)
		Staurosporine
		Irinotecan
		5-Fluorouracil (ROS generation, mtDNA damage)
		Cisplatin (ROS generation)
		Betulinic acid (disrupts membrane potential)
		Imexon, parthenolide, mangafodipir, menadione, motexafine gadolinium, and β-lapachone (oxidative stress and ROS generation)

16.3 MITOCHONDRIAL TARGETING

There are four strategies for achieving mitochondrial targeting; two of these strategies mimic endogenous mitochondrial directed proteins: (1) the use of mitochondrial leader sequences and (2) mitochondriotropic peptides, while two of the strategies exploit the high negative membrane potential of mitochondria: (3) delocalized cations and (4) DQASomes. Mimicking endogenous mitochondrial targeting is a very rational approach to mitochondrial drug delivery as most mitochondrial proteins are nuclear encoded and imported into mitochondria.[7] The translocase of the outer membrane (TOM) complex is the primary mitochondrial importer in the OMM and the main translocase of this complex is the TOM40 protein.[29] As depicted in Figure 16.2, there are two mechanisms of mitochondrial protein import with either N-terminal mitochondrial leader sequences (MLS) or internal MLS which requires chaperone delivery to mitochondria.[29] The proteins with internal MLS are hydrophobic IMM proteins that would aggregate and misfold in the cytosol without chaperone stabilization and protection.[29] Similarly, chaperones in the IMS assist delivery of these proteins into the IMM.[29] This strategy is highly effective and mimicking endogenous MLS is assisted with databases and tools such as Mitofates[30] (Figure 16.3).

Similarly, mitochondriotropic peptides are modeled on endogenous MLS but encompass an entire peptide, not just a fragment of the peptide. These peptides are also referred to as mitochondrial penetrating peptides (MPPs) and a common group of these peptides are the Szeto-Schiller peptides.[31–34] The two design principles of these peptides are (1) high positive charge and (2) lipophilicity[33] Mitochondria have the most negative membrane potential (–170 mV) of any cellular and subcellular compartment; as such, positive residues accumulate at the site of mitochondria. Likewise, the IMM is hydrophobic and lipophilic peptides are able to enter mitochondria.[33] The Szeto-Schiller peptides are a group of MPPs designed by Hazel Szeto in 2006; although there are current and past clinical trials of these peptides the efficacy for treating mitochondrial myopathies has not been demonstrated.[35]

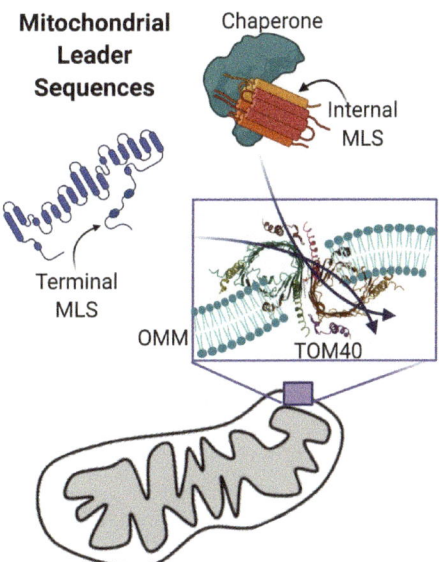

FIGURE 16.3 Mitochondrial leader sequences. The mitochondrial leader sequences (MLS) can be terminal or internal. Peptides with internal MLS require chaperones. Once at the OMM the MLS guides translocation into mitochondria through TOM40. The three other approaches for mitochondrial targeting include the use of mitochondriotropic peptides, delocalized cations, or DQAsomes. Reprinted with permission and credited to Biorender.com.

Targeting mitochondria with delocalized lipophilic cations (DLC) and highly positively charged molecules exploits the negative membrane potential of mitochondria. The most common DLC used for targeting molecules and particles to mitochondria is triphenylphosphonium (TPP).[7,36] DLCs accumulate preferentially in cancer cells and cardiomyocyctes and are useful for tumor targeting or cardiovascular targeting; however, they do tend to be substrates for drug efflux pumps such as P-glycoprotein.[37] The fourth strategy for achieving mitochondrial targeting is with DQASomes, self-assembled bolaform dequalinium structures.[38] Dequalinium is a bactericidal quaternary ammonium cation. DQASomes also exploit the negative membrane potential of mitochondria and have been used for drug and DNA delivery in preclinical cancer models.[39,40]

16.4 MITOCHONDRIAL NANOMEDICINE

The four mitochondrial targeting strategies are necessary for mitochondrial accumulation; coupling these targeting strategies with nanomedicine enables the delivery of diverse therapeutics. As illustrated in Figure 16.4, the desired nanoparticle behavior can be achieved through nanoparticle design. Mitochondrial targeting via one of the four strategies is one aspect of mitochondrial delivery, but before a formulation can reach mitochondria in a target cell it must transverse systemic circulation or the biological barriers associated with the route of administration, must enter target tissue and accumulate in target cells, and must have low residual toxicity. Nanoparticle shape and size can help avoid immune recognition; smaller spherical particles that are less resemblant of bacteria are less likely to be cleared. Likewise, excessive charge can induce immune clearance and toxicity; the nanoparticles must be compatible with physiological pH. The surface modification will dictate how the nanoparticles avoid immune recognition and how they enter cells. The internalization mechanism will determine the rate and limitation of uptake kinetics. Finally, the

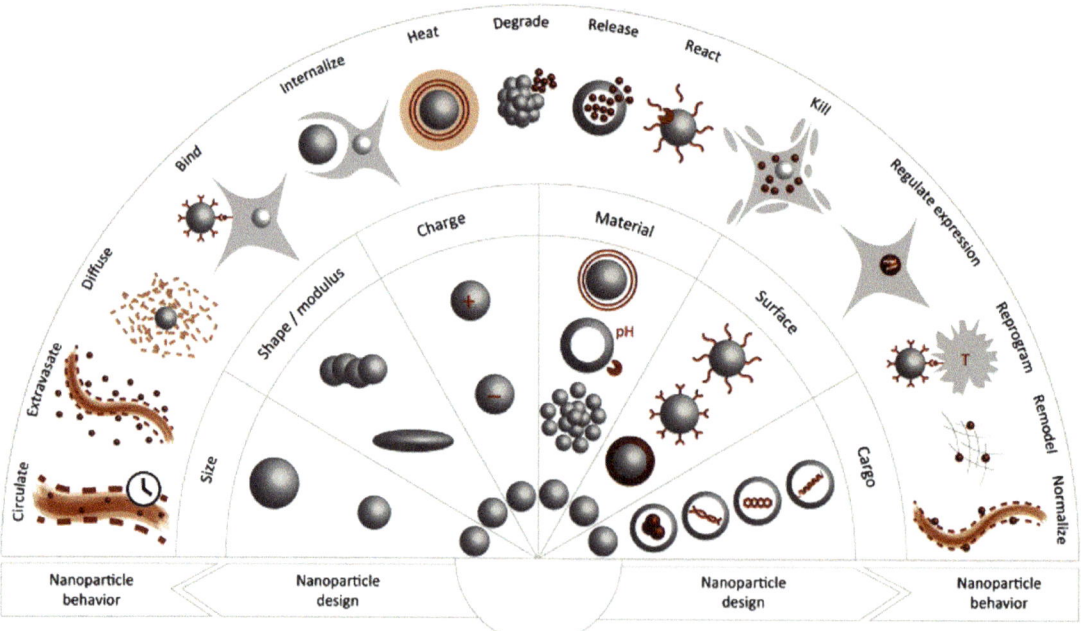

FIGURE 16.4   Nanomedicine design. Reprinted with Permission from: Hauert, S. & Bhatia, S. N. Mechanisms of cooperation in cancer nanomedicine: towards systems nanotechnology. Trends in biotechnology 32, 448–455, doi:https://doi.org/10.1016/j.tibtech.2014.06.010 (2014). Copyright © 2014 Elsevier Ltd.[41]

nanoparticle payload will determine the biological response. Table 16.1 details some mitochondriotropic molecules that target and affect mitochondria and are ideal cargos for mitochondrial nanomedicines.

The development of platform systems such as DQASomes is very pivotal to the clinical translation of mitochondrial nanomedicine as the more applications and data a system can acquire, the greater the translational potential. These platform systems can interchange drugs for different applications and may even be capable of altering the surface modification. One such platform system is MITO-Porter.[42] MITO-Porter was designed as a versatile platform that can fuse with the OMM.[42] The system is composed of a mitochondrial fusogenic lipid consisting of 1,2-dioleoyl-sn-glycero-3-phosphatidyl ethanolamine (DOPE) and sphingomyelin (SM).[42] The surfaces of the nanoparticles are studded with cell-penetrating peptide octaarginine residues to enable macropinocytosis.[42] Figure 16.5 illustrates the MITO-Porter strategy. This system is ideal for multiple applications; even the cell-penetrating peptide could be exchanged for a different cell targeting residue. The liposome formulation would enable the delivery of hydrophobic therapeutics (in the lipid bilayer of the nanoparticle) and hydrophilic therapeutics (in the aqueous core). As a proof of concept the researchers loaded the MITO-Porter nanoparticles with Co-enzyme Q_{10}, a ubiquinol antioxidant, for treating hepatic ischemia/reperfusion in a mouse model.[42] MITO-Porter nanoparticles improved the drug delivery of Co-enzyme Q_{10}, and increased the efficacy.[42] The researchers also evaluated the MITO-Porter system for cancer therapy and separately evaluated the delivery of gentamicin, doxorubicin, and rTA, a pi-extended porphyrin-type photosensitizer.[42] The MITO-Porter system demonstrated improved efficacy in cellular and animal models of human cancers.[42] Developing flexible platforms such as MITO-Porters for mitochondrial drug delivery is important for advancing mitochondrial nanomedicine; the more safety and efficacy studies that are completed in one system, the stronger the data for clinical translation.

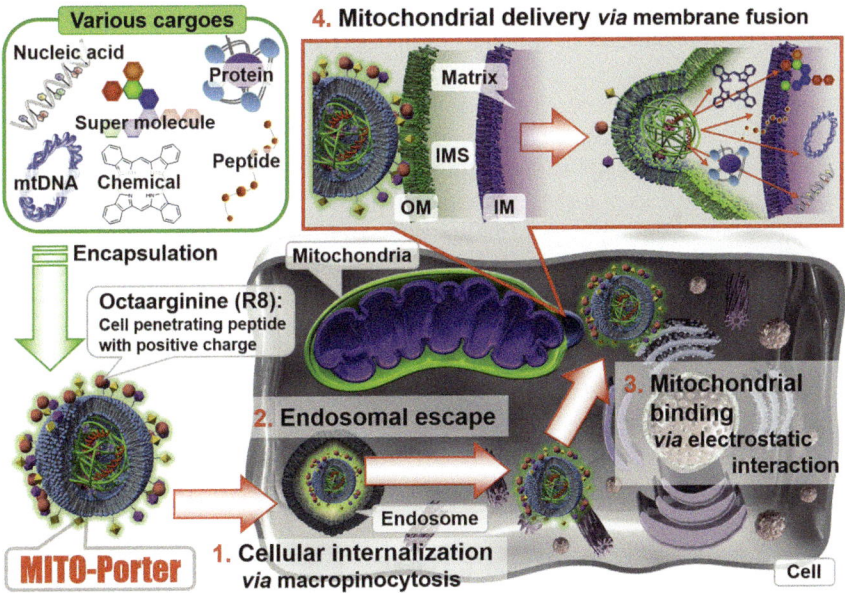

FIGURE 16.5 MITO-Porter nanoparticles. MITO-Porter nanoparticles are nanoparticles that have been designed to fuse with the mitochondrial OMM. This is a platform technology where the drug payload can be interchanged for different applications. The surfaces of the nanoparticles are coated with octoarginine to enable cell penetration, they are internalized via micropinocytosis, and they escape endosomal clearance and interact with mitochondria via electrostatic interactions before nanoparticle-OMM membrane fusion. Reprinted with permission from Yamada, Y. et al. Power of mitochondrial drug delivery systems to produce innovative nanomedicines. *Advanced Drug Delivery Reviews* **154–155**, 187–209, doi:https://doi.org/10.1016/j. addr.2020.09.010 (2020). Copyright © 2020 Elsevier.[42]

ROS scavenging, as with Co-enzyme Q_{10}, is an important approach for reversing ROS-induced damage and cell death. TPP has actually been conjugated to co-enzyme Q_{10} to direct the antioxidant to mitochondria; mitoquinol 10 is commercially available as a dietary supplement.[43] ROS-scavenging liposomes have been evaluated for the treatment of type II diabetes mellitus using mitochondrial-PBN (ROS scavenger).[27] The ROS-scavenging nanoparticles were able to reduce ROS, improve mitochondrial function, and reverse insulin resistance in a diabetic mouse model.[27] ROS scavenging is also relevant to developing therapies for treating neurodegenerative disease. An example of ROS-scavenging nanoparticles for CNS disease is the application of curcumin loaded TPP-polymeric (PLGA) nanoparticles.[44] Researchers overloaded cells with excessive (20 µM) β-amyloid protein and observed that treatment with the curcumin-loaded TPP-PLGA nanoparticles reduced β-amyloid protein neurotoxicity.[44] ROS-activated nanomedicines have also been developed for treating rheumatoid arthritis (RA).[45] In this very unique approach, investigators exploited the excessive ROS in RA synovial joints by using ROS-cleavable linkers in PLGA-PEG micelles loaded with berberine.[45] Upon accumulation in drug-resistant synoviocytes with high ROS, the linkers of the micelles were cleaved, releasing berberine which decreased complex 1 activity and ROS accumulation.[45]

One of the most explored applications of mitochondrial nanomedicine is for treating cancer. Our group designed actively targeted, combination therapy polymeric nanoparticles for inhibiting the Warburg effect in cancer and for inducing apoptosis.[46–49] The polymeric nanoparticles were surface modified with an Epidermal Growth Factor Receptor (EGFR) specific peptide which is overexpressed in multi-drug-resistant (MDR) triple negative breast cancer (TNBC).[46–49] The nanoparticles were loaded with lonidamine, a hexokinase 2 (HXK2) inhibitor, and with paclitaxel, a common chemotherapeutic agent that hyper-stabilizes microtubules.[46–49] A complete *in vitro* and *in vivo* preclinical study was performed in cellular models of MDR TNBC and orthotopic models of human MDR TNBC in nude mice.[46–49] The EGFR targeted nanoparticles improved the tumor pharmacokinetics of lonidamine, reduced the markers of aerobic glycolysis in tumors, and significantly decreased tumor volumes relative to treatment with drug solutions and single agent treatment.[46–49] Mitochondrial targeted nanomedicines are important for treating MDR cancer.

Mitochondrial targeting in cancer cells seems to have efficacy without any drug payload, suggesting that the mitochondria in cancer are sensitized to the effects of targeting. A study evaluating the use of sclareol loaded TPP liposomes demonstrated that TPP liposomes alone (with no drug) increased cell death relative to non-targeted nanoparticles.[50] Sclareol is a direct apoptotic activator through caspase 8, 9, and 3 induction.[50] Although drug-free TPP liposomes resulted in less than 30% cell death, non-targeted drug free liposomes resulted in no significant cell death and sclareol loaded TPP liposomes resulted in 60% cell death in COLO205 human colon adenocarcinoma cells after 24 hours of treatment, the effect of mitochondrial targeting alone should be significantly considered in cancer.[50] Targeting mitochondria may enable a drastically lower dose of drug to be administered relative to non-targeted treatments, and our studies support this as well. This is a very exciting benefit of mitochondrial targeting in cancer.

REFERENCES

1. Paupe, V., and J. Prudent. "New Insights into the Role of Mitochondrial Calcium Homeostasis in Cell Migration." *Biochemical and Biophysical Research Communications* 500, no. 1 (2018): 75–86. doi:10.17863/CAM.12394.
2. Mishra, P., and D. C. Chan. "Metabolic Regulation of Mitochondrial Dynamics." *Journal of Cell Biology* 212, no. 4 (2016): 379–87. doi:10.1083/jcb.201511036.
3. Wang, T. S., I. Coppens, A. Saorin, N. R. Brady, and A. Hamacher-Brady. "Endolysosomal Targeting of Mitochondria Is Integral to BAX-Mediated Mitochondrial Permeabilization During Apoptosis Signaling." *Developmental Cell* 53, no. 6 (2020): 627–645 e627. doi:10.1016/j.devcel.2020.05.014.

4. Tan, Y. Q., X. Zhang, S. Zhang, T. Zhu, M. Garg, P. E. Lobie, and V. Pandey. "Mitochondria: The Metabolic Switch of Cellular Oncogenic Transformation." *Biochimica & Biophysica Acta (BBA): Reviews on Cancer* (2021), 188534. doi:10.1016/j.bbcan.2021.188534.

5. Hüttemann, M., I. Lee, L. Samavati, H. Yu, and J. W. Doan. "Regulation of Mitochondrial Oxidative Phosphorylation Through Cell Signaling." *Biochimica & Biophysica Acta (BBA): Molecular Cell Research* 1773, no. 12 (2007): 1701–20. doi:10.1016/j.bbamcr.2007.10.001.

6. Bonora, M., and P. Pinton. "The Mitochondrial Permeability Transition Pore and Cancer: Molecular Mechanisms Involved in Cell Death." *Frontiers in Oncology* 4 (2014). doi:10.3389/fonc.2014.00302.

7. Milane, L., M. Trivedi, A. Singh, M. Talekar, and M. Amiji. "Mitochondrial Biology, Targets, and Drug Delivery." *Journal of Controlled Release* 207 (2015): 40–58. doi:10.1016/j.jconrel.2015.03.036.

8. Carrington, E. M., Y. Zhan, J. L. Brady, J. G. Zhang, R. M. Sutherland, N. S. Anstee, R. L. Schenk, I. B. Vikstrom, R. B. Delconte, D. Segal, N. D. Huntington, P. Bouillet, D. M. Tarlinton, D. C. Huang, A. Strasser, S. Cory, M. J. Herold, and A. M. Lew. "Anti-Apoptotic Proteins BCL-2, MCL-1 and A1 Summate Collectively to Maintain Survival of Immune Cell Populations Both In Vitro and In Vivo." *Cell Death & Differentiation* 24, no. 5 (2017): 878–88. doi:10.1038/cdd.2017.30.

9. Peña-Blanco, A., and A. J. García-Sáez. "Bax, Bak and Beyond: Mitochondrial Performance in Apoptosis." *FEBS Journal* 285, no. 3 (2018): 416–31. doi:10.1111/febs.14186.

10. Wang, C., and R. J. Youle. "The Role of Mitochondria in Apoptosis*." *Annual Review of Genetics* 43 (2009): 95–118. doi:10.1146/annurev-genet-102108-134850.

11. Dan Dunn, J., L. A. Alvarez, X. Zhang, and T. Soldati. "Reactive Oxygen Species and Mitochondria: A Nexus of Cellular Homeostasis." *Redox Biology* 6 (2015): 472–85. doi:10.1016/j.redox.2015.09.005.

12. Abate, M., A. Festa, M. Falco, A. Lombardi, A. Luce, A. Grimaldi, S. Zappavigna, P. Sperlongano, C. Irace, M. Caraglia, and G. Misso. "Mitochondria as Playmakers of Apoptosis, Autophagy and Senescence." *Seminars in Cell & Developmental Biology* 98 (2020): 139–53. doi:10.1016/j.semcdb.2019.05.022.

13. Ferro, F., S. Servais, P. Besson, S. Roger, J. F. Dumas, and L. Brisson. "Autophagy and Mitophagy in Cancer Metabolic Remodelling." *Seminars in Cell & Developmental Biology* 98 (2020): 129–38. doi:10.1016/j.semcdb.2019.05.029.

14. Whitworth, A. J., and L. J. Pallanck. "PINK1/Parkin Mitophagy and Neurodegeneration: What Do We Really Know In Vivo?." *Current Opinion in Genetics & Development* 44 (2017): 47–53. doi:10.1016/j.gde.2017.01.016.

15. Chan, N. C., A. M. Salazar, A. H. Pham, M. J. Sweredoski, N. J. Kolawa, R. L. Graham, S. Hess, and D. C. Chan. "Broad Activation of the Ubiquitin–Proteasome System by Parkin Is Critical for Mitophagy." *Human Molecular Genetics* 20, no. 9 (2011): 1726–37. doi:10.1093/hmg/ddr048.

16. Pickrell, Alicia M., and Richard J. Youle. "The Roles of PINK1, Parkin, and Mitochondrial Fidelity in Parkinson's Disease." *Neuron* 85, no. 2 (2015): 257–73. doi:10.1016/j.neuron.2014.12.007.

17. Hoshino, A., Y. Mita, Y. Okawa, M. Ariyoshi, E. Iwai-Kanai, T. Ueyama, K. Ikeda, T. Ogata, and S. Matoba. "Cytosolic p53 Inhibits Parkin-Mediated Mitophagy and Promotes Mitochondrial Dysfunction in the Mouse Heart." *Nature Communications* 4 (2013): 2308. doi:10.1038/ncomms3308.

18. Hanahan, D., and Robert A. Weinberg. "Hallmarks of Cancer: The Next Generation." *Cell* 144, no. 5 (2011): 646–74. doi:10.1016/j.cell.2011.02.013.

19. Fadeel, B., A. Ottosson, and S. Pervaiz. "Big Wheel Keeps on Turning: Apoptosome Regulation and Its Role in Chemoresistance." *Cell Death & Differentiation* 15, no. 3 (2008): 443–52. doi:10.1038/sj.cdd.4402265.

20. López-Lázaro, M. "The Warburg Effect: Why and How Do Cancer Cells Activate Glycolysis in the Presence of Oxygen?." *Anti-Cancer Agents in Medicinal Chemistry* 8, no. 3 (2008): 305–12. doi:10.2174/187152008783961932.

21. Mathupala, S. P., Y. H. Ko, and P. L. Pedersen. "Hexokinase II: Cancer's Double-Edged Sword Acting as Both Facilitator and Gatekeeper of Malignancy When Bound to Mitochondria." *Oncogene* 25, no. 34 (2006): 4777–86. doi:10.1038/sj.onc.1209603.

22. Pedersen, P. L. "Warburg, Me and Hexokinase 2: Multiple Discoveries of Key Molecular Events Underlying One of Cancers' Most Common Phenotypes, the 'Warburg Effect' i.e., Elevated Glycolysis in the Presence of Oxygen." *Journal of Bioenergetics & Biomembranes* 39, no. 3 (2007): 211–22. doi:10.1007/s10863-007-9094-x.

23. Benn, S. C., and C. J. Woolf. "Adult Neuron Survival Strategies: Slamming on the Brakes." *Nature Reviews. Neuroscience* 5, no. 9 (2004): 686–700. doi:10.1038/nrn1477.

24. Van Giau, V., S. S. A. An, and J. P. Hulme. "Mitochondrial Therapeutic Interventions in Alzheimer's Disease." *Journal of the Neurological Sciences* 395 (2018): 62–70. doi:10.1016/j.jns.2018.09.033.

25. Devi, L., B. M. Prabhu, D. F. Galati, N. G. Avadhani, and H. K. Anandatheerthavarada. "Accumulation of Amyloid Precursor Protein in the Mitochondrial Import Channels of Human Alzheimer's Disease Brain Is Associated with Mitochondrial Dysfunction." *Journal of Neuroscience* 26, no. 35 (2006): 9057–68. doi:10.1523/jneurosci.1469-06.2006.

26. Panga, V., A. A. Kallor, A. Nair, S. Harshan, and S. Raghunathan. "Mitochondrial Dysfunction in Rheumatoid Arthritis: A Comprehensive Analysis by Integrating Gene Expression, Protein-Protein Interactions and Gene Ontology Data." *PLOS ONE* 14, no. 11 (2019): e0224632. doi:10.1371/journal.pone.0224632.

27. Wu, M., L. Liao, L. Jiang, C. Zhang, H. Gao, L. Qiao, S. Liu, and D. Shi. "Liver-Targeted Nano-mitoPBN Normalizes Glucose Metabolism by Improving Mitochondrial Redox Balance." *Biomaterials* 222 (2019), 119457. doi:10.1016/j.biomaterials.2019.119457.

28. Ishikita, A., T. Matoba, G. Ikeda, J. Koga, Y. Mao, K. Nakano, O. Takeuchi, J. Sadoshima, and K. Egashira. "Nanoparticle-Mediated Delivery of Mitochondrial Division inhibitor 1 to the Myocardium Protects the Heart from Ischemia-Reperfusion Injury Through Inhibition of Mitochondria Outer Membrane Permeabilization: A New Therapeutic Modality for Acute Myocardial Infarction." *Journal of the American Heart Association* 5, no. 7 (2016): e003872. doi:10.1161/JAHA.116.003872.

29. Schmidt, O., N. Pfanner, and C. Meisinger. "Mitochondrial Protein Import: From Proteomics to Functional Mechanisms." *Nature Reviews. Molecular Cell Biology* 11, no. 9 (2010): 655–67. doi:10.1038/nrm2959.

30. Fukasawa, Y., J. Tsuji, S. C. Fu, K. Tomii, P. Horton, and K. Imai. "MitoFates: Improved Prediction of Mitochondrial Targeting Sequences and Their Cleavage Sites." *Molecular & Cellular Proteomics* 14, no. 4 (2015): 1113–26. doi:10.1074/mcp.M114.043083.

31. Mitchell, W., E. A. Ng, J. D. Tamucci, K. J. Boyd, M. Sathappa, A. Coscia, M. Pan, X. Han, N. A. Eddy, E. R. May, H. H. Szeto, and N. N. Alder. "The Mitochondria-Targeted Peptide SS-31 Binds Lipid Bilayers and Modulates Surface Electrostatics as a Key Component of Its Mechanism of Action." *Journal of Biological Chemistry* 295, no. 21 (2020): 7452–69. doi:10.1074/jbc.RA119.012094.

32. Szeto, H. H. "Cell-Permeable, Mitochondrial-Targeted, Peptide Antioxidants." *AAPS Journal* 8, no. 2 (2006): E277–E83. doi:10.1007/BF02854898.

33. Horton, K. L., K. M. Stewart, S. B. Fonseca, Q. Guo, and S. O. Kelley. "Mitochondria-Penetrating Peptides." *Chemistry & Biology* 15, no. 4 (2008): 375–82. doi:10.1016/j.chembiol.2008.03.015.

34. Chen, W. H., X. D. Xu, G. F. Luo, H. Z. Jia, Q. Lei, S. X. Cheng, R. X. Zhuo, and X. Z. Zhang. "Dual-Targeting Pro-Apoptotic Peptide for Programmed Cancer Cell Death via Specific Mitochondria Damage." *Science Report* 3 (2013): 3468. doi:10.1038/srep03468.

35. U.S. National Library of Medicine. 2020. https://www.clinicaltrials.gov/ct2/show/NCT03323749?term=elamipretide&draw=2&rank=5.

36. Zielonka, J., J. Joseph, A. Sikora, M. Hardy, O. Ouari, J. Vasquez-Vivar, G. Cheng, M. Lopez, and B. Kalyanaraman. "Mitochondria-Targeted Triphenylphosphonium-Based Compounds: Syntheses, Mechanisms of Action, and Therapeutic and Diagnostic Applications." *Chemical Reviews* 117, no. 15 (2017): 10043–120. doi:10.1021/acs.chemrev.7b00042.

37. Kurtoglu, M., and T. J. Lampidis. "From Delocalized Lipophilic Cations to Hypoxia: Blocking Tumor Cell Mitochondrial Function Leads to Therapeutic Gain with Glycolytic Inhibitors." *Molecular Nutrition & Food Research* 53, no. 1 (2009): 68–75. doi:10.1002/mnfr.200700457.

38. Weissig, V., J. Lasch, G. Erdos, H. W. Meyer, T. C. Rowe, and J. Hughes. "DQAsomes: A Novel Potential Drug and Gene Delivery System Made from Dequalinium." *Pharmaceutical Research* 15, no. 2 (1998): 334–7. doi:10.1023/a:1011991307631.

39. Shi, M., J. Zhang, X. Li, S. Pan, J. Li, C. Yang, H. Hu, M. Qiao, D. Chen, and X. Zhao. "Mitochondria-Targeted Delivery of Doxorubicin to Enhance Antitumor Activity with HER-2 Peptide-Mediated Multifunctional pH-Sensitive DQAsomes." *International Journal of Nanomedicine* 13 (2018): 4209–26. doi:10.2147/IJN.S163858.

40. Weissig, V. "DQAsomes as the Prototype of Mitochondria-Targeted Pharmaceutical Nanocarriers: Preparation, Characterization, and Use." *Methods in Molecular Biology* 1265 (2015): 1–11. doi:10.1007/978-1-4939-2288-8_1.

41. Hauert, S., and S. N. Bhatia. "Mechanisms of Cooperation in Cancer Nanomedicine: Towards Systems Nanotechnology." *Trends in Biotechnology* 32, no. 9 (2014): 448–55. doi:10.1016/j.tibtech.2014.06.010.

42. Yamada, Y., M. Satrialdi, M. Hibino, D. Sasaki, J. Abe, and H. Harashima. "Power of Mitochondrial Drug Delivery Systems to Produce Innovative Nanomedicines." *Advanced Drug Delivery Reviews* (2020): 154–5, 187–209. doi:10.1016/j.addr.2020.09.010.

43. Li, Y., J. P. Fawcett, H. Zhang, and I. G. Tucker. "Transport and Metabolism of MitoQ10, a Mitochondria-Targeted Antioxidant, in Caco-2 Cell Monolayers." *Journal of Pharmacy & Pharmacology* 59, no. 4 (2007): 503–11. doi:10.1211/jpp.59.4.0004.

44. Marrache, S., and S. Dhar. "Engineering of Blended Nanoparticle Platform for Delivery of Mitochondria-Acting Therapeutics." *Proceedings of the National Academy of Sciences* 109, no. 40 (2012): 16288. doi:10.1073/pnas.1210096109.

45. Fan, X.-X., M. Z. Xu, E. L. Leung, C. Jun, Z. Yuan, and L. Liu. "ROS-Responsive Berberine Polymeric Micelles Effectively Suppressed the Inflammation of Rheumatoid Arthritis by Targeting Mitochondria." *Nano-Micro Letters* 12, no. 1 (2020). doi:10.1007/s40820-020-0410-x.

46. Milane, L., Z. F. Duan, and M. Amiji. "Pharmacokinetics and Biodistribution of Lonidamine/Paclitaxel Loaded, EGFR-Targeted Nanoparticles in an Orthotopic Animal Model of Multi-Drug Resistant Breast Cancer." *Nanomedicine* 7, no. 4 (2011): 435–44. doi:10.1016/j.nano.2010.12.009.

47. Milane, L., Z. Duan, and M. Amiji. "Development of EGFR-Targeted Polymer Blend Nanocarriers for Combination Paclitaxel/Lonidamine Delivery to Treat Multi-Drug Resistance in Human Breast and Ovarian Tumor Cells." *Molecular Pharmacology* 8, no. 1 (2011): 185–203. doi:10.1021/mp1002653.

48. Milane, L., Z. Duan, and M. Amiji. "Role of Hypoxia and Glycolysis in the Development of Multi-Drug Resistance in Human Tumor Cells and the Establishment of an Orthotopic Multi-Drug Resistant Tumor Model in Nude Mice Using Hypoxic Pre-Conditioning." *Cancer Cell International* 11 (2011): 3. doi:10.1186/1475-2867-11-3.

49. Milane, L., Z. Duan, and M. Amiji. "Therapeutic Efficacy and Safety of Paclitaxel/Lonidamine Loaded EGFR-Targeted Nanoparticles for the Treatment of Multi-Drug Resistant Cancer." *PLOS ONE* 6, no. 9 (2011): e24075. doi:10.1371/journal.pone.0024075.

50. Patel, N. R., S. Hatziantoniou, A. Georgopoulos, C. Demetzos, V. P. Torchilin, V. Weissig, and G. G. D'Souza. "Mitochondria-Targeted Liposomes Improve the Apoptotic and Cytotoxic Action of Sclareol." *Journal of Liposome Research* 20, no. 3 (2010): 244–9. doi:10.3109/08982100903347931.

Directed Therapies to Nucleic Acid and Cytoplasmic RNA

17

Mitali Ghose

Contents

DOI: 10.1201/9781003092773-19

17.1 INTRODUCTION

Directed therapies also known as targeted therapies have emerged as an important tool in the treatment of various diseases including the likes of cancer, rheumatoid arthritis, and multiple sclerosis, among many others.[1] There are many organelles in cells to which drugs and therapies can be targeted for effective treatment outcomes, but in this chapter, we will focus on subcellular organelles, more importantly the various nucleic acids present in the cells.

But why target subcellular organelles? The subcellular compartments in eukaryotic cells have specialized roles that aid in the overall cellular function. A few important subcellular organelles include mitochondria which is involved in the ATP production in cells, plasma membrane that separates cellular contents from the extracellular space, the nucleus that houses the DNA important in cell survival, proliferation, etc., lysosomes that are involved in phagocytosis and apoptosis, and the Golgi apparatus involved in post-translational modifications of protein after synthesis,[2] among many others. If there is dysregulation of function of any of these organelles, it directly affects the overall functioning of the cell and may lead to cell death.[3] Aberrant functioning of the cells and their organelles can also lead to the onset of various diseases like MS or cancer.

Cancer is one of the most prevailing diseases in the world. According to the American Cancer Society, it is estimated that there will be around 1.9 million new cases in 2021 in the USA alone with an estimated death of more than 600,000 patients.[4] Cancer can be characterized by the uncontrolled growth of cells with no differentiation, invasion, and metastasis.[1] There are various therapies used to target and treat cancer cells including chemotherapy, photodynamic therapy (PDT), surgery, radiation, gene therapy, hyperthermal therapy, etc.[3] Causes of cancer include genetic changes, exposure to carcinogens, heavy metals, and cancer-causing chemicals and pollution.[5] Along with this, increased risk factors including family history, lifestyle factors, and exposure to radiation and chemotherapy also increase the chance of developing cancer.[6]

17.2 DNA AND NUCLEUS

17.2.1 Nucleus

The nucleus, only found in the cells of eukaryotes, is a highly specialized organelle that stores DNA, the genetic material of a cell, and is involved in the processes of reproduction metabolism and protein synthesis of a cell.[7] The nucleus is made up of a double membrane structure called the nuclear envelope which is in continuation with the endoplasmic reticulum. The nuclear envelope also contains structures called the nuclear pore complexes or NPCs.[8] The NPCs are used for active and passive transport of various molecules across the nuclear membrane. The size of the central channel of the NPC is only 9 nm and only allows the transport of molecules with a size less than 50 kDa through passive transport. Any molecule larger than the size requires the use of NLS and NPC.[1] Nuclear localization signal (NLS) is a protein with a few amino acids that helps in the transport of larger proteins into the nucleus. The transportation of proteins through NLS requires recognition of NLS by the NLS receptor. Recognition leads to docking of the protein at the NPC. This process is energy dependent. The translocation of the protein via the NPC and its release into the nucleus are also energy dependent.[9] The nuclear envelope is made up of two concentric layers of lipid bilayers. The nuclear envelope is supported by the nuclear lamina which forms a meshwork on the inner side of the inner nuclear membrane and on the outer side of the outer nuclear membrane. The nuclear envelope is important to separate the cytosol from the nucleus and to maintain the biochemical environment of the nucleus to help maintain the high concentration of substrates and enzymes that work on nucleic acids.[10]

17.2.2 DNA

17.2.2.1 Structure of DNA

DNA or deoxyribonucleic acid is a double-stranded molecule with two long polynucleotide chains. It is made up of four types of nucleotide subunits: adenine (A), guanine (G), cytosine (C), and thymine (T). Each strand of this polynucleotide chain is called a DNA strand. Hydrogen bonds hold the two polynucleotide chains together. Each nucleotide of DNA is composed of a five-carbon deoxyribose sugar with one phosphate group and a nitrogen-containing base. Each nucleotide is linked to the other one through alternating sugar-phosphate bonds. These forms make up the backbone of the DNA. The chemical polarity of a DNA strand is due to the way nucleotides are linked together. Due to this linking of the bases, one end of a DNA strand is the 3' hydroxyl end while the other is the 5' phosphate end. Due to the presence of hydrogen bonds between the two polynucleotide chains, all the bases are on the inside of the chains, leaving the backbone on the outside which leads to the formation of the double helix structure of the DNA. Adenine and guanine are purines while thymine and cytosine are pyrimidines. Adenine pairs with thymine, and guanine always pairs with cytosine which leads to complementary base pairing. This helps DNA to have the most energetically favorable arrangement in the nucleus and holds the backbone at an equal distance throughout the DNA.[10]

17.2.2.2 Function of DNA

DNA carries the genetic information of the cell which is passed down to the daughter cells when the parent cell divides. The genetic materials or genes are parts of DNA that encode information for the functioning and survival of the cell. The gene is a sequence of nucleotides (A, T, G, or C) that generally codes for a single protein. Since proteins are responsible for the functioning of the cell and the 3-D structure of the protein is responsible for the functioning of the cell, the amino acid sequence of the protein becomes very important. The sequence of amino acids is determined by the nucleotide sequence of a gene. The process of generating a functioning protein from nucleotides sequences is called protein synthesis and involves transcription and translation.[10]

The part of an organism's DNA that has all the information for all the proteins an organism can make is called the genome and is a small part of the total DNA in a cell. Each cell has the complete genome in the nucleus, and this genome is passed from parent cell to daughter cell during cell division.[10]

17.2.2.3 DNA and Mitochondria

Mitochondria, classically known as the powerhouse of the cell, are cytosolic organelles involved in oxidative phosphorylation, ATP production in cells, and multiple processes spanning from intrinsic apoptosis to thermoregulation.[11] These organelles contain a circular genome with 16,569 base pairs.

Mitochondria are found in all eukaryotic cells except RBCs.[12] Mitochondria consist of two membranes: an inner mitochondria membrane known as IMM and an outer mitochondrial membrane known as OMM. The inner membrane forms tubular pleomorphic structures called cristae that are involved in membrane fusion and fission.[13] The outer membrane of mitochondria connects the organelle to the cytosol of the cell and is involved in maintaining the morphology, biogenesis, and inheritance of the mitochondria.[14] Mitochondria are involved in a variety of physiological functions in the cell including ATP production, calcium homeostasis, cell cycle and growth, metabolism regulation, neurotransmission, and cellular signaling and apoptosis.[12]

The mitochondrial DNA or mtDNA is double-stranded DNA and encodes genes. But when compared to nuclear DNA, mtDNA is circular and has fewer DNA base pairs thanthe nuclear genome.[15] The mtDNA only has 37 genes which and codes for 13 proteins, 22 tRNAs, and 2 rRNAs. The proteins encoded by the mitochondrial genome are involved in the process of oxidative phosphorylation which helps in the ATP production in cells. Not all the proteins needed for the process of oxidative phosphorylation are produced in the mitochondria and the use of the nuclear genome is required as well. Unlike the nuclear genome, the mitochondrial genome has several copies of itself in a mitochondrion. Since there are many mitochondria present in a cell, there are multiple copies of the mitochondrial genome in comparison to one copy of the nuclear genome in each cell. The mitochondrial genome is also not packed into an envelope with chromatin and has fewer noncoding DNA sequences than the nuclear genome. The mitochondrial genome inheritance is strictly from the maternal side whereas the nuclear genome is inherited equally from the paternal and the maternal side.[16]

Since there are multiple copies of the mitochondrial genome in a cell and the mitochondrial genome has a higher mutation rate than the nuclear genome, it leads to the presence of a heterogeneous population of mitochondrial DNA within the same cell and even within the same mitochondrion. During cellular division mitochondria are segregated in a random manner which leads to much less organized mitochondrial genome segregation leading to similar but not identical copies of the mitochondrial DNA in daughter cells. The higher rate of mutation in mtDNA might be due to a nucleotide imbalance leading to a lower functioning DNA polymerase protein (encoded by PLOG gene) and thus higher mtDNA mutation rates.[17] Some syndromes due to mutations in the mtDNA are Leber hereditary optic neuropathy (LHON) and post-lingual deafness. LHON is a mitochondrion-associated disease causing loss of vision in both eyes and post-lingual deafness is deafness that occurs after three years of age and is caused by a mutation in the RNR1 gene of the mitochondrial genome encoded ribosomal RNA.[18] mtDNA mutations have also been thought to contribute to many diseases like diabetes, Alzheimer's disease, and Parkinson's disease, etc.

Due to advances in the field of medicine, it has now been shown that mitochondria are involved in the process of aging as well as cancer. One of the by-products of oxidative phosphorylation is the generation of reactive oxygen species (ROS). These reactive species can lead to mutations in the mtDNA which can proliferate and generate large numbers of cancer-causing cells. Mutations in the protein coding region and ribosomal RNA genes are seen in cells of colon cancer.[19] It has now been established that mtDNA mutations are linked to solid tumors and leukemias. Clearly the mitochondrial genome is involved in various disease conditions in humans like aging and neurodegeneration and thus can make viable targets for the treatment of diseases.[15]

17.3 RNA AND IMPORTANCE OF TARGETING CYTOPLASMIC RNA

Ribonucleic acid (RNA) can be found in most living organisms. It is also found in many viruses as their genetic material. Like DNA, RNA is also made up of sugars, nitrogen bases, and phosphate groups. The sugar molecules in RNA are ribose sugars, hence the name ribonucleic acid. The nitrogenous bases are like the ones found in DNA. Adenine (A), guanine (G), and cytosine (C) are the three nitrogenous bases shared by DNA and RNA. The fourth nitrogen base thymine (T) in DNA is replaced by uracil (U) in RNA.[20]

RNA exists in single-strand form and has varied length and structures. There are also many viral RNAs that exist in double-stranded structures. RNA is mostly involved in protein synthesis in cells and can also act as a regulator of gene expression. The process of formation of RNA from DNA is called transcription and the process of synthesis of proteins from RNA is called translation. Together, transcription and translation make up the process of protein synthesis from DNA.[20]

There are three main types of RNA involved in protein synthesis: messenger RNA (mRNA), transfer RNA (tRNA), and ribosomal RNA (rRNA).

mRNA: RNA transcribed from DNA is called mRNA. It contains the blueprint of the DNA to synthesize proteins. In eukaryotes, after the process of transcription, the mRNA is called pre-mRNA and contains introns (non-coding regions) and exons (coding regions). The introns are then spliced from the pre-mRNA and the exons are joined in a process called maturation to give the final mRNA that is translated into the proteins. After joining of the exons, a

7-methylguanosine is added to the 5' end of the RNA and a chain of adenine nucleotides called a poly(A) chain is added to the 3' end of the RNA. 7-methylguanosine protects RNA from degradation and the poly(A) tail helps in stability during transport.[20]

tRNA: transfer RNAs help translate mRNA sequence into proteins. tRNA has a cloverleaf structure with a 3' end and 5' end. The 3' end has an acceptor site and the 5' end has the terminal phosphate. Other than these structures, tRNA also consists of a D arm, T arm, and an anticodon arm.[20] A codon is a set of three nucleotides that code for one amino acid. There are 64 sets of codons out of which 61 codons are specific for the 21 amino acids and 3 codons are stop codons.[21] When the anti-codon arm of tRNA corresponds to the codon on the mRNA, enzyme aminoacyl-tRNA synthetase helps load the appropriate amino acid on the 3' arm of the free tRNA. Once the amino acid binds to the 3' end, the tRNA is considered to be an aminoacyl tRNA. Once this complex forms, the tRNA carries the amino acid to the ribosomal complex for protein synthesis.[20]

rRNA: ribosomal RNA is involved in the assembly of amino acids into proteins. The eukaryotic 80S ribosome comprises a large 60S and a small 40S ribosomal subunit. Each ribosome also has three specific sites E (exit), P (peptidyl), and A (acceptor) that bind the amino acid containing tRNA and assemble the proteins. This completes the process of translation and protein synthesis.[20]

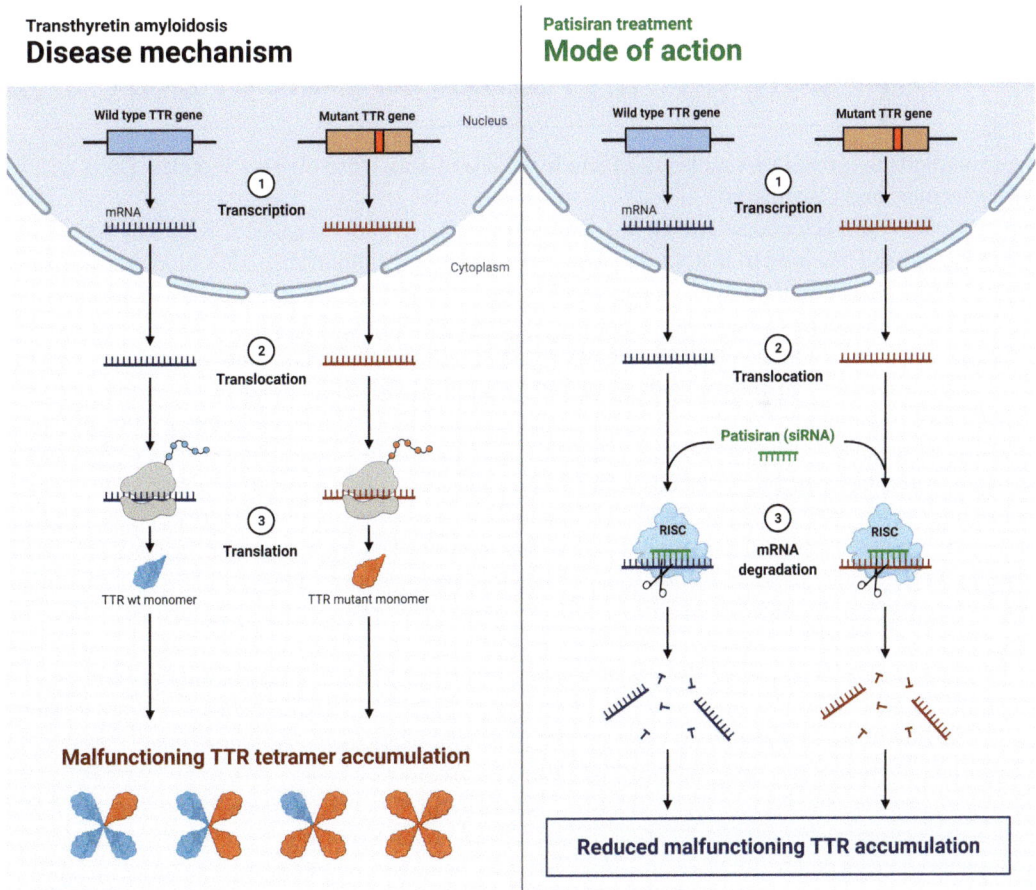

FIGURE 17.1 Mechanism of patisiran RNAi. RNA interference is an excellent tool for the post-transcriptional regulation of protein translation. In transthyretin amyloidosis there is accumulation of a mutant transthyretin tetramer. Patisiran "silences" the expression of this mutant protein by leading to mRNA degradation. Created using Biorender.com.

Other than the three RNA types described above, there are many subcategories of RNA found in the eukaryotic cells. For example, microRNA or miRNA are small regulatory RNAs involved in gene regulation. Another type of small regulatory RNA is small nuclear RNA or snRNAs that are involved in RNA splicing and thus in gene regulation. Small RNAs like small interfering RNAs (siRNAs) are involved in the inhibition of gene expression. Patisiran is an interfering RNA drug for the treatment of transthyretin amyloidosis. The mechanism of patisiran RNAi is demonstrated in Figure 17.1. Another set of small RNAs are small nucleolar RNAs which are involved in the processing of rRNA molecules.[22] Apart from these, RNA regulatory elements like riboswitches are also present in eukaryotic cells. Riboswitches or RNA switches act like sensors and change gene expression based on environmental or cellular signals. Another type of RNA found in eukaryotic cells is catalytic RNA or ribozymes. These enzymes are RNAs with enzyme activity and are involved in the process of splicing, and mRNA processing.[22]

Since different types of RNA are involved in different stages of gene expression, they become an important target for nucleic acid therapies. Mutations in RNA lead to various disease conditions like prostate cancer and neuromuscular disorders like myotonic dystrophy, and spinal muscular atrophy, etc. Myotonic dystrophy is caused by a CTG nucleotide repeat leading to a gain of function mutation.[20] Mutations in the miRNA can also lead to cancers like Burkitt's lymphoma wherein there is an abundance of miR-155.[22] tRNA is also involved in the regulation of apoptosis, acting as a scavenger for cytochrome c.

17.4 CURRENT METHODS TO TARGET DNA

Current methods to target DNA molecules include the use of anti-sense oligonucleotides, DNA aptamers, small molecules, and gene therapy.

Anti-sense oligonucleotides (ASOs) are single-stranded and short sequences with lengths between 8 and 50 base pairs. They bind to mRNA sequences and cause steric hindrance, thus blocking the function of the mRNA. Another method through which mRNA function is blocked is due to ASO-mRNA complex degradation by endogenous RNase H immediately after ASO binding.[23]

First-generation ASOs were susceptible to degradation by nuclease enzymes since they were mostly in their unmodified form. However, with second-generation ASOs modifications were made in the structural backbone of the molecules and the ribose sugar component of the molecule. These changes made the second-generation ASOs more stable and improved their specificity and binding strength. The modifications made in the ASOs included the addition of a phosphodiester or a phosphorothioate in the backbone with the latter being most common. Phosphorothioate in ASOs helps improve stability and specificity and leads to longer time of action due to gradual uptake by target cells. Modification of the ribose sugar in the 2' position helps reduce degradation by nucleases. ASOs are currently being studied for the treatment of various neurodegenerative diseases and two ASO therapies have been approved by the FDA for clinical use.[23]

Aptamers are single-stranded RNA or DNA molecules that bind to the nucleotide coding region and act as a decoy. The aptamers are about 16–120 nucleotides long. Like the anti-sense oligonucleotides, aptamers bind strongly to the nucleic acid target by structural recognition. Aptamers can be used as a better alternative to mono-clonal antibodies as they are non-immunogenic, have no toxicity, have better tissue penetration properties, and can be easily modified for *in vitro* and *in vivo* systems. The process of isolation of aptamers is called systematic evolution of ligands by exponential enrichment (SELEX) which requires a large pool of nucleic acids. Another process of aptamer generation is called AptaBind.[23] Currently only one aptamer is FDA approved for clinical use. However, many aptamer molecules are currently being tested to treat various diseases like many cancers, AMD, macular degeneration, diabetes, etc.[24]

One popular field of drug development that targets nucleic acids especially DNA is gene therapy. Gene therapy is used to replace a non-functioning or abnormal functioning gene with a proper functioning variant. To deliver the therapeutic gene of interest, a vector is used. The most common vectors used today are either retroviruses or adenoviruses. These vectors are then delivered either to the germ line which is heritable in nature or to the somatic cell line which is not heritable. The therapeutic gene delivered needs to be composed of the following: a promoter, the transgene, and the termination signal. The promoter gene drives the process of gene transcription, the transgene is the actual gene that restores cellular function, and the termination signal ends the process of gene transcription. Gene therapy can be used to treat many diseases such as hemophilia, cystic fibrosis, Gaucher's disease, etc., but to date only two gene therapies have been FDA approved for clinical use with many more being tested in clinical trials.

17.5 CURRENT METHODS TO TARGET CYTOPLASMIC RNA

Ever since it was identified that RNA plays an important role during protein synthesis, these molecules have also been targeted to treat several disease conditions. In this chapter we will be discussing a few methods used to target cytoplasmic RNA.

The first method named RNA interference (RNAi) was identified in the 1980s by Fire et al.[25] in *Caenorhabditis elegans*. RNA interference uses RNA molecules with complementary sequences to that of a gene's coding sequence to degrade the corresponding mRNA, thereby blocking the translation process of mRNA to protein. RNAi used siRNA molecules to block the mRNA of genes. siRNA are double-stranded short sequences only 21–23 nucleotides long. They can be synthesized chemically and are delivered as duplexes making them more stable than DNA oligonucleotides. Since they act on mRNA in the cytoplasm, they also don't have the need to cross the nuclear envelope, making them a better option than DNA oligonucleotides. Currently there are four drugs approved by the FDA for patient use.

MicroRNAs are short single-stranded sequences, part of the non-coding RNA. They are 15–22 nucleotides in length and are associated with many human diseases like cancer. MicroRNAs act as negative regulators in post-translational function. When used as a therapeutic agent microRNAs target multiple molecules and are efficient in regulating distantly related biological processes. Diseases such as Alzheimer's disease, cardiovascular diseases, and immunological diseases see an increased expression of microRNAs. MicroRNA therapeutics are of two types, namely miRNA antagonists and miRNA replacements or miRNA mimics.[23] miRNA antagonists can be used to block endogenous miRNAs that acquire a gain of function mutation while miRNA mimics can be used to restore miRNA function in diseased cells.[26] Many miRNA therapeutics are currently in clinical trials but none of them have been approved to date.

Another method to target RNA is the use of RNA aptamers. They are also known as RNA "decoys". RNA aptamers are small RNA molecules that fold into a three-dimensional structure and bind to proteins to inhibit their function. These three-dimensional structures can also be used to deliver other RNA therapeutics into cells. Like DNA aptamers, RNA aptamers too are sensitive to nuclease function and require modifications in the terminal region to prevent degradation. Modified nucleotides like 2′-O-modified pyrimidines or 2′-fluoro pyrimidines can be used. The advantage of RNA aptamers over other RNA therapeutics is that they can bind directly to extracellular targets and carry out their function and do not need to be present inside the cell. These molecules are also better at reaching their intracellular targets than other RNA therapeutics. The first aptamer received FDA approval in 2004 for clinical use.[23]

Catalytic RNAs or ribozymes are another class of RNA therapeutics. These molecules are a subset of RNA that are enzymatically active in the absence of proteins. Ribozymes have high specificity and a huge range of targets they act on. Since they act before the process of protein translation, ribozymes can be used for gene suppression in disease conditions. Many ribozymes can also be designed artificially for gene activity suppression making them an attractive field in RNA therapeutics. Ribozymes act by cleaving mRNA before the process of protein synthesis begins. Another use of ribozymes is that they can be used to validate disease-related genes. Ribozymes have many structures, but the hammerhead model is most widely studied due to its efficacy and specificity. Currently many ribozymes are under clinical trials but none of them have been approved.[23]

17.6 DELIVERY OF NUCLEIC ACID THERAPIES

Targeting nucleic acids and cytoplasmic RNA is not the only step in the successful delivery of the therapies to the cell. DNA and RNA in their naked forms can be easily degraded by the extracellular DNAses and RNAses present in the cells. In order to protect these therapeutic molecules, they need to be delivered using other components that can prevent their degradation and help increase their delivery to the target. This is where formulations come in.

The most commonly used form of nucleic acid delivery to targeted cells is nanoparticles. Nanoparticles are particles with size in the nanometer range for at least one of their measurements. Nucleic acids are encapsulated in these nanoparticles, and these NPs can help prevent degradation by providing a physical block between the enzymes and DNA/RNA, and by modifying their chemistry, NPs can help target DNA/RNA and increase their uptake in cells.[27] The materials used for making the nanoparticles include cationic polymers like poly-L-lysine, polyethyleneimine, chitosan, etc., poly (B-amino esters), lipids like lecithin, DOPC, etc., micelles and lipid CaP, etc.[27,28] Other than these lipids, various molecules are used to modify the properties of nanoparticles, molecules such as cholesterol, PEG, calcium, phosphate. These molecules can be used to modify the toxicity and stability while helping the NPs escape endosomes and increase efficacy. The addition of adjuvants to NPs helps increase the immunogenicity of nucleic acid therapies especially when the therapy is to induce an inflammatory reaction in the body like vaccines. Common adjuvants include various types of alums and PEG among many others to increase immunogenicity.[27,28]

Another way to deliver nucleic acids other than using nanoparticles is conjugating a bioactive ligand to RNA/DNA which helps increase uptake in the cells of interest. The most common form of conjugation used is GalNAc (N-acetylgalactosamine) to increase uptake in hepatocytes. GalNAc is conjugated to siRNA to target the asialoglycoprotein receptor and increase uptake of siRNA. Other molecules that can also be used for conjugation are cholesterol, vitamin E, cell-penetrating peptides, and antibodies.[27]

17.7 DIRECTED THERAPIES IN CLINIC

There are many drugs for various diseases that are currently being used in clinics. Many other drugs are under various stages of clinical trials. In this section we will discuss some of the drugs approved and some that are under clinical trials.

17.7.1 DNA

17.7.1.1 Fomivirsen

Fomivirsen was the first ASO drug that was approved for the management of cytomegalovirus (CMV) retinitis in 1998. Manufactured by Isis Pharmaceuticals, this was a first-generation ASO that binds to the IE2 fragment of mRNA. This region is involved in the replication process of CMV. The drug was discontinued after the advent of antiretroviral therapies for HIV treatment which caused a reduction of cytomegalovirus retinitis. Fomivirsen administration is through intravitreal injection. The drug has a long duration of action in the eye and has negligible plasma level concentrations. It also has no significant drug interactions except with cidofovir, and no serious side effects are seen with the drug. The drug is metabolized locally in the eye by the exonuclease enzyme.[23]

17.7.1.2 Mipomersen

Mipomersen is an ASO used for the treatment of homozygous familial hypercholesterolemia (HoFH).[23] This is a genetic disorder that causes high levels of low-density lipoprotein cholesterol (LDL-C) in the blood and leads to advanced and premature atherosclerotic cardiovascular disease (ACVD).[29] This disease is highly life-threatening if left untreated.[29] HoFH is an autosomal dominant disorder. Mutations are seen in the LDL-C receptor, PCSK9 protein (pro-protein convertase subtilisin/kexin 9), and in apolipoprotein B. Mipomersen inhibits the synthesis of apolipoprotein B-100 which is an essential component of LDL and VLDL. Mipomersen binds to mRNA of the abnormal apo B and prevents its synthesis which helps remove the excess LDL-C. Mipomersen also binds to plasma proteins in the blood and thus has a long half-life of 20–30 days. Mipomersen is administered as a subcutaneous injection, and its side effects include pain and erythema at the site of injection along with chills, fatigue, and some hepatic impairment.[23]

17.7.1.3 Gendicine

Used for the treatment of squamous cell carcinoma of head and neck, gendicine is an engineered adenovirus expressing p53, the tumor suppressor gene. It is used in combination with chemotherapy and radiation. It can also be used for the treatment of pancreatic cancer. Gendicine also can reduce the toxicity of chemotherapy when administered together.[23]

17.7.1.4 Alipgene

Used for the treatment of a rare disease called lipoprotein lipase deficiency, Alipgene is an adeno-associated virus that has the lipase gene. This drug is currently approved for use in the EU.[23]

17.7.2 RNA

17.7.2.1 Patisiran

Patisiran (Onpattro®) is an interfering RNA drug for the treatment of transthyretin amyloidosis (see Figure 17.1).

17.7.2.2 Miravirsen

Miravirsen is a miRNA drug that targets microRNA-122 in the liver. The drug is a β-d-oxy-locked nucleic acid-modified phosphorothioate antisense oligonucleotide that acts as an antagonist. This drug has been used for the treatment of hepatitis C in clinical trials. The drug is currently under trials to be used as a broad-spectrum antiviral along with existing anti-viral therapy.[23]

17.7.2.3 Angiozyme™

Angiozyme is a ribozyme currently being evaluated in clinical trials. It is used for reducing angiogenesis. The drug cleaves the mRNA required for the synthesis of vascular endothelial growth factor (VEGF) receptors KDR and FLt-. It is administered as an IV infusion and is well tolerated in healthy subjects.[23]

17.7.2.4 Pegaptanib

Pegaptanib is an RNA aptamer used for the treatment of age-related macular degeneration (AMD).[23] It acts on VEGF which is a mitogenic protein having a critical role in angiogenesis and the permeability of blood vessels. This causes vision loss in patients with AMD. Pegaptanib binds to the 165 isoform of VEGF, blocking the interaction with cognate receptor, and stops the intraocular blood vessel growth. Pegaptanib is nuclease resistant due to the addition of PEG. It was approved by the FDA in 2004. It is administered as an intravitreal injection every six weeks and is metabolized in the intravitreal region itself.[24]

17.7.2.5 mRNA Vaccines for COVID-19

The emergence of the SARS-CoV-2-caused pandemic COVID-19 has led to the development of many different vaccinations in the past year. Figure 17.2 depicts the lifecycle of the virus. The major focus during the development of vaccinations has been on developing mRNA-based vaccines as they are similar to DNA vaccines but skip the transcription step to express the viral protein.[30] These vaccines are delivered to their

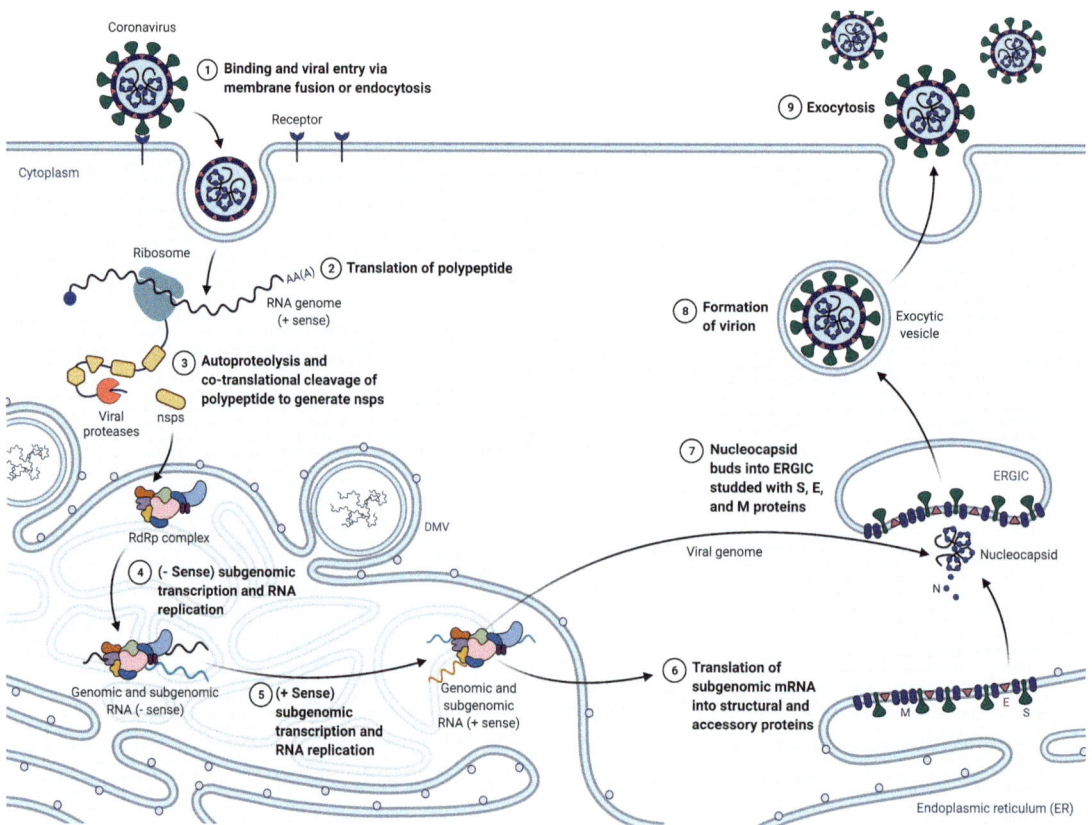

FIGURE 17.2   The lifecycle of SARS-CoV-2. (1) The SARS-CoV-2 coronavirus enters a host cell when the viral spike protein binds to the host ACE2 receptor which is expressed at a high level in the lung. (2) The positive-sense RNA is translated by host ribosomes. (3) Co-translational cleavage of the polypeptide generates negative-sense progeny subgenomes (NSPS) and the RNA-dependent RNA polymerase (RdRp) complex is formed. (4) Negative sense transcription and replication and (5) positive sense transcription and translation occur in the host endoplasmic reticulum in convoluted and double membrane vesicles. (6) Translation of subgenomic mRNA into structural and accessory proteins occurs as the endoplasmic reticulum continues to form convoluted vesicles and (7) the nucleocapsid (N) buds into the endoplasmic reticulum Golgi intermediate compartment (ERGIC) with the viral spike (S), envelope (E), and membrane (M) proteins. The enveloped virus is formed and (9) exocytosed. Acknowledgment: Jessica M Tucker, Britt A Glaunsinger et al. created using Biorender.com.

site of action using lipid nanoparticles. The first two vaccines to be approved by the US FDA were mRNA vaccines delivered using nanoparticles developed by Pfizer/BioNTech and Moderna respectively.[31]eptor which is expressed at a high level in the lung. (2) The positive-sense RNA is translated by host ribosomes. (3) Co-translational cleavage of the polypeptide generates negative-sense progeny subgenomes (NSPS) and the RNA-dependent RNA polymerase (RdRp) complex is formed. (4) Negative sense transcription and replication and (5) positive sense transcription and translation occur in the host endoplasmic reticulum in convoluted and double membrane vesicles. (6) Translation of subgenomic mRNA into structural and accessory proteins occurs as the endoplasmic reticulum continues to form convoluted vesicles and (7) the nucleocapsid (N) buds into the endoplasmic reticulum Golgi intermediate compartment (ERGIC) with the viral spike (S), envelope (E), and membrane (M) proteins. The enveloped virus is formed and (9) exocytosed. Acknowledgment: Jessica M Tucker, Britt A Glaunsinger et al. created using Biorender.com.

The structure of the SARS-CoV-2 spike protein (main vaccine target) is depicted in Figure 17.3. The Pfizer/BioNTech mRNA vaccine uses a modified nucleoside mRNA that codes for the full spike protein of the virus which, when presented to the cells, leads to the formation of antibodies against the virus. Apart from the currently approved BNT162b2 variant of the vaccine, Pfizer/BioNTech is currently developing three additional vaccines: BNT162a1 having the uridine mRNA, BNT162b1 having the receptor binding domain (RBD) mRNA, and BNT162c2 having a self-amplifying mRNA.[30,31]

The Moderna vaccine uses mRNA that codes the full-length spike protein which is perfusion stabilized. The Moderna vaccine mRNA1273 uses lipid nanoparticles (LNPs) for the delivery of the mRNA to the cells.[30,31]

LNP formulations are currently being used as the delivery method of RNA vaccines as they help protect the mRNA from degradation by extracellular RNAses and help increase the uptake efficiency of the vaccine.[30] These formulations can also be surface modified to increase target specificity in the body. The current LNP formulation of both these vaccines uses an adjuvant to increase the immunogenicity of the vaccines and produce a better immune response. The Moderna vaccine LNP formulation uses PEG 2000

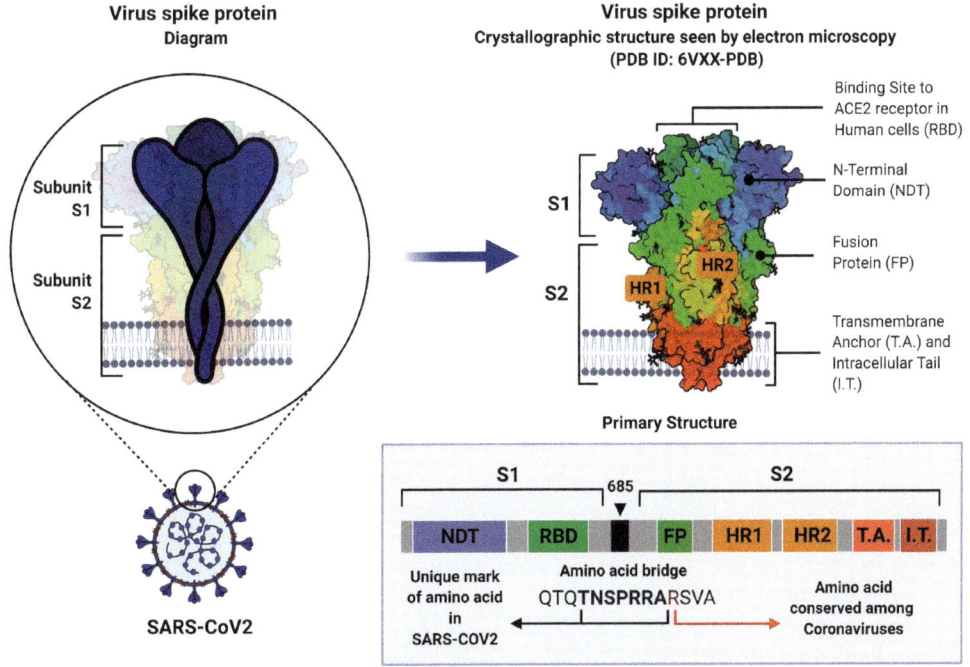

FIGURE 17.3   SARS-CoV-2 spike glycoprotein structure. The spike protein is the primary target for vaccine development. Acknowledgment to Diana Sofia Mollocana Yanez, created using Biorender.com.

(polyethylene glycol), dimyristoyl glycerol (DMG), DSPC (cholesterol, 1,2-distearoyl-sn-glycero-3-ph osphocholine), acetic acid, tromethamin hydrochloride, sucrose, sodium acetate, and a proprietary lipid termed Proprietary Ionic lipid SM-102. The Pfizer/BioNTech vaccine formulation uses the lipids cholesterol and ((4-hydroxybutyl)azanediyl)bis(hexane-6,1-diyl)bis(2-hexyldecanoate) among others, along with potassium chloride, sodium chloride, monobasic potassium phosphate, dibasic sodium phosphate dihydrate, and sucrose.[31]

Other vaccination strategies employed for vaccine development include DNA vaccines, protein and peptide vaccines, inactivated and live attenuated viruses, virus-like particles (VLPs), replicating vectored vaccines, and non-replicating vector vaccines among many others.[30] Even though various DNA vaccines are being developed, RNA vaccines have been given more importance because the expression of RNA vaccines begins when they enter the cytosol of the cell unlike DNA vaccines that need to enter the cell nucleus to begin expression. Other advantages of using RNA vaccines are that they have self-adjuvating properties, and their expression can be modified by changing the delivery formulation. RNA vaccines tend to create a greater IFN response in the body which can downregulate protein expression of the vaccine. But by modifying the formulations and the nucleotides of the mRNA, an siRNA can be created that has a balanced expression while triggering the inflammatory responses of the body.[30] Nevertheless, the development of different vaccination platforms is just as important in mitigating the severity of COVID-19 as is the development of RNA-based vaccines.

17.8 CONCLUSION

Nucleic acids are genetic material present in most cells of eukaryotic organisms. Since many aspects of a disease can be traced back to abnormalities with the proteins or genes themselves, using nucleic acids as a target for treatment and symptom alleviation is the next step in drug discovery and development. Targeting nucleic acids in cells using traditional methods becomes very difficult. But with the advent of modern techniques, increased understanding of the working of the cell, and development of better delivery systems and molecules, targeting nucleic acids has become a very important field in pharmaceutics. Even though there are many drugs and small molecules that are currently under clinical trials for various diseases, very few have been approved for patient use. Key challenges in the clinical translation of drugs include delivery to the site of action, pharmacokinetics, mass production issues, immunogenicity, and toxicity issues. But even with these challenges, nucleic acid therapies have the capacity to target a broad spectrum of diseases and that makes it a compelling target for future therapeutics.

REFERENCES

1. Sakhrani, N. M., and H. Padh. "Organelle Targeting: Third Level of Drug Targeting." *Drug Design, Development & Therapy* 7 (2013): 585–99. doi:10.2147/DDDT.S45614.
2. Cooper, G. M. *The Cell: A Molecular Approach* vol. 2. Sunderland, MA: Sinauer Associates, 2000.
3. Chen, W.-H., G.-F. Luo, and X.-Z. Zhang. "Recent Advances in Subcellular Targeted Cancer Therapy Based on Functional Materials." *Advanced Materials* 31, no. 3 (2019): 1802725. doi:10.1002/adma.201802725.
4. Bandari, S. K., A. Purushothaman, V. C. Ramani, G. J. Brinkley, D. S. Chandrashekar, S. Varambally, J. A. Mobley, Y. Zhang, E. E. Brown, I. Vlodavsky, and R. D. Sanderson. "Chemotherapy Induces Secretion of Exosomes Loaded with Heparanase That Degrades Extracellular Matrix and Impacts Tumor and Host Cell Behavior." *Matrix Biology* 65 (2018): 104–18. doi:10.1016/j.matbio.2017.09.001.
5. Faik, A. *Cancer Causing Substancesnull*. London: IntechOpen, 2018.

6. Chen, C., X. Yao, Y. Xu, Q. Zhang, H. Wang, L. Zhao, G. Wen, Y. Liu, L. Jing, and X. Sun. "Dahuang Zhechong Pill Suppresses Colorectal Cancer Liver Metastasis via Ameliorating Exosomal CCL2 Primed Pre-Metastatic Niche." *Journal of Ethnopharmacology* 238 (2019): 111878. doi:10.1016/j.jep.2019.111878.

7. Davidson, M. W. *Molecular Expressions*, 1995. Tallahassee, FL: Florida State University

8. Görlich, D., and U. Kutay. "Transport Between the Cell Nucleus and the Cytoplasm." *Annual Review of Cell & Developmental Biology* 15 (1999): 607–60. doi:10.1146/annurev.cellbio.15.1.607.

9. Chan, C. K., and D. A. Jans. "Using Nuclear Targeting Signals to Enhance Non-Viral Gene Transfer." *Immunology & Cell Biology* 80, no. 2 (2002): 119–30. doi:10.1046/j.1440-1711.2002.01061.x.

10. Alberts, B., A. Johnson, J. Lewis, Martin Raff, Keith Roberts, and Peter Walter. *Molecular Biology of the Cell*. 4th ed. New York: Garland Publishing Science, 2002.

11. Green, D. R., L. Galluzzi, and G. Kroemer. "Mitochondria and the Autophagy-Inflammation-Cell Death Axis in Organismal Aging." *Science* 333, no. 6046 (2011): 1109–12. doi:10.1126/science.1201940.

12. Panchal, K., and A. K. Tiwari. "Mitochondrial Dynamics, a Key Executioner in Neurodegenerative Diseases." *Mitochondrion* 47 (2019): 151–73. doi:10.1016/j.mito.2018.11.002.

13. Mannella, C. A. "The Relevance of Mitochondrial Membrane Topology to Mitochondrial Function." *Biochimica & Biophysica Acta (BBA): Molecular Basis of Disease* 1762, no. 2 (2006): 140–7. doi:10.1016/j.bbadis.2005.07.001.

14. Walther, D. M., and D. Rapaport. "Biogenesis of Mitochondrial Outer Membrane Proteins." *Biochimica & Biophysica Acta (BBA): Molecular Cell Research* 1793, no. 1 (2009): 42–51. doi:10.1016/j.bbamcr.2008.04.013.

15. Chial, H. C. *mtDNA and Mitochondrial Diseases* vol. 1, 217. London: Nature Publishing Education, 2008.

16. Taylor, R. W., and D. M. Turnbull. "Mitochondrial DNA Mutations in Human Disease." *Nature Reviews. Genetics* 6, no. 5 (2005): 389–402. doi:10.1038/nrg1606.

17. Song, S., Z. F. Pursell, W. C. Copeland, M. J. Longley, T. A. Kunkel, and C. K. Mathews. "DNA Precursor Asymmetries in Mammalian Tissue Mitochondria and Possible Contribution to Mutagenesis Through Reduced Replication Fidelity." *Proceedings of the National Academy of Sciences of the United States of America* 102, no. 14 (2005): 4990–5. doi:10.1073/pnas.0500253102.

18. Yu-Wai-Man, P., P. G. Griffiths, D. T. Brown, N. Howell, D. M. Turnbull, and P. F. Chinnery. "The Epidemiology of Leber Hereditary Optic Neuropathy in the North East of England." *American Journal of Human Genetics* 72, no. 2 (2003): 333–9. doi:10.1086/346066.

19. Polyak, K., Y. Li, H. Zhu, C. Lengauer, J. K. Willson, S. D. Markowitz, M. A. Trush, K. W. Kinzler, and B. Vogelstein. "Somatic Mutations of the Mitochondrial Genome in Human Colorectal Tumours." *Nature Genetics* 20, no. 3 (1998): 291–3. doi:10.1038/3108.

20. Wang, D., and A. Farhana. *Biochemistry, RNA Structure*. Treasure Island, FL: StatPearls Publishing, 2020.

21. Lodish, H., A. Berk, S. L. Zipursky, S. Lawrence Zipursky, Paul Matsudaira, David Baltimore, and James Darnell. *Molecular Cell Biology*. 4th ed. Treasure Island, FL: W. H. Freeman, 2000.

22. Clancy, S. R. N. A. *Functions*. 2008.

23. Sridharan, K., and N. J. Gogtay. "Therapeutic Nucleic Acids: Current Clinical Status." *British Journal of Clinical Pharmacology* 82, no. 3 (2016): 659–72. doi:10.1111/bcp.12987.

24. Kaur, H., J. G. Bruno, A. Kumar, and T. K. Sharma. "Aptamers in the Therapeutics and Diagnostics Pipelines." *Theranostics* 8, no. 15 (2018): 4016–32. doi:10.7150/thno.25958.

25. Fire, A., S. Xu, M. K. Montgomery, S. A. Kostas, S. E. Driver, and C. C. Mello. "Potent and Specific Genetic Interference by Double-Stranded RNA in Caenorhabditis elegans." *Nature* 391, no. 6669 (1998): 806–11. doi:10.1038/35888.

26. Das, N., N. Tripathi, and S. Khurana. "Micro RNA Mimics and Antagonists." *International Journal of Scientific & Technology Research* 4 (2015): 176–80.

27. Kaczmarek, J. C., P. S. Kowalski, and D. G. Anderson. "Advances in the Delivery of RNA Therapeutics: From Concept to Clinical Reality." *Genome Medicine* 9, no. 1 (2017): 60. doi:10.1186/s13073-017-0450-0.

28. Zhou, S., W. Chen, J. Cole, and G. Zhu. "Delivery of Nucleic Acid Therapeutics for Cancer Immunotherapy." *Medicine in Drug Discovery* 6 (2020): 100023.

29. Cuchel, M., E. Bruckert, H. N. Ginsberg, F. J. Raal, R. D. Santos, R. A. Hegele, J. A. Kuivenhoven, B. G. Nordestgaard, O. S. Descamps, E. Steinhagen-Thiessen, A. Tybjærg-Hansen, G. F. Watts, M. Averna, C. Boileau, J. Borén, A. L. Catapano, J. C. Defesche, G. K. Hovingh, S. E. Humphries, P. T. Kovanen, L. Masana, P. Pajukanta, K. G. Parhofer, K. K. Ray, A. F. Stalenhoef, E. Stroes, M. R. Taskinen, A. Wiegman, O. Wiklund, M. J. Chapman, and European Atherosclerosis Society Consensus Panel on Familial Hypercholesterolaemia. "Homozygous Familial Hypercholesterolaemia: New Insights and Guidance for Clinicians to Improve Detection and Clinical Management. A Position Paper from the Consensus Panel on Familial Hypercholesterolaemia of the European Atherosclerosis Society." *European Heart Journal* 35, no. 32 (2014): 2146–57. doi:10.1093/eurheartj/ehu274.

30. Tregoning, J. S., E. S. Brown, H. M. Cheeseman, K. E. Flight, S. L. Higham, N. M. Lemm, B. F. Pierce, D. C. Stirling, Z. Wang, and K. M. Pollock. "Vaccines for COVID-19." *Clinical & Experimental Immunology* 202, no. 2 (2020): 162–92. doi:10.1111/cei.13517.

31. Milane, L., and M. Amiji. "Clinical Approval of Nanotechnology-Based SARS-CoV-2 mRNA Vaccines: Impact on Translational Nanomedicine." *Drug Delivery & Translational Research* 11, no. 4 (2021): 1–7. doi:10.1007/s13346-021-00911-y.

Considerations for Engineering Nanoparticles for Achieving Subcellular Organelle Targeting

18

Ketki Bhise, Katyayani Tatiparti, Somrita Dey,
Kushal Vanamala, Ayatakshi Barari,
Samaresh Sau, and Arun K. Iyer

Contents

DOI: 10.1201/9781003092773-20

459

18.1 INTRODUCTION

One of the main bottlenecks to the successful delivery of anticancer agents is the undesirable off-target specificity of the drug. Many drugs are rendered ineffective by chemical breakdown or metabolized to be inactivated before they reach their intended targets. Some drugs may face challenges in crossing the biological barriers, often limited by poor solubility and poor bioavailability. Traditionally, these issues can be mitigated by administering larger or repeated dosing of drugs [1]. However, from the perspective of potent anticancer drugs, administering large or repeated drug doses may translate to systemic toxicity or resistance to treatment, both of which limit the treatment outcome [2]. Hence, drugs that specifically target the desired tissues, while minimizing off-target toxicity and undesirable side effects are the most rational approach to anticancer therapy. Novel drug delivery systems like dendrimers, liposomes, polymerosomes, etc., provide higher drug accumulation in target tissues as compared to conventional drugs [3–5].

The delivery of these systems can be improved by tagging them with suitable targeting ligands that specifically carry the cargo to the tissue of interest, in pursuit of binding to the complementary receptors. These targeting strategies can be based on receptor expression on the surface of cells, or even at the subcellular level by exploiting the biological characteristics of these organelles. Intracellular organelle targeting at the level of the nucleus, mitochondria, endoplasmic reticulum, and Golgi bodies may be a desirable approach to specifically ferry and consequently trigger the release of the drug cargo in the organelles. This approach may offer the advantages of reduced toxicity, higher drug accumulation, lower systemic dose, and avoiding unwanted drug inactivation. It may also help in overcoming multi-drug resistance, which is a major hurdle to drug delivery.

This chapter intends to cover the most recent research on organelle targeting, starting from broad platforms for organelle targeting, followed by approaches to achieve delivery to specific organelles including nanoparticle systems, and lastly closing the discussion with techniques to characterize intracellular delivery of nanomaterials.

18.2 BROAD PLATFORMS FOR ORGANELLE TARGETING

18.2.1 Chemotherapy

Chemotherapy is the most widely used treatment type for cancer as it is more convenient and has a wide range of applications. Most of the cancer treatments are highly dependent on chemotherapy although it is accompanied by a lot of side effects including high dosage, non-selectivity, faster systemic clearance, drug resistance, etc. [6]. Years of research have contributed to finding better chemotherapeutic agents for superior cancer killing activity and to reduce side effects. Newer chemotherapeutic agents are majorly focused on selectively targeting the tumor site by targeting tumor-specific mechanisms. These include small molecule drugs and monoclonal antibodies which can target the overexpression of certain proteins in the tumor microenvironment [7]. One of the advancements towards targeted therapy is nano drug delivery systems which are proving to have a significant rise in therapeutic activity over free drug delivery and also overcoming the side effects. Due to their ultra-small size, they can deliver drugs to the subcellular organelles which are the primary site of action for many therapeutics to initiate cell apoptotic mechanisms [8]. For example, the first line chemotherapeutic drug, cisplatin, can cross-link the tumor DNA and reduce the gene replication of a wide range of cancer cells. Directing cisplatin into the nucleus of a cancer cell by administering it in a nucleus-targeted nanocarrier can show a better therapeutic outcome compared to free drug which has difficulty in diffusing into the cytoplasm [9]. Therefore, side effects and recurrence could be avoided. Similarly, organelle dysfunction by chemotherapy can activate specific cell death signal, and nano drug delivery is a promising approach to deliver these therapeutics, bypassing the systemic barriers, and showing better therapeutic activity [10]. Organelle-targeted nano drug delivery is an emerging field which employs nanoparticles surface coated with organelle-targeting moieties such as nuclear localization signal (NLS), TAT peptide, or mitochondrial targeting sequence (MTS) to localize the therapeutics at their subcellular/organelle site of action and provide protection from systemic degradation factors [11–13].

18.2.2 Radiotherapy

Radiotherapy in cancer is to deliver high-intensity ionization radiations (X-rays or γ-rays) with high accuracy to the tumor tissue resulting in the killing of tumor cells. It occurs by direct or indirect (generation of free radicals) destruction of DNA and other cell components triggering tumor cell lysis [14]. Radiotherapy is a non-invasive, better tissue penetrating, and controlled (in terms of dose and duration) treatment, however it has concerning limitations including radiation resistance, insignificant malignant tumor killing, and high dosage resulting in the killing of surrounding healthy cells [15]. The efficacy and safety can be improved by applying multiple approaches including enhancing the radio sensitization of tumor tissue, the reversal of radiation resistance, and enhancing the radio resistance of healthy tissue [16]. Typically, selected high atomic number metal elements (Au or Ag) possess high radiation absorption capacity and by delivering metal nanoparticles into the tumor site can reduce the dosage of radiation drastically [17]. Furthermore, subcellular organelles have definite function in maintaining cell energy and regulating cell apoptosis which can be the target for radiosensitizers to maximize the therapeutic outcomes. In this way, organelle-targeted radiotherapy proves to be a promising approach to achieve elevated therapeutic outcomes with minimized side effects.

18.2.3 Photodynamic Therapy

Photodynamic therapy is a form of light (photo) therapy involving the use of a photoactivated photosensitizing drug which generates reactive oxygen species (ROS) and, through a series of reactions, induces cell death [18]. Some of its drawbacks include inadequate tissue penetration of light, inability to treat metastasizing tumor cells, and the hydrophobicity of the photosensitizer drugs which causes aggregation. The use of nanomaterials and monoclonal antibodies has significantly improved these drawbacks by targeting specific subcellular organelles [19]. Cell-adhering (RGD) and cell-penetrating (TAT) peptides are conjugated with nanomaterials to recognize tumor cells and are in charge of nuclear targeting [20]. The better permeability with short duration irradiation and irreversible cell death with longer duration irradiation is addressed by the dual stage light ray method for rupturing the mitochondrial cell membrane through a self-delivery system with a complex chemical structure of PpIX-PEG-(KLAKLAK)$_2$ which breaks into nanoparticles for tumor accumulation [21]. Metal complex nanoparticles conjugated with pH activable photosensitizers are used to efficiently target lysosomes because of the highly acidic environment [22].

18.2.4 Photothermal Therapy

Photothermal therapy is a type of photodynamic therapy, but it does not need oxygen to react with target cells. Instead, a photothermal agent (PTA) is stimulated by near infrared light to release heat into selectively targeted abnormal tissues and cells [23]. The main challenge of this therapy is that after a certain time, heat from the target cell will leak out into surrounding healthy cells. Since diseased cells are distinguishable from normal cells, targeted therapy was developed to target only the diseased cells. But even single targeted PTA could not properly control that effect [24]. One advancement to overcome the issue is the development of dual targeted photothermal agents modified with two different targeting groups [25].

It has a highly precise locating capability to target tumor sites, the tumor microenvironment, and specific organelle sites. For organelle targeting, the PTA is conjugated with an organelle targeted ligand to efficiently induce apoptosis in organelles after endocytosis. These aggregate in the organelle and destroy it at low-dose irradiation because of the presence of heat-sensitive proteins and genetic material, with negligible damage to surrounding tissue [26]. With this strategy, organelles like the nucleus, mitochondria, endoplasmic reticulum, and lysosomes can be targeted using specific targeted ligands conjugated with PTA made of gold nanoshells, carbon nanomaterials, or organic polymers [27].

18.2.5 Gene Therapy

Gene therapy utilizes the approach of inserting a genetic material directly into the cell using a genetically engineered vector to compensate, replace, or correct problematic genes, triggering cell death [28]. Strategies to do this include using vectors that have efficient cellular uptake, can escape the endosome to shield enzyme from being degraded, can rapidly release genes, and can transport genes to specific targeted organelles. Genes used in this regard are plasmid DNA, messenger RNAs (mRNAs), small interfering RNA (siRNA), and microRNA (miRNA) [29]. Nuclear targeted gene delivery systems are nanoparticles that have multiple functional groups to increase the chances of crossing different physiological barriers and with the help of nuclear localization sequences can transport DNA into the nucleus [10]. Mitochondria targeted delivery usually requires dicationic dequalinium molecules (DQAsomes) and mitochondria targeting sequences for the transport of DNA [30]. Lipid-based vectors and cationic polymers with disulfide bonds have been effective in transporting siRNA for cytoplasm targeted delivery [31].

18.3 ENHANCED PERMEABILITY AND RETENTION (EPR) EFFECT AND PASSIVE TARGETING VERSUS ACTIVE TARGETING

The rapidly multiplying tumor cells require their own conduit of blood vessels to provide for their growing demands for nutrients and oxygen. To satisfy this, angiogenesis is induced in solid tumors, prompted by the secretion of vascular endothelial growth factors (VEGF) [32, 33]. The tumor vasculature is markedly different from the normal tissue vasculature, in the sense that it is leaky, disorganized, lacking basement membrane, and with a poor lymphatic drainage. The vascular permeability and tumor growth are sustained by the secretion of bradykinin, prostaglandins [34]. The increased vascular permeability would imply greater leakage of macromolecules into the tumor interstitium, and poor drainage would mean greater retention of the drug molecules in the tumors. This phenomenon, called the enhanced permeability and retention (EPR) effect, was discovered by Dr. Hiroshi Maeda and marks a baseline theory about passive or non-targeted delivery of macromolecules, including nanoparticles, to solid tumors [35].

Many nanoparticles and macromolecular drug delivery systems can be thought to exploit the EPR effect for delivery of the therapeutic or imaging payload to solid tumors. Nanoparticles may include polymeric, lipid-based systems [36–38]. Although passive targeting via the EPR effect can be thought to selectively deliver drugs to the tumor milieu, it is unconvincing to rely upon such strategies to achieve intracellular targeting. Passive targeting lacks the cues to localize the drugs to specific target sites, which is where active targeting strategies come into the picture.

Active targeting strategy is guided by ligand-receptor interaction rather than passive accumulation at the target tissue site. This strategy is demonstrated to improve the accumulation of macromolecules at the tumor site [39]. Tumor retention is largely dictated by receptor-mediated endocytosis owing to the presence of targeting ligands. In cases of nanoparticles delivering biomacromolecules or siRNA, the nature and physicochemical properties of the nanoparticles (for example, polymer used for complexation with siRNA) along with the targeting ligand will be judged for improved delivery [40]. Targeted nanoparticles designed for cellular delivery may unload the cargo in the cell cytoplasm. Cancer cells often overexpress certain biomarkers like folate, CD44, lactoferrin, etc. [41–43]. Recent advances in cancer immunotherapy on PD-1, PD-L1, CTLA-4, A2A adenosine receptor antagonists, etc., have opened avenues to target interactions between cancer and immune cells, thereby retarding tumor growth [44–46]. To target at the subcellular level, strategies beyond cell-surface targeting are being studied. Nanoparticles can be engineered on a dual-targeting modality, where one targeting ligand directs the nanoparticle to the cancer cell, and the other ligand helps to efficiently internalize the nanoparticle to the desired subcellular organelle. Examples include dual-targeting with transferrin-arginase [47], cell-specific peptides [48], and carbonic anhydrase antibody-CPP33 [49].

18.4 DESIGN CONSIDERATIONS OF NANOPARTICULATE DRUG DELIVERY SYSTEMS FOR ORGANELLE TARGETING

Once the nanoparticles are extravasated to the tumor tissue, they are taken up by endocytosis inside the cancer cells. On entering the cellular milieu, the nanoparticles are further trafficked to their predetermined targeting organelles depending on the way they are engineered to do so. However, there are many factors that may hinder the otherwise impeccable subcellular delivery, and they are discussed below. Overcoming the challenges to subcellular delivery is a promising step towards achieving higher drug accumulation and promoting better therapeutic outcomes.

18.4.1 Physicochemical and Biological Barriers to Delivery

i. Effect of size and shape of nanoparticles: in general, nanoparticles less than 200 nm have a higher tendency to accumulate in the tumors. A size greater than ~200 nm makes the nanoparticles destined for uptake by the liver and spleen. Conversely, nanoparticles that are very small in size (~<10 nm) may be filtered through the kidneys [50]. The shape of the nanoparticles also has a pronounced role in the uptake by cancer cells. Spherical nanoparticles will have a higher tendency for uptake as compared to rod-shaped nanoparticles [51].

ii. Effect of surface modification and charge of nanoparticles: surface coating of the nanoparticles with PEG improves the circulation half-life and serum stability of nanoparticles [52]. Hence, most of the nanoparticles in research and those that have achieved market status, for example Doxil, are engineered with a PEG coating. Since the cellular surface has a slight negative charge, it would be logical to engineer positively charged nanoparticles to achieve maximum internalization of the nanoparticles. However, positively charged nanoparticles are often accompanied with toxicity issues because of higher non-specific cellular internalization and short circulation time [53]. Nanoparticles with a slightly negative zeta potential tend to strike the balance between good specific uptake, while minimizing toxicity issues [54].

iii. Mode of cellular uptake: macromolecules can be taken by the cell either by direct permeation, adsorption, receptor-mediated clathrin-coated endocytosis, phagocytosis, macropinocytosis, or caveolae-mediated endocytosis [55]. Direct permeation is suitable for small molecules but not for larger-sized nanoparticles, the only exception being if they are nanoparticles decorated with cell-penetrating peptides on the surface [56]. Nanoparticles taken up via clathrin-coated pits enter the acidic lysosome/endolysosome system where they undergo degradation and eventually the receptors are recycled. On the other hand, those nanoparticles taken up by caveolae-mediated endocytosis do not undergo degradation in the acidic lysosomes [57]. Such differences in the mode of nanoparticle uptake may offer variability in the mechanism of downstream organelle targeting. For those nanoparticles that enter the lysosomes, they have to encounter an additional step of lysosomal escape before they can ferry themselves to the subcellular organelles they are engineered for.

18.5 NANOPARTICULATE STRATEGIES TO TARGET SUBCELLULAR ORGANELLES

Although the nanoparticles deliver the drugs into the cytoplasm by cellular targeting, the drug needs to reach the site of action at the subcellular level or organelles such as the nucleus, mitochondria, endoplasmic reticulum, microtubules, and so on (Figure 18.1). Subcellular delivery of drugs is expected to be multistage with specific localization of the drug delivery system in the targeted organelles. This understanding of the importance of the organelle has begun highly focused research efforts on organelle-targeted delivery to enhance the therapeutic efficacy of the targeted delivery systems. The goal of such subcellular targeting is to improve the therapeutic efficacy and safety of the drugs and reduce resistance to them. A brief discussion on some of the strategies applied in the organelle targeting ensues henceforth.

18.5.1 Strategies for Targeting the Nucleus

The nucleus is the main organelle that is targeted for subcellular drug delivery for the primary reason that it is the control center of the cell. It holds the genetic information of the cells and hence is responsible for the synthesis of the functional proteins of the cells by transcription and translation machinery. Targeting the nucleus is especially useful in the case of drugs that directly modify the functioning of DNA that leads to cell death [58–60]. Even with nanoparticles loaded with drugs that induce DNA damage, it is reported that a very small percentage of the loaded drug actually enters the nucleus, and a vast majority remains trapped in the lysosomes for destruction [61]. Hence, in the context of nanoparticles targeting the nucleus, it may be beneficial to have a deeper targeting approach. Especially when the therapeutic moiety is a plasmid DNA (pDNA), introducing it to the tumor milieu with a pin-pointed targeting approach would

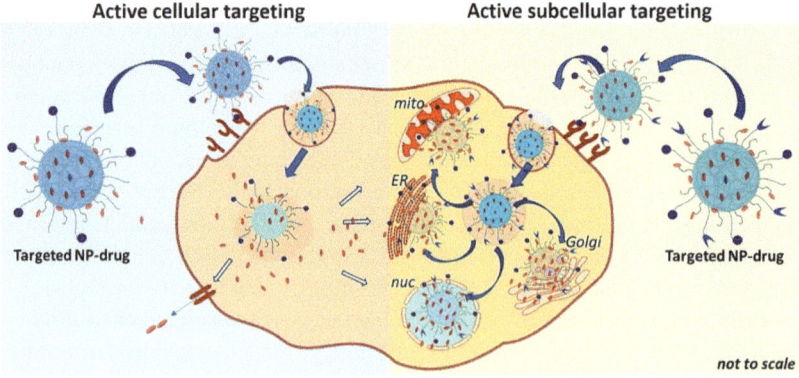

FIGURE 18.1 Active cellular targeting is primarily achieved by interactions between the ligand and the targeted delivery system into which it is incorporated. The targeted delivery system is internalized by endocytosis to release the drug payload into the cytoplasm. Similarly, the active subcellular targeting is achieved by decorating the delivery systems with ligands that target specific organelles. Figure taken from open access reference [1].

be beneficial. An example would be complexation of the pDNA with a polymer with high transfection efficacy, and further, for the fulfilment of nuclear delivery, conjugating the binary complex system with hyaluronan (specific to CD44 on the cell surface) and R8-RGD [62]. Further, some researchers have developed nanoparticle systems comprising of two different drugs tethered together: one that targets the mitochondria and the other that targets the nucleus. Such simultaneous targeting of two subcellular organelles opens a myriad of possibilities to efficient anticancer therapy [63].

There are several strategies introduced to target the nucleus. A reduction in cytotoxicity and higher nuclear accumulation is a good indicator of a successful targeted delivery. One of the techniques is the direct delivery of therapeutic moieties through the nuclear pores complex (NPC) which forms channels through the nuclear membrane, or disrupts nuclear membrane during cell division [7]. These are associated with importins β proteins and nucleoporins. The NPC is the primary gate for the delivery of macromolecules inside and outside of the nucleus, be it passive or active targeting. While small molecules pass through the nucleus via passive diffusion, molecules larger than 45 kDa need to take advantage of the nuclear localization signals (NLS) to be able to actively be transported into the nucleus [64, 65].

Another means is the utilization of the nuclear localization signals (NLS) transport system that works in conjunction with the NPC to deliver macromolecules inside the nucleus. This system uses small peptide sequences that can be anchored on the surface of the nanoparticles to be used for the delivery of the therapeutic moiety [66]. Larger molecules utilize this pathway to enter the nucleus. Together, the NPC-NLS transport system can be of great value while designing the nano-delivery systems. Some of these include the magnetic NLS tagged nanoparticles, gold-based nanoparticles, and so on [67–72]. Optimum density of the NLS on the nanoparticle surface and the overall size of the nanoparticle are pertinent factors in the context of nuclear delivery. Accordingly, it was found that intermediate density of NLS on larger nanoparticles improved the nuclear accumulation, whereas the same density of NLS on smaller nanoparticles resulted in a poorer nuclear uptake [73]. PEGylation is a technique used to increase the circulation of nanoparticles in the blood stream by preventing untimely opsonization. A 5% NLS sequence (GGFSTSLRARKA) appended to the ligand shell of nanoparticles resulted in the uptake of the nanoparticles in endosomes and the nucleus, but not in the cytoplasm [74]. This shows that a minor fraction of NLS sequence used as the targeting ligand may be sufficient to facilitate nuclear delivery.

More recently investigated is the transport of nanoparticles by TAT peptides [75]. TAT can be classified as a cell-penetrating peptide (CPP), other examples of which include penetratin, R8, transportan, xentry, TAT-HA, cTAT, etc. [76]. This came into limelight after the discovery of an NLS peptide, the HIV TAT protein, that can efficiently penetrate through the cell into the nucleus [77]. The TAT peptide can efficiently translocate nanoparticles into the nucleus by binding to import receptors importins α and β. As an example, TAT peptide was covalently attached on the surface of mesoporous silica nanoparticles and further loaded with doxorubicin destined for release in the nucleoplasm. The researchers of this study found a strong red signal in the nucleus corresponding to doxorubicin for TAT-modified nanoparticles as opposed to the unmodified nanoparticles, indicating the efficacy of TAT-mediated nuclear delivery [78]. The TAT peptide can be modified to suit delivery requirements. The tumor microenvironment is mildly acidic. Thioketal crosslinked polyphosphoester (PPE) nanoparticles modified with pH-sensitive TAT were shown to be activated only in the acidic tumor milieu, leading to the eventual release of the drug payload in the perinuclear region [79].

Active targeting can be achieved by modifying the surface charge of the nanoparticles by cations such as gold, silver, etc., on the carriers [80]. Yet another means of delivery is the glyco-dependent nuclear transport system involving lectins that transport glycosylated molecules in the nucleus [81, 82]. It has been found that such transport is specific to the class of the sugar being transported. Using this mechanism of transport, several nano-delivery systems have been designed decorated with glycosylated carrier groups [83]. Nuclear receptors such as estrogen receptors, glucocorticoid receptors, and so on also serve as good nuclear targets. Further, irradiation for photodynamic therapy has been employed as a strategy to deliver the therapeutics inside the nucleus. For this purpose, photosensitizers have been used [84]. Light is used to activate photosensitizers that generate ROS that are cytotoxic. This technique is applied in a non-invasive manner at the site/vicinity of therapy, i.e., nucleus [20]. On similar lines, photothermal therapy can be used that converts light into heat in a non-invasive manner upon irradiation of photothermal agents that can kill cancer cells [85–87]. Gene delivery to the nucleus was initiated around 1998 using liposomes [88]. These main routes used to deliver chemotherapy, radiotherapy, photothermal and photodynamic therapy, or gene therapy along with others allow the delivery of drugs effectively to the nucleus by active targeting and passive diffusion [89]. Several studies have shown that the use of these mechanisms has greatly improved the efficacy of the therapeutic modalities [90, 91]. However, there is more research required to tap the potential of nuclear targeting for application in disease-modification and therapy (Figure 18.2).

18.5.2 Strategies to Target Mitochondria

Mitochondria are responsible for the generation of energy in the form of ATP by oxidative phosphorylation mechanisms (OXPHOS) involving several metabolic enzymes. Mitochondria have their own DNA (16,500 base pairs) and hence are autonomous [93]. In disease states such as cancer, mitochondrial function may change and encourage the Warburg effect. This can occur due to the mutations in mitochondrial DNA effecting the mechanism and the enzymes involved in energy production [94–96]. Mitochondria participate in the intrinsic pathway of apoptosis by regulating the translocation of pro-apoptotic proteins from the mitochondrial intermembrane space to the cytosol [97]. The role of mitochondria is also implicated in other forms of cell-death, including necroptosis [98]. This evidence suggests that mitochondria can be a potential target for cancer treatment. There are several avenues in targeting mitochondria that have been explored recently including targeting the metabolic mechanisms of the organelle by reversing the Warburg effect and blocking the uptake of glucose via the glucose transporter GLUT1. ROS generation is one of the important functions of mitochondria that can be unbalanced in disease states leading to ROS accumulation. Hence, it is a potential mechanism that can be targeted [99, 100]. The permeability transition pore complex (PTPC) of this organelle is a very important target that could be explored as a target for drug delivery because it is responsible for the transport of materials across the mitochondrial membrane. PTPC includes the voltage gated anion channels of the outer mitochondrial membrane, adenine nucleotide translocase (ANT) of the inner membrane, and cyclophilin D in the mitochondrial matrix that be manipulated by either blocking these pathways using inhibitors or altering their functions such as Ca^{2+} homeostasis and ROS generation in mitochondria. The goal of both approaches is to increase the organelle's membrane permeability allowing targeted drug delivery [101]. Mitochondrial outer membrane permeabilization (MOMP) system is another good target for drug delivery to mitochondria. MOMP is responsible for the cellular apoptosis mechanisms controlled by the Bcl2 protein family that inhibit proapoptosis mediators Bax and Bak. Drugs that can inhibit the activity of the Bcl2 class of prosurvival proteins can be used to increase tumor cell death [102, 103]. Several strategies to deliver drugs have been explored recently to improve the accumulation of therapeutic agents in mitochondria and their subsequent safety profile in the organelle including the use of lipophilic cations (which use the mitochondrial membrane potential as the driving force) [104–106], ligands such as mitochondria targeting sequence (MTS)-containing peptides for mitochondrial membrane receptors [104, 105, 107, 108], and so on. Chemotherapeutic agents specific to mitochondrial activity that are explored include classes of drugs such as metabolic inhibitors (dichloroacetate), Bcl2 inhibitors (obotoclax), transport mechanism modulators (GSAO), ROS regulators (menadione), retinoids (CD437), heat-shock protein 90 inhibitors (gamitrinibs), and other drugs such as resveratrol, and so on [97]. These drugs coupled with the nanotechnological advances in designing targeted drug delivery systems that can be augmented using other non-invasive targeting techniques discussed in this article may be a good research strategy for mitochondrial delivery.

Inducing cell death by triggering either one or many pathways of mitochondrial activation as described above is a vital step towards achieving targeted anticancer therapy. Towards this end, nanoparticles targeting mitochondria are studied by many groups. Positively charged nanoparticles tend to have a better targeting ability for mitochondria owing to the hydrophilicity and strong negative membrane potential of the mitochondrial inner membrane. Graphene oxide-based spherical nanoparticles coated with cationic polyethylene amine (PEI) and loaded with cisplatin/topotecan induced the formation of mitochondrial

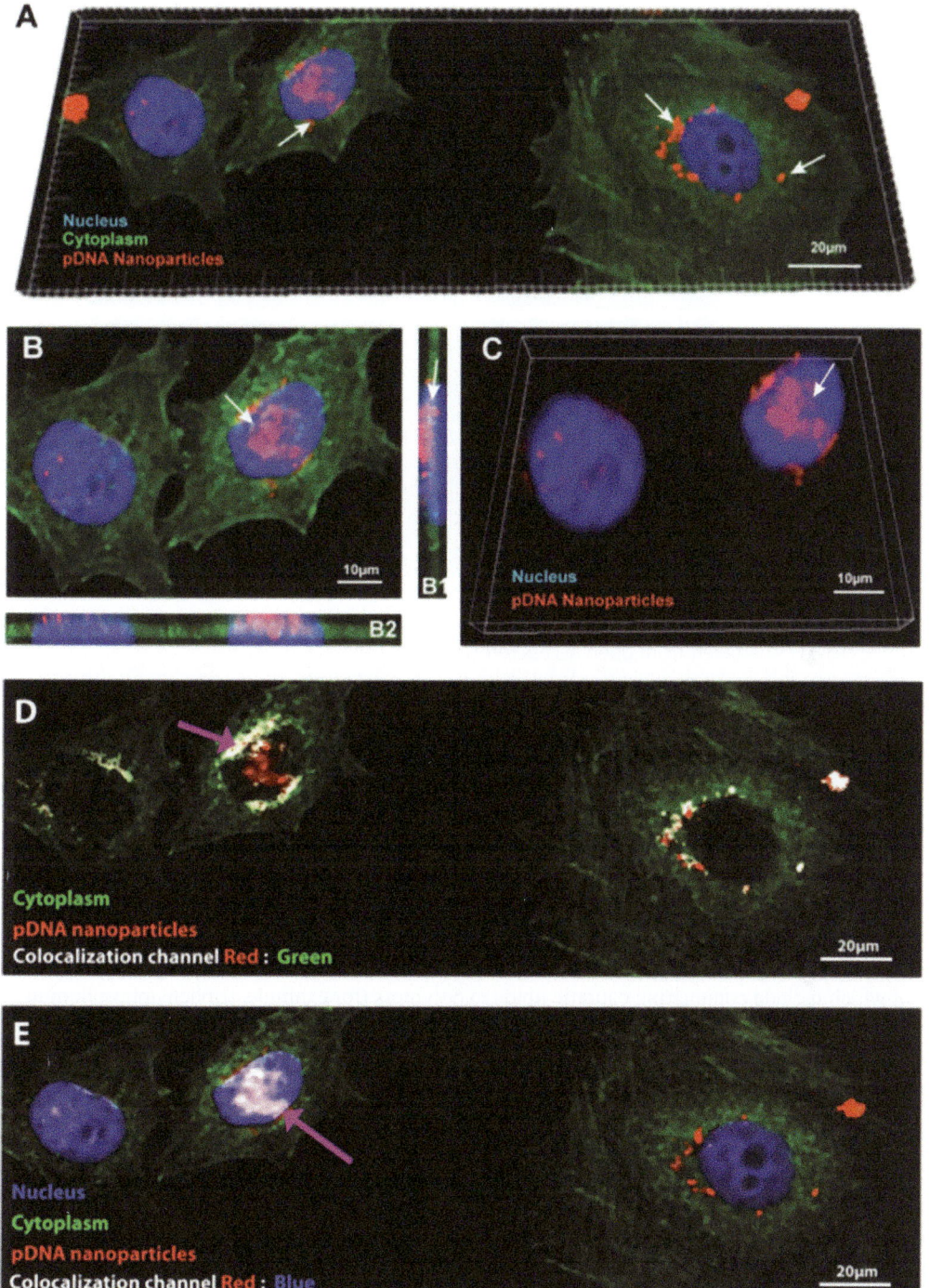

FIGURE 18.2   Chitosan-histidine-arginine/pDNA (CH-H-R/pDNA) nanoparticles were formulated for specific targeting to the nucleus. Figure shows strong nuclear uptake on the nanoparticles after 4 h incubation. Figure taken from open access reference [92].

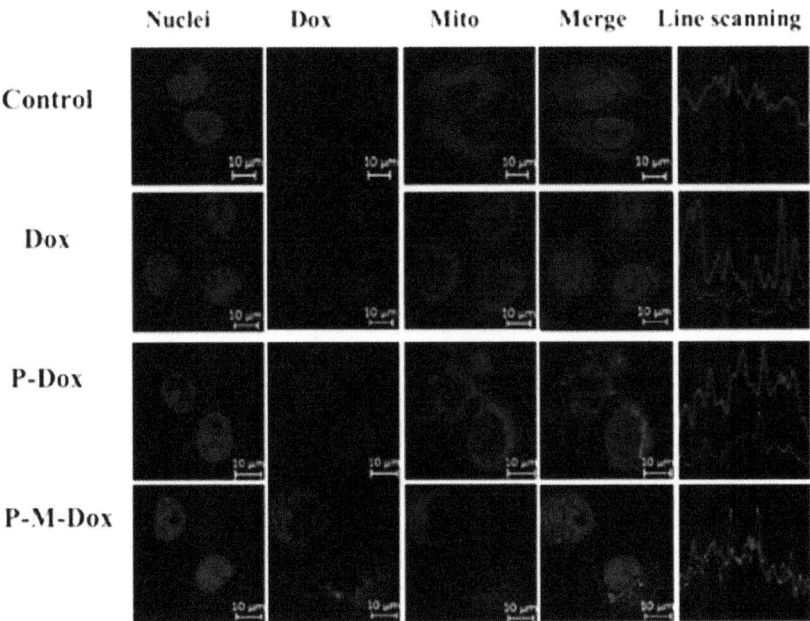

FIGURE 18.3 Mitochondrial colocalization of polymeric doxorubicin nanoparticles analyzed by CLSM in MCF-7/ADR cells. Figure taken from open access reference [115].

transition pores (MTP), triggering MOMP. The damage to mitochondria mediated by this system induced ROS generation thus kickstarting the process of cancer cell death [109]. Polydopamine-coated gold/silver alloy nanoparticles irreversibly accumulate in the mitochondria, leading to cell cycle arrest at the S-phase. The researchers of this study showed that these inorganic nanoparticles had the ability to partially diminish the mitochondrial crista [110]. In another study, gold nanoparticles conjugated non-covalently to green fluorescent protein tagged with amino-terminal mitochondrial signal were studied for uptake by cancer cells. These nanoparticles induced a partial rupture of the mitochondrial outer membrane, triggering downstream events leading to cell death [111].

Apart from inorganic nanoparticles, there are various other strategies to target the mitochondria, some of which include conjugating cationic lipids to polymers (for example, triphenylphosphonium), liposomes of dequalinium, mitochondrial penetrating peptides (for example, Szeto-Schiller-31), liposomes modified with R8 and sphingomyelin, and mitochondrial import protein machinery [112]. Nanosystems composed of polycaprolactone (PCL) modified by PEG and TPP and loaded with CoQ10 were efficiently trafficked to the mitochondria. These systems offered the advantage of controlled and stable size, efficient drug loading, prolonged circulation due to PEG, and mitochondrial targeting with the help of TPP [113]. Liposomes encapsulating a combination of drugs and targeted with dequalinium for mitochondrial delivery were able to provoke release of the drugs in the mitochondria [114]. Such strategies are robust in ensuring delivery of the drugs to the mitochondria (Figure 18.3).

18.5.3 Strategies to Target Other Cellular Organelles

Endoplasmic reticulum (ER) controls the transport of molecules in the cells. It has a role in signaling pathways and is one of the sources of stress responses in the cells. These roles are fulfilled by the maintenance of homoeostasis and ion balances along with lipid synthesis in the cells. Any disturbances in these factors can lead to stress responses that include ROS generation, misfolding of proteins, chemical imbalances, and hypoxia [116]. Hence, it is unnecessary to say that the ER and the cellular stress developed by it have a major role in several diseases including cancer [117]. Researchers have recently found that ER can also be used as a target for drug delivery specifically to this organelle to modify disease states by applying several ER-specific drugs, treatment strategies, and designing targeted nanoparticles [118, 119]. Gene therapy, peptide delivery including vaccination, and siRNA have been researched specifically for ER targeting.

Lysosomes are other organelles that are responsible for cellular homeostasis, degradative processes of the cell, plasma membrane maintenance, cholesterol level regulation, apoptosis, and cell signaling. They are a major known digestive organelle of the cell. However, their utility as a suitable target for drug delivery and disease therapy has been identified recently [120] which is attributed to the fact that they have an acidic environment and enzymatic functions [121]. It has been observed that lysosomal targeting is much easier than targeting other organelles because of the propensity of nanoparticles to accumulate in the lysosomes making it easier to design stimuli-responsive nano-delivery systems for lysosomal delivery [1, 23, 27, 66, 86, 120–123].

Recently, dendritic cells, exosomes, and other extracellular vesicles have been gaining much attention in terms of organelle targeting for disease-modifying therapeutics. This rising importance is because of the new understanding that these extracellular vesicles are not just cell debris but possess the ability to elicit immune responses and regulate the functions of the cellular target receptors. The advantage of such vesicles is their small size that does not impede transcellular transport. Hence, they are believed to be potential carriers of therapeutic agents for cellular and subcellular targeted delivery. These vesicles are found in the biological fluids of different origins [124], and are of varied sizes ranging from 30 nm to 2 μm [125]. Further, they have the ability to cross the biological barriers making them a good avenue as delivery systems that do not require vast surface modifications and show excellent stability [124, 126, 127].

18.6 CHARACTERIZATION OR EVALUATION OF SUBCELLULAR LOCALIZATION OF NANOMATERIALS

The *in vitro* tools which define the characteristics of nanoparticles like size, chemical composition, morphology, surface area, surface chemistry, and reactivity in solution are mainly performed using transmission electron (TEM) and atomic force microscopy (AFM) along with tip-enhanced Raman spectroscopy which is sensitive to the single molecule level. These tools are ineffective once the particles reach the intracellular compartment, because of the intense molecular environment imposed by proteins, nanomachines, protein complexes, vesicles, and organelles [128]. This plethora of macromolecules insert a transient or covalent charge on the nanoparticles which may change the hydrodynamic radius (R_h) as well as surface chemistry [129]. Thus, the effects of nanoparticles may depend on the subcellular localization and interaction, understanding of which requires analysis of physicochemical NP-properties in the living cell [130].

18.6.1 Fluorescence-Tagged Systems

To quantitatively analyze the subcellular localization of nanoparticles (NPs), living cells are incubated with fluorescence-tagged NPs like fluorescent FITC and fluorescent yellow orange for a predetermined time, followed by analyses and quantification of the fluorescence signals. Tools like confocal microscopy are widely used for detection. Fluorescence-tagged NPs strongly accumulate in the cytoplasm; however additional fluorescence is observed in the cell nucleus as a diffuse pattern [131]. These fluorescent systems can also be used to characterize the nano-bio-interface in living cells by a system called fluorescence recovery after photobleaching (FRAP). In this system a high-intensity light beam is applied which destroys the fluorescent property of the fluorophores in a particular region termed photobleaching, following which the fluorescence in the photobleached region will start to recover, allowing other fluorescent molecules to enter. This recovery is monitored by means of a fluorescence microscope, followed by a suitable mathematical model for analysis, generally yielding the fraction of molecules that are mobile. This method is fast and reveals a complete exchange of the investigated nanoparticles at the levels of the mitochondria, the cytoplasmic vesicles, or the nuclear envelope. Nuclear translocation is observed within minutes by free diffusion and active transport [132]. Further fluorescence correlation spectroscopy (FCS) and raster image correlation spectroscopy (RICS) can be used to measure the diffusion coefficients of polystyrene and silica nanoparticles as well as hydrodynamic radii in the nucleus and the cytoplasm that are consistent with particle motion in living cells based on diffusion [133, 134].

18.6.2 Fluorescence Lifetime Imaging Microscopy

Fluorescence lifetime imaging (FLIM) is a fluorescence imaging technique. It is a current innovative method which has been recently used in various biomedical and life science applications. FLIM is usually a combination of conventional laser scanning confocal microscopy with time correlated single photon counting, thus, enabling the recording of fluorescence lifetime decay traces for each pixel. By simplifying we can say that FLIM depends on the lifetime of individual fluorophores rather than their emission spectra. The fluorescence lifetime can be described as the average time that a molecule remains in an excited state prior to returning to the ground state by emitting a photon. The fluorescence lifetime decay curve represents the excited-state decay behavior of a fluorochrome, and it typically decays within the nanosecond range [135], and can be approximately calculated by a single or summation of several exponential functions [136]. FLIM is very advantageous as it is not influenced by concentration, absorption by the sample, sample thickness, photobleaching, or excitation intensity, and the local environment of the fluorochrome can be monitored independently of these factors, which makes it more robust than the intensity-based methods.

FLIM can be used to study protein interactions in living cells. FLIM image analysis allows for a fast and reliable localization of target molecules, and this discrimination of NP against the background has recently been shown for zinc oxide NP along with indocarbocyanine (ICC)-labeled core–multishell nanoparticles in the skin, as well as indocarbocyanine-labeled dPGS in the liver. FLIM has also been found effective for visualizing subcutaneously injected silica-based NPs. Recent developments of both hard- and software have further contributed to the advancement of FLIM that seems to hold great potential for use in a number of biomedical applications [137].

18.6.3 Rotor-Based Organelle Viscosity Imaging (ROVI)

Rotor-based organelle viscosity imaging (ROVI) is a current technique used for characterizing parameters within the organelles of living cells, dependent on microscopic viscosity like diffusion-controlled reactions and the correct folding of nascent proteins. Real-time dynamic measurement of microscopic viscosity is carried out by molecular rotors which are small synthetic fluorophores, environment-sensitive fluorescent dyes which are directed via active targeting to specific intracellular compartments of live cells. Viscosity and the molecular crowding environment affect the photophysical properties of molecular rotors. Quantitative determination of the microviscosity of the local environment, namely the cytosol, nucleus, ER, and mitochondria, can be done by measuring the fluorescence lifetime of molecular rotors via time-correlated single photon counting fluorescence lifetime imaging (TCSPC FLIM) [138]. In addition to providing measurements of microviscosity in multiple compartments of the cell with a single "molecular rotor" probe, ROVI can also be used to analyze striking variation of microviscosity between and within each organelle. ROVI certainly explores new avenues to study the biophysical mechanisms within the biological process of the cell.

18.7 CONCLUDING REMARKS

The intention of targeted delivery would be to ensure the maximum therapeutic benefit to the subject while minimizing toxic side effects. This is made possible by engineering delivery systems that have the propensity to selectively accumulate the drug in the target tissue. Many biological impediments limit the potential of nanoparticles in active targeting, including but not limited to renal clearance, splenic uptake, serum instability, burst release, and immunogenic response to the injected biomaterials. Although nanoparticles like doxil (liposomal doxorubicin) and abraxane (albumin paclitaxel) have been on the market for a long time, studies have shown the suboptimal uptake of the encapsulated drugs at the organelle level. These organelles are the primary targets of drug action most of the time, and lower levels of drugs may hinder the therapeutic outcome. Hence, although organelle-targeted delivery systems are yet to face the market, they offer great potential in improving anticancer medicine. Nanoparticles engineered with the ultimate aim of targeting subcellular organelles are widely being researched, and these combine the intrinsic advantages of nanoparticles with the means to target subcellular organelles. The current level of appreciation for the ongoing research in organelle targeting will help develop a better understanding of the means to improve the outcome of nanoparticle-mediated therapeutics.

REFERENCES

1. Nag, O. K., and J. B. Delehanty. "Active Cellular and Subcellular Targeting of Nanoparticles for Drug Delivery." *Pharmaceutics* 11, no. 10 (2019): 543.
2. Vasan, N., J. Baselga, and D. M. Hyman. "A View on Drug Resistance in Cancer." *Nature* 575, no. 7782 (14-Nov-2019): 299–309.
3. Bhise, K., S. K. Kashaw, S. Sau, and A. K. Iyer. "Nanostructured Lipid Carriers Employing Polyphenols as Promising Anticancer Agents: Quality by Design (QbD) Approach." *International Journal of Pharmacy* 526, no. 1–2 (2017): 506–15.
4. Bhise, K., S. Sau, R. Kebriaei, S. A. Rice, K. C. Stamper, H. O. Alsaab, M. J. Rybak, and A. K. Iyer. "Combination of Vancomycin and Cefazolin Lipid Nanoparticles for Overcoming Antibiotic Resistance of MRSA." *Materials* 11, no. 7 (Jul. 2018): 1245.
5. Bhise, K., S. Sau, H. Alsaab, S. K. Kashaw, R. K. Tekade, and A. K. Iyer. "Nanomedicine for Cancer Diagnosis and Therapy: Advancement, Success and Structure-Activity Relationship." *Therapeutic Delivery* 8, no. 11 (2017): 1003–18.
6. Gao, P., W. Pan, N. Li, and B. Tang. "Boosting Cancer Therapy with Organelle-Targeted Nanomaterials." *ACS Applied Materials & Interfaces*, 11, no. 30 (31-Jul-2019): 26529–58.
7. Sakhrani, N. M., and H. Padh. "Organelle Targeting: Third Level of Drug Targeting." *Drug Design, Development & Therapy* 7 (2013): 585–99.
8. Guo, X., X. Wei, Z. Chen, X. Zhang, G. Yang, and S. Zhou. "Multifunctional Nanoplatforms for Subcellular Delivery of Drugs in Cancer Therapy." *Progress in Materials Science* 107 (01-Jan-2020): 100599.
9. Zhang, Y., F. Wang, M. Li, Z. Yu, R. Qi, J. Ding, Z. Zhang, and X. Chen. "Self-Stabilized Hyaluronate Nanogel for Intracellular Codelivery of Doxorubicin and Cisplatin to Osteosarcoma." *Advancement of Science* 5, no. 5 (May 2018): 1700821.
10. Chen, W. H., G. F. Luo, and X. Z. Zhang. "Recent Advances in Subcellular Targeted Cancer Therapy Based on Functional Materials." *Advanced Materials* 31, no. 3 (18-Jan-2019).
11. Flierl, A., C. Jackson, B. Cottrell, D. Murdock, P. Seibel, and D. C. Wallace. "Targeted Delivery of DNA to the Mitochondrial Compartment via Import Sequence-Conjugated Peptide Nucleic Acid." *Molecular Therapy* 7, no. 4 (Apr. 2003): 550–7.
12. De La Fuente, J. M., and C. C. Berry. 2005. "Tat Peptide as an Efficient Molecule to Translocate Gold Nanoparticles into the Cell Nucleus." *Bioconjugate Chemistry* Sep–Oct 16 (5): 1176–80.

13. Kang, B., M. A. Mackey, and M. A. El-Sayed. "Nuclear Targeting of Gold Nanoparticles in Cancer Cells Induces DNA Damage, Causing Cytokinesis Arrest and Apoptosis." *Journal of the American Chemical Society* 132, no. 5 (Feb. 2010): 1517–9.

14. Hogle, W. P. "The State of the Art in Radiation Therapy." *Seminars in Oncology Nursing* 22, no. 4 (Nov. 2006): 212–20.

15. Chen, Y., P. Gao, T. Wu, W. Pan, N. Li, and B. Tang. "Organelle-Localized Radiosensitizers." *Chemical Communications* 56, no. 73 (Sep. 2020): 10621–30.

16. Kwatra, D., A. Venugopal, and S. Anant. "Nanoparticles in Radiation Therapy: A Summary of Various Approaches to Enhance Radiosensitization in Cancer." *Translational Cancer Research* 2, no. 4 (2013): 330–42.

17. Her, S., D. A. Jaffray, and C. Allen. "Gold Nanoparticles for Applications in Cancer Radiotherapy: Mechanisms and Recent Advancements." *Advanced Drug Delivery Reviews* 109 (15-Jan-2017): 84–101.

18. Yang, Z., Z. Sun, Y. Ren, X. Chen, W. Zhang, X. Zhu, Z. Mao, J. Shen, and S. Nie. "Advances in Nanomaterials for Use in Photothermal and Photodynamic Therapeutics (Review)." *Molecular Medicine Reports* 20, no. 1 (Jul. 2019): 5–15.

19. Li, S.-Y., W.-X. Qiu, H. Cheng, F. Gao, F.-Y. Cao, and X.-Z. Zhang. "A Versatile Plasma Membrane Engineered Cell Vehicle for Contact-Cell-Enhanced Photodynamic Therapy." *Advanced Functional Materials* 27, no. 12 (Mar. 2017): 1604916.

20. Pan, L., J. Liu, and J. Shi. "Intranuclear Photosensitizer Delivery and Photosensitization for Enhanced Photodynamic Therapy with Ultralow Irradiance." *Advanced Functional Materials* 24, no. 46 (Dec. 2014): 7318–27.

21. Han, K., Q. Lei, S. Wang, J. Hu, W. Qiu, J. Zhu, W. Yin, X. Luo, and X. Zhang. "Dual-Stage-Light-Guided Tumor Inhibition by Mitochondria-Targeted Photodynamic Therapy." *Advanced Functional Materials* 25, no. 20 (May 2015): 2961–71.

22. Tian, J., L. Ding, H. J. Xu, Z. Shen, H. Ju, L. Jia, L. Bao, and J. S. Yu. "Cell-Specific and pH-Activatable Rubyrin-Loaded Nanoparticles for Highly Selective Near-Infrared Photodynamic Therapy Against Cancer." *Journal of the American Chemical Society* 135, no. 50 (Dec. 2013): 18850–8.

23. Zou, L., H. Wang, B. He, L. Zeng, T. Tan, H. Cao, X. He, Z. Zhang, S. Guo, and Y. Li. "Current Approaches of Photothermal Therapy in Treating Cancer Metastasis with Nanotherapeutics." *Theranostics* 6, no. 6 (2016): 762–72.

24. Son, J., G. Yi, J. Yoo, C. Park, H. Koo, and H. S. Choi. "Light-Responsive Nanomedicine for Biophotonic Imaging and Targeted Therapy." *Advanced Drug Delivery Reviews* 138 (01-Jan-2019): 133–47.

25. Wen, Y., C. L. Schreiber, and B. D. Smith. "Dual-Targeted Phototherapeutic Agents as Magic Bullets for Cancer." *Bioconjugate Chemistry* 31, no. 3 (Mar. 2020): 474–82.

26. Ma, X., N. Gong, L. Zhong, J. Sun, and X. J. Liang. "Future of Nanotherapeutics: Targeting the Cellular Sub-Organelles." *Biomaterials* 97 (01-Aug-2016): 10–21.

27. Wang, K., Y. Xiang, W. Pan, H. Wang, N. Li, and B. Tang. "Dual-Targeted Photothermal Agents for Enhanced Cancer Therapy." *Chemical Science* 11, no. 31 (21-Aug-2020): 8055–72.

28. Kerr, D. "Clinical Development of Gene Therapy for Colorectal Cancer." *Nature Reviews. Cancer* 3, no. 8 (Aug. 2003): 615–22.

29. Yin, H., R. L. Kanasty, A. A. Eltoukhy, A. J. Vegas, J. R. Dorkin, and D. G. Anderson. "Non-Viral Vectors for Gene-Based Therapy." *Nature Reviews. Genetics* 15, no. 8 (15-Jul-2014): 541–55.

30. Weissig, V., and V. P. Torchilin. "Towards Mitochondrial Gene Therapy: DQAsomes as a Strategy." *Journal of Drug Targeting* 9, no. 1 (2001): 1–13.

31. Son, S., R. Namgung, J. Kim, K. Singha, and W. J. Kim. "Bioreducible Polymers for Gene Silencing and Delivery." *Accounts of Chemical Research* 45, no. 7 (Jul. 2012): 1100–12.

32. Leung, D. W., G. Cachianes, W. J. Kuang, D. V. Goeddel, and N. Ferrara. "Vascular Endothelial Growth Factor Is a Secreted Angiogenic Mitogen." *Science* 246, no. 4935 (1989): 1306–9.

33. Marme, D. "Tumor Angiogenesis: The Pivotal Role of Vascular Endothelial Growth Factor." *World Journal of Urology* 14, no. 3 (Jun. 1996): 166–74.

34. Iyer, A. K., G. Khaled, J. Fang, and H. Maeda. "Exploiting the Enhanced Permeability and Retention Effect for Tumor Targeting." *Drug Discovery Today* 11, no. 17–18 (01-Sep-2006): 812–8.

35. Maeda, H. "Tumor-Selective Delivery of Macromolecular Drugs via the EPR Effect: Background and Future Prospects." *Bioconjugate Chemistry* 21, no. 5 (19-May-2010): 797–802.

36. Maeda, H. "SMANCS and Polymer-Conjugated Macromolecular Drugs: Advantages in Cancer Chemotherapy." *Advanced Drug Delivery Reviews* 46, no. 1–3 (Mar. 2001): 169–85.

37. Matsumura, Y., T. Hamaguchi, T. Ura, K. Muro, Y. Yamada, Y. Shimada, K. Shirao, T. Okusaka, H. Ueno, M. Ikeda, and N. Watanabe. "Phase I Clinical Trial and Pharmacokinetic Evaluation of NK911, a Micelle-Encapsulated Doxorubicin." *British Journal of Cancer* 91, no. 10 (Nov. 2004): 1775–81.

38. Iyer, A. K., K. Greish, T. Seki, S. Okazaki, J. Fang, K. Takeshita, and H. Maeda. "Polymeric Micelles of Zinc Protoporphyrin for Tumor Targeted Delivery Based on EPR Effect and Singlet Oxygen Generation." *Journal of Drug Targeting* 15, no. 7–8 (Aug. 2007): 496–506.

39. Shi, J., Z. Xiao, N. Kamaly, and O. C. Farokhzad. "Self-Assembled Targeted Nanoparticles: Evolution of Technologies and Bench to Bedside Translation." *Accounts of Chemical Research* 44, no. 10 (18-Oct-2011): 1123–34.

40. Farokhzad, O. C., and R. Langer. "Impact of Nanotechnology on Drug Delivery." *ACS Nano* 3, no. 1 (Jan. 2009): 16–20.

41. Bahrami, B. *et al.* "Folate-Conjugated Nanoparticles as a Potent Therapeutic Approach in Targeted Cancer Therapy." *Tumor Biology* 36, no. 8 (24-Aug-2015): 5727–42.

42. Huang, W. Y., J. N. Lin, J. T. Hsieh, S. C. Chou, C. H. Lai, E. J. Yun, U. G. Lo, R. C. Pong, J. H. Lin, and Y. H. Lin. "Nanoparticle Targeting CD44-Positive Cancer Cells for Site-Specific Drug Delivery in Prostate Cancer Therapy." *ACS Applied Materials & Interfaces* 8, no. 45 (Nov. 2016): 30722–34.

43. Kondapi, A. K. "Targeting Cancer with Lactoferrin Nanoparticles: Recent Advances." *Nanomedicine* 15, no. 21 (01-Sep-2020): 2071–83.

44. Carosella, E. D., G. Ploussard, J. LeMaoult, and F. Desgrandchamps. "A Systematic Review of Immunotherapy in Urologic Cancer: Evolving Roles for Targeting of CTLA-4, PD-1/PD-L1, and HLA-G." *European Urology.* 68, no. 2 (01-Aug-2015): 267–79.

45. Alsaab, H. O., S. Sau, R. Alzhrani, K. Tatiparti, K. Bhise, S. K. Kashaw, and A. K. Iyer. "PD-1 and PD-L1 Checkpoint Signaling Inhibition for Cancer Immunotherapy: Mechanism, Combinations, and Clinical Outcome." *Frontiers in Pharmacology* 8, no. Aug. (23-Aug-2017): 561.

46. Hatfield, S. M., and M. Sitkovsky. "A2A Adenosine Receptor Antagonists to Weaken the Hypoxia-HIF-1α Driven Immunosuppression and Improve Immunotherapies of Cancer." *Current Opinion in Pharmacology* 29 (01-Aug-2016): 90–6.

47. Deshpande, P., A. Jhaveri, B. Pattni, S. Biswas, and V. Torchilin. "Drug Delivery Transferrin and Octaarginine Modified Dual-Functional Liposomes with Improved Cancer Cell Targeting and Enhanced Intracellular Delivery for the Treatment of Ovarian Cancer." *Drug Delivery* 25, no. 1, no.v (2018): 517–32.

48. Sun, W., L. Li, L. J. Li, Q. Q. Yang, Z. R. Zhang, and Y. Huang. "Two Birds, One Stone: Dual Targeting of the Cancer Cell Surface and Subcellular Mitochondria by the Galectin-3-Binding Peptide G3-C12." *Acta Pharmacologica Sinica* 38, no. 6 (Jun. 2017): 806–22.

49. Lin, C., X. Zhang, H. Chen, Z. Bian, G. Zhang, M. K. Riaz, D. Tyagi, G. Lin, Y. Zhang, J. Wang, A. Lu, and Z. Yang. "Dual-Ligand Modified Liposomes Provide Effective Local Targeted Delivery of Lung-Cancer Drug by Antibody and Tumor Lineage-Homing Cell-Penetrating Peptide." *Drug Delivery* 25, no. 1 (Jan. 2018): 256–66.

50. Alexis, F., E. Pridgen, L. K. Molnar, and O. C. Farokhzad. "Factors Affecting the Clearance and Biodistribution of Polymeric Nanoparticles." *Molecular Pharmaceutics* 5, no. 4 (2008): 505–15.

51. Kumar, A., A. Ahmad, A. Vyawahare, and R. Khan. "Membrane Trafficking and Subcellular Drug Targeting Pathways." *Frontiers in Pharmacology* 11 (27-May-2020): 629.

52. Suk, J. S., Q. Xu, N. Kim, J. Hanes, and L. M. Ensign. "Pegylation as a Strategy for Improving Nanoparticle-Based Drug and Gene Delivery." *Advanced Drug Delivery Reviews* 99, no. A (01-Apr-2016): 28–51.

53. Yamamoto, Y., Y. Nagasaki, Y. Kato, Y. Sugiyama, and K. Kataoka. "Long-Circulating Poly(Ethylene Glycol)-Poly(D,L-Lactide) Block Copolymer Micelles with Modulated Surface Charge." *Journal of Controlled Release* 77, no. 1–2 (Nov. 2001): 27–38.

54. Kommareddy, S., and M. Amiji. "Biodistribution and Pharmacokinetic Analysis of Long-Circulating Thiolated Gelatin Nanoparticles Following Systemic Administration in Breast Cancer-Bearing Mice." *Journal of Pharmaceutical Sciences* 96, no. 2 (Feb. 2007): 397–407.

55. Kievit, F. M., and M. Zhang. "Cancer Nanotheranostics: Improving Imaging and Therapy by Targeted Delivery Across Biological Barriers." *Advanced Materials* 23, no. 36 (22-Sep-2011): H217.

56. Veiseh, O., F. M. Kievit, H. Mok, J. Ayesh, C. Clark, C. Fang, M. Leung, H. Arami, J. O. Park, and M. Zhang. "Cell Transcytosing Poly-Arginine Coated Magnetic Nanovector for Safe and Effective siRNA Delivery." *Biomaterials* 32, no. 24 (Aug. 2011): 5717–25.

57. Kumari, S., S. Mg, and S. Mayor. "Endocytosis Unplugged: Multiple Ways to Enter the Cell." *Cell Research* 20, no. 3 (02-Mar-2010): 256–75.

58. Hua, Q., Z. Qiang, M. Chu, D. Shi, and J. Ren. "Polymeric Drug Delivery System with Actively Targeted Cell Penetration and Nuclear Targeting for Cancer Therapy." *ACS Applied Bio Materials* 2, no. 4 (Apr. 2019): 1724–31.

59. Chen, X., X. Zhang, Y. Guo, Y. Zhu, X. Liu, Z. Chen, and F. Wu. "Smart Supramolecular 'Trojan Horse'-Inspired Nanogels for Realizing Light-Triggered Nuclear Drug Influx in Drug-Resistant Cancer Cells." *Advanced Functional Materials* 29, no. 13 (Mar. 2019): 1807772.

60. Cai, Y., H. Shen, J. Zhan, M. Lin, L. Dai, C. Ren, Y. Shi, J. Liu, J. Gao, and Z. Yang. "Supramolecular 'Trojan Horse' for Nuclear Delivery of Dual Anticancer Drugs." *Journal of the American Chemical Society* 139, no. 8 (Mar. 2017): 2876–9.

61. Seynhaeve, A. L. B., B. M. Dicheva, S. Hoving, G. A. Koning, and T. L. M. Ten Hagen. "Intact Doxil Is Taken up Intracellularly and Released Doxorubicin Sequesters in the Lysosome: Evaluated by In Vitro/In Vivo Live Cell Imaging." *Journal of Controlled Release* 172, no. 1 (2013): 330–40.

62. Li, L., X. Li, Y. Wu, L. Song, X. Yang, T. He, N. Wang, S. Yang, Y. Zeng, Q. Wu, Z. Qian, Y. Wei, and C. Gong. "Multifunctional Nucleus-Targeting Nanoparticles with Ultra-High Gene Transfection Efficiency for In Vivo Gene Therapy." *Theranostics* 7, no. 6 (2017): 1633–49.

63. Mallick, A., P. More, S. Ghosh, R. Chippalkatti, B. A. Chopade, M. Lahiri, and S. Basu. "Dual Drug Conjugated Nanoparticle for Simultaneous Targeting of Mitochondria and Nucleus in Cancer Cells." *ACS Applied Materials & Interfaces* 7, no. 14 (Apr. 2015): 7584–98.

64. Feldherr, C. M. "The Nuclear Annuli as Pathways for Nucleocytoplasmic Exchanges." *Journal of Cell Biology* 14, no. 1 (Jul. 1962): 65–72.

65. Pouton, C. W., K. M. Wagstaff, D. M. Roth, G. W. Moseley, and D. A. Jans. "Targeted Delivery to the Nucleus." *Advanced Drug Delivery Reviews* 59, no. 8 (10-Aug-2007) 698–717.

66. Torchilin, V. P. "Tat Peptide-Mediated Intracellular Delivery of Pharmaceutical Nanocarriers." *Advanced Drug Delivery Reviews* 60, no. 4–5 (01-Mar-2008): 548–58.

67. Xu, C., J. Xie, N. Kohler, E. G. Walsh, Y. E. Chin, and S. Sun. "Monodisperse Magnetite Nanoparticles Coupled with Nuclear Localization Signal Peptide for Cell-Nucleus Targeting." *Chemistry: An Asian Journal* 3, no. 3 (Mar. 2008): 548–52.

68. Nitin, N., L. Laconte, W. J. Rhee, and G. Bao. "Tat Peptide Is Capable of Importing Large Nanoparticles Across Nuclear Membrane in Digitonin Permeabilized Cells." *Annals of Biomedical Engineering* 37, no. 10 (2009): 2018–27.

69. Panté, N., and M. Kann. "Nuclear Pore Complex Is Able to Transport Macromolecules with Diameters of ~39 nm." *Molecular Biology of the Cell* 13, no. 2 (Jan. 2002): 425–34.

70. Yang, C., J. Uertz, D. Yohan, and B. D. Chithrani. "Peptide Modified Gold Nanoparticles for Improved Cellular Uptake, Nuclear Transport, and Intracellular Retention." *Nanoscale* 6, no. 20 (Oct. 2014): 12026–33.

71. Liu, H., Y. Sun, L. Lang, T. Yang, X. Zhao, C. Cai, Z. Liu, and P. Ding. "Nuclear Localization Signal Peptide Enhances Transfection Efficiency and Decreases Cytotoxicity of Poly(Agmatine/ N , N '-Cystamine-Bis-Acrylamide)/pDNA Complexes." *Journal of Cellular Biochemistry* 120, no. 10 (Oct. 2019): 16967–77.

72. Battistella, C., and H.-A. Klok. "Controlling and Monitoring Intracellular Delivery of Anticancer Polymer Nanomedicines." *Macromolecular Bioscience* 17, no. 10 (Oct. 2017): 1700022.

73. Tammam, S. N., H. M. E. Azzazy, H. G. Breitinger, and A. Lamprecht. "Chitosan Nanoparticles for Nuclear Targeting: The Effect of Nanoparticle Size and Nuclear Localization Sequence Density." *Molecular Pharmaceutics* 12, no. 12 (Oct. 2015): 4277–89.

74. Nativo, P., I. A. Prior, and M. Brust. "Uptake and Intracellular Fate of Surface-Modified Gold Nanoparticles." *ACS Nano* 2, no. 8 (Aug. 2008): 1639–44.

75. Jeang, K. T., H. Xiao, and E. A. Rich. "Multifaceted Activities of the HIV-1 Transactivator of Transcription, Tat." *Journal of Biological Chemistry* 274, no. 41 (08-Oct-1999): 28837–40.

76. Patel, S. G., E. J. Sayers, L. He, R. Narayan, T. L. Williams, E. M. Mills, R. K. Allemann, L. Y. P. Luk, A. T. Jones, and Y. H. Tsai. "Cell-Penetrating Peptide Sequence and Modification Dependent Uptake and Subcellular Distribution of Green Florescent Protein in Different Cell Lines." *Scientific Report* 9, no. 1 (Dec. 2019): 1–9.

77. Green, M., M. Ishino, and P. M. Loewenstein. "Mutational Analysis of HIV-1 Tat Minimal Domain Peptides: Identification of Trans-Dominant Mutants That Suppress HIV-LTR-Driven Gene Expression." *Cell* 58, no. 1 (Jul. 1989): 215–23.

78. Pan, L., Q. He, J. Liu, Y. Chen, M. Ma, L. Zhang, and J. Shi. "Nuclear-Targeted Drug Delivery of Tat Peptide-Conjugated Monodisperse Mesoporous Silica Nanoparticles." *Journal of the American Chemical Society* 134, no. 13 (Apr. 2012): 5722–5.

79. Cao, Z., D. Li, J. Wang, M. Xiong, and X. Yang. "Direct Nucleus-Targeted Drug Delivery Using Cascade pH $_e$ /photo Dual-Sensitive Polymeric Nanocarrier for Cancer Therapy." *Small* 15, no. 36 (Sep. 2019): 1902022.

80. Ojea-Jiménez, I., L. García-Fernández, J. Lorenzo, and V. F. Puntes. "Facile Preparation of Cationic Gold Nanoparticle-Bioconjugates for Cell Penetration and Nuclear Targeting." *ACS Nano* 6, no. 9 (Sep. 2012): 7692–702.

81. Wagstaff, K. M., and D. A. Jans. "Importins and Beyond: Non-Conventional Nuclear Transport Mechanisms." *Traffic* 10, no. 9 (01-Sep-2009): 1188–98.

82. Duverger, E., C. Pellerin-Mendes, R. Mayer, A. C. Roche, and M. Monsigny. "Nuclear Import of Glycoconjugates Is Distinct from the Classical NLS Pathway." *Journal of Cell Science* 108, no. 4 (1995): 1325–32.

83. Wijagkanalan, W., S. Kawakami, and M. Hashida. "Glycosylated Carriers for Cell-Selective and Nuclear Delivery of Nucleic Acids." *Frontiers in Bioscience* 16, no. 1 (Jun. 2011): 2970.

84. Zhu, Y. X., H. R. Jia, G. Y. Pan, N. W. Ulrich, Z. Chen, and F. G. Wu. "Development of a Light-Controlled Nanoplatform for Direct Nuclear Delivery of Molecular and Nanoscale Materials." *Journal of the American Chemical Society* 140, no. 11 (Mar. 2018): 4062–70.

85. Li, N., Q. Sun, Z. Yu, X. Gao, W. Pan, X. Wan, and B. Tang. "Nuclear-Targeted Photothermal Therapy Prevents Cancer Recurrence with Near-Infrared Triggered Copper Sulfide Nanoparticles." *ACS Nano* 12, no. 6 (Jun. 2018): 5197–206.

86. Li, J., X. Zu, G. Liang, K. Zhang, Y. Liu, K. Li, Z. Luo, and K. Cai. "Octopod PtCu Nanoframe for Dual-Modal Imaging-Guided Synergistic Photothermal Radiotherapy." *Theranostics* 8, no. 4 (2018): 1042–58.

87. Pan, L., J. Liu, and J. Shi. "Nuclear-Targeting Gold Nanorods for Extremely Low NIR Activated Photothermal Therapy." *ACS Applied Materials & Interfaces* 9, no. 19 (May 2017): 15952–61.

88. Wu, M., Q. Meng, Y. Chen, Y. Du, L. Zhang, Y. Li, L. Zhang, and J. Shi. "Large-Pore Ultrasmall Mesoporous Organosilica Nanoparticles: Micelle/Precursor Co-Templating Assembly and Nuclear-Targeted Gene Delivery." *Advanced Materials* 27, no. 2 (Jan. 2015): 215–22.

89. Tammam, S. N., H. M. E. Azzazy, and A. Lamprecht. "How Successful Is Nuclear Targeting by Nanocarriers?." *Journal of Controlled Release* 229 (10-May-2016): 140–53.

90. Pan, L., J. Liu, and J. Shi. "Cancer Cell Nucleus-Targeting Nanocomposites for Advanced Tumor Therapeutics." *Chemical Society Reviews* 47, no. 18 (21-Sep-2018) 6930–46.

91. Huang, Z., W. Li, J. A. MacKay, and F. C. Szoka. "Thiocholesterol-Based Lipids for Ordered Assembly of Bioresponsive Gene Carriers." *Molecular Therapy* 11, no. 3 (Mar. 2005): 409–17.

92. Costa, E. C., V. M. Gaspar, J. G. Marques, P. Coutinho, and I. J. Correia. "Evaluation of Nanoparticle Uptake in Co-Culture Cancer Models." *PLOS ONE* 8, no. 7 (Jul. 2013): e70072.

93. Pustylnikov, S., F. Costabile, S. Beghi, and A. Facciabene. "Targeting Mitochondria in Cancer: Current Concepts and Immunotherapy Approaches." *Translational Research: the Journal of Laboratory & Clinical Medicine* 202 (01-Dec-2018): 35–51.

94. Liu, V. W. S., Y. Wang, H. J. Yang, P. C. Tsang, T. Y. Ng, L. C. Wong, P. Nagley, and H. Y. Ngan. "High frequency of mitochondrial genome instability in human endometrial carcinomas." *British Journal of Cancer* 89, no. 4 (2003): 697–701. doi:10.1038/sj.bjc.6601110.

95. Hao, Y., R. Ruiz, L. Yang, A. G. Neto, M. R. Amin, D. Kelly, S. Achlatis, S. Roof, R. Bing, K. Kannan, S. M. Brown, Z. Pei, and R. C. Branski. "Mitochondrial Somatic Mutations and the Lack of Viral Genomic Variation in Recurrent Respiratory Papillomatosis." *Scientific Report* 9, no. 1 (Dec. 2019).

96. Canter, J. A., A. R. Kallianpur, F. F. Parl, and R. C. Millikan. "Mitochondrial DNA G10398A polymorphism and invasive breast cancer in African-American women." *Cancer Research* 65, no. 17 (2005): 8028–33. doi:10.1158/0008-5472.CAN-05-1428.

97. Fulda, S., L. Galluzzi, and G. Kroemer. "Targeting Mitochondria for Cancer Therapy." *Nature Reviews. Drug Discovery* 9, no. 6 (14-Jun-2010): 447–64.

98. Galluzzi, L., and G. Kroemer. "Necroptosis: A Specialized Pathway of Programmed Necrosis." *Cell* 135, no. 7 (2008): 1161–3.

99. Weinberg, S. E., and N. S. Chandel. "Targeting Mitochondria Metabolism for Cancer Therapy." *Nature Chemical Biology* 11, no. 1 (01-Jan-2015): 9–15.

100. Nogueira, V., and N. Hay. "Molecular Pathways: Reactive Oxygen Species Homeostasis in Cancer Cells and Implications for Cancer Therapy." *Clinical Cancer Research* 19, no. 16 (Aug. 2013): 4309–14.

101. Marchetti, P., P. Guerreschi, L. Mortier, and J. Kluza. "Integration of Mitochondrial Targeting for Molecular Cancer Therapeutics." *International Journal of Cell Biology* 2015 (2015): 283145.

102. Hong, J. R., H. V. Wang, J. R. Hong, Y. C. Su, and J. R. Hong. "Anti-Apoptotic Genes Bcl-2 and Bcl-xL Overexpression Can Block Iridovirus Serine/Threonine Kinase-Induced Bax/Mitochondria-Mediated Cell Death in GF-1 Cells." *Fish & Shellfish Immunology* 61 (Feb. 2017): 120–9.

103. Murphy, M. P. "Selective Targeting of Bioactive Compounds to Mitochondria." *Trends in Biotechnology* 15, no. 8 (01-Aug-1997): 326–30.

104. Kelso, G. F., C. M. Porteous, C. V. Coulter, G. Hughes, W. K. Porteous, E. C. Ledgerwood, R. A. Smith, and M. P. Murphy. "Selective Targeting of a Redox-Active Ubiquinone to Mitochondria Within Cells: Antioxidant and Antiapoptotic Properties." *Journal of Biological Chemistry* 276, no. 7 (Feb. 2001): 4588–96.

105. Ross, M. F., A. Filipovska, R. A. J. Smith, M. J. Gait, and M. P. Murphy. "Cell-Penetrating Peptides Do Not Cross Mitochondrial Membranes Even When Conjugated to a Lipophilic Cation: Evidence Against Direct Passage Through Phospholipid Bilayers." *Biochemical Journal* 383, no. 3 (Nov. 2004): 457–68.

106. Lu, P., B. J. Bruno, M. Rabenau, and C. S. Lim. "Delivery of Drugs and Macromolecules to the Mitochondria for Cancer Therapy." *Journal of Controlled Release* 240 (Oct. 2016): 38–51.

107. Mukhopadhyay, A., L. Ni, C. S. Yang, and H. Weiner. "Bacterial Signal Peptide Recognizes HeLa Cell Mitochondrial Import Receptors and Functions as a Mitochondrial Leader Sequence." *Cellular & Molecular Life Sciences* 62, no. 16 (Aug. 2005): 1890–9.

108. Vestweber, D., and G. Schatz. "DNA-Protein Conjugates Can Enter Mitochondria via the Protein Import Pathway." *Nature* 338, no. 6211 (1989): 170–2.

109. Mallick, A., A. Nandi, and S. Basu. "Polyethylenimine Coated Graphene Oxide Nanoparticles for Targeting Mitochondria in Cancer Cells." *ACS Applied Bio Materials* 2, no. 1 (2018) 2019: 14–9.

110. Wang, W., J. Liu, W. Feng, S. Du, R. Ge, J. Li, Y. Liu, H. Sun, D. Zhang, H. Zhang, and B. Yang. "Targeting Mitochondria with Au-Ag@polydopamine Nanoparticles for Papillary Thyroid Cancer Therapy." *Biomaterials Science* 7, no. 3 (Mar. 2019): 1052–63.

111. Mkandawire, M. M., M. Lakatos, A. Springer, A. Clemens, D. Appelhans, U. Krause-Buchholz, W. Pompe, G. Rödel, and M. Mkandawire. "Induction of Apoptosis in Human Cancer Cells by Targeting Mitochondria with Gold Nanoparticles." *Nanoscale* 7, no. 24 (Jun. 2015): 10634–40.

112. Wang, Z., W. Guo, X. Kuang, S. Hou, and H. Liu. "Nanopreparations for Mitochondria Targeting Drug Delivery System: Current Strategies and Future Prospective." *Asian Journal of Pharmaceutical Sciences* 12, no. 6 (01-Nov-2017): 498–508.

113. Sharma, A., G. M. Soliman, N. Al-Hajaj, R. Sharma, D. Maysinger, and A. Kakkar. "Design and Evaluation of Multifunctional Nanocarriers for Selective Delivery of Coenzyme Q10 to Mitochondria." *Biomacromolecules* 13, no. 1 (Jan. 2012): 239–52.

114. Zhang, L., H. J. Yao, Y. Yu, Y. Zhang, R. J. Li, R. J. Ju, X. X. Wang, M. G. Sun, J. F. Shi, and W. L. Lu. "Mitochondrial Targeting Liposomes Incorporating Daunorubicin and Quinacrine for Treatment of Relapsed Breast Cancer Arising from Cancer Stem Cells." *Biomaterials* 33, no. 2 (Jan. 2012): 565–82.

115. Li, Q., and Y. Huang. "Mitochondrial Targeted Strategies and Their Application for Cancer and Other Diseases Treatment." *Journal of Pharmaceutical Investigation* 50, no. 3 (01-May-2020): 271–93.

116. Sukumaran, P., A. Schaar, Y. Sun, and B. B. Singh. "Functional Role of TRP Channels in Modulating ER Stress and Autophagy." *Cell Calcium* 60. 2, no. 2 (01-Aug-2016): 123–32.

117. Ozcan, L., and I. Tabas. "Role of Endoplasmic Reticulum Stress in Metabolic Disease and Other Disorders." *Annual Review of Medicine* 63 (2012): 317–28.

118. Yasui, H., R. Takeuchi, M. Nagane, S. Meike, Y. Nakamura, T. Yamamori, Y. Ikenaka, Y. Kon, H. Murotani, M. Oishi, Y. Nagasaki, and O. Inanami. "Radiosensitization of Tumor Cells Through Endoplasmic Reticulum Stress Induced by Pegylated Nanogel Containing Gold Nanoparticles." *Cancer Letters* 347, no. 1 (May 2014): 151–8.

119. Wang, J., X. Fang, and W. Liang. "Pegylated Phospholipid Micelles Induce Endoplasmic Reticulum-Dependent Apoptosis of Cancer Cells but Not Normal Cells." *ACS Nano* 6, no. 6 (Jun. 2012): 5018–30.

120. Appelqvist, H., P. Wäster, K. Kågedal, and K. Öllinger. "The Lysosome: From Waste Bag to Potential Therapeutic Target." *Journal of Molecular Cell Biology* 5, no. 4 (01-Aug-2013): 214–26.

121. Bae, Y. M., Y. I. Park, S. H. Nam, J. H. Kim, K. Lee, H. M. Kim, B. Yoo, J. S. Choi, K. T. Lee, T. Hyeon, and Y. D. Suh. "Endocytosis, Intracellular Transport, and Exocytosis of Lanthanide-Doped Upconverting Nanoparticles in Single Living Cells." *Biomaterials* 33, no. 35 (Dec. 2012): 9080–6.

122. Han, S. S., Z. Y. Li, J. Y. Zhu, K. Han, Z. Y. Zeng, W. Hong, W. X. Li, H. Z. Jia, Y. Liu, R. X. Zhuo, and X. Z. Zhang. "Dual-pH Sensitive Charge-Reversal Polypeptide Micelles for Tumor-Triggered Targeting Uptake and Nuclear Drug Delivery." *Small* 11, no. 21 (Jun. 2015): 2543–54.

123. Du, Y., W. Chen, M. Zheng, F. Meng, and Z. Zhong. "PH-Sensitive Degradable Chimaeric Polymersomes for the Intracellular Release of Doxorubicin Hydrochloride." *Biomaterials* 33, no. 29 (Oct. 2012): 7291–9.

124. Aryani, A., and B. Denecke. "Exosomes as a Nanodelivery System: A Key to the Future of Neuromedicine?." *Molecular Neurobiology* 53, no. 2 (2016): 818–34.

125. Sousa, C., I. Pereira, A. C. Santos, C. Carbone, A. B. Kovačević, A. M. Silva, and E. B. Souto. "Targeting Dendritic Cells for the Treatment of Autoimmune Disorders." *Colloids & Surfaces, Part B: Biointerfaces* 158 (01-Oct-2017): 237–48.

126. Pinheiro, A., A. M. Silva, J. H. Teixeira, R. M. Gonçalves, M. I. Almeida, M. A. Barbosa, and S. G. Santos. "Extracellular Vesicles: Intelligent Delivery Strategies for Therapeutic Applications." *Journal of Controlled Release* 289 (10-Nov-2018): 56–69.

127. Liao, W., Y. Du, C. Zhang, F. Pan, Y. Yao, T. Zhang, and Q. Peng. "Exosomes: The Next Generation of Endogenous Nanomaterials for Advanced Drug Delivery and Therapy." *Acta Biomaterialia* 86 (01-Mar. 2019): 1–14.

128. Dix, J. A., and A. S. Verkman. "Crowding Effects on Diffusion in Solutions and Cells." *Annual Review of Biophysics* 37, no. 1 (Jun. 2008): 247–63.

129. Cedervall, T., I. Lynch, S. Lindman, T. Berggård, E. Thulin, H. Nilsson, K. A. Dawson, and S. Linse. "Understanding the Nanoparticle-Protein Corona Using Methods to Quntify Exchange Rates and Affinities of Proteins for Nanoparticles." *Proceedings of the National Academy of Sciences of the United States of America* 104, no. 7 (Feb. 2007): 2050–5.

130. Hemmerich, P. H., and A. H. von Mikecz. "Defining the Subcellular Interface of Nanoparticles by Live-Cell Imaging." *PLOS ONE* 8, no. 4 (Apr. 2013): e62018.

131. Deschout, H., K. Raemdonck, J. Demeester, S. C. De Smedt, and K. Braeckmans. "FRAP in Pharmaceutical Research: Practical Guidelines and Applications in Drug Delivery." *Pharmaceutical Research* 31, no. 2 (Feb. 2014): 255–70.

132. Bacia, K., S. A. Kim, and P. Schwille. "Fluorescence Cross-Correlation Spectroscopy in Living Cells." *Nature Methods* 3, no. 2 (Feb. 2006): 83–9.

133. Digman, M. A., C. M. Brown, P. Sengupta, P. W. Wiseman, A. R. Horwitz, and E. Gratton. "Measuring Fast Dynamics in Solutions and Cells with a Laser Scanning Microscope." *Biophysical Journal* 89, no. 2 (2005): 1317–27.

134. Bastiaens, P. I. H., and A. Squire. "Fluorescence Lifetime Imaging Microscopy: Spatial Resolution of Biochemical Processes in the Cell." *Trends in Cell Biology* 9, no. 2 (01-Feb. 1999): 48–52.

135. Ostrowski, A., D. Nordmeyer, A. Boreham, C. Holzhausen, L. Mundhenk, C. Graf, M. C. Meinke, A. Vogt, S. Hadam, J. Lademann, and E. Rühl. "Overview About the Localization of Nanoparticles in Tissue and Cellular Context by Different Imaging Techniques." *Beilstein Journal of Nanotechnology* 6, no. 1 (2015): 263–80.

136. Rosenblum, L. T., N. Kosaka, M. Mitsunaga, P. L. Choyke, and H. Kobayashi. "Molecular Membrane Biology In Vivo Molecular Imaging Using Nanomaterials: General In Vivo Characteristics of Nano-Sized Reagents and Applications for Cancer Diagnosis (Review) In Vivo Molecular Imaging Using Nanomaterials: General In Vivo Characteristics of Nano-Sized Reagents and Applications for Cancer Diagnosis (Review)." *Molecular Membrane Biology* 27, no. 7 (2010): 274–85.

137. Thorek, D. L. J., A. K. Chen, J. Czupryna, and A. Tsourkas. "Superparamagnetic Iron Oxide Nanoparticle Probes for Molecular Imaging." *Annals of Biomedical Engineering* 34, no. 1 (Jan. 2006): 23–38.

138. Chambers, J. E., M. Kubánková, R. G. Huber, I. López-Duarte, E. Avezov, P. J. Bond, S. J. Marciniak, and M. K. Kuimova. "An Optical Technique for Mapping Microviscosity Dynamics in Cellular Organelles." *ACS Nano* 12, no. 5 (May 2018): 4398–407.

Index